International Travel
Health Guide

2006-2007

nternational Travel Health Guide

2006-2007

— 13th Edition —

Stuart R. Rose, MD, FACEP
Jay S. Keystone, MD, Msc(CTM), FRCPC

Contributing Editors:
Bradley A. Connor, MD
Peter Hackett, MD
Phyllis E. Kozarsky, MD
Dr. Doug Quarry, MD, MBBS, MSC

MOSBY

1600 John F. Kennedy Blvd.
Ste 1800
Philadelphia, PA 19103-2899

INTERNATIONAL TRAVEL HEALTH GUIDE   ISBN-13: 9-7803-2304-0501
                                           ISBN-10: 0-323-04050-0

Notice

Knowledge and best practice in this field are constantly changing. As new research and experience broaden our knowledge, changes in practice, treatment and drug therapy may become necessary or appropriate. Readers are advised to check the most current information provided (i) on procedures featured or (ii) by the manufacturer of each product to be administered, to verify the recommended dose or formula, the method and duration of administration, and contraindications. It is the responsibility of the practitioner, relying on their own experience and knowledge of the patient, to make diagnoses, to determine dosages and the best treatment for each individual patient, and to take all appropriate safety precautions. To the fullest extent of the law, neither the Publisher nor the Authors assume any liability for any injury and/or damage to persons or property arising out of or related to any use of the material contained in this book.

Acquisitions Editor: Tom Hartman
Editorial Assistant: Dennis DiClaudio
Publishing Services Manager: Frank Polizzano
Project Manager: Jeff Gunning
Design Direction: Nancy Sharkey

Printed in the United States of America

Working together to grow
libraries in developing countries
www.elsevier.com | www.bookaid.org | www.sabre.org

ELSEVIER   BOOK AID International   Sabre Foundation

Last digit is the print number: 9   8   7   6   5   4   3   2   1

To my wife Waltraud, my sons John and Justin, and my stepson Nick.

Stuart Rose

I dedicate this book to my children, Danielle (and Amos), Kathryn, Jen (and Sara), David, and Kevin, and to my first granddaughter Lylah . . . may you always maintain your love of travel . . . and may your travels always be in good health.

Jay Keystone

Preface

The *International Travel Health Guide* is unique. It is the only travel health book in the United States to be published annually. Until this guide became available, travelers had no concise source of updated travel health advice and information.

I wrote the first edition of the *International Travel Health Guides* out of sheer frustration. In counseling my patients who traveled, I often didn't have enough time to tell them how to prepare for their trip or how to stay healthy abroad. Even when I did spend additional time reviewing the risks, how much, I wondered, did they remember later on?

I knew I couldn't recommend reading an entire textbook on tropical medicine for my patients who traveled, and travel books that gave health advice often didn't cover the necessary information in sufficient detail. Furthermore, all of these books are soon outdated—with important information possibly misleading. If only I could give my patients a book that summarizes the latest advice . . . and so in 1989, the first edition of the *International Travel Health Guide* was born.

This 13th edition of the *Health Guide* continues to focus on those topics that are the most important, the most common, or the most interesting to a great many travelers, especially those going to less developed countries. The *Health Guide* contains the very latest medical information on diseases and their prevention. This information is presented in an easy-to-understand, concise format. And if the *Health Guide* doesn't provide the information you need, it tells you where to find it.

Perhaps the most unique feature of the *International Travel Health Guide* is the World Medical Guide section. This section gives you quick reference to disease risks in over 200 countries worldwide.

The 13th edition of the *International Travel Health Guide* is co-authored with Dr. Jay Keystone from the University of Toronto. Dr. Keystone is a leading authority in travel medicine, especially in the fields of malaria and parasitic diseases. For several aspects of this project, Dr. Keystone and I were fortunate to have the expert assistance of our medical advisers: Dr. Phyllis Kozarsky from Emory University (Travel and Pregnancy, AIDS/HIV, Trip Preparation); Dr. Bradley Connor, President, International Society of Travel Medicine (Hepatitis); Dr. Peter Hackett, University of Colorado Health Science Center (Altitude Illness); and Dr. Doug Quarry, Medical Director, International SOS (Travel Assistance, Emergency Medical Transport, Medical Care Abroad). We thank them for their advice.

Stuart R. Rose
Jay S. Keystone

Acknowledgments

I wish to express my appreciation to all of those in the travel medicine community who have told me over the years how much they have relied on the *International Travel Health Guide* to help them counsel travelers.

I especially wish to thank Tom Hartman and his team at Elsevier for now introducing the *International Travel Health Guide* to a wider audience—the millions of everyday travelers who need access to accurate, concise, up-to-date information on safe travel.

Stuart Rose

I would like to thank Lori Kalata for her superb editing, excellent suggestions, and incredible, logical approach to problem solving.

Jay Keystone

About the Authors

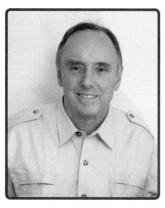

Stuart R. Rose, MD, FACEP

Dr. Rose is a graduate of Columbia University College of Physicians and Surgeons. He is board certified in internal medicine and emergency medicine and Assistant Clinical Professor of Emergency Medicine, Tufts University School of Medicine. Dr. Rose is Founder and President of Travel Medicine, Inc.

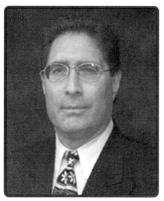

Jay S. Keystone, MD, MSc(CTM), FRCPC

Dr. Keystone is Professor of Medicine, Department of Medicine, and Immediate Past President, Medical Alumni Association at the University of Toronto. He also is a senior staff physician (and former director) of the Centre for Travel and Tropical Medicine at Toronto General Hospital.

Dr. Keystone received his medical degree from the University of Toronto Faculty of Medicine in 1969. He completed his internship at Toronto General Hospital and his residency at Sunnybrook Hospital, Toronto, as well as at the University of Michigan Medical Center, Ann Arbor. He received his Master's Degree in Clinical Tropical Medicine at the London School of Hygiene and Tropical Medicine. He has carried out his field work in sub-Saharan Africa, South America, and India. He is a past president of the International Society of Travel Medicine, the clinical division of the American Society of Tropical Medicine, and The Canadian Society of International Health.

Dr. Keystone has more than 150 scientific publications to his credit and is the senior author of a recently published textbook on travel medicine.

His claim to fame is being the first and last attending physician to make rounds at Toronto General Hospital on rollerblades.

Contents

HEALTH AND INTERNATIONAL TRAVEL

Overview of Travelers' Health

KEY POINTS:

▶ Health risks vary according to destination, itinerary, and medical history of the traveler.

▶ As many as 70% of travelers report an illness or impairment during their trip. Most self-reported health problems are minor.

▶ Fewer than 1% of travelers required hospital admission abroad.

▶ Accidents and injuries cause most deaths in travelers younger than age 55, and most are preventable.

▶ Cardiovascular disease is the cause of most deaths in older travelers.

▶ Education, combined with common sense, can prevent most illness or injury during travel.

▶ All individuals traveling frequently, or planning an extended trip abroad, should have a pre-travel evaluation, preferably in a travel clinic.

The Risk of Illness While Traveling

How risky is foreign travel? People tend to exaggerate unlikely dangers such as terrorism or the potential for transmission of Ebola virus, and disregard or minimize more common perils such as motor vehicle accidents and malaria. Disasters, like the Indonesian earthquake and resultant tsunami of December 2004, killed thousands of tourists, but such catastrophic events are often unpredictable. Large disasters often divert attention from the simple day-to-day precautions that travelers can take to stay healthy and safe.

The chances of acquiring certain diseases, or of having an accident, depend largely on where you travel and what you do while traveling. Out of 30 million Americans who go abroad each year, approximately 8 million go to less developed countries where the incidences of tropical and infectious diseases are often high. Almost 7 million U.S. citizens travel to countries where there is risk of malaria. Surveys of travelers show that:

- There is a 60% to 70% possibility of illness when traveling in less developed countries for up to 90 days (median trip duration—19 days). Most of these illnesses are minor.
- There is a 5% to 8% chance you will seek medical care while traveling in a developing country.
- Your chance of being hospitalized will be less than 1%.
- The most common reported illnesses are: diarrhea (34%); a respiratory disease (26%); a skin disorder (8%); acute mountain sickness (6%); motion sickness (5%); an accident and injury (5%); an illness with fever (3%).

- On return home, there is a 26% chance that you will have a bout of diarrhea, a respiratory illness, a skin problem, or a fever related to your trip.

Your individual risk, however, may vary considerably. For example, if visiting the Indian subcontinent, (and particularly friends and relatives) your risk of typhoid fever may be as high as 18 times greater than for any other geographic region. Other variables that can affect your health include (1) the duration of your trip; (2) your use (or nonuse) of preventive antimalarial drugs; (3) your use of prevention measures against insect bites; (4) your vaccination status; (5) your risk-taking (or avoidance) behavior; and (6) your underlying health status.

Bear in mind, though, that traveling is usually good for one's physical and emotional health. Aside from seeking holiday pleasures, some people travel to improve their lifestyle, perhaps to change harmful personal habits, "get in shape"—or temporarily (perhaps permanently) leave a stressful job, a bad relationship, a harsh climate, or other adverse life events.

Prevention of Illness

Preventing illness abroad involves learning as much as possible about the countries you will be visiting, consulting with a travel medicine provider to receive immunizations and medications and taking the necessary clothing, equipment, or devices (such as a water filter or mosquito net) to deal with local health conditions and climate. Your own health status should also be evaluated.

Most travel-related diseases can be prevented. Hepatitis, meningitis, yellow fever, and rabies are some of the diseases that can be prevented by vaccination. Chemoprophylaxis, combined with protective measures against mosquito bites, can prevent virtually all cases of malaria, as well as many other insect-transmitted diseases. Sexually transmitted diseases, including HIV, can be avoided with behavior modification.

Types of Illnesses

Diarrhea (see Chapter 6) This is the most common malady affecting travelers. There is a 35% to 60% chance that you will acquire travelers' diarrhea during a month-long trip to a less developed country. Adhering to safe food and drink practices can reduce your risk (but most travelers have trouble sticking to the guidelines). Prompt treatment with antibiotics and loperamide quickly resolves most cases of travelers' diarrhea.

Malaria (see Chapter 7) This mosquito-transmitted illness, which can be fatal, is the most important parasitic disease to avoid overseas. Malaria is a serious health problem in many tropical and subtropical countries. Check your itinerary carefully to assess your risk of exposure.

Hepatitis (see Chapter 12) The viruses hepatitis A and hepatitis B pose a serious risk for travelers. Although both are rarely fatal, hepatitis A can ruin a carefully planned vacation and result in weeks or months of disability; contracting hepatitis B can have serious long-term consequences. You can prevent hepatitis A with the appropriate vaccine and hepatitis B with vaccination and/or limiting your exposure to potentially contaminated blood and secretions. Although there are no vaccines against hepatitis C and E, Chapter 12 outlines measures you can take to reduce your risk of these illnesses.

Other Illnesses Colds and respiratory infections, skin rashes, ear infections, sunburn, sprains, contusions, and superficial injuries account for the majority of less serious problems.

Fatalities During Travel

Although it is quite possible you will have some type of minor illness while abroad, the chance that your illness will be fatal is reassuringly small. In 1984, out of 30 million travelers overseas, just 1,298 deaths were recorded. Mortality abroad is due mainly to heart

Figure 1.1   **Monthly Incidence Rates of Health Problems During Stays in Developing Countries**

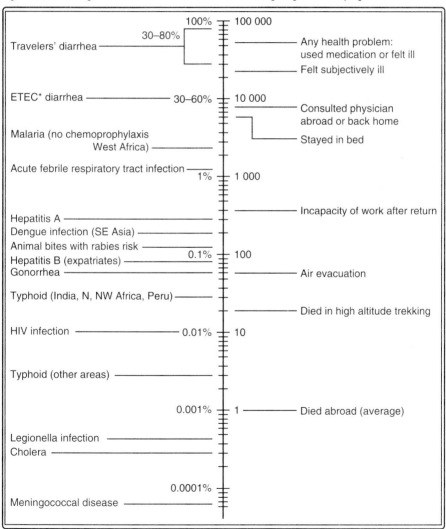

*ETEC = Enterotoxigenic E. coli. ETEC is usually responsible for 30–60% of all cases of travelers' diarrhea.

attacks, motor vehicle accidents, and other injuries. Cardiovascular disease causes about 50% of all deaths abroad, but most of these occur in older travelers. Cardiovascular death rates, however, are not increased by travel. Other points include the following:

- Injuries are the most common cause of death in younger travelers. Fatal injuries are mostly due to motor vehicle accidents or drowning.
- The number of accidental deaths in 15- to 44-year-old travelers is higher by a factor of 2 to 3 as compared with rates among the same age group back at home in the United States or Canada. "Excess mortality" abroad, therefore, is mainly due to accidental injuries.
- Infections cause fewer than 4% of deaths abroad.

ACCIDENTS AND TRAVEL

Accidents are the leading cause of death among travelers younger than the age of 55. Death rates from motor vehicle accidents, according to The Association for Safe International Road Travel, are 20 to 80 times higher in some countries than in the

Table 1.1   Reported Deaths of U.S. Citizens Abroad by Cause of Death*

Vehicle-related accidents	569
Homicide	287
Drowning	213
Other accidents	207
Suicide	204
Air accident	74
Drug-related	60
Natural disaster	42
Terrorist action	51
Train accident	11
Maritime accident	10
Under investigation	1
Unknown	1

*From October 1, 2002 to December 31, 2004.
NOTE: This chart does not represent a statistically complete account of U.S. citizen deaths abroad. The chart depicts only deaths that were reported to the Department of State for which it was possible to establish that death was not due to natural causes. Most U.S. citizens who die abroad are resident abroad. Also, it is difficult to establish how many deaths go unreported to the Department of State. Note also that deaths attributed to "Terrorist action" do not include deaths of U.S. military and government personnel in Iraq.

United States, illustrating one reason why "excess mortality" abroad is primarily injury related. The majority of deaths in younger travelers are from motor vehicle and motorcycle accidents, and drowning; air crashes (usually nonscheduled carries), suicides/homicides, burns, and electrocution are less frequent causes.

Each year, an estimated 750 Americans die of injuries on foreign roads, and at least 25,000 are injured. One study has revealed that many road accidents involving tourists do not involve a collision between two vehicles but are often due to loss of driver control caused by fatigue, alcohol intoxication, unfamiliar road conditions, or other factors. In many developing countries, vehicles are in disrepair; drivers are inexperienced; roads are not well maintained; and common-sense rules of the road are disregarded.

The Bethesda, Maryland-based Association for Safe International Road Travel (ASIRT; Tel: 301-983-5252; website: www.asirt.org) can provide a report on road safety conditions in 70 foreign countries. Their road travel reports also contain information about seasonal hazards; city, rural, and interstate traffic; and the most dangerous roads in various countries. ASIRT currently cites Egypt, Kenya, India, South Korea, Turkey, and Morocco as some of the most dangerous countries. (ASIRT, a nonprofit organization, requests a small donation in exchange for the information it provides.)

Preventing Traffic Accidents and Injuries

If you follow the recommendations below, you will decrease your chances of having an accident or being injured while driving overseas.

- Always wear a seat belt (if one is present).
- Bring a car seat for infants, and place them in the back seat.

Table 1.2 Global Road Toll Fact Sheet

1.7 million people die annually on roads worldwide.
30 million people are injured annually on roads worldwide.
Road crashes are the single greatest cause of premature death and injury in men ages 15-45.
Road crashes are the fifth leading cause of death in women.
Twenty percent of fatal accidents in developing countries involve children younger than the age of 15.
Road accidents will soon become the third greatest health burden worldwide.
More than 80% of all road deaths and serious injuries occur in developing countries in Africa, Asia, Latin America, and the Middle East.
More than 40% of the accidents occur in countries in the Asian-Pacific region.
Road accidents cost developing countries 100 billion U.S. dollars annually.

From the Association for Safe International Road Travel, www.asirt.org. Used with permission.

- Consider hiring a qualified guide or driver.
- Do not be afraid to tell your driver to slow down or use more caution.
- Rent a larger rather than a smaller vehicle.
- Know the meaning of all road sign symbols (found inside the back cover of this book).
- Be sure you have collision/liability insurance.
- Know that a driver approaching a traffic circle must yield the right of way to those already in the circle.
- Know the route to your destination. Study road maps thoroughly in advance of your trip.
- The two most important rules to follow are:
    - Do not drive at night in rural areas.
    - Do not ride a motorcycle, moped, or bicycle (even if you are experienced).

PERSONAL SAFETY GUIDELINES

Although you can't escape the remote possibility that you simply may find yourself "in the wrong place at the wrong time," you can take steps to enhance your personal safety while traveling: plan your trip carefully, be reasonably cautious, obey common-sense rules of behavior, and don't panic! Remember that the vast majority of travelers arrive home unscathed.

The following guidelines will be helpful in ensuring your travel safety:
- Carefully select swimming areas. Don't swim alone, while intoxicated, or at night.
- Avoid small, nonscheduled airlines in less developed countries.
- Don't travel by road at night outside urban areas. If you are out at night, stay in a group.
- Don't go out alone on beaches at night.
- Don't hitchhike or pick up hitchhikers.
- Don't sleep in your car or RV at the roadside at night.
- Camp only in legal campsites.
- If you are drinking alcohol, don't relax by sitting on the railing of your hotel balcony. Falls and serious injuries often occur this way.
- Review hotel fire safety rules. Locate nearest exits.
- If possible, book a room between the second and seventh floors—high enough to prevent easy entrance by an intruder and low enough for fire equipment to reach.
- Lock your hotel room at all times.
- Keep valuables and travel documents in your room (in-room safe) or hotel safe.
- Avoid countries or regions where there is drug-related violence and drug trafficking. Avoid excursions into remote areas of certain countries such as Mexico, Colombia, or Peru, where you might be mistaken for a drug agent or a rival drug dealer.
- Never purchase, transport, or use illegal drugs.
- Don't accept drinks or rides from a stranger you have just met.
- Familiarize yourself with the local laws and customs of the countries to which you are traveling and abide by them. Know the laws about exchanging money and deal only with authorized agents when you exchange money or purchase art or antiques.

- Put identifying markings on your luggage. Don't, however, put your home address or telephone number on your luggage tags. Instead, put a business card in the tag, or a use a P.O. box address and a business, mobile telephone, or third-party telephone number for contact.
- Do not put all your valuables in luggage you check; e.g., jewelry, cameras, watches. Besides your luggage possibly being lost, there is, unfortunately, increasing theft occurring during security searches of checked luggage. The best course is not to travel with any item of significant value.

There are numerous publications that provide specific advice on personal safety and security. Suggested titles include *The Safe Travel Book—A Guide for the International Traveler* by Peter Savage (Lexington Books: 800-462-6420) and *The Security Minute; How to Be Safe in the Streets, at Home, and Abroad So You Can Save Your Life!* by Robert L. Siciliano (Safety Zone Press: 800-438-6223).

CORPORATE SECURITY

Risk Management Companies

In times of geopolitical turmoil and terrorist activity, corporate interests are often targeted and advising corporations on matters of safety and security has become increasingly important. The companies listed below provide a variety of services that include the following: crisis management and contingency planning; hostage-release negotiation; counter-terrorism education/training; defensive driving training; executive protection; travel advisories and warnings; country-specific political analyses and risk assessments.

International SOS Assistance, Inc.
3600 Horizon Boulevard, Suite 300
Trevose, PA 19053
215-942-8000 or 1-800-523-8930
http://www.internationalsos.com/

iJET Travel Risk Management
910F Bestgate Road
Annapolis, MD 21401
410-573-3860
http://www.ijet.com

Kroll International
900 Third Ave., 8th floor
New York, NY 10022
800-212-593-1000
http://www.krollworldwide.com

State Department Security Advisories

You can obtain in-depth advice about specific security issues in any country by contacting the Regional Security Officer (RSO) at the embassy of the country to which you will be traveling. Here is the procedure:

- Contact the Department of State at 202-647-4000 and ask to be connected to the Country Desk covering the destination country.
- Request the name and overseas telephone number of the Regional Security Officer (RSO) stationed at the embassy. Some of this information is also available on the Department of State website (http://www.state.gov/www/about_state/contacts/keyofficer_index.html).
- Telephone the RSO during embassy business hours in the destination country. Inquiries often include questions about:
  - The safest taxi cab/route to take from the airport
  - Street crime or terrorism problems
  - Neighborhoods to avoid
  - Recent incidents involving tourists or corporate executives
  - Safety of public transportation

OSAC

The **Overseas Security Advisory Council (OSAC)** was established in 1985 by the U.S. Department of State to foster the exchange of security-related information between the U.S. Government and American private sector operating abroad. Administered by the Bureau of Diplomatic Security, OSAC has developed into a successful joint venture for effective security cooperation. Through OSAC, the American private sector, including colleges and universities, is provided timely information on which to make informed corporate decisions on how best to protect their investment, facilities, and personnel abroad.

The criteria for access to the website include the following:

- OSAC services are available to any American enterprise with overseas interests (business, religious, educational, nongovernmental, etc.) incorporated in the United States.
- Access to OSAC's website is available to federal, state, and local law enforcement or security agencies.

To locate the OSAC website go to www.travel.state.gov, click on "International Travel" then click "Safety Issues" on the sidebar, then click on the "Overseas Security Advisory Council" link. Chapter 19 has additional information on health and security related to business and corporate travel.

BUREAU OF CONSULAR AFFAIRS

How the Government Can Help

There is a vast amount of information available from the U.S. Department of State, Bureau of Consular Affairs, including passport and visa requirements, foreign country entry requirements, emergency services for U.S. citizens abroad, and much more. The Bureau of Consular Affairs also issues travel warnings, consular information sheets, and public announcements on more than 200 countries.

- Consular information sheets include the location and telephone number of the embassy and each consulate, information on health conditions, political disturbances, currency, entry regulations, and crime and security activities.
- Travel warnings list countries the State Department believes should be avoided, except for essential travel.
- Public announcements disseminate information about terrorist threats and other relatively short-term and/or trans-national conditions posing significant risks to the security of travelers.

    Information can be obtained by telephone or the Internet.

    The website of the Bureau of Consular affairs (www.travel.state.gov) is an extensive, and convenient, source of information. Browse the website to see what's offered. You may need to spend some time getting familiar with it, but here are some quick steps to finding useful information: Click on "International Travel" then go to the side bar and click on "Emergencies and Crises" then "Crisis Management." Now click on "Emergency Services for U.S. Citizens Overseas." You now have several choices. Scroll down this page and you will come to a listing of doctors and hospitals in more than 40 countries. There many other useful links, including "Help for Americans Abroad A-Z" and "Medical Information for Americans Traveling Abroad."

Emergency Services to U.S. Citizens Abroad

The Overseas Citizen's Service (OCS) is a division of the Bureau of Consular Affairs (www.travel.state.gov) that is responsible for issues concerning the welfare and whereabouts of U.S. citizens traveling and residing abroad. By calling their telephone number, you can be connected to an OCS case officer who will assist in matters involving services for Americans abroad, including:

- Arrest/detention of an American citizen abroad
- Robbery of a citizen abroad
- Death of an American citizen abroad
- American citizen missing abroad; welfare and whereabouts inquiries
- Legal services; document issuance; help with financial emergencies
- Disaster assistance
- Crises abroad that involve a U.S. citizen
- Medical emergencies. If emergency medical transport or an air ambulance is needed, the OCS may refer you (or the people helping you) to an assistance company. The U.S. government won't pay the costs of transport, but the OCS can facilitate transfer of funds. Working with the embassy or consulate, the OCS will help coordinate stretcher transport on a commercial airliner to bring a sick traveler home to the United States. In event of death, they will assist with returning the remains.
- Overseas Citizens Services Telephone Assistance—888-407-4747 (From Canada and overseas—317-472-2328)

    The U.S. Department of State also has another website, www.state.gov.travel, which has overlapping links with the website of the Bureau of Consular Affairs.

TRAVEL HEALTH INFORMATION

Almost all health problems related to travel are preventable or can be minimized, but most travelers are often unaware of the actual health risks they may encounter. A travel clinic is an excellent source for this information, but time constraints limit the amount of advice a practitioner can dispense in one or two office visits. And if given printed material, how much will you remember? And is the information you are given sufficient? An additional amount of pre-departure reading and data gathering is usually essential. The Internet can provide the most current information, if you know where to locate it, but books that are updated on a regular basis remain your best references (and can be brought along on your trip, as well). However, no single resource, printed or electronic, will provide all the information that you may need, so numerous resources are listed in this chapter. Be aware that these sources of information may not always be in agreement. For example, the Centers for Disease Control and Prevention (CDC) recommends that malaria prophylaxis be taken in *all* malarious areas, whereas many travel clinics and other information sources usually advise that low-risk, short-term travelers may rely instead on insect bite-prevention measures, or carry standby malaria treatment medication. And some literature in travel medicine advises that children with diarrhea not be treated with quinolone antibiotics, when in fact this treatment is now usually preferred. NOTE: Information is sometimes available from retail travel agents, tour operators, and airlines and other common carriers, but the quality of this information varies and may be unreliable.

Travel Health Information from the CDC

The United States Public Health Service Centers for Disease Control and Prevention (CDC) has expanded its International Fax Information Service and Internet information systems. You can get current malaria advisories, immunization schedules, disease risk and prevention information by regions (but not by countries) of the world, bulletins on disease outbreaks and epidemics, guidelines for the HIV-infected traveler, lists of countries where yellow fever is endemic or active (and where a yellow fever vaccination certificate may be required), and much more.

CDC's Travelers' Health website www.cdc.gov/travel
Voice information: 888-232-3228
Information by fax: 888-232-3299. The directory lists a six-digit number for each document. You then call back and order, by number, as many as five documents at once.

Health Information Online from the United States, Canada, the United Kingdom, and Europe

United States

- MD Travel Health—www.mdtravelhealth.com
- Shoreland, Inc.—www.tripprep.com
- Travel Medicine, Inc.—www.travmed.com

Canada
- HEALTH CANADA—http://www.phac-aspc.gc.ca/tmp-pmv

United Kingdom
- The Travel Doctor—www.traveldoctor.co.uk
- MASTA (The Medical Advisory Society to Travellers)-http://www.masta.org

Europe
- Fit For Travel-http://www.fit-for-travel.de/en

TRAVEL CLINICS

Before you depart you'll want to consult with your health-care provider if you have medical problems, are traveling to a less-developed country (where there is often the risk of tropical and infectious diseases), or planning an extended trip abroad. Specialized immunizations and prophylactic medications may be recommended or required. Although your own doctor may be able to administer some routine immunizations, most physicians' offices don't stock specialized vaccines, such as typhoid, rabies, or meningitis, and they are not authorized to stock and administer yellow fever vaccine, or issue the International Certificate of Vaccination. (Public health departments can administer yellow fever vaccines.) More importantly, your health-care provider may not have the expertise or resources to advise you about safe travel, or what to do if you get sick abroad. There are more than 220 different countries with evolving and varying disease-risk patterns, and providing travelers with accurate health information can be complex and time consuming. Most physicians are not prepared, or willing, to give this type of consultation.

Fortunately, the specialty of travel medicine has expanded rapidly over the past 15 years and there are now many physicians and nurse practitioners that either specialize in this field, or have added it to their regular practice. Although no specialty board certification is required to practice travel medicine, most travel medicine practitioners have received further training under the auspices of the International Society of Travel Medicine (www.istm.org) and/or the American Society of Tropical Medicine and Hygiene (www.astmh.org). Both of these organizations have developed specialty examinations that award a Certificate of Knowledge.

Types of Travel Clinics Travel clinics vary in their ranges of services and professional staffing. Sometimes a medical facility is dedicated solely to this specialty, but often a travel clinic is from a doctor's private practice, an ambulatory care clinic, an HMO or group practice, an occupational health clinic, or the infectious disease department of a university teaching hospital. These clinics, unlike regular physician's offices, are almost all tied into Internet and electronic databases that provide them with updated travel/health information and conditions worldwide.

Travel clinics supervised by physicians trained in infectious and/or tropical diseases are usually better able to counsel travelers with special needs, or who have returned from abroad with a suspected or undiagnosed tropical or infectious disease. Such clinics are often, but not invariably, associated with a university hospital or a medical school.

Finding a Travel Clinic

If you need to locate a travel clinic, visit one of the websites listed below. They have extensive listings, but no one website lists all clinics currently operational. The ISTM, ASTM&H, and Travel Medicine, Inc., websites also list travel clinics in many countries worldwide. This can be helpful if a travel/tropical disease specialist needs to be contacted for an illness occurring abroad.

Travel Medicine, Inc.
(www.travmed.com and www.travelinghealthy.com)

Shoreland, Inc., Travel Health Online
(www.tripprep.com)

International Society of Travel Medicine (ISTM)
(www.istm.org)

American Society of Tropical Medicine and Hygiene (ASTM&H)
(www.astmh.org)

HEALTH CANADA
(http://www.phac-aspc.gc.ca/tmp-pmv/travel/clinic_e.html)

Travel Clinics in the United Kingdom
The Travel Doctor
http://www.traveldoctor.co.uk/clinics.htm

MASTA
http://www.masta.org

Hospitals and Doctors Overseas

The **International Association for Medical Assistance to Travellers** (IAMAT) publishes a booklet listing English-speaking physicians and healthcare facilities worldwide. IAMAT also provides information on tropical diseases such as malaria and schistosomiasis. IAMAT is a tax-free foundation, and there is no charge for their publications; a donation, however, is requested. IAMAT, 417 Center Street, Lewiston, NY 14092; 716-754-4883. In Canada: 40 Regal Road, Guelph, Ontario, N1K 1B5; 519-836-0102.

The **Bureau of Consular Affairs** website (www.travel.state.gov) has a listing of doctors and hospitals in more than 40 countries. The lists have been submitted by various embassies or consulates, and vary in their completeness. From the home page, click on the "International Travel" link; next, click on "Health Issues" on the sidebar. Scroll down and click on "Lists of Doctors/Hospitals Abroad." The "Health Issues" section also contains updates on SARS and Avian flu. Further scrolling brings you down to a listing of domestic and international air ambulance providers.

Travel insurance policies with assistance. Companies such as the International SOS (http://www.internationalsos.com) and Medex (http://www.medexassist.com)

provide policyholders with access to an extensive network of doctors and hospitals worldwide. Physician referrals and monitoring of hospital care are parts of the assistance package provided.

Embassies and Consulates overseas also have listings of local health-care providers. **Hotels and resorts** can usually refer you to a local English-speaking doctor.

TRAVEL MEDICINE PUBLICATIONS

Travelers' Health Publications

Travel Medicine, edited by Jay Keystone, M.D., et al. (Mosby 2004.) A comprehensive textbook in the field of travel medicine, with contributions from over 70 internationally recognized experts.

Textbook of Travel Medicine and Health edited by Herbert L. DuPont, M.D. and Robert Steffen, M.D., (B.C. Decker 2001). A concise textbook focusing on all aspects of travel medicine.

Travel Medicine Advisor—A comprehensive source of travel health information from an online database with bimonthly newsletter updates in both print and electronic formats. Editor: Frank Bia, MD, MPH; American Health Consultants, Atlanta, GA; 800-688-2421—(www.ahcpub.com).

The Travel and Tropical Medicine Manual, edited by Elaine C. Jong, M.D. and Russell McMullen, M.D. (WB Saunders, 2000. Paperback). A comprehensive source of information on tropical medicine and travel-related infectious diseases.

Traveller's Health—How to Stay Healthy Abroad by Dr. Richard Dawood (Random House, 2002). A well-known source of travel health information compiled primarily by British experts.

Health Information for International Travel (The "CDC Yellow Book"). This is a primary travel medicine reference manual published biannually. The Yellow Book can be ordered from Elsevier at www.US.Elsevierhealth.com. The Yellow Book is written primarily for health-care providers, but travelers may find it useful.

Wilderness Medicine and First-Aid

Wilderness Medicine—Management of Wilderness and Environmental Emergencies, 2001. Paul S. Auerbach, M.D., editor (Mosby, 2001). The primary reference for anyone seriously involved in outdoor and wilderness medicine.

A Comprehensive Guide to Wilderness and Travel Medicine by Eric A. Weiss, M.D. (Adventure Medical Kits; 800-324-3517). Also available from Amazon.com.

Common Sense First Aid for Travel and Home by Alan Spira, M.D. (2000). Available from Amazon.com.

Underwater Medicine/Decompression Chambers

For a guide to hyperbaric and decompression chamber facilities worldwide, contact the Undersea and Hyperbaric Medical Society, 9650 Rockville Pike, Bethesda, MD; 301-571-1817.

High Altitude Illness

Medicine for Mountaineering & Other Wilderness Activities, by James A. Wilkerson (Paperback, 2001). Available from Amazon.com.

Internet-based altitude illness information: www.high-altitude-medicine.com. This website also contains a listing of numerous publications on mountaineering medicine, altitude illness, wilderness medicine, and first-aid.

Travel Medicine Databases

During the past decade, there have been dramatic increases in the amount of travel health information available electronically, either via the Internet or distributed on PC disks or CD-ROMs. The advantage of these systems lies in their ability to provide updated, organized, itinerary-specific information in a format that can be printed out for the traveler. This is of great help in pre-travel counseling and trip preparation. In addition, some systems can also alert overseas travelers via e-mail about evolving emergency conditions—be they medical or safety/security related. Other systems allow a company to check on an employee's whereabouts and current status—a feature especially used by corporate medical and security departments tracking overseas employees who may be at risk.

TRAVEL CARE—International SOS Assistance, Inc., 3600 Horizon Boulevard, Suite 300, Trevose, PA 19053; 215-942 8000 or 1-800-523-8930. www.internationalsos.com (or www.travelcare.com for a free demonstration).

Online travel health program designed for the medical professional conducting pre-travel medical consultations. TRAVEL CARE's sophisticated but easy-to-use databases help the practitioner decide on appropriate vaccinations and malaria prophylaxis and also evaluate current health risks for any itinerary. Detailed country reports and advisories include comprehensive medical and disease-risk information, as well as nonmedical information—such as safety and security issues, cultural tips, and types of electrical plugs (including photos). Updated health and security advisories can be sent by e-mail to the overseas traveler. The "Traveler Locator Service" from the International SOS consolidates a company's airline booking data into one database and allows company executives to search this data online to track employee travel. These searches can be current, prospective or historic, with data searched by continent, country, city, hotel, flight number, or country risk rating.

TRAVAX-Shoreland, Inc., 2401 N. Mayfair Road, Suite 309, Milwaukee, WI 53226; 800-433-5256; 414-290-1900; e-mail: sales@shoreland.com; Internet: www.shoreland.com. Basic travel health recommendations, including country-by-country disease-risk information, vaccine recommendations, and current disease outbreak alerts. Disease-by-disease fact sheets. Very detailed malaria, yellow fever, and cholera risk maps by country. Health-related entry requirements. Detailed country profiles, including geography and climate. Crime, security, and other associated information. Contact information for U.S., Australian, and Canadian embassies and consulates. List of Internet URLs for U.S. State Department resources. Itinerary maker feature considers order of travel and presents summary recommendations for entire itinerary.

Printout for each country can be customized to allow physician-added comments and allows deletion of sections not of use to an individual patient.

Travax EnCompass, an expanded (detailed overseas medical facility data) wholly Internet-based version, is available to corporations under a licensing agreement.

CATIS-Computerized-Assisted Travel Information System (CATIS). Dr. David Lawee; Travel Information & Supplies; PO Box 41003, 2795 Bathurst St. Toronto, Ontario, Canada M6B 4J6. Tel/fax: 416-785-6219.

Content: Country-by-country vaccine recommendations, plus disease risk information both textual or illustrated with colored maps. Brief disease and vaccine fact sheets. Comparison maps for the CDC, WHO, CATMAT; malaria recommendations. Itinerary maker feature requires responses to a multiscreen detailed questionnaire even if patient and itinerary are uncomplicated. Requires patient to have detailed knowledge of in-country itinerary. Printout generated accounting for traveler health status. Printed prescription for malaria prophylaxis with calculation of dosage, number of tablets required, and schedule of administration. No country background or emergency contact information.

Kidney Dialysis Abroad

Dialysis and Transplantation: The List (Creative Age Publications: 800-442-5667 or 818-782-7328). Worldwide listing of dialysis clinics.

Dialysis at Sea Cruises. They have contracts with a number of cruise lines and provide onboard dialysis. Tel: 800-544-7604 for further information on schedules and destinations.

CHAPTER 2

Trip Preparation

KEY POINTS:

Most travelers are advised to:

▶ Visit a travel clinic prior to departure. Travel clinics can provide specialized immunizations and prescriptions for medications, as well as providing essential advice about how to prevent or treat illness abroad.

▶ Learn about the availability and quality of health care available at their destination.

▶ Know how to obtain the names of qualified, English-speaking doctors and which facilities provide the best care at their destination.

▶ Purchase a travel health policy that directly pays doctors and hospitals abroad and that also coordinates and pays for emergency medical evacuation.

▶ Carry standby antibiotics to treat travelers' diarrhea, and bring at least a basic medical kit.

▶ Have available copies of key portions of their medical records (e.g., a recent ECG) and a list of their medications, if health problems are a concern.

▶ See a physician immediately if a fever develops during a trip to the tropics, or soon after return. Malaria is a medical emergency, and must be considered.

When preparing for your trip, list the countries you will be visiting (in order) and the length of time you plan to spend in each one. There are five questions you need to answer about your trip, which will determine the degree of detail needed in planning ahead.

What is My Destination?

You should ask yourself the following questions: What illnesses are prevalent in the region I will be visiting? What is the general level of sanitation? How competent, and close by, is medical care? How harsh is the climate? How safe are the roads? Is the country politically stable?

Also, remember that a trip to Western Europe, for example, doesn't require as much preparation as an extended stay in a remote village in a less developed region. Because some countries and cities are much safer than others, be careful not to overdo precautions. You don't need a typhoid shot if you are going to London or Tokyo, nor do you necessarily need a whole series of immunizations if you're taking a brief trip to a less developed country but staying exclusively in a deluxe hotel in a large city. For updated information on country-by-country disease risks, consult the World Medical Guide section of this book.

What Will I Be Doing?

Staying in rural areas of less developed countries puts you at greater risk of contact with unsanitary food and drink and usually brings greater exposure to disease-carrying insects. (However, some diseases, such as dengue fever, are also transmitted in urban areas. There is also the risk of malaria in most cities in sub-Saharan Africa.)

Traveling on a tour and staying only in air-conditioned, deluxe hotels, typically carries less risk than traveling in rural areas off the usual tourist routes. Planning an adventure or wilderness itinerary with exposure to extremes of heat, cold, or altitude also takes additional preparation, as does trekking or camping in a remote area far from medical care. Driving a car, motorcycle, or moped in a less developed country may be quite hazardous as motor vehicle accidents account for most preventable fatalities among travelers. Higher risk activities also include swimming in unfamiliar, possibly treacherous, waters, or wading/rafting in freshwater ponds, lakes, or streams. Engaging in casual, unprotected sex is another potential health problem. Therefore, a close analysis of your activities is critical in helping you avoid illness and injury.

How Long Will I Be There?

A brief trip usually means less exposure to diseases and less opportunity for an accident. Longer trips increase the likelihoods of side trips and excursions that may place you at an unforeseen risk, perhaps for a mosquito-transmitted disease such as malaria. Longer travel may also cause you to discontinue prophylactic antimalarial medication, abandon safe food and drink practices, or neglect insect protection measures. Long-stay travel also brings with it the risk of "culture shock" and the need to know more about local customs, traditions, and history. Therefore, if you will be working overseas, you must also consider what psychological stresses you, and perhaps your family, will experience while adjusting to life abroad and what resources you will need beforehand to help make a smooth adjustment.

What Should I Bring?

Your itinerary, the climatic conditions you expect to encounter, the duration of your trip, and the disease risks in the countries you will be visiting all influence what you should bring. For example, many travelers to tropical and subtropical regions neglect to take precautions against insect bites necessary to prevent malaria and other insect-transmitted diseases. Be sure you have the necessary supplies (DEET repellents, permethrin insecticide, mosquito netting) described in Chapter 7. Your health status may also require you to take additional precautions.

When traveling overseas, take an ample supply of any medication that you use regularly, as well as copies of your prescriptions and the generic names of the medications; brand names are usually different overseas. Do not carry a mixture of pills in unmarked vials. To avoid problems with customs officers who might suspect that your pills are recreational drugs or illegal narcotics, keep each medication in its labeled original container. NOTE: Certain countries deny entry to HIV-positive travelers. If you are HIV-positive, be prudent when packing your medications.

Carry legally prescribed narcotics and controlled drugs (tranquilizers, sleeping pills, etc.) only if medically necessary. If you are a diabetic taking insulin and carrying needles and syringes, you may also arouse suspicion at customs checkpoints. Obtain a letter on a professional letterhead from your doctor certifying the need for these medications and certifying your diagnosis and treatment. The same applies if you will be carrying needles and syringes in an HIV/hepatitis prevention kit.

Preparation Checklists

Use the following checklists as general guidelines and modify them according to your itinerary and specific travel and health needs. A nylon or canvas pack (e.g., the Wallaby Trip Kit by Eagle Creek) or a first aid kit (see page 22 for a list of suppliers of medical kits) are useful for carrying medications and other healthcare items. Any medical kit containing sharp objects, such as scissors or a scalpel, should be in your checked baggage to avoid possible confiscation at an airline security checkpoint. Medications and other items needed en route should always be carried on your person.

Medical and Personal Care Items

- An adequate supply of your prescription medications—Carry copies of your prescriptions by generic names. Determine how much of each medication you will need for the duration of your trip, and if you will need refills. Check local availability of medications, but know that regionally manufactured drugs may be substandard or counterfeit. The illicit market in bogus, copied, relabeled, adulterated, and look-alike drugs is burgeoning; therefore, be careful. It may be prudent to bring enough medications for your entire trip—or make arrangements for additional drugs to be shipped to you from home.
- Antibiotics for treating travelers' diarrhea—Quinolone antibiotics are the most effective and include ofloxacin (Floxin), levofloxacin (Levaquin), and ciprofloxacin (Cipro). Azithromycin (Zithromax) is the best alternative. Ciprofloxacin and azithromycin are available in liquid forms for children.
- Antibiotics for self-treatment of other infections—Levofloxacin is probably the best choice because of it broad spectrum of activity against common, as well as uncommon, infections. It is effective against acute bacterial bronchitis, many pneumonias, urinary tract infections, typhoid fever, skin infections (cellulitis, skin abscesses), and uncomplicated pelvic inflammatory disease (PID) due to gonorrhea and chlamydia. Azithromycin is the best alternative multipurpose antibiotic.
- Loperamide (Imodium-AD, Diamode)—Use to treat mild to moderate travelers' diarrhea, or use in combination with an antibiotic to treat more severe diarrhea.
- An antimalarial drug—Use especially if you are going to an area where falciparum malaria is a threat (see Chapter 7). These drugs are usually taken for prophylaxis; occasionally, they are carried for self-treatment.
- Medical kit—Carry at the minimum a first-aid kit that contains a thermometer, Band-Aids, gauze pads, and 1 or 2 roller gauzes, antibiotic ointment, scissors, and tape. Blister pads (moleskin) should be included. The size of the medical kit de-

pends on the number of travelers, length of stay, and the availability of local health care. Some travelers (especially those with multinational corporations) also carry kits with suture supplies and intravenous fluids.

- Water filtration/purification supplies—MicroPur tablets, Katadyn filter, and the Extreme water purification bottle are popular.
- Oral rehydration salts (e.g., CeraLyte)—Use to treat dehydration caused by severe diarrhea. A 1 liter plastic bottle is adequate for storing water or rehydration solution.
- Epinephrine kit—If you have a history of severe bee sting reactions or severe food or drug allergies, have your doctor prescribe an emergency epinephrine self-injection kit (EpiPen). Be sure you are instructed in its use before you travel.
- Sterile needle/syringe kit—These are often recommended when traveling to countries where hepatitis and HIV transmission are potential threats and where the sterility of medical supplies is questionable.
- Analgesics, such as ibuprofen (e.g., Motrin, Advil) or acetaminophen (Tylenol)— Acetaminophen with codeine, besides being an effective pain medication, also has antidiarrheal properties. Aspirin can lose potency when exposed to humidity and heat. Acetaminophen is not affected by these conditions.
- Antacids—Maalox or Mylanta are useful.
- Pepto-Bismol—Useful for the prevention and treatment of diarrhea (Chapter 6).
- Cathartics and/or stool softeners. Constipation is not uncommon, especially in the elderly.
- Motion/sea sickness drugs—TransDerm Scōp patch (for sea sickness on cruises); SCOPACE (scopolamine tablets), Dramamine, and Phenergan are shorter-acting agents.
- Drugs to prevent or treat altitude illness (see Chapter 15)—These should be considered when ascending above 8,000 feet.
- Jet lag—Sleeping pills, e.g., triazolam (Halcion) are helpful for some people who find insomnia the most troublesome symptom of jet lag. Zolpidem (Ambien) and zaleplon (Sonata) are alternatives. A new drug, Lunesta, which helps prevent early awakening, may also be helpful. Melatonin has limited effectiveness, and has not been approved by the FDA.
- Contact lens wearers—Antibiotic eye drops containing a quinolone (levofloxacin or ciprofloxacin) for treating an infected corneal ulcer should be carried. Untreated bacterial infections can cause corneal scarring.
- Hand sanitizer gel or disinfecting skin towelettes—These are convenient when soap and water are not available. Good hand hygiene helps prevent the transmission of travelers' diarrhea, as well as viruses and respiratory infections.
- Nasal decongestant spray—Afrin or Neo-Synephrine.
- EarPlanes—Pressure-regulating earplugs will reduce pain associated with air travel. Especially recommended if you have trouble clearing your nasal passages during flight.
- Antihistamine tablets—Useful for allergic reactions and rhinitis (hay fever). Zyrtec and Claritin-D are long acting and less sedating. Check with your pharmacist about

any possible drug interactions with medications you may be already taking for a chronic condition.

- V̄o Sol solution (2% acetic acid)—This prevents or treats swimmer's ear.
- Corticosteroid cream, such as Cortaid or Topicort—The steroid creams available by prescription are more effective for treating rashes than the over-the-counter products.
- Antifungal foot powder—Lotrisone and Tinactin are good choices. These are essential when traveling in the heat and humidity of the tropics.
- Antifungal tablets—A single, oral 150-mg tablet of fluconazole (Diflucan) will eradicate a vaginal yeast infection. (These infections can result from using an antibiotic.)
- Extra pair of prescription glasses or contact lenses—Bring a copy of lens prescription.
- Other useful items:
  - Tweezers (good for tick removal), small knife, scissors, or Swiss Army knife (keep out of carry-on luggage). Large safety pins are also very useful.

For Rain, Sun, Heat, and Insects

- Hat, sunglasses, umbrella
- Sunscreens—Broad-spectrum sunscreen, minimum SPF 30.
- Insect repellent—Important when traveling to a country where insect-transmitted diseases, such as malaria, are a threat. Travelers should use a skin repellent that contains at least 30% DEET. A good choice is Ultrathon, which provides 12-hour protection against mosquitoes, as well as ticks and biting flies.
- Clothing insecticide—Permethrin is an insecticide that kills insects that touch the treated fabric (e.g., clothing, gear, tents, mosquito nets). Against ticks, it is more effective than DEET. When used in combination with a DEET repellent (as is done by the U.S. military), up to 100% protection against mosquito and tick bites can be achieved.
- Mosquito bed net (preferably permethrin-treated)
- Insecticide spray (e.g., Raid Flying Insect Spray) to rid sleeping quarters of night-biting insects

  Medical kits and other supplies: Sources include Travel Medicine, Inc., 369 Pleasant Street, Northampton, MA 01060, 800-TRAVMED (800-872-8633); on-line catalog www.travmed.com and Chinook Medical Gear, Durango, CO (800-766-1365). On-line catalog www.chinookmed.com

Checking the Weather at Your Destination

Global Weather Information: http://www.weather.yahoo.com

Wilderness Travel

Adequate pre-trip planning is essential. If you're on an adventure itinerary, determine what exposure you will have to heat, cold, or altitude. If you are on a trek, most tour organizers will advise you of what to bring, but you may need to consult experts in outdoor/wilderness travel to determine if what is recommended is truly adequate. A Comprehensive Guide to Wilderness & Travel Medicine, 3rd ed., AMK Publishers, Oakland, CA 2000, by Eric A. Weiss, M.D., is a recommended resource and can be ordered from the publisher (Adventure Medical Kits: 800-324-3517) or amazon.com.

Checklist for campers, hikers, and trekkers—You need to anticipate sudden changes in weather, in particular, high winds, rain, and temperature drops. For your comfort and safety, be sure always to carry an outer shell or parka that is waterproof and breathable, fleece vest or jacket, cap and gloves. Multiple layers of clothing should be worn in more extreme conditions. Review the following checklist for additional items your trip may require.

- Sleeping bag
- Bivouac bag
- Ground cloth and pad
- Vapor barrier
- Tent
- Thermal blanket
- Radiant heat barrier
- Fuel, fire starter
- Fire and camping permits
- Stove
- Matches
- First-aid kit
- Sleep sack/sleeping bag liner
- Cooking gear, dehydrated food
- Candle and candle lantern
- Maps and travel guides
- Compass
- GPS
- Mobile phone
- Two-way radio
- Binoculars
- Wrist compass/altimeter/barometer
- Flashlight
- Extra batteries and bulbs
- Rope
- Trowel and shovel
- Chemical hand and feet warmers
- Washcloth, soap, toiletry kit

Travel Documents You May Need

- Passports—The Bureau of Consular Affairs' website (http://www.travel.state.gov) provides comprehensive information about applying for, or renewing, a passport or visa. Passport application forms can be downloaded from this site.

Make two copies of your passport identification page. This will facilitate replacement if your passport is lost or stolen. Leave one copy at home with friends or relatives. Carry the other with you in a separate place from your passport. Be sure to fill in the emergency contact information section of your passport.

What if I need a passport in a hurry, or I have lost my passport? Normally, it takes about 6 weeks to get your passport from the U.S. Passport Agency. The Agency will expedite the process for an additional $60, plus overnight shipping, and your passport will arrive in about 2 weeks. Passport/visa service companies, however, can obtain a passport for you in as little as one business day, plus overnight shipping. This assumes you have all your documents in order. Also, if this is a first-time passport, the application must be witnessed and sealed by an authorized passport acceptance agent (found at federal, state and probate courts, post offices, some public libraries, and a number of county and municipal offices) before the passport/visa service company is able to process the application. This expediting can be expensive—you pay the passport government's passport fee, plus as much as $180, plus shipping for next-day service. Standard expedited service (6 to 9 business days) is about $60 plus the other charges. Contact one of the following:

- American Passport Express, 800-841-6778 (www.americanpassport.com)
- Passport Plus, New York, NY, 212-759-5540 or 800-367-1818 (www.passportplus.net)
- Passport and Visa Expeditors, Washington, DC, 800-237-3270
- Travisa, Washington, DC, 202-463-6166 or 800-222-2589 (www.travisa.com)
- TravelSeeker (www.passportnow.com). Lists numerous online companies that can expedite getting a new or renewed passport.
- Lost Passport Overseas—Go to the nearest American consulate and bring the following:
  - A police report that documents the loss or theft
  - Four passport-sized photos (2″ × 2″ size)
  - Application fee in U.S. currency, traveler's checks, or local currency. Bring the exact amount of currency.
  - If you have a photocopy of the lost passport showing the passport number and the date and place of issue, it will speed the process. Bring any other proof of identity available.

  You will need to complete a new passport application. The consular officer taking an application for replacement of a lost, stolen, or misplaced passport must be reasonably satisfied as to your identity and citizenship before issuing the replacement. In virtually all cases this can be done through examination of whatever citizenship and identity documents are available, conversations with the applicant, close observation of demeanor, replies to questions, and discussions with the applicant's traveling companions or contacts in the United States.

  U.S. embassies and consulates will continue to issue passports that are needed for urgent travel, but these are temporary documents, without the digitized images and other security features introduced in 2002. Such passports will be limited in validity, and cannot be extended. Bearers will be required to exchange, at no additional cost, their limited-validity passports for a full-validity digitized passport on completion of their urgent travel.
- Visas—The best source to obtain up-to-date visa requirements for travel to other countries is the website of the Bureau of Consular Affairs (http://www.travel.state.gov).

  After verifying the need for a visa, contact the embassy or consulate of the country or countries of your destination to verify information regarding the documents you will need and the processing time required. You can also use one of the passport expeditor companies listed on the previous page to file the application. Go to their websites to view the process and fees.
- HIV testing requirements for entry into foreign countries—Go to the State Department's Bureau of Consular Affairs website: http://travel.state.gov. Click on "American Citizen Traveling Abroad?" link, then "Foreign Entry requirements." Not all HIV testing requirements are found here, or the requirements may have changed, so check with the embassy or consulate of the country that you plan to visit to verify the requirement for entry, *if any.* The HIV test is usually required only for those applying for a foreign work permit, prolonged residence, or immigration—not for tourist visits of less than 1 to 3 months. Tests done in the United States or Canada may not be accepted.

- International Certificate of Vaccination (Yellow Card)—Yellow fever vaccinations must be given at official Yellow Fever Vaccination Centers (e.g., a travel clinic, local health department) as designated by respective state health departments. The international certificate of vaccination (the Yellow Card) must be validated with the "Uniform Stamp" and signed by the physician or the physician's designee. The Centers for Disease Control and Prevention website (www.cdc.gov/travel) lists clinics within the United States, by state, that are licensed to administer the yellow fever vaccine and the certificate. You need to have in your possession a validated Yellow Card when entering countries that require proof of yellow fever vaccination. You should carry the yellow card with your passport. The yellow card has useful sections where you can also list all of your other vaccinations and medications, as well as any exemptions from vaccination.

Note: Currently no country "officially" requires cholera vaccination as a condition of entry. Local authorities in some (usually sub-Saharan) countries, however, may require documentation of vaccination. This tactic may be used to extract a bribe to waive the "requirement." Depending on your itinerary (and because the cholera vaccine is no longer available in the United States), you may have your health-care provider state on your Yellow Card "Exempt from cholera vaccine" and have the exemption stamped and signed. NOTE: There is no section for cholera vaccination on the new Yellow Cards. Some travel clinics routinely state that the vaccine is contraindicated; in some cases the clinic will create a cholera stamped area while being sure that the traveler knows that they did not receive the injection.

- Extra photos—Obtain at least eight (8) additional 2″ x 2″ photos when applying for your passport or visa(s). These extra photos will come in handy if you need additional visas or an international driver's permit or if you need to replace a lost passport or other document.
- Personal health records—Consider carrying photocopies of your health and hospital records, recent electrocardiogram (ECG), laboratory test results, list of current medications, allergies, etc. Or, you may wish to subscribe to a service that can assemble all of your pertinent medical records, store them in a computer, and fax or e-mail them anywhere in the world within minutes. Contact Global Med-Net (800-650-SAVE) for further information.
- Travel health insurance—It is always a good idea to purchase a travel insurance policy (Chapter 18). These policies pay overseas doctors and hospitals at the time of the visit, and they also cover emergency medical transport. Check your existing health insurance policy to see what benefits are provided in case of illness overseas. Normally, only emergencies are covered. Medicare does not pay for out-of-country illnesses or accidents, so anyone with Medicare should also have MediGap coverage.
- Doctors and hospitals abroad—The International Association for Assistance to Travelers (IAMAT) publishes a booklet listing hospitals and English-speaking physicians overseas. 417 Center Street, Lewiston, NY 14092; 716-754-4883.
- Medic Alert bracelet—If you have a serious or chronic medical condition, a history of severe drug allergy, etc., you should consider wearing a Medic Alert bracelet. Call 1-800-ID-ALERT to order.

- Prescription drugs abroad—Worldwide delivery of non-controlled (non-narcotic) medications sent via Federal Express or DHL. Contact: Global RX, 4024 Carrington Lane, Efland, NC 27243; Tel: 919-304-4278; Fax: 919-304-4405; E-mail: info@globalrx.com; www.globalrx.com
- Divers Alert Network (DAN)—For non-emergency medical questions and general information, scuba divers can call (919) 684-2948 for DAN'S Dive Safety and Medical Information Line. (Website: www.diversalertnetwork). For scuba diving emergencies, DAN'S Diving Emergency Hotline is (919) 684-4DAN (4326) or (919) 684-8111. These lines are open to all divers.
- Mobile phones overseas—Unless you have a multi-band GSM phone, your own mobile (cell) phone is probably useless overseas, so you may want to buy or rent a phone for your trip. A low-cost option is buying a cheap, prepaid phone on arrival. You can also buy a phone before departure, or at your destination, whose SIM card can be reloaded with airtime purchased locally. Good resources for mobile phones overseas include Telestial (www.telestial.com) and Cellular Abroad (www.cellularabroad.com). NOTE: Camera phones are not allowed in Saudi Arabia and their use in some other countries may arouse suspicion.
- Telephone number and e-mail address of your personal physician
- Foreign language telephone assistance—When dealing with medical problems long distance, there may be language barriers. Call AT&T's Language Line at 800-628-8486 for assistance. The service costs vary per minute, depending on the language being interpreted.
- Traveler's checks—Make a photocopy of the numbers. Leave the photocopy at home and carry with you the list of numbers that you get with the checks. Copy the date and place of purchase and where to call if the checks are lost or stolen.
- Credit cards—Know your charge card credit limits. U.S. citizens have been arrested in some countries for exceeding credit limits. Keep a copy of your card numbers in case they are lost or stolen. Report the loss immediately.
- Money—ATM facilities in other countries are becoming more prevalent; they offer convenience and usually the best exchange rates. Foreign banks usually will advance cash against your credit card. Be sure you have your PIN number.
- Birth certificate and photo ID—These documents can sometimes be used in lieu of a passport for entry into certain countries. They're also useful to have if you lose your passport. If you are living overseas or getting married in a foreign country, be sure to have these documents with you.
- Green card for resident aliens—Don't leave home without it.
- Doctor's letter—You may want a doctor's letter describing and authorizing the prescription medications you will be taking on your trip, including needles/syringes if you are a diabetic. The letter should contain the generic names of the medications and the dosages.
- International driver's permit—This is available at any AAA office. When applying you'll need two passport-sized photos, your driver's license, and $10 for the fee. The international driver's permit is printed in nine languages and serves as a translation for your license, which is valid in many countries. A few countries (China, Egypt, Nepal) do not allow tourists to drive.

- Notarized parental consent—Necessary when a minor child is traveling with the noncustodial parent. This permission letter may even be required when one parent is traveling internationally alone with his/her child. You may not be able to board the aircraft or enter a country (e.g., Mexico) without this document.

Vaccinations
See Chapter 3 for travel vaccination guidelines.

TRAVELERS WITH SPECIAL NEEDS

Heart Disease
If you have a history of coronary heart disease, and your condition is stable, travel is generally low risk, and airline travel is considered safe. Heart disease, per se, is not a contraindication for travel to high altitudes (see Chapter 15, Altitude Illness). No matter where you go, be sure you have:

- An adequate supply of your medications
- A copy of your most recent ECG and any relevant medical records

Pacemakers A pacemaker or an implanted defibrillator/cardioverter is not a contraindication to air travel, and these devices are not affected by walk-through airport security magnetometers. However, the handheld security magnetometers should never be used on someone with an implanted defibrillator. Electronic telephone checks of pacemaker function cannot be transmitted by international satellite.

Chronic Lung Disease and Air Travel
If you have chronic obstructive pulmonary disease (COPD, emphysema), air travel is considered safe if you can walk a block or climb a flight of stairs without becoming breathless. In-flight oxygen may be indicated if your sea level arterial oxygen level (PaO_2) on room air is 72 mm Hg or less. This corresponds to an in-flight PaO_2 of 55 mm Hg when the cabin is pressurized to 8,000 feet.

If your doctor advises in-flight oxygen, contact the airline medical department at least 48 to 72 hours prior to departure. There may be a $50 to $75 charge for oxygen for each flight/plane change. The airline may request a physician's letter stating your medical condition and a prescription for the oxygen. Be sure to carry copies of these documents with you. Unlike foreign airlines, U.S. carriers must legally supply all in-flight oxygen. You will not be allowed to use your personal oxygen supply en route, and if you have a portable unit, it must be empty when checked in. Unfortunately, on-board oxygen delivery systems (mask or nasal cannula) are not standardized, and you may need to use a system other than your own. In addition, the airline will not provide oxygen for ground use. You'll need to make arrangements yourself if you need ground oxygen between flights.

Diabetes
- If you take pills to control blood sugar, no time zone adjustment of dosage is necessary when flying. Take your medication according to the local time.

- If you are a diabetic using insulin, take enough insulin and U-100 syringes to last the entire trip. (Many countries still use U-80 syringes.)
- If traveling by air, call the carrier 72 hours before departure to order a diabetic menu.
- Hand carry your insulin at airport security checkpoints.
- Consider carrying all diabetic supplies in a specially designed case, such as the DIA-PAK. Insulin will keep its full potency for several months even if it's not refrigerated, but its temperature should be kept below 86° F. The DIA-PAK (two models available) has a refreezable cold pack for keeping insulin cool in hot climates. The company also carries glucose gel packets and other accessories. Contact B & A Products at 918-696-5998 or www.baproducts.com.
- Test blood glucose at 6-hour intervals or before each meal during the flight.
- Carry sugar cubes, glucose gel, or a snack in case an insulin reaction (hypoglycemia) occurs.

Figure 2.1   Nomogram for Predicting In-Flight Arterial Oxygen Tension from Cabin Altitude and Preflight Arterial Oxygen Tension

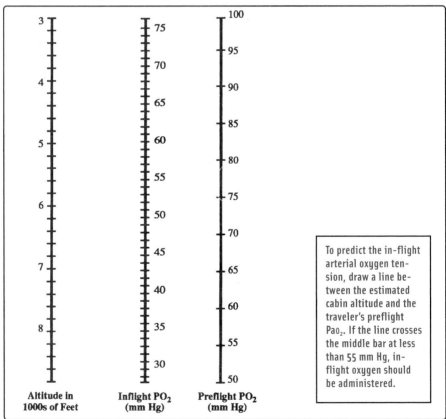

Altitude in 1000s of Feet

Inflight PO₂ (mm Hg)

Preflight PO₂ (mm Hg)

To predict the in-flight arterial oxygen tension, draw a line between the estimated cabin altitude and the traveler's preflight Pao₂. If the line crosses the middle bar at less than 55 mm Hg, in-flight oxygen should be administered.

Teeth, Eyes, and Feet

- Schedule a dental checkup—Allow enough time for corrective work. Avoid dental work and injections in countries where HIV and hepatitis B infections are threats. Consider carrying an emergency dental kit to treat broken or lost fillings—a DenTemp kit (for example see Fig. 2.2.)
- Check your feet—Proper foot care is essential, especially for hikers and diabetics. Carefully trim nails, corns, and calluses. Use foot powder to keep feet dry and fungus free. Be sure shoes and hiking boots are broken in and fit properly. Don't let a painful, infected blister or another preventable foot problem ruin your trip or jeopardize your health.
- Schedule an eye examination—Carry an extra set of eyeglasses. Contact-lens wearers should also carry a pair of eyeglasses. Keep a copy of your eyeglass prescription with you. Also, if you wear contact lenses, carry antibacterial eye drops (Ciloxan, containing ciprofloxacin, is a good choice). Contact-lens wearers, especially those who wear their lenses overnight, are at increased risk for developing bacterial keratitis (infected corneal ulcers, which may be caused by *Pseudomonas* or *Serratia* bacteria). These infections may cause permanent corneal scarring or perforation if not treated promptly. NOTE: Even daily-wear soft contact lenses are three times more likely to cause bacterial keratitis as are the daily-wear, rigid, gas-permeable lenses.

The HIV-Positive Adult Traveler

Pre-travel evaluation   Pre-travel medical screening should include (just as with all travelers) a medical history, immunization history, allergy history, and a history of any problems during previous travel. Those whose CD4+ cell counts are normal or greater than $500/\mu L$ are usually at no greater risk than noninfected travelers for travel-related problems, but those whose CD4+ cell counts are less than 200 cells/μL, or who are symptomatic, are at a greater risk of acquiring infections.

Figure 2.2   The DenTemp dental repair kit is available at most pharmacies.

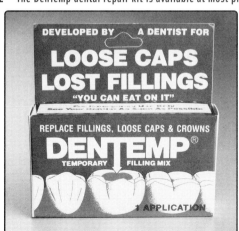

Travelers' Diarrhea   In HIV-positive travelers, this disorder can occur more frequently, be more severe, and be more difficult to treat. Infections with *Salmonella, Shigella,* and *Campylobacter* species are more protracted and more often associated with bacteremia. The usual 1- to 3-day course of antibiotic treatment for travelers' diarrhea may need to be extended to 7 days.

Cryptosporidium, a common cause of diarrhea in the tropics, produces severe chronic diarrhea, malabsorption, and, occasionally, inflammation of the gallbladder (cholecystitis). *Cyclospora* parasites cause similar symptoms. *Isospora belli* infections are also common and cause malabsorption and weight loss. There is no apparent increased risk for gastrointestinal infections caused by viruses, *Entamoeba histolytica, Giardia lamblia,* or enterotoxigenic *Escherichia coli* (the most common cause of travelers' diarrhea).

Other Infections   Respiratory illnesses, such as bacterial pneumonia and fungal infections (e.g., histoplasmosis and coccidiomycosis), cause greater mortality in HIV-positive patients. Tuberculosis is a serious risk for those living or working in lower socioeconomic populations in the developing world. Short-term business travelers and tourists are at low risk for acquiring tuberculosis. Visceral leishmaniasis is difficult to diagnose and treat, and the mortality is high. Even short-term travelers to Spain, southern Europe, and other risk areas have acquired this illness. Increased severity of malaria has not been demonstrated conclusively in HIV-infected patients, but this infection must be prevented by chemoprophylaxis and insect-bite prevention measures.

Preventive Measures   Food and drink precautions should be carefully followed. Undercooked meat, fish, shellfish, eggs, raw and unpeeled fruits, raw vegetables and salads, tap water, and unpasteurized dairy products should be avoided. Hands should be washed, or a hand sanitizer gel applied, before meals to reduce the spread of gastrointestinal and respiratory diseases. Consideration should be given to giving prophylactic antibiotics to short-term travelers with low CD4+ cell counts to prevent travelers' diarrhea. All other travelers, including those travelers taking prophylactic sulfa drugs to prevent pneumocystis pneumonia, should carry a standby self-treatment course of a quinolone antibiotic. Taking precautions against insect bites is important to prevent diseases such as malaria, dengue, and leishmaniasis.

Sexually Transmitted Diseases   HIV-infected travelers should be counseled against engaging in sexual behavior that might infect others or that will increase their own risks of acquiring infections such as syphilis, herpes simplex, or an intestinal microorganism. Hepatitis B is likely to be more severe as is the chance of becoming a chronic carrier of the virus.

Immunization (vaccination)   All HIV-positive travelers should be appropriately immunized, but the antibody response to immunization may be impaired, especially when the CD4+ cell counts are less than 200 cells/μL. Increased doses of hepatitis B vaccine, for example, may be needed in immunosuppressed individuals. Because the antibody response to vaccines is higher in individuals with early HIV disease and higher CD4+ counts, it is best to immunize such individuals at the earliest opportunity. This applies to any HIV-positive person who contemplates possible future travel, as well as any person who has imminent travel plans. In general, live vaccines are contraindicated in those who are symptomatic or who have low CD4+ cell counts.

POST-TRAVEL ILLNESS

Evaluation of Illness Acquired Abroad

If you have traveled abroad, especially to rural tropical areas, you may be at risk for developing a serious illness—or for harboring a bacterial or parasitic organism in your intestine that could later cause medical problems and possibly infect others who have had close contact with you. If you have any of the following post-travel symptoms, you should consult a physician.

Important Post-Travel Symptoms

The most common symptoms of a tropical or infectious disease are the following:

- Fever
- Abdominal pain
- Diarrhea
- Weight loss
- Fatigue
- Cough or shortness of breath
- Skin rash

It is beyond the scope of this book to consider every diagnostic possibility, but fever, which is the most important post-travel symptom, should always be carefully and promptly evaluated. Your doctor must determine if your fever is possibly caused by a travel-related illness or is due to an illness that you may have acquired after returning home. However, in about 25% of travelers, no cause of the fever can be found, and it is assumed in these instances that the fever is due to a self-limited viral infection.

Key point: All travelers who become sick after returning from a trip overseas should ask their primary care physician to consult with a travel medicine specialist if there is any possibility that their illness might be caused by a tropical disease.

Diagnosing the Cause of Fever

The length of time after returning home and the length of time after possible disease exposure have diagnostic implications. Some diseases cause symptoms only a few days after exposure, whereas others become evident after weeks to months. Table 2.1 lists many travel-related diseases with fever and their incubation periods.

Your travel itinerary helps the clinician determine what illness may be causing the fever. Certain diseases, such as malaria, can immediately be eliminated if they don't exist in any of the countries you visited. Also, being vaccinated against a disease makes it much less likely to contract it. Consult the World Medical Guide in this book to see which infectious or tropical diseases are present in the countries on your itinerary. Then combine the knowledge of possible disease exposure (e.g., insect bites, exposure to potentially contaminated food or water) with the incubation period data in Table 2.1 to narrow the diagnostic possibilities. Finally, laboratory testing can often clinch the diagnosis.

For example, if you have returned from East Africa and 1 month later you develop a high fever, malaria may be the most likely diagnosis; however, a blood smear may show a high eosinophil count, indicating another type of parasitic disease, and another blood test may confirm the diagnosis of schistosomiasis, a common disease in that region.

CDC Malaria Hotline	770-488-7788

Table 2.1 Incubation Periods for Select Infections with Fever

	Acute (0-14 Days)	Subacute (2 Weeks to 6 Months)	Chronic (More than 6 Months)
Protozoal	Malaria	Malaria	Malaria
	Trypanosomiasis	Amebic colitis/abscess	Amebic abscess
		Leishmaniasis	Leishmaniasis
		Trypanosomiasis	
Bacterial	Typhoid fever	Brucellosis	Brucellosis
	Leptospirosis	Tuberculosis	Tuberculosis
	Meningitis		
	Legionellosis		
	Bacterial enteritis		
Rickettsial	Boutonneuse fever*		
	Rocky Mt. spotted fever		
	Typhus		
Viral	Dengue, West Nile	Hepatitis A, B, E	
	Other arboviruses	HIV seroconversion	HIV
	Viral hemorrhagic fever	CMV, E-B virus	
Helminths (Flukes)	Schistosomiasis	Schistosomiasis Filariasis	Filariasis

*Also known as Mediterranean spotted fever and African tick typhus. Other tick-borne rickettsial diseases include North Asian tick-borne rickettsiosis and Queensland tick typhus. CMV, cytomegalovirus. (From Wiselka MJ, et al: Travel Medicine International, October 1992.)

THE POST-TRAVEL MEDICAL CHECKLIST

Although you might have traveled in countries where certain diseases exist, this doesn't necessarily mean you had any exposure; therefore, a detailed history of your actual activities is essential to assess your risks. Your immunization status is also important. Questions a clinician should ask you are the following:

- Your itinerary: What countries did you visit and for how long? Were you in a disease-endemic area in that country?
- What were your arrival and departure dates? When did you return home?
- Which vaccinations did you receive prior to departure? For example, if you were given the hepatitis A or yellow fever vaccine, these diseases could virtually be eliminated as diagnostic possibilities. The typhoid fever vaccine, however, is not 100% effective, so vaccination will not entirely eliminate the risk of this disease.
- Did you travel in rural areas of tropical/semitropical countries?
- Did you take measures to prevent insect/mosquito bites?
- Did you adhere to your malaria prophylaxis schedule (if prescribed) and was the drug appropriate?
- Did you adhere to safe food and drink guidelines? Did you eat snails, crabs, prawns, raw fish, or inadequately cooked exotic foods made from beef, pork, bear, walrus, or fish?
- Did you have contact with sick people with respiratory illnesses, such as tuberculosis?
- Did you get sick during your trip? Were you treated by a doctor? Was your illness diagnosed? What medications were you given? Did you receive any injections or blood transfusions?

Table 2.2   Physical Findings in Select Tropical Infections with Fever

Physical Finding	Disease
Rash	Dengue fever, typhoid, typhus, syphilis, HIV, cutaneous leishmaniasis, brucellosis, Lyme disease
Jaundice	Malaria, hepatitis, yellow fever, leptospirosis, relapsing fever
Lymphadenopathy	Dengue fever, brucellosis, visceral leishmaniasis, HIV, rickettsial infections, mononucleosis, CMV, EBV
Hepatomegaly	Malaria, typhoid, hepatitis, leptospirosis, amebiasis
Splenomegaly	Malaria, brucellosis, typhoid, relapsing fever, visceral leishmaniasis, typhus, dengue fever, trypanosomiasis
Eschar	Rickettsial diseases, e.g., tick typhus or scrub typhus, cutaneous anthrax

CMV, cytomegalovirus; EBV, Ebola virus.

- When was the onset of your post-travel symptoms—days, weeks, months, after return?
- What was your exposure to the following:
  - Unsafe food and drink—Did you eat undercooked or raw meat or fish (e.g., sushi); cold food from salad bars; street vendor food not piping hot?
  - Insect and animals bites—Were you bitten by mosquitoes, flies, or ticks? Were you bitten by a dog or other animal?
  - Walking barefoot on beaches or moist soil?
  - Freshwater swimming, wading, or bathing?
  - Unprotected sex with a new partner?
  - Recreational drugs (especially by injection), tattooing, body piercing, or plastic surgery procedures?
  - People with infectious diseases?

It is only after a detailed history has been taken that a physical examination should be performed and select laboratory tests obtained.

Table 2.3   Laboratory Tests

The basic laboratory tests available to evaluate post-travel illness include the following:

- Complete blood count to screen for anemia, eosinophilia, elevated white blood cell count and/or low platelets

- Thick and thin blood films to screen for malaria (3 times over 24 hours)

- Dip stick malaria assay, if available

- Stool culture. Smear for fecal leukocytes.

- Microscopic examination of stool for ova and parasites

- Liver function tests

- Blood culture × 2

- Serology testing (for dengue, brucella, typhus, parasites, etc.)

- Chest x-ray

- Urinalysis and urine culture

IMPORTANT ALERT

Malaria is the most important illness to consider if you develop a fever after having been in a malaria-endemic area, especially one in sub-Saharan Africa or Oceania. If you develop a fever after returning home, be sure to tell your doctor that you have traveled abroad and that a tropical illness, especially malaria, is a possibility. If malaria is a consideration, request thick and thin blood films and have them repeated two to three times over 24 hours if the initial result is negative.

CHAPTER 3

Vaccines for Travel

KEY POINTS:

▶ Although the cholera vaccine is not usually recommended because the infection is rare in travelers, it may be beneficial for aid workers and healthcare providers working in highly endemic areas.

▶ Influenza vaccine should be considered for all travelers, including pregnant women, because this infection is more common than previously suspected.

▶ Hepatitis A is one of the most frequent vaccine-preventable diseases in travelers; the vaccine provides rapid and lifetime protection.

▶ Hepatitis B is a risk to *all* travelers to developing countries because of the widespread prevalence of poorly sterilized injection equipment that might be used in the event of a serious illness or accident. Immunization with the combined hepatitis A and B vaccine (Twinrix) is an excellent lifetime investment for people who travel internationally.

▶ Immune globulin is no longer necessary to protect against hepatitis A except in immune compromised individuals who are unable to mount an immune response to the vaccine.

▶ Typhoid vaccine is highly recommended for travelers returning to their country of origin to visit friends and relatives (VFRs).

▶ The new meningococcal conjugate vaccine (Menactra) appears to be more effective and longer lasting than the polysaccharide vaccine (Menomune). Neither vaccine, however, protects against serogroup B meningitis.

▶ Polio, eradicated from much of the western world and Europe, has resurged in Africa, and is active in Saudi Arabia and Yemen; polio is also an on-going threat in Afghanistan, Pakistan, the Indian sub-Continent, and Indonesia.

Being up-to-date on your "shots," or completing a vaccination (immunization) schedule before departure, is one of the most important steps you can take to prevent a travel-related disease. Immunizing travelers, however, has become increasingly complex because new vaccines (e.g., Menactra, for meningitis; Dukoral for travelers' diarrhea and cholera) are being brought to market, whereas others (e.g., injectable cholera) are being phased out. In the meantime, new diseases for which vaccines are not yet available, such as SARS and avian influenza, have emerged.

Travelers may complicate the situation by not allowing enough time to be immunized according to established vaccination schedules or requirements. Of course, in some cases, their departures may be unscheduled, perhaps for business or personal reasons.

Although some vaccines, such as the combined hepatitis A and B vaccine (Twinrix), may be administered "off label" in an accelerated schedule over 3 weeks, some travelers may be forced to delay their trip, or forgo essential protection, if they are scheduled to depart on short notice. Therefore, travelers planning an itinerary should seek pre-travel health advice 6 to 8 weeks before departure to be sure there is enough time for multiple doses of one or more vaccines, if these are needed. Business travelers, or others, who have unpredictable schedules, should have their travel immunizations updated regularly to ensure that they are prepared for last minute travel, regardless of the destination.

Planning Vaccinations

Vaccination recommendations are determined by a host of factors:

- The traveler's age, past medical history, vaccination history, travel history, country of birth, and country where he or she was raised.
- The duration of planned travel, lifestyle activities during travel (e.g., possible unsafe sexual contact or drug use), high-risk occupational exposure (e.g., health-care or relief worker).
- The traveler's present health status. Individuals who have immunodeficiency diseases (such as AIDS) or who are taking immunosuppressive medications may be more susceptible to vaccine-preventable diseases, are at increased risk of dangerous virus replication from live vaccines and may have a diminished immune response to vaccines.
- The current disease patterns in the *specific localities* of the country to be visited.
- The types of accommodations and restaurants to be frequented.
- The likely extent of close contact with local people. This may favor, for example, administering meningitis vaccine.
- The traveler's budget for vaccines. Unfortunately, for "budget" travelers, the cost of vaccines, in the United States in particular, can approach the budget for the entire trip. Although the cost of some vaccines may be covered by health insurance, most travel clinics operate on a cash payment basis.
- Pregnancy: Vaccinating pregnant women requires expertise regarding the effect of the vaccine, if any, on the fetus, and the magnitude of the risk of exposure to the disease. In general, live-virus vaccines are not given to pregnant women. However, in the case of yellow fever, the risk of disease may outweigh the possible risk of vaccination.

The standard approach to travel immunization is to consider the "3 Rs:" (1) Routine, (2) Required, and (3) Recommended immunizations. *Routine* immunizations are childhood or adult immunizations that should be updated regardless of travel (e.g., tetanus, polio, diphtheria, measles, mumps, rubella, etc.). *Required* immunizations are those required by destination countries for entry according to international health regulations (e.g., yellow fever, meningococcal meningitis) and *Recommended* immunizations are those recommended according to risk of infection (e.g., hepatitis A and B, typhoid, Japanese encephalitis, yellow fever, etc.) Travel medicine advisors carry out an individual risk assessment for each client in these three areas of immunization, taking into consideration the factors discussed above. A risk management program of immunization is then constructed to meet the needs, time available before departure, and financial resources of the traveler.

Vaccines for routine use and specialized vaccines for international travel are described subsequently. Table 3.2 contains specific information on dosing schedules, indications, booster doses, and precautions. Table 3.3 contains HIV immunization guidelines. Childhood immunization schedules for the United States are found in Figure 3.2. Immunization during pregnancy is discussed in Chapter 20.

VACCINE AND DISEASE SUMMARY

Chickenpox (Varicella)

Chickenpox is a viral infection caused by *Varicella zoster*. It is highly contagious and usually quite mild, although serious complications, even fatalities, may result, especially when the infection occurs in an adult. It is primarily a disease of children; in North America 90% of children will have been infected or vaccinated by age 10. New immigrants from Latin America and South Asia should be tested for varicella antibodies if the history of infection is unknown because in these areas of the world chickenpox tends to occur at an older age. The infection is spread by contact with infected objects and the respiratory route. Those who have had this disease have lifelong immunity and do not need the vaccine.

Chickenpox vaccine is now a routine immunization for all children in the United States. All children should receive one dose of chickenpox vaccine between 12 and 18 months of age, or at any age after that, if they have never had chickenpox. Adults and adolescents 13 years of age or older should receive two doses of the vaccine, 4 to 8 weeks apart. Chickenpox vaccine, which is a live virus vaccine, should not be given during pregnancy, and female patients should not become pregnant for at least 1 month after immunization.

International travelers of any age who have had neither the disease nor the vaccine should receive this vaccine prior to departure. This applies especially to female travelers of childbearing age who may become pregnant because varicella zoster may cause severe injury to the fetus. See Table 3.2 for a summary of the varicella vaccine schedule, indications, precautions, and booster recommendations.

Cholera

The manufacture of the injectable cholera vaccine in the United States ceased in June 2000. Currently, a cholera vaccine is not available in this country. However, oral cholera vaccines are available in a number of other countries, including Canada. Cholera vaccine is no longer listed in the *International Certificate of Vaccination* booklet and is not "officially" required for entry into, or exit from, any country. However, because of the risk of large-scale outbreaks during the Hajj or Umra, Saudia Arabia may require proof of cholera vaccination from travelers before entry is permitted. Anticipating such a situation, travelers may need a medical exemption letter from their health-care provider that contains an official-looking stamp. It may be advisable to contact the embassy or consulate at a destination country to confirm the requirement for cholera vaccination and the acceptability of a medical exemption letter.

Oral Cholera Vaccines Two recently developed oral cholera vaccines provide good protection for up to 3 years. Both vaccines appear to provide better immunity and fewer side effects than the previously available injectable vaccine.

- A live attenuated vaccine (Mutachol, Orochol) is available in Europe. This vaccine provides 90% protection against severe diarrhea for six months and 86% against any diarrhea.
- An inactivated bacterial vaccine (Dukoral) is available in Canada and some European countries. It provides 85% protection against cholera for at least three years. This vaccine also gives 50% to 60% protection against enterotoxigenic *E. coli* (ETEC), the most frequent bacterial cause of travelers' diarrhea.

Cholera vaccine is not recommended for the typical international traveler because the risk of disease is so low; however, the vaccine may be beneficial for subgroups of travelers who may be at increased risk:

- Travelers with increased susceptibility to the disease due to decreased stomach acid—the result of medication, disease, or previous surgery.
- Relief and healthcare workers in refugee camps who live and work under unsanitary conditions in a high-risk environment.

Diphtheria-Tetanus-Pertussis

Diphtheria, caused by the bacterium *Corynebacteria diphtheriae*, manifests with a severe sore throat (pharyngitis) and sometimes toxin-induced heart damage (myocarditis). Diphtheria is spread person-to-person through close contact and respiratory secretions. Pertussis commonly called whooping cough, is caused by the bacterium *Bordetella pertussis* and is also spread by the respiratory route. Pertussis is now the most frequent cause of persistent cough lasting longer than 3 weeks. It is also under-reported and under-diagnosed because most people believe, as they do about diphtheria, that the disease doesn't occur after childhood.[*]

Tetanus is not spread person-to-person; it is caused by a toxin secreted by *Clostridium tetani* a bacterium that is found in soil and acquired by contamination of an open wound or sore. It may be present as a localized infection commonly termed "lockjaw"—so-called because of the paralysis and spasm of muscles, including those of respiration.

The DTaP vaccine, which protects against diphtheria, tetanus, and pertussis, is a routine childhood immunization in the United States and Canada. It is a 5-dose series starting at 2 months of age and finishing at 4 to 6 years of age. It is frequently given in combination with the *Haemophilus influenzae* (Hib) vaccine. Following completion of the childhood DTaP series, the bivalent tetanus/diphtheria (Td) vaccine is used to maintain immunity against tetanus and diphtheria in adolescents and adults, with boosters every 10 years. The Td vaccine, however, provides no on-going protection against pertussis, a disease that is making a resurgence among adolescents and young adults. Until recently, DTaP vaccines were not administered after the seventh birthday; now, however, an acellular dTap vaccine is available in Canada for children over six years of age

---

[*]Adult pertussis is often unrecognized because of its different clinical and laboratory features. Although generally milder than the childhood form, severe illness in adults may occur. Pertussis remains a significant threat that requires on-going public health measures for control.

and adults who have not completed their basic immunization series; also, a single dose is recommended for pre-adolescents, adolescents, and adults who have never had a dose of acellular pertussis vaccine. In the United States, the Food and Drug Administration (FDA) has recently approved an acellular pertussis Tdap vaccine (ADACEL) for a single booster immunization against pertussis, in combination with tetanus and diphtheria, for adolescents and adults 11 to 64 years of age. (ADACEL contains the same components as the DTaP vaccine for infants and children, but the diphtheria toxoid and one of the pertussis components are in reduced quantities.) Introduction of trivalent Tdap vaccines will soon make it possible to maintain immunity after childhood against all three of these diseases with a single vaccine.

Haemophilus Influenzae Type b (Hib)

Haemophilus influenzae Type b is a bacterial infection of children that is spread by the respiratory route and that causes meningitis. Hib vaccine is a routine childhood immunization in the United States. This is a four-dose series (it may be a three-dose series depending on the brand of Hib vaccine used) starting at 2 months of age and finishing at 12 to 15 months of age. Many pediatricians give this vaccine in combination with the DTaP vaccine. Because infection with *H. influenzae* is rare after 5 years of age, older children and adults do not routinely need this vaccine. *H. influenzae* type b disease is common in many countries of the world. Every child should be vaccinated against this disease before international travel.

NOTE: *Haemophilus influenza* type b disease and viral influenza ("the flu") are different illnesses. The similarity of their names acknowledges their historical association. See Figure 3.2 for Hib vaccine schedule recommendations.

Hepatitis A

Hepatitis A is a viral infection of the liver that is acquired by ingestion of contaminated food and water. It is highly endemic in developing countries where personal hygiene and sanitation are substandard. Poorly cooked shellfish are an important source of infection because they may be grown in water that is contaminated by raw sewage.

Hepatitis A vaccine is recommended for all nonimmune international travelers older than 2 years of age (1 year in Canada) going to lesser-developed countries. Hepatitis A is one of the most frequent vaccine-preventable diseases of travelers, and there are three vaccines available in the United States: Vaqta (Merck), Havrix (GlaxoSmithKline) and Twinrix (GlaxoSmithKline)—a combination of the hepatitis A and B vaccines. In Canada Avaxim (Sanofi-Pasteur) and Epaxal (Berna) are available. They all give rise to measurable antibody levels within 2 weeks after a single injection. A second dose, recommended 6 to 12 months later, dramatically boosts antibody levels and provides virtually 100% immunity—probably for life. If a person's hepatitis A immune status is unknown, he or she may choose to be vaccinated or blood may be tested for existing immunity. People who have had the disease do not need vaccination; vaccinating people who are already immune causes no harm.

Hepatitis A vaccine becomes effective in about 2 weeks, which is soon enough to protect against symptomatic disease even if travelers are exposed to the hepatitis A virus immediately on arrival at their destination. In other words, vaccination, even at the last minute is effective and immune globulin (see later) is not necessary. It is important to know that experts at the Centers for Disease Control and Prevention (CDC in Atlanta, Georgia) recommend immune globulin for those who do not receive hepatitis A vaccine 2 weeks before departure. This recommendation is not in agreement with those of national advisors in all other industrialized countries who recommend the vaccine alone right up to the day of departure. See Table 3.2 for hepatitis A vaccine schedule, indications, precautions, and booster recommendations.

Hepatitis B

Hepatitis B is a viral infection that attacks the liver. It is transmitted by contact with blood and body fluids through sexual activity, contaminated injection equipment (primarily needles and syringes), handling of blood products, and from an infected mother to child at birth.

Hepatitis B vaccine is a routine immunization for all infants, children, and adolescents in the United States who are 18 years of age and younger. The vaccines now used in the United States and Canada are produced by recombinant DNA technology. The duration of protection after three doses of vaccine is considered to be lifelong. Serum antibody levels are not routinely measured when the vaccine is administered for travel. However, if antibody levels are tested, and a traveler does not develop hepatitis B antibodies 1 month after the immunization series has been completed, he or she is considered to be a "non-responder." If time is available, the administration of extra vaccine doses should be considered. It is important to understand that one-third of those who develop immunity (antibody levels >10 IU/mL) will lose their antibodies within 5 years and still be protected for life because of the presence of immune memory cells.

- Increasingly, travel medicine advisors feel that *all* travelers to high-risk areas should be immunized against this infection because immunity is lifelong and one cannot predict when a serious illness or accident will necessitate an injection potentially administered with unsterilized equipment.

The highest risk groups include:

- Long-term/expatriate travelers (3 months or more)
- Travelers likely to engage in unsafe sex or recreational drug-sharing activities
- Travelers, especially young children, exposed to locals in high-risk areas who have open skin sores
- Travelers with underlying health problems who may require medical or dental treatment involving injections and/or transfusions
- Health-care and aid workers

Immune Globulin (IG)

Immune globulin (also known as IG, immune serum globulin, ISG, or gamma globulin) is not a vaccine but rather a high concentration of antibodies against a variety of infections, particularly hepatitis A. Although IG contains pooled human blood products, it has never been shown to transmit infectious disease, such as HIV. It is effective for the prevention of hepatitis A for international travelers (for 3 to 5 months, depending on the amount given), and it is also effective if used for the prevention of measles or hepatitis A immediately after a known exposure. Since the introduction of hepatitis A vaccine in 1995, the use of IG has markedly decreased.

Travelers younger than 2 years of age (1 year in Canada) who should not be given hepatitis A vaccine, and who need protection against hepatitis A should receive a single dose of IG.* Immunocompromised travelers who are not likely to respond to the vaccine should also receive IG. However, currently there is a shortage of IG making it very difficult to obtain.

IG can interfere with replication of live viruses in vaccines. Experience has shown that this occurs only with measles, mumps, and rubella vaccine (MMR) and with the varicella vaccine. Therefore, these vaccines should not be administered in the period from 2 weeks before IG is administered until several months after the IG. If IG must be given soon after MMR or varicella, these vaccines must be repeated at a later date. See Table 3.2 for immune globulin schedule, indications, precautions, and booster recommendations.

Influenza

Influenza is a contagious viral disease that occurs worldwide, and travel increases exposure. Because the influenza viruses change continually and vary geographically, vaccines need to be reconstituted each year to reflect this change. In the Northern and Southern hemispheres influenza outbreaks occur during the cool winter months—whereas in the tropics, infection occurs year-round.

The influenza vaccine is now a routine immunization in the United States for children ages 6 to 23 months, adults 50 years of age and older, those with underlying medical problems—such as chronic obstructive lung disease, heart disease, diabetes, and malignancy, and women who expect to be pregnant during the flu season—but travelers of any age going to countries where influenza activity is reported should be immunized. In North America and Europe, the optimum time to receive this vaccine is annually from mid-October through November.

Southern Hemisphere Vaccine Travelers to Australia, New Zealand, South America, and South Africa between April and October, should consider vaccination at their destination site with the influenza vaccine formulated for the Southern Hemisphere. This vaccine is not licensed in the United States and has a slightly different formulation. See Table 3.2 for influenza vaccine schedule, indications, precautions, and booster recommendations.

Japanese Encephalitis (JE)

Japanese encephalitis, a severe viral infection of the brain, is transmitted by an evening and night-biting mosquito in rural areas of South and Southeast Asia. Seasonal transmission occurs in northern areas (summer); whereas in the south, year-round transmission occurs.

Three doses of JE vaccine, administered over a 30-day period (at 0, 7, and 30 days), are recommended for travelers who will be at risk (see Chapter 9). A two-dose schedule

*Almost all children under 2 years will remain asymptomatic when they become infected with hepatitis A; the main threat is that they can transmit the infection to others.

Table 3.1 Antiviral Agents for Influenza

Generic Name	Trade Name	Indications	Dosage	Comments
M2 Inhibitors—Influenza A				
Amantadine	Symmetrel	Treatment > age 1	100 mg bid × 7 days	CNS side effects
		Prophylaxis > age 1	100 mg qd	>age 65–dose decreased to 100 mg qd
			Decrease if kidney function impaired	If CrCl < 80 mL/min– decrease dose
Rimantidine	Flumadine	Treatment > age 14	100 mg bid × 7 days	If CrCl < 20 mL/min– decrease dose
		Prophylaxis > age 1	100 mg qd	
Neuraminidase Inhibitors—Influenza A and B				
Zanamivir	Relenza	Treatment > age 7	2 blisters bid × 5 days	Diskhaler inhalation device
				Pending indication: Prophylaxis > age 7
				Caution with history of bronchospasm
Oseltamivir	Tamiflu	Treatment > age 18	75 mg bid × 5 days	Pending indications: treatment > age 1
		Prophylaxis *(Adult)	75 mg daily × 1–6 weeks	Prophylaxis > age 1 Mild GI side effects
There is no vaccine against avian influenza, but oseltamivir (Tamiflu) may be effective.				

*1 week–close contact; 6 weeks–community outbreak.

(at 0 and 14 days) may be used when the 30-day schedule is impractical. Two doses will give about 80% protection. If neither schedule is possible, two doses of vaccine, administered 1 week apart, will offer some protection. It is advisable to receive the last injection of vaccine a minimum of 10 days before departure to (1) allow time for immunity to develop and (2) have access to medical care if any side effects occur.

Severe side effects from this vaccine include urticaria (hives), angioedema (edema of the face or other body parts), and hypotension (low blood pressure). These symptoms are quite rare (less than six cases per 100,000 doses of vaccine) and usually occur within a few days following immunization, but may be delayed 7 to 10 days. Because of the risk of delayed side effects, if possible, travelers should avoid international travel within 10 days of their last dose of JE vaccine. Travelers at risk should not forgo the immunization because they have fewer than 10 days before departure. The adverse effects of immunization need to be weighed against the risk of infection, which can be fatal in 10% to 25% or lead to permanent brain damage in as many as one third of symptomatic people. See Table 3.2 for Japanese encephalitis vaccine schedule, indications, precautions, and contraindications.

Lyme Disease

A Lyme disease vaccine (LYMErix, GlaxoSmithBeecham) was licensed in the United States in 1998 but was withdrawn from the market in 2001.

Measles

Measles (rubeola) is a viral infection, spread by the respiratory route, that has the potential to cause severe illness in young children, especially those who are malnourished; it is one of the leading causes of death among children worldwide.

The World Health Organization is hopeful that measles (rubeola) will be eradicated worldwide by the year 2010. All cases now occurring in the United States originate abroad, brought in by travelers, many of them foreign students attending U.S. secondary schools and colleges. Measles continues to be a major health problem in many developing countries, especially in sub-Saharan Africa and on the Indian subcontinent. Travelers to less developed countries should be immune to measles, either by having had the disease, or by immunization. Occasionally, there are reports of measles in developed countries—such as recent outbreaks in Holland and Ireland. Many adult travelers, however, may not be immune to measles. Measles vaccination in the United States began in the late 1950s. People born before 1957 (before 1970 in Canada) are assumed to have had the disease during childhood and therefore have lifelong immunity. In fact, even when measles was prevalent and "everyone got it," some individuals escaped the disease and remain susceptible. This number is higher than is generally appreciated. The same is true for mumps, rubella, and varicella (chickenpox.). It should be noted that all of these diseases are far more severe when they occur in adults—making immunity especially important for older people.

In the mid-1960s, when effective live virus vaccines were introduced, experts believed that one dose would provide lifelong immunity. But experience has shown that immunity from measles vaccine is all or none—a "take" or a "no take"—and one dose immunizes only about 90% of those vaccinated; the second dose immunizes most of the rest. Therefore, travelers born after 1957 in the U.S. or between 1970 and 1996 in Canada should have a second dose of measles vaccine if they have not already received two doses.

Measles vaccine (given as MMR—measles, mumps, rubella combination) is a two-dose series given on or after the first birthday and again at 4 to 6 years of age, but it is acceptable to give the two doses any time with as little as 1 month between them. The MMR vaccine should not be given during pregnancy, and female patients should not become pregnant for at least 3 months after immunization.

NOTE: It is not contraindicated to give MMR to a breastfeeding mother. For babies ages 6 to 11 months traveling to countries where measles is endemic (e.g., India), a single dose of monovalent measles (MMR is acceptable) is recommended. If the vaccine is given at ages 6 to 11 months, a routine MMR is still recommended at age 1 year or as soon after as practicable. Maternal-derived antibodies protect infants younger than 6 months of age. See Table 3.2 for measles vaccine schedule, indications, precautions, and booster recommendations.

Meningococcal

Meningococcal disease, which usually presents clinically as meningitis, is caused by the bacterium *Neisseria meningitidis*. There are five meningococcal serogroups. A, B, C, Y, and W135 that can cause disease, and these vary geographically in their worldwide distribution. There is currently no vaccine that protects against serogroup B.

The quadrivalent polysaccharide vaccine Menomune (Sanofi Pasteur), available in the United States, protects for 3 years against four serogroups: A, C, Y, and W135. In January 2005 the Food and Drug Administration licensed Menactra (Sanofi Pasteur), a quadrivalent conjugate vaccine which is more immunogenic and lasts longer, perhaps for 8 years. The Menactra vaccine also eliminates the nasal carriage of meningococcal bacteria, a critical factor in breaking the chain of disease transmission. Currently, Menactra is recommended by the manufacturer only for ages 11 to 55 years, but there is no reason why the vaccine can't be administered "off-label" to both younger and older travelers. Unlike Menomune, the conjugate vaccine Menactra may be effective in children under 2 years of age.

A bivalent meningococcal vaccine against serogroups A and C is available in Europe and the United Kingdom and two conjugate group C vaccines (Menjugate, Neisvac) are available in Canada. Because of their limited coverage (one or two serogroups only), these vaccines are not ideal for travelers. A quadrivalent vaccine (Menomune or Menactra), covering all four serogroups is recommended for travelers going to countries within the meningitis belt of sub-Saharan Africa (serogroups A, C, W-135 prevalent), or to outbreak areas, and is a requirement for travel to Saudi Arabia during the Hajj.

Meningococcal serogroup W-135 has recently emerged as an important cause of meningitis in Saudi Arabia. All travelers to Hajj or Umrah will be asked by the Saudi Arabian embassy for proof of meningitis ACYW-135 vaccination on applying for their visa. The embassy requires that the vaccine should be administered at least 10 days before travel. Proof of vaccination is currently valid for a period of three years, but this is likely to change with the introduction of the longer-lasting conjugate vaccine.

Two doses of meningococcal ACWY vaccine are required for children ages six months to two years, with an interval of three months between the two doses.

The vaccinating center must provide a vaccination booklet or letter completed with the traveler's name, vaccine, date of administration, and signature.

NOTE: Meningococcal vaccine is usually not recommended for children under two years of age but under special circumstances (e.g., travel to Saudi Arabia) may be administered to infants as young as 3 months. The conjugate vaccine should be used.

The CDC no longer recommends the meningococcal vaccine for routine travel to Nepal, India, Mongolia, Kenya, Burundi, or Tanzania. In June 2005, however, an outbreak of meningococcal meningitis was reported in Delhi, India. Travelers to India should check current vaccination recommendations to this country on the CDC website www.cdc.gov/travel. See Table 3.2 for meningococcal vaccine schedule, indications, precautions, and booster recommendations.

Pertussis (Whooping Cough)

Pertussis, caused by *Bordetella pertussis* is a bacterial infection transmitted by the respiratory route that produces whooping cough. Pertussis infects an estimated 60 million people worldwide annually, causing 600,000 deaths, mostly children in developing countries. It can be a serious disease, especially in infants, and it is highly contagious. Pertussis is characterized by choking and coughing—often prolonged for many weeks.

Pertussis vaccine is administered to children as the DTaP vaccine (diphtheria, tetanus, and acellular pertussis). However, the vaccine is not 100% protective, and vaccinated children may still become infected (although the disease tends to be milder), making it important to limit exposure to the disease. Immunity from vaccination lasts about 10 years, making older teenagers and adults susceptible, but for a generally milder form of the disease. See Table 3.2 for DTaP vaccine schedule, indications, precautions, and booster recommendations. See p. 38 for an update on pertussis vaccines for adolescents and adults.

Polio (Poliomyelitis)

Poliomyelitis is a highly contagious infection caused by poliovirus, which is transmitted person-to-person through exposure to fecal material or respiratory secretions containing the virus. Polio has been eradicated from much of the world, including the Western Hemisphere, Europe, and Southeast Asia, but there has been a recent resurgence of polio in Africa, chiefly in Nigeria. Polio has been spreading from northern Nigeria since 2003, when vaccination campaigns there were halted because of rumors that the vaccine could make people sick, or cause AIDS. Most cases from the outbreak have been in the Muslim Sahel, the band of arid land south of the Sahara stretching from Mali to Ethiopia. Polio has now appeared in Saudi Arabia and Yemen. The remaining pockets of polio in the world are in Pakistan, northern India, Afghanistan, Egypt, and Indonesia.

Persons who have received a complete series of polio vaccine, either IPV (inactivated polio vaccine) or OPV (oral polio vaccine) should receive an additional single dose of vaccine if they are 18 years of age or older and are traveling to a polio-endemic area. These areas include Africa, the Middle East, and the Indian subcontinent. This additional (booster) dose of polio vaccine is necessary only once in adulthood. Only inactivated polio vaccine (IPV) should be used for this dose.

OPV can, very rarely, cause paralytic polio in the recipient, or nonimmune persons in contact with the recipient. Therefore, OPV is no longer manufactured or administered in the United States—only injectable polio vaccine (IPV) is used. OPV, however, is still widely used in the rest of the world. The only circumstances in which OPV should be used are the following:

- For an unvaccinated child who will be traveling in fewer than 4 weeks to areas of the world where wild poliovirus still exists.
- For the third or fourth dose of polio vaccination series for children whose parents will not accept the additional number of injections required to complete the series with IPV.
- In mass vaccination campaigns to control outbreaks.

See Table 3.2 for polio vaccine schedule, indications, precautions, and booster recommendations.

Rabies

Rabies is a uniformly fatal viral infection of the brain transmitted by the bite of an animal, usually a dog or monkey in the developing world, and by bats, skunks, foxes, and raccoons in North America. Rabies vaccine is recommended for long-stay travelers to endemic areas, particularly children, who are often attracted to animals and who are less likely to report a bite or scratch.

The primary series of rabies vaccine is a total of three injections given at intervals of 0, 7, and 21 or 28 days. For travelers, two boosters are required *only* when an individual is potentially exposed to the virus. Veterinarians and spelunkers should receive a booster every 2 to 3 years. The main advantage of giving pre-exposure rabies vaccine is to eliminate the need for rabies immune globulin (to inject into the bite-site) at the time of the exposure. Rabies immune globulin is often very scarce in the developing world, whereas rabies vaccine is usually readily available. Therefore, an animal bite could be a trip-ending experience if one is forced to fly to another city or country, or even home, to obtain rabies immune globulin. Also, pre-exposure vaccination reduces the number of doses of post-exposure vaccine, and possibly lengthens the safe interval between animal exposure and the onset of treatment. It does not preclude the essential step of proper wound cleansing with soap and water.

Rabies intradermal vaccine is not recommended when travelers are taking chloroquine or mefloquine for malaria prevention. The intramuscular formulation should be used. The intradermal rabies vaccine series, if used, should be started 30 days before the administration of either chloroquine or mefloquine. Three types of rabies vaccine, all equally effective, are available in the United States. See Table 3.2 for rabies vaccine schedule, indications, precautions, and booster recommendations.

Rubella (German measles)

Rubella, or German measles, caused by the rubella virus, is usually a mild infection in children but a very serious infection if it occurs during pregnancy because of severe damage to the developing fetus. Most Americans and Canadians are immune to rubella, either by having had the disease, or by vaccination with the measles-mumps-rubella (MMR—Merck) vaccine. For the past 2 decades, nearly all children have been receiving two doses of MMR vaccine. The only travelers who need the rubella component of the vaccine are women who may become pregnant and whose rubella immunity status is unknown. These women should consider receiving one dose of MMR. One dose of the rubella component immunizes virtually 100% of recipients for life.

Rubella Vaccine and Arthritis   About 10% to 25% of postpubertal women report joint pain after receiving rubella vaccine and about 10% report arthritis-like signs and symptoms. When joint symptoms occur, they generally begin 1 to 3 weeks after vaccination, persist for 1 day to 3 weeks, and rarely recur.

Tetanus/Diphtheria (Td)

Tetanus is an infectious complication of wounds, caused by the toxin of *Clostridium tetani* bacteria. This organism is found worldwide in the soil and in the feces of various animals and some humans. When wounds become contaminated with soil containing the spores of *C. tetani*; the spores germinate and the resulting bacteria produce a toxin that is absorbed into the central nervous system, resulting in severe muscle contractions and spasms, respiratory paralysis, and sometimes death. Tetanus is a global health problem, occurring particularly among infants and young children in developing countries. In the United States, most infections are seen in the elderly who have never received a primary series of injections.

The tetanus/diphtheria vaccine (Td vaccine) is a routine immunization in the United States. Following completion of the DTaP (Diphtheria, Tetanus, and acellular Pertussis) series (by the seventh birthday), Td is given at 11 to 12 years of age if at least 5 years have elapsed since the last dose of DTaP. Subsequent Td boosters are recommended every 10 years. The schedule for tetanus immunization is identical to that for diphtheria, and the two vaccines are generally combined in one product.

See Table 3.2 for Td vaccine schedule, indications, precautions, and contraindications.

Tick-Borne Encephalitis (TBE)

Tick-borne encephalitis is a serious viral infection of the brain transmitted by tick bites, usually after travel to rural or forested areas from spring to fall. The disease may also be acquired by ingesting unpasteurized dairy products.

There are two subtypes of TBE:

- Western subtype (or Central European encephalitis) transmitted by *Ixodes ricinus* ticks. This subtype occurs in the forested areas of Central, Eastern, and Northern Europe.
- Eastern subtype (or Russian spring/summer encephalitis) transmitted by *Ixodes persulcatus* ticks. This subtype occurs in the former USSR, east of the Ural Mountains, and also in areas of China, Japan, and Korea.

There are three vaccines for tick-borne encephalitis:

- FSME Immun (Baxter) is an inactivated viral vaccine manufactured in Austria and available in Europe but not in the United States. In Canada, the vaccine may be obtained through the Emergency Drug Release Program at 613-941-2108 or at the Bureau of Biologics at 613-941-2114. A full series consists of three doses over a 1-year period (at intervals of 0, 1, and 12 months).
- Encepur (Chiron) is manufactured in Germany and also available in Europe. Three doses are administered over a 1-year period.
- A third vaccine for tick-borne encephalitis is produced in Russia.

Accelerated Schedule   Two doses of vaccine, 1 week apart, probably give adequate protection. A third dose should be given 3 to 4 weeks later, followed by a fourth dose in 1 year's time.

The vaccine is recommended for travelers to endemic forested areas during warm months where they are likely to be exposed to ticks during extensive outdoor activities— such as camping, cycling, or work. Even a brief trip may put a traveler at risk.

Travelers' Diarrhea (Enterotoxigenic *E. coli*)

Travelers' diarrhea is the most frequent cause of illness among travelers, affecting up to 80% of international travelers depending on the destination. Although travelers' diarrhea is self-limited in most cases, nearly 40% of affected individuals will be forced to change their itinerary and 20% will be confined to bed. The most frequent cause of travelers' diarrhea is a toxin-producing *E. coli* bacteria, known as enterotoxigenic *E. coli* (ETEC). This bacterium accounts for up to 60% of the causes of travelers' diarrhea in some parts of the world, particularly in Latin America, Africa, and the Indian subcontinent.

Recently introduced in Canada and Europe, the oral cholera vaccine Dukoral (Sanofi-Pasteur) provides approximately 60% protection against ETEC and 85% protection against cholera; the latter rarely occurring in travelers. To protect against ETEC the vaccine is administered in two doses, 1 week apart, and is protective for 3 months. If a booster dose is not given within 5 years, the two-dose schedule must be repeated. Even if one is vaccinated, it is still advisable for travelers to carry Imodium and an antibiotic for self-treatment of diarrhea. Travelers who would most benefit from this vaccine are those with underlying health problems such as diabetes mellitus, kidney disease, bowel problems, and immune deficiencies.

Tuberculosis (BCG–Bacille Calmette Guérin)

Tuberculosis (TB), a bacterial infection spread by cough and caused by *Mycobacterium tuberculosis*, is now recognized as the most frequent infectious cause of death globally. It is estimated that more than one-third of the world's population are infected with the bacterium, the majority of whom have a silent (latent) infection that will never cause disease. However, tuberculous lung disease is very common in AIDS patients as their immunity further wanes.

BCG vaccine is used very rarely in travelers; the risk for acquiring the disease while traveling is low. The CDC states: "To become infected, a person usually would have to spend a long time in a closed environment where the air was contaminated by a person with untreated tuberculosis (TB) who is coughing and has numerous TB bacteria in secretions from the lung." Recent studies have shown that the risk of tuberculosis in travelers is approximately 3% per year of stay in a high-risk area. BCG is routinely given to children in many countries, both developed and developing. In the United States, TB control is based on identifying and treating infected individuals and BCG vaccine is not given.

BCG may be appropriate for children (children of missionaries, for example) who have prolonged and close contact with local populations in remote areas of developing countries with high incidences of TB. In children younger than 5 years of age, BCG is more effective in preventing severe complications (meningitis and disseminated infection) than in preventing the infection itself. In the United States, current recommendations for individuals at risk are not to use BCG vaccine but to perform TB skin testing before and after exposure (including travel) and to treat individuals who convert their skin test from negative to positive. The ideal time to perform a TB skin test is 3 months after the last possible exposure.

Typhoid

Typhoid fever, a bacterial infection caused by *Salmonella typhi*, is a potentially serious systemic illness characterized by prolonged fever, headache, cough, and constipation. Infection occurs from ingestion of contaminated food and water, or close contact with an infected person (fecal-oral transmission).

Two typhoid vaccines are available. The efficacy of both vaccines is 55% to 72% in different studies.

- Type 21a oral live typhoid vaccine is available in two forms: a capsule form that is available in the United States and Canada as well as in Europe, and a suspension form (sachets) that is currently available in Europe and Canada. In the United States, a four-dose regimen is followed (1 capsule on alternate days). In Europe and Canada, a three-dose regimen of either capsules or suspension is followed—1 sachet (packet) on alternate days for a total of 3 doses. A booster dose is recommended in 3 to 7 years, depending on country labeling. The capsules and sachets must be refrigerated and taken with a cool liquid approximately 1 hour before eating. Protection is achieved seven days after the last dose. Side effects are uncommon and may include abdominal discomfort, nausea, and rash or hives. Oral typhoid vaccine should not be taken with antibiotics, because they may interfere with effectiveness. If all doses are not taken, the entire series must be restarted to achieve protection.

- Typhim Vi is a single-dose (0.5 mL intramuscular injection) vaccine used in persons 2 years of age or older. Side effects, which are uncommon, may include discomfort at the injection site, fever, and headache. A booster dose is recommended in 2 years in the United States and 3 years in Canada.

Because the majority of cases of typhoid fever in the United States originate in immigrants from developing countries, the vaccine is strongly recommended for VFRs (immigrants returning to their country of birth to visit family, friends, and relatives), particularly those returning to Latin America, South Asia, and Southeast Asia. See Table 3.2 for typhoid vaccine schedule, indications, precautions, and booster recommendations.

Yellow Fever

Yellow fever is a severe viral infection of the liver found only in Sub-Saharan Africa, South America, and Panama; transmission occurs from a day-biting mosquito that feeds primarily at dusk and dawn. The risk of yellow fever (in unvaccinated people) in both urban and rural areas of Africa ranges from 1:250 per two-week stay during epidemics to 1:2,500 between epidemics. In South America the risk is primarily in rural areas and is lower at 1:25,000 per 2-week stay.

Yellow fever is the only vaccine that may be required for entry into certain countries. (visit http://www.cdc.gov/travel/yelfever.htm for a comprehensive listing of vaccination certificate requirements worldwide.) After vaccination (by a travel clinic or the local health department) an *International Certificate of Vaccination* is issued which will meet entry requirements for all persons traveling to or arriving from countries where there is active, or a potential for, yellow fever transmission. If there is a medical reason (e.g., infants younger than 4 months old, pregnant women, persons hypersensitive to eggs, and those who are thymectomized or have an immunosuppressed condition) not to receive the vaccine, most countries will accept a medical waiver. The CDC recommends obtaining the waiver from a consulate or embassy before departure.

Yellow fever vaccine is a live attenuated viral vaccine. A single dose confers immunity lasting 10 years or more. The vaccine is considered to be protective 10 days after the initial dose and immediately after booster doses. If the first dose of vaccine has not been given 10 days before entry to a country that requires the vaccine for entry, travelers may be refused entry until the 10 days are completed.

Vaccine Precautions   The vaccine generally is associated with few side effects: fewer than 5% of vaccinees develop mild headache, muscle pain, or other minor symptoms 5 to 10 days after vaccination. However, several groups of individuals should not receive the vaccine, while others should be closely evaluated.

The vaccine is contraindicated for three groups:

- Yellow fever vaccine should never be given to infants under 4 months of age due to a risk of developing viral encephalitis. In most cases, vaccination should be deferred until 9 to 12 months of age.
- Pregnant women should not be vaccinated because of a theoretical risk that the developing fetus may become infected from the vaccine. However, the vaccine should be offered to pregnant women planning to travel in endemic areas because studies have shown that the vaccine was safe when it was inadvertently given to pregnant women during mass vaccination campaigns in the tropics.
- Persons hypersensitive to eggs should not receive the vaccine because it is prepared in embryonated eggs.
   Other groups that should be closely evaluated before administering the vaccine include:
- Persons with an immunosuppressed condition associated with AIDS or HIV infection, or those with immune systems altered by other diseases, such as thymectomy, leukemia and lymphoma, or receiving drugs and/or radiation. People with asymptomatic HIV infection who have CD4 counts above 250 cells/mL may be vaccinated if they are at risk.

- Elderly travelers (>65 years of age). Recent studies have shown that this group may be at significantly greater risk of severe adverse reactions to the vaccine. Therefore, a careful risk/benefit assessment should be carried out in this group. The risk in the elderly of severe reactions increases to 1:50,000 from 1:350,000 in younger-aged groups. However, it should be noted that this risk occurs *only* with the first dose and not with booster doses.

Figure 3.1A South America—Yellow Fever Endemic Zones

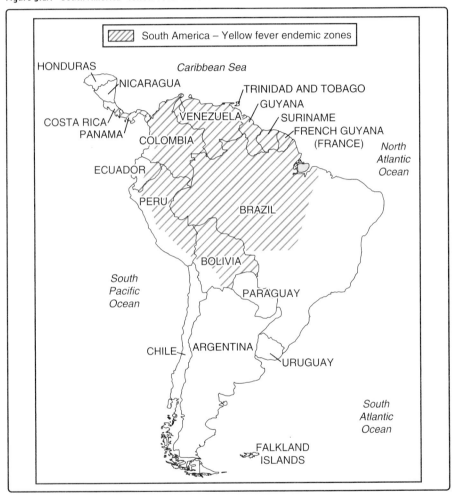

Figure 3.1B Africa—Yellow Fever Endemic Zones

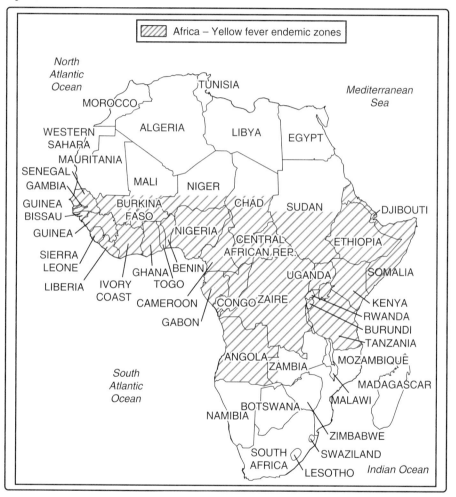

Figure 3.2 Recommended Childhood and Adolescent Immunization Schedule (United States 2005)

Vaccine ▼ / Age ▶	Birth	1 month	2 months	4 months	6 months	12 months	15 months	18 months	24 months	4–6 years	11–12 years	13–18 years
Hepatitis B[1]	HepB #1	HepB #2	HepB #2			HepB #3					HepB Series	
Diphtheria, Tetanus, Pertussis[2]			DTaP	DTaP	DTaP			DTaP		DTaP	Td	Td
Haemophilus influenzae type b[3]			Hib	Hib	Hib	Hib						
Inactivated Poliovirus			IPV	IPV		IPV				IPV		
Measles, mumps, rubella[4]						MMR #1				MMR #2	MMR #2	
Varicella[5]						Varicella				Varicella		
Pneumococcal Conjugate[6]			PCV	PCV	PCV	PCV	PCV		PCV		PPV	
Influenza[7]					Influenza (Yearly)	Influenza (Yearly)				Influenza (Yearly)		
Hepatitis A[8]										Hepatitis A Series		

Vaccines below this line are for select populations

Legend:
- Range of recommended ages
- Catch-up immunization
- Preadolescent assessment
- Only if mother HBsAg (–)

Indicates age groups that warrant special effort to administer those vaccines not previously administered. Additional vaccines may be licensed and recommended during the year. Licensed combination vaccines may be used whenever any components of the combination are indicated and other components of the vaccine are not contraindicated. Providers should consult the manufacturers' package inserts for detailed recommendations. Clinically significant adverse events that follow immunization should be reported to the Vaccine Adverse Event Reporting System (VAERS). Guidance about how to obtain and complete a VAERS form is available at www.vaers.org or by telephone, 800-822-7967.

This schedule indicates the recommended ages for routine administration of currently licensed childhood vaccines, as of December 1, 2004, for children through age 18 years. Any dose not administered at the recommended age should be administered at any subsequent visit when indicated and feasible.

1. **Hepatitis B (HepB) vaccine.** All infants should receive the first dose of HepB vaccine soon after birth and before hospital discharge; the first dose may also be administered by age 2 months if the mother is hepatitis B surface antigen (HBsAg) negative. Only monovalent HepB may be used for the birth dose. Monovalent or combination vaccine containing HepB may be used to complete the series. Four doses of vaccine may be administered when a birth dose is given. The second dose should be administered at least 4 weeks after the first dose, except for combination vaccines which cannot be administered before age 6 weeks. The third dose should be given at least 16 weeks after the first dose and at least 8 weeks after the second dose. The last dose in the vaccination series (third or fourth dose) should not be administered before age 24 weeks.

   Infants born to HBsAg-positive mothers should receive HepB and 0.5 mL of hepatitis B immune globulin (HBIG) at separate sites within 12 hours of birth. The second dose is recommended at age 1–2 months. The final dose in the immunization series should not be administered before age 24 weeks. These infants should be tested for HBsAg and antibody to HBsAg (anti-HBs) at age 9–15 months.

   Infants born to mothers whose HBsAg status is unknown should receive the first dose of the HepB series within 12 hours of birth. Maternal blood should be drawn as soon as possible to determine the mother's HBsAg status; if the HBsAg test is positive, the infant should receive HBIG as soon as possible (no later than age 1 week). The second dose is recommended at age 1–2 months. The last dose in the immunization series should not be administered before age 24 weeks.

2. **Diphtheria and tetanus toxoids and acellular pertussis (DTaP) vaccine.** The fourth dose of DTaP may be administered as early as age 12 months, provided 6 months have elapsed since the third dose and the child is unlikely to return at age 15–18 months. The final dose in the series should be given at age ≥4 years. Tetanus and diphtheria toxoids (Td) is recommended at age 11–12 years if at least 5 years have elapsed since the last dose of tetanus and diphtheria toxoid–containing vaccine. Subsequent routine Td boosters are recommended every 10 years.

3. *Haemophilus influenzae* **type b (Hib) conjugate vaccine.** Three Hib conjugate vaccines are licensed for infant use. If PRP-OMP (PedvaxHIB® or ComVax® [Merck]) is administered at ages 2 and 4 months, a dose at age 6 months is not required. DTaP/Hib combination products should not be used for primary immunization in infants at ages 2, 4, or 6 months but can be used as boosters after any Hib vaccine. The final dose in the series should be administered at age ≥12 months.

4. **Measles, mumps, and rubella vaccine (MMR).** The second dose of MMR is recommended routinely at age 4–6 years but may be administered during any visit, provided at least 4 weeks have elapsed since the first dose and both doses are administered beginning at or after age 12 months. Those who have not previously received the second dose should complete the schedule by age 11–12 years.

5. **Varicella vaccine.** Varicella vaccine is recommended at any visit at or after age 12 months for susceptible children (i.e., those who lack a reliable history of chickenpox). Susceptible persons aged ≥13 years should receive 2 doses administered at least 4 weeks apart.

6. **Pneumococcal vaccine.** The heptavalent **pneumococcal conjugate vaccine (PCV)** is recommended for all children aged 2–23 months and for certain children aged 24–59 months. **Pneumococcal polysaccharide vaccine (PPV)** is recommended in addition to PCV for certain high-risk groups. See *MMWR* 2000;49(RR-9):1–35.

7. **Influenza vaccine.** Influenza vaccine is recommended annually for children aged ≥6 months with certain risk factors (including, but not limited to, asthma, cardiac disease, sickle cell disease, human immunodeficiency virus [HIV], and diabetes), healthcare workers, and other persons (including household members) in close contact with persons at high risk (see *MMWR* 2004;53[RR-6]:1–40). In addition, healthy children aged 6–23 months and close contacts of healthy children aged 0–23 months are recommended to receive influenza vaccine because children in this age group are at substantially increased risk for influenza-related hospitalizations. For healthy persons aged 5–49 years, the intranasally administered, live, attenuated influenza vaccine (LAIV) is an acceptable alternative to the intramuscular trivalent inactivated influenza vaccine (TIV). See *MMWR* 2004;53(RR-6):1–40. Children receiving TIV should be administered a dosage appropriate for their age (0.25 mL if aged 6–35 months or 0.5 mL if aged ≥3 years). Children aged ≤8 years who are receiving influenza vaccine for the first time should receive 2 doses (separated by at least 4 weeks for TIV and at least 6 weeks for LAIV).

8. **Hepatitis A vaccine.** Hepatitis A vaccine is recommended for children and adolescents in selected states and regions and for certain high-risk groups; consult your local public health authority. Children and adolescents in these states, regions, and high-risk groups who have not been immunized against hepatitis A can begin the hepatitis A immunization series during any visit. The 2 doses in the series should be administered at least 6 months apart. See *MMWR* 1999;48(RR-12):1–37.

Table 3.2   Immunizations for International Travel

Vaccine	Type/Brand	Primary Series	Booster	Indications for Travelers	Comments and Precautions
Cholera, Oral*	Live, attenuated bacterial (Orachol, Mutachol)	Single dose orally for persons 2 years and older	Every 6 months	High-risk travelers, e.g., relief workers living in endemic/epidemic areas under unsanitary conditions	The live, attenuated vaccine should not be given to immune-compromised people or those with liver disease.
Cholera, Oral	Killed whole-cell (Dukoral)	2-dose series, 1-6 weeks apart, in persons >6 years of age	Every 2 years	Same	Killed vaccine, safe in pregnancy; oral cholera vaccines are not available in the U.S.
ETEC** (Oral)	Killed, whole-cell bacterial (Dukoral)	2 doses, 1 week apart	Every 3 months. Repeat 2-dose series if there is a gap > 5 years since last dose	Travelers who need to reduce the risk of travelers' diarrhea	Reduces by 50%-60% travelers' diarrhea caused by enterotoxigenic *E. coli* (ETEC).
Hepatitis A	Inactivated viral (VAQTA) (Havrix) (AVAXIM) (EPAXAL)	Two-dose series, 6-12 mos apart	None	All non-immune travelers, regardless of destination, should probably be vaccinated	Ages 2 yrs and older in the U.S.; age >1 year in Canada Off-label use over 2 mos: 3 doses at 2, 4, 6 months or 2 doses at 6-18 mos.

*No longer manufactured or available in the United States: An oral 3-dose vaccine is available in Canada.
**ETEC = Enterotoxigenic E. coli

Table 3.2 Immunizations for International Travel, cont'd

Vaccine	Type/Brand	Primary Series	Booster	Indications for Travelers	Comments and Precautions
Hepatitis B	Inactivated viral (Recombivax) (Engerix-B)	Three-dose series, at 0, 1, and 6 mos; Engerix-B may be given at 0, 1, and 2 mos; booster at 12 mos.	Not routinely given (May be needed in immune-compromised patients)	Routine immunization for children 0-18 years; medium- to high-risk travel to endemic areas	Accelerated schedule: 0, 7, 21 days, and 12 mos; TwinRix effective for those departing immi-nently and who need pro-tection against both Hepatitis A and B.
Hepatitis A & B	Inactivated viral (TwinRix)	3-dose series at 0, 1, 6 mos.	None	Travel to developing countries	Convenient formulation (0, 7, 21 days, and 12 mos—see above)
Immune globulin (IG)	Pooled human immunoglobulins	One dose 0.02 mL/kg IM for 3-month protection; 0.06 mL/kg IM for 5-mo protection	3-5 mo intervals, depending on initial dose	Single visit <5 mos to en-demic area, used when im-mediate protection is needed	Give measles >2 wks before or >3 mos after IG; give varicella >3 wks before or >5 mos after IG
Influenza	Inactivated viral, whole and split	One dose annually	None	All travelers, including pregnant women, may ben-efit, regardless of age	Consider Southern Hemi-sphere vaccine for sum-mer travel to Australia, New Zealand, S. Africa

Continued

Table 3.2 Immunizations for International Travel, cont'd

Vaccine	Type/Brand	Primary Series	Booster	Indications for Travelers	Comments and Precautions
Japanese B encephalitis	Inactivated viral (JE-VAX)	Three doses at 0, 7, and 30 days	3 yrs	>30 days to rural SE Asia, especially near rice paddies and pig farms	Contraindicated: pregnancy; age <1 yr
Measles, mumps, rubella	Live viral monovalent or combined MMR	Two doses, at least one mo apart	None	Routine childhood immunization; travelers to endemic countries should be fully immunized	Contraindicated: immunocompromised; pregnancy; immunoglobulins;
Meningococcal *Serogroups* A,C,Y,W-135	Inactivated bacterial (Menomune) (Menactra)	One dose	3-5 yrs (Menomune) ~8 years (Menactra)	Travel to meningitis belt of Africa; travel to new epidemic areas; travel to Saudi Arabia for Hajj; absence of spleen	Neither vaccine protects against Group B meningococcal meningitis
Pneumococcal *(PPV-23)*	Inactivated bacterial	One dose	Consider dose if >5 yrs since primary dose and primary dose given < age 65	Routine immunization age ≥65; absence of spleen; immunocompromised	Also boost immunedeficient and aspelenic people

Table 3.2 Immunizations for International Travel, cont'd

Vaccine	Type/Brand	Primary Series	Booster	Indications for Travelers	Comments and Precautions
Poliomyelitis, oral* (OPV)	Oral live viral	Three-dose series; 2nd dose 6-8 wks after 1st, 3rd dose 8-12 mos after 2nd	One-time booster for foreign travel in adult if >10 years since primary series	Single dose of either OPV or IPV may be used when <4 weeks before departure	No longer in use in the U.S. For use when IPV is not available. Contraindicated in immune-deficient people.
Poliomyelitis, injectable (IPV)	Inactivated viral	As above	As above	Travel to countries where polio is epidemic or endemic	Use for immune-deficient people and their close contacts. Either IPV or OPV can be given to the pregnant traveler.
Rabies	Inactivated viral HCDV (available in ID & IM formulations); PCEC; RVA	Three-dose series at 0, 7, and 21-28 days	None for most travelers; 2 yrs for high-risk groups (spelunkers) if antibodies decline	>30 days in risk areas	If ID rabies vaccine is not completed before starting chloroquine or mefloquine, use IM vaccine
Tetanus-diptheria	Bacterial toxoid	Three-dose series, 2nd dose 4-8 wks after 1st dose, 3rd dose 6-12 mos later	Every 10 yrs or 5 yrs with dirty wound	Routine immunization; nonimmune	Diptheria protection also important, especially in older travelers

Continued

Table 3.2 Immunizations for International Travel, cont'd

Vaccine	Type/Brand	Primary Series	Booster	Indications for Travelers	Comments and Precautions
Typhoid, oral	Attenuated live bacterial Ty21a (Vivotif)	One capsule at 0, 2, 4, and 6 days (3 sachets at 0, 2, and 4 days in Canada)	3-7 yrs Varies by country labeling	Travel to a developing country, especially Indian sub-continent.	Contraindicated: immunocompromised; pregnancy; concurrent antibiotic use; age
Typhoid, injectable	Bacterial polysaccharide (Typhim Vi)	Single dose	2-3 yrs Varies by country labeling	Travel in developing country	Contraindicated: pregnancy; age <2 yrs
Tick-borne encephalitis	Inactivated viral (FMSE-IMMUN), Encepur)	3-dose series on day 0, 3 weeks-3 months, 9-12 months; accelerated schedule—administer 2nd dose at 2 weeks	Every 3 yrs	Rural travel with high-risk tick exposure in endemic areas in late spring and summer.	Not available in the United States.
Varicella	Live viral	One dose at 12 mos—12 yrs, 2 doses 4-8 wks apart, ages 13 and older	None	Routine childhood immunization <13 yrs old; likely exposure in nonimmune adolescent or adult	Contraindicated: immunocompromised; pregnancy; concurrent aspirin use; neomycin; immunoglobulins

Table 3.2 Immunizations for International Travel, cont'd

Vaccine	Type/Brand	Primary Series	Booster	Indications for Travelers	Comments and Precautions
Yellow fever	Live viral	Single dose	10 yrs	Travel to endemic areas of Africa and South America; required for entry by some countries	Contraindications: thymectomy; immuno-compromised; preg-nancy; age <9 mos; use with caution over age 65

Table 3.3   Immunizations for the HIV-Positive Traveler

Vaccine	Recommendation	Comments
Cholera (oral)	Probably safe	Use only inactivated bacterial
H. influenza type b	Recommended	Consider one dose of conjugated vaccine
Hepatitis A	Recommended	The expected immune response may not be obtained
Hepatitis B	Recommended	Test for preexisting immunity
Influenza	Recommended	Administer annually
Japanese encephalitis	Recommended	Mosquito-bite prevention
Measles (MMR)	Recommended for persons not severely compromised	Not recommended for persons severely compromised
Meningococcal	Recommended	Booster in 3-5 years
Pneumococcal (PPV-23 vaccine)	Recommended	Booster after 5 years
Polio	Use only inactivated vaccine (IPV)	The live oral polio vaccine (OPV) is contraindicated
Rabies	Recommended	Administer by IM route only
Tetanus/diphtheria	Booster every 10 years	Diphtheria immunity may be diminished or absent
Typhoid	Use Typhim Vi	Avoild live oral typhoid vaccine
Varicella	Recommended for some asymptomatic individuals	Not recommended for symptomatic persons
Yellow fever	Recommended for asymptomatic patients if risk of disease is unavoidable (7250 CD4 count)	Letter of waiver if vaccine not administered. Strict mosquito-bite protection advised

*Medical waivers—Most countries will accept a medical waiver for persons with a health reason for not receiving the yellow fever vaccination. The CDC recommends obtaining written waivers from consular or embassy officials before departure, but travel clinics hardly ever recommend doing this. Instead, a physician's letter that states the reason for withholding the vaccination and that is written on letterhead stationery usually suffices. The letter should bear the stamp used by a health department or official immunization center to validate the *International Certificate of Vaccination* (Yellow Card).

CHAPTER 4

Jet Lag and Motion Sickness

KEY POINTS:

▶ Insomnia is the primary symptom of jet lag.

▶ Jet lag diets and formulas are not effective.

▶ Short-acting sleeping pills may be helpful for some travelers.

▶ Contrary to popular belief, drinking lots of fluids doesn't prevent jet lag.

▶ Antihistamines are somewhat effective for motion sickness.

▶ Traveler's thrombosis is a potentially fatal, but very rare condition.

Most travelers have experienced jet lag. The common symptoms—insomnia, fatigue, change in appetite, irritability—are due in part to your body's cyclical hormone production being temporarily out of synch with your activities. After several days at your destination, your body's biological clock (circadian rhythm) becomes reset, and the symptoms subside. In general, it takes the body 1 day to adjust for each time zone crossed.

Like many disorders that have no cure, there are lots of proposed jet lag remedies and preventatives. Numerous travelers have tried jet lag "diets." More recently, exposures to artificial light sources and melatonin have been touted as being effective in resetting the body's clock. NOTE: For short stays of 3 days or less, adjustment of the body clock is not possible and should not be attempted.

Jet Lag Diets

Food has no effect on jet lag. There has never been any scientific evidence that jet lag diets do any good, and they have declined in popularity. Many travelers find these diets too complex and tedious to follow. Any claimed benefits most likely are psychological, due to a placebo effect.

Jet Lag Formulas

These vitamin-amino acid formulas or homeopathic preparations supposedly help reset your biorhythms, but like jet lags diets, they are not scientifically proved and work primarily by placebo effect. Some jet lag formulas previously contained the amino acid L-tryptophan, which has proved mild sedative qualities, but the purified substance is now banned. The amino acids and vitamins in jet lag preparations are the same as those available in any drugstore.

Light Exposure

Light exposure seems to play a role in resetting circadian rhythms. The mechanism involves suppression of the hormone melatonin, which is secreted by the brain's pineal gland. The current dogma is that for eastward travel additional morning sunlight (whether cloudy or not) is beneficial, whereas for westward travel, afternoon light is important. Special high-intensity lights (>10,000 lux) are available to help accomplish this end. Regardless of travel destination and arrival time, recent studies suggest that exposure to outdoor light at any time of day assists in readjustment of your circadian rhythm.

Melatonin

Ten years of placebo-controlled studies have shown that the hormone melatonin can reset your body's internal clock. In one study, travelers were given 3 to 5 mg of melatonin at the "destination nighttime" for 3 days before travel, then for 3 days after arrival. They experienced much less fatigue, required less time to normalize their sleep patterns, and scored better on a visual analog scale. Some other studies, however, have shown no significant beneficial effect in about 25% of recipients, and up to 10% of travelers taking melatonin have adverse side effects (e.g., headache and excessive drowsiness). In summary, melatonin appears to be somewhat beneficial, but there is much individual variation in response to this hormone. Although there is little evidence of toxicity, concerns have been raised about melatonin's safety because the drug's strength, quality, and purity are not standardized. Also, there are little data on optimal dosing and timing of administration.

Researchers point out that little is known about melatonin's long-term safety, its effects on reproduction, and its possible dangers to people with autoimmune diseases. Because melatonin is a hormone, it is not recommended for children or during pregnancy. It should also be noted that unidentified chemical impurities have been detected in some melatonin preparations.

Sleeping Pills

Insomnia is one of the most troublesome symptoms of jet lag. While you're trying to fall asleep, your internal clock is saying "wake up." If you need to adapt more rapidly to the new time zone, and you have a problem with insomnia, ask your doctor to prescribe a sleeping pill. The first of the nonbarbiturate, short-acting sleeping pills was Halcion (triazolam), a benzodiazepine (similar to Valium). Although safe and rapidly effective, there were reports (albeit extremely rare) of next-day memory impairment or amnesia associated with this drug, especially after long-haul flights and the consumption of alcohol.

For travelers who want an alternative to Halcion and similar (benzodiazepine) hypnotics (e.g., Dalmane, Restoril) newer agents are now available; they include the following:

- Ambien (zolpidem): Dose: 5 to 10 mg for adults
- Sonata (zaleplon): Dose: 10 to 20 mg for adults
- Lunesta (eszopiclone): Dose: 1 to 3 mg for adults

Ambien, Sonata, and Lunesta are chemically unrelated to the benzodiazepines. Lunesta is the newest of these drugs and is approved for longer-term (up to 6 months) use. These drugs have rapid onset, adequate duration of action, and claim minimum or no residual effect on daytime performance. Transient memory impairment, however, has been reported with all of these drugs, albeit with a very low incidence.

Are sleeping pills safe? Generally yes, especially if they are used for only a short time and in the lowest effective dose. According to the Harvard Medical School Health Letter (May 1990), "Taking sleeping pills for a short period—perhaps a few days—can be quite helpful . . . and there is little controversy about prescribing them to help people through a crisis."

So, What to Do?

Before taking medication or using techniques to prevent jet lag, consider the following:
- Is the treatment safe? Are there side effects?
- Is the treatment effective?
- Is the treatment practical and cost effective?

What Really Causes Jet Lag Anyway?

Feeling tired and irritable after a long trip is not due entirely to changes in your circadian rhythms. The issue is more complex. Consider the typical scenario:

For several days before departure, you are frantically taking care of what seems like a thousand and one last minute errands and details.
- You are probably too keyed up to get enough sleep.
- Your normal eating and drinking patterns are disrupted.
- You are somewhat apprehensive about flying.
- You are anxious about leaving home and/or your family.
- You fight heavy traffic getting to the airport.
- You park your car, but wonder if it will be safe.
- You carry a heavy suitcase a half a mile to the check-in point and hope it won't get lost.
- You catch a connecting flight and you stand in line again at check-in.
- You clear security checkpoints.
- Then you wait in a crowded airport lounge because your overseas flight is delayed by hours.

It's no surprise that you're feeling stressed out even before takeoff. Add to this a lack of sleep en route, cramped seating, further dehydration, and even constipation. Then, after arrival in a foreign country, you face still more hassles simply getting to your hotel. No wonder you've got jet lag.

The *Health Guide* takes the following view: Jet lag is not a single entity and the symptom complex will probably never be completely alleviated by a single treatment. The symptoms you experience are usually a combination of travel-related physical and emotional stresses, sleep deprivation, plus the biological effect of your circadian rhythm being out of synch.

En-Route Strategies to Reduce Jet Lag

- Don't drink too much alcohol—If you are a drinker, there's no reason not to have your cocktail, but remember that although alcohol is a depressant drug, it may cause rebound nervous stimulation, interfering with sleep.

- Don't drink too much coffee—Excess caffeine may cause nervousness and possibly insomnia. Excess caffeine stimulates gastric acid production, which can cause heartburn. However, if you habitually drink many cups of coffee each day, missing your "caffeine fix" during your flight may not be a good idea. You might get symptoms of caffeine withdrawal and feel even worse (e.g., headache)! Coffee-drinker strategy: Reset your watch to the destination time when you board the aircraft. Drink your coffee en-route at the destination time that corresponds to your regular "caffeine fix" time at home.
- Drink water and fruit juices—They are good substitutes for (or complements to) alcoholic drinks and coffee. You may be somewhat dehydrated at the beginning of the flight due to disrupted eating and drinking habits before departure, and your sense of thirst may also be increased by breathing low-humidity cabin air.
- Sleep en-route?—This may be hard to avoid, especially if your flight is to Australia or Asia from North America. No studies have been done to assess whether sleeping en-route significantly alters the symptoms of jet lag. You'll probably feel better on arrival, but falling asleep later might be more difficult.

After Arrival at Your Destination

- The most important principle is to begin all activities, including eating and sleeping, at destination times as soon as possible. If you have an evening arrival, have a light dinner and go to bed late. The next day try to eat and sleep according to the local time.
- If you have a morning arrival, stay active during the day and get as much exposure to natural light as possible, if your schedule and the weather permit. If possible, don't nap, but overpowering fatigue should not be resisted. If you do nap, keep it to under 45 minutes to avoid Stage IV (REM) sleep, which causes grogginess on awakening. NOTE: For trips less than 3 days, short naps should be taken when you feel most tired.
- Take a sleeping pill if you have troubling insomnia. Discontinue sleeping medication after 3 to 5 nights.

The Myth of Dehydration

For many years it has been touted by the travel media that dry cabin air in jet airliners causes dehydration, which presumably could aggravate jet lag. The recommended remedy is usually to drink extra fluids en route, sometimes as much as a glass of water every hour. However, the Medical Director of British Airways Aviation Medical Services has found (as reported in the medical journal *Lancet*) that low cabin humidity causes, at most, only a 3-ounce water loss during an 8-hour trip. The reason you think you are dehydrated is because your mouth is dry from breathing dry air, not because you actually are dehydrated. In fact, the stress of travel causes your body to retain water.

Also advised: "Avoid caffeine and alcohol, these will also dehydrate you." This advice is not true. According to a study from the University of Nebraska Medical Center, healthy adults showed the same "hydration status" (as determined from urine analyses and other tests) when they drank caffeinated beverages, such as coffee or caffeinated co-las as when they drank only water and/or fruit drinks. There is no net loss of water from drinking coffee. Concentrated alcoholic drinks, in excess, may cause a mild diuresis, but beer, wine, and many mixed drinks contain lots of water and won't cause dehydration. Therefore, dehydration from dry cabin air, aggravated by certain beverages, appears to be a myth, and compulsively drinking extra water en route is both inconvenient and unnecessary.

Keep the Problem of Jet Lag in Perspective

Enjoying your vacation is more important than fighting jet lag. Don't waste your time following complex jet lag diets and cures that have not been shown to work. Try not to worry too much about jet lag. Less than one half of travelers report significant symptoms.

Business Travelers   If you are traveling on important business, you probably have more need than others to reduce the symptoms of jet lag. Consider the following strategies: (1) reserve a sleeperette (reclining airline seat) to improve the chances of sleeping en route; (2) budget, if possible, 1 or 2 extra days after arrival to rest and recuperate before business activities; or (3) break up a long trip (>6 time zones) along the way for 1 or 2 days.

MOTION SICKNESS

Strictly speaking, motion sickness is neither an illness nor a "sickness" but a normal, albeit exaggerated, response to unfamiliar motion of increased intensity and duration. Nausea, sweating, salivation, and vomiting are the usual symptoms. If vomiting does occur, it is frequently followed by drowsiness and lethargy.

Motion sickness occurs most commonly with acceleration in a direction perpendicular to the longitudinal axis of the body, which is why head movements away from the direction of motion are so provocative. Vertical oscillatory motion (appropriately called heave) at a frequency of 0.2 Hertz is most likely to cause motion sickness. (This frequency would be experienced on board a ship with a roll rate of 5 seconds.) The incidence of motion sickness falls quite rapidly at higher frequencies. The apparent protection at these higher frequencies helps explain why motion sickness is commonly experienced on camelback, but not on horseback, and on board ships, but not while windsurfing.

Risk Factors

- Sea > Air > Car > Train
- Women > Men
- Inexperienced travelers > Experienced travelers
- Young age > Older age
- Passengers > Crew
- Passengers > Driver

Motion sickness occurs in about 1% of airline passengers. Symptoms are rare in children younger than age 2 and peak between the ages of 3 and 12. The elderly are less susceptible.

Preventing/Treating Motion Sickness

Don't travel on an empty stomach; this seems to promote symptoms. If you feel yourself becoming nauseated, keep your head stationary. Don't read, but do listen to music if you have a portable radio, iPod, or airline headset. A stable head position is very important in controlling motion sickness because your inner ears contain the balance "gyroscopes" that monitor and coordinate motion and body position.

Increasing ventilation, decreasing food intake, and avoiding alcohol are other techniques to reduce motion sickness. For those interested in natural remedies, ginger root may offer some benefit.

Body Position On a boat, try to stay amidships. Lie supine with your head supported on pillows. Keep your head still and your eyes closed. If on deck, look out at the horizon. One trick: pretend you are "dancing with the ship." On airliners, either (1) press your head against the seat in front of you, or (2) lean back in the seat, keep your head still, and look straight ahead. In cars, sit in the front seat. Look forward at the horizon, rather than out the side windows.

Acupressure bands (Sea-Bands)—Some people swear by these wrist bands with the plastic beads, but a study conducted by Condé Nast Traveler magazine (October 1991) found no measurable effect on the symptoms of seasickness.

Drugs

Stimulation of nerve fibers in the balance center of the inner ear (the labyrinth) causes the symptoms of motion sickness. The drugs used to control motion sickness not only reduce the activity of these nerve fibers but also appear to act directly on the body's vomiting center located in the brainstem. The drugs commonly used to prevent motion sickness are the scopolamine preparations and the antihistamines.

Scopolamine

Scopolamine is a drug extract (alkaloid) of the nightshade plant. It is similar to another extract, popularly called belladonna, and known in medicine as atropine. The most frequent side effect of these drugs is dryness of the mouth, but blurred vision, drowsiness, and urinary retention can also occur.

TRANSDERM SCŌP The Transderm Scōp System (Fig. 4.1) is a circular flat patch that delivers 1.0 mg of scopolamine at a constant rate over 3 days. Because of its prolonged action, it is especially useful for seasickness. Travelers may want to try it for a few days before departure to identify any adverse effects.

SCOPACE (scopolamine hydrobromide) This drug is an oral form of scopolamine with a duration of 6 to 8 hours. It acts more rapidly than the scopolamine patch. The more rapid onset and shorter action make it better suited for airline or automobile travel. The dosage range is 0.4 to 0.8 mg. You should take it on an empty stomach 1 hour before departure. The dosage can be titrated for best effect.

Ginger This natural motion sickness remedy is safe and moderately effective and is readily available in health food stores.

Figure 4.1 The small patch placed behind the ear releases minute amounts of scopolamine that permeate the intact skin at a preprogrammed rate over a 72-hour period. The scopolamine is directly absorbed into the blood stream. Scopolamine acts on the nerve fibers of the inner ear and brainstem to reduce nausea and vomiting. The transdermal patch should not be used by children, travelers with glaucoma, or men with prostate enlargement. Confusion in the elderly may occur.

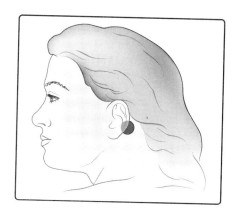

Antihistamines

Although scopolamine is considered to be the more effective drug for the treatment of motion sickness, many physicians prefer antihistamines because they produce fewer adverse effects (e.g., dry mouth, blurred vision) than scopolamine. Drowsiness is the most common antihistamine side effect, which can be troublesome if you need to drive a car. Drowsiness, on the other hand, can help you sit or lie quietly and thus may be beneficial on a boat or a plane.

Antivert (meclizine) The initial adult dose is 25 to 50 mg. Take 1 hour before departure. Repeat every 12 to 24 hours, as needed, for the duration of the journey. Available by prescription only.

Dramamine (dimenhydrinate) Available without prescription. This drug has a rapid onset of action, and you can use it for either prevention or treatment of symptoms. Adults and children older than 12 years should take one or two tablets every 4 to 6 hours, as needed. Start 1 hour before embarkation. Follow package instructions for younger children.

Phenergan (promethazine) The average adult dose is 25 mg taken twice daily. Take the first dose 30 minutes to 1 hour before embarkation and repeat in 8 to 12 hours, as necessary. Suppositories are quite helpful. For children: Phenergan tablets, syrup, or rectal suppositories, 12.5 to 25 mg (for larger children), twice daily may be administered. This drug, available by prescription, may be the most effective of the antihistamines for the treatment of motion sickness. Contraindicated for children under age 2.

Which One to Choose?   Given the choice of motion sickness medications, how is one to choose? A recent comparative trial of seven commonly used agents to prevent motion sickness showed that they all performed equally well.

SINUSES AND EARS

When traveling by commercial airliner, you will be cruising at an altitude of 30,000 to 45,000 feet above sea level. Your cabin will be pressurized to an altitude of 6,000 to 8,000 feet above sea level. The air contained in your middle ear and sinuses will expand by about 25% and will usually escape without causing any symptoms. During descent, however, cabin air pressure starts to increase and exceeds the pressure in the middle ear. To allow equalization of pressure on either side of the eardrum, the eustachian tube must open to allow air to enter from the back of your nose. If necessary, clearing the tube can usually be accomplished by yawning or swallowing. Pinching your nostrils and slowly forcing air into the ears can assist this process. Chewing gum can also help contract the muscles at the end of the tube to allow passage of air up into the middle ear.

If the pressure difference between your middle ear and the nasopharynx (back of the throat) becomes too great during descent, the end of the eustachian tube might collapse completely, making further ventilation of the middle ear impossible (Fig. 4.2). If this occurs, pressure will continue to rise outside the eardrum (tympanic membrane), causing painful stretching and inward bulging of this structure. You might experience dizzi-

Figure 4.2   Descent from cruising altitude increases pressure on the canal side of the drum (A), which must be equalized in the middle ear (B). This can be effected only by airflow via the nasopharynx through the eustachian tube (C). If the latter is not open, airflow is impeded (D), and the relative negative pressure in the middle ear sets in motion a chain of damaging effects—beginning with pain due to the stretching of the tympanic membrane. (Adapted from Schley WS: Airflight and the middle ear. Hosp Med, 1998, pp 85,86, 95. Copyright Hospital Publications, Inc.)

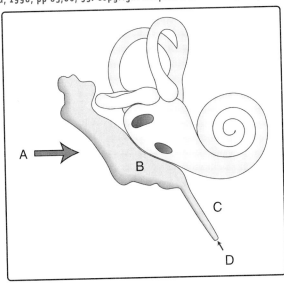

ness, vertigo, and decreased hearing. There could be bleeding into the middle ear from ruptured blood vessels. More commonly, you might experience several hours, rarely days, of pain and pressure in the ear. During this period of inadequate middle ear ventilation, an acute middle ear infection requiring antibiotics might develop.

If your sinus openings are blocked, pressure symptoms will develop over that particular sinus where air is trying to enter. You may feel a headache over the lower forehead or eyebrows, or over your cheek and around your eyes.

Prevention and Treatment   Your ear structure may be such that you may have difficulty adapting to the pressure changes described. (You would probably also note similar symptoms when scuba diving, traveling in high-speed elevators, or even driving in the mountains.) In this case, you may benefit from a decongestant. A recent study concluded that taking the oral decongestant (pseudoephedrine—Sudafed) decreases the incidence of ear pain and discomfort associated with air travel, but that using a popular decongestant nasal spray (oxymetazoline—Afrin) is only minimally effective. The *Health Guide*, however, sees no reason why these drugs shouldn't be taken together. NOTE: There are reports of pseudoephedrine (which is similar to the recently banned stimulant, ephedrine) triggering heart attacks and stroke even in otherwise healthy young people. Be sure not to exceed the recommended dose.

EarPlanes   These devices regulate the air flowing into and out of the ear thereby alleviating ear pain caused by rapid changes in cabin pressure. Inside, porous ceramic ele-

Figure 4.3   EarPlanes are recommended for travelers who must fly with colds, allergies, or sinus conditions.

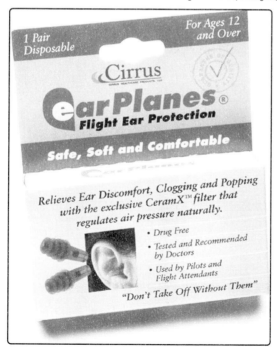

ments slow down rapid pressure changes, giving the eustachian tubes more time to equalize pressure between your middle ear and the cabin.

If you are suffering from an acute ear infection, sinusitis, or an upper respiratory infection, you might have too much swelling and edema of the nasal mucous membranes to allow equalization of pressure during air travel. You probably should not fly under these conditions. If in doubt, consult your physician or an ear-nose-throat specialist.

Here is a summary of the steps you can take to reduce ear and sinus discomfort when traveling by air:

- If you are suffering from hay fever (allergic rhinitis), have your doctor prescribe a nasal steroid spray such as Vancenase or Beconase plus the nonsedating antihistamine Zyrtec. In addition, take an oral decongestant such as pseudoephedrine (Sudafed). Start treatment several days before departure.
- If your problem is simple congestion from a head cold, or if you have a history of trouble equalizing middle-ear pressure, start decongestants. Use an oral decongestant, plus a nasal spray, such as oxymetazoline (Afrin) or phenylephrine (Neosynephrine). Start Sudafed at least one day before departure. Use the nasal spray 1 to 2 hours before landing.
- Have your doctor prescribe an antibiotic if you have signs of a serious sinus infection (facial pain, fever, thick nasal discharge, or postnasal drip). Most cases of sinusitis, however, are caused by viruses and don't respond to antibiotics.
- Blow your nose frequently to remove mucus.
- Remain awake during descent to keep up with pressure changes. Pinch your nose and blow air up into the eustachian tube, as necessary.
- Infants: During descent, they should be in a sitting position only when given their bottles, which should contain only water.

CABIN AIR

Contrary to popular belief, the cabin air in airliners is not a major source of contamination. Although cabin air contains varying amounts of carbon dioxide, ozone, volatile organic compounds, dust particles, and microbial aerosols, the risk of contamination (especially the risk of acquiring an infectious disease) is practically eliminated by the filtering and air exchange mechanisms used in today's airliners. According to Thomas Bettes, M.D., M.P.H., former regional medical director for American Airlines, there are fewer microbial aerosols in an airliner than in any other public location. In fact, the heating and filtration to which cabin air is subjected maintain their qualities to those of an operating room with the exception of increased carbon dioxide.

The risk of airborne illness is not related to inadequate filtration of cabin air but rather to being in close contact with a passenger who happens to have a communicable disease (such as tuberculosis or the flu) that can be transmitted directly to you when that person coughs in your direction and you happen to inhale the infected droplets.

TRAVELER'S THROMBOSIS

Sitting and traveling for long periods put you at a slight risk for developing a blood clot in your leg. Called deep vein thrombosis (DVT), the clot can break off and move to the lungs, possibly causing a fatal pulmonary embolism. But how many travelers get a DVT in the first place? Estimates of the incidence of traveler's thrombosis vary dramatically, from a handful of cases to perhaps tens of thousands annually.

One problem is defining the condition. The vast majority of blood clots dissolve on their own, and the passenger is never the wiser. Problems (like a swollen leg) sometimes don't arise for days after the flight, and the traveler doesn't realize the two events are related. A study published in the medical journal *Lancet*, where the authors used ultrasound as the screening method, found that as many as 10% of the subjects studied developed asymptomatic deep vein thrombosis in the calf during flights of 8 hours or longer. But other investigators have found a lower incidence. The LONFLIT study series, for example, found an incidence of only 4% to 5% using ultrasound screenings, and that was among high-risk subjects.

Another report (*Lancet*, October 2000) downplays the risk. Of 788 patients with DVT that were studied and compared with a control group, there was no association of travel (by air, bus, automobile, train, or boat) with DVT. These authors concluded that "these results do not lend support to the widely accepted assumption that long traveling time is a risk factor for venous thrombosis. Even for journeys lasting more than 5 hours no association was apparent."

What about pulmonary embolism, the complication of DVT that threatens lives? A study in 2001, found just 56 cases of confirmed pulmonary embolism among the 135 million passengers who arrived at Charles de Gaulle airport. The authors also discovered that the risk of pulmonary embolism does increase with the distance traveled. For those flying 3,000 miles, the risk was 1.5 cases per million. At 6,000 miles, the risk grew to 4.8 cases per million.

Basing their opinion on these and other studies, the World Health Organization has concluded that there is a definite link between long-distance air travel and deep vein thrombosis, but they say it is small, and mostly affects people who are already at risk for blood clots.

Symptoms and Diagnosis

Pain and swelling of a leg are typically noted, but some DVTs are silent, or cause swelling without any pain. If a DVT results in a pulmonary embolus (PE), shortness of breath and/or chest pain usually occur, but sometimes fainting is the first symptom. A blood test called D-dimer assay (which measures blood clot fragments) can be used to screen for DVT, but if there is a high suspicion of DVT or a PE based on symptoms, an ultrasound examination of the leg, or a computed tomogram (CT) of the chest, should be done—even if the D-dimer test is not elevated.

Risk/Prevention

In 2004, the American College of Chest Physicians (ACCP) issued recommendations for travelers on long-distance flights lasting at least 6 hours. The ACCP came up with measures that are applicable to (1) all travelers and (2) those who are at increased risk.

Basic preventive measures for all travelers sitting for at least 6 hours:

- Avoid constrictive clothing around the lower extremities and waist;
- Drink plenty of fluids to maintain hydration;
- Exercise and stretch the calf muscles*;
- Take frequent walks up and down the aisle.

For travelers at increased risk. These are travelers with the following risk factors:

- Previous DVT or phlebitis
- Varicose veins
- Obesity
- Older age
- Recent surgery, especially knee, hip, or abdominal surgery
- Recent leg fracture
- Pregnancy—especially during the third trimester and first month postpartum
- Recent serious illness, such as cancer or congestive heart failure
- High-estrogen contraceptives or hormone replacement therapy
- Inherited or acquired blood clotting disorders

If you have one or more of the risk factors listed above, consult your doctor. There are two other options that can help to prevent DVT:

- Support stockings. These compression stockings must be properly fitted so they won't decrease circulation to your leg.
- Anticoagulants: These drugs are reserved for people at very high risk.
  - An injection of low molecular weight heparin (LMWH) or the newer anticoagulant, fondaparinux (Arixtra), can be administered shortly before departure. Fondaparinux is more effective than LMWH and also has a longer half-life, a more predictable response, and fewer side effects than LMWH.
  - Low-dose warfarin (Coumadin) is highly effective, without significant adverse effects.
- Aspirin is no longer recommended to prevent travel-related DVT.

Traveler's Thrombosis in Perspective

In their report, *Air Travel and Health*, the British House of Lords Select Committee on Science and Technology commented:

"For healthy individuals, the risk of getting a clinically significant DVT solely because they are taking a flight seems to be exceedingly small. For those who are already at risk because they are subject to predisposing factors, there may be additional risk from flying, but it is not currently quantifiable. The current lack of sound information makes it difficult for individuals to make reasoned judgments about their personal DVT risk and, consequently, the precautions to take."

---

*Point foot downward, clench toes, and hold for three seconds. Point toes upward, clench toes, hold for three seconds. Do ten repetitions with each foot every one-half hour.

CHAPTER 5

Food and
Drink Safety

▶ Chlorine, in doses recommended for wilderness and foreign travel, is not effective in eradicating *Cryptosporidium* cysts from water, and may be poorly effective in eliminating *Giardia*.

▶ Chlorine dioxide, however, is effective against these parasites, and will also eliminate bacteria and viruses.

▶ Chlorine dioxide is an oxidizing chemical—it does not use chlorine as the disinfectant.

▶ Boiling is unnecessary to purify water—heating water for 2 minutes at 149° F (65° C) or 20 minutes at 113° F (45° C) will make it safe to drink.

▶ Hand washing is an effective and underused method of reducing disease transmission.

▶ Travelers should take measures to eliminate bacteria and parasites from their drinking water. Healthy, fully immunized travelers shouldn't worry too much about viruses in drinking water.

▶ Infants and young children, the elderly, pregnant women, and people with decreased immunity should take precautions against viruses.

Most Americans take for granted the safety of their food and water. If we do worry, we may focus on sugar, salt, cholesterol, saturated fat, food additives—and now carbohydrates! We forget that modern methods of food preparation, packaging, refrigeration, and the use of preservatives—combined with efficient municipal water purification and sanitation—have given the United States and other developed countries unparalleled safety and freedom from infectious diseases transmitted by contaminated food and water. Probably the main health hazard we face from food is its abundance. We eat too much. Obesity, not food-borne illness, is the greater health threat.

Food and Drink in the United States and Canada

Despite our excellent safety record, hundreds of sporadic outbreaks of food- and water-borne illnesses are officially reported each year in the United States. Undercooked food—contaminated eggs, meat, and chicken transmit most cases of disease. The most common illnesses are enterocolitis (usually caused by *Salmonella* and *Campylobacter* bacteria) and hepatitis A. Outbreaks often affect hospital patients, nursing home residents, or school children. Cases of hemolytic-uremic syndrome (HUS), associated with the consumption of undercooked hamburger meat containing *Escherichia coli* bacteria,

Health and International Travel **75**

have received extensive publicity, but HUS has also been associated with consuming raw cider, person-to-person contact, as well as bathing in the "kiddie pool" at water parks. Gastroenteritis caused by various *Vibrio* species of bacteria is occasionally reported from the Gulf of Mexico; most cases are related to the consumption of raw shellfish. Botulism, caused by the improper home canning of food, is sporadically reported, and giardiasis, a water-borne parasitic illness, sometimes afflicts hikers and wilderness campers who drink from contaminated ponds, lakes, or streams. Giardiasis and cryptosporidiosis outbreaks have also resulted from breakdowns in municipal water treatment plants. In addition, we have suffered from "travelers' diarrhea" without even traveling. In 1995 to 1997, multistate outbreaks of cyclosporiasis were traced to raspberries and mesclun lettuce imported from Central America!

Food and Drink Overseas

Outside of the United States, Canada, Europe, Australia, and parts of Asia, the situation is far more serious. Most less developed countries don't have our standard of living, our sanitation technology, or our cultural attitudes toward the disposal of human fecal material. Raw sewage may drain into the sources of drinking water, and agricultural fields may be contaminated with various bacteria, viruses, and parasites because human feces (night soil) are often used as fertilizer.

Many countries have only rudimentary water treatment facilities and water distribution systems, and where these facilities do exist there are often breakdowns in the system. Public health regulations and inspections may not be enforced or nonexistent. The hygiene of restaurant personnel is usually below Western standards. The importance of hand washing may not be emphasized to kitchen workers. Refrigeration of food in restaurants may be inadequate, or totally lacking, and countertops and cutting surfaces may not be cleaned as required. Such practices not only promote the transmission of diarrheal diseases caused by bacteria and viruses, but also help spread hepatitis A, typhoid fever, trichinosis, tapeworm, and other bacterial and parasitic diseases rarely found in this country.

FOOD SAFETY

Sources of Risk

When you choose foods to eat, evaluate each item in terms of its ability to harbor dangerous organisms or harmful toxins. Eating undercooked, raw, or unpasteurized products is potentially hazardous. Remember that thorough cooking will destroy bacteria, parasites, and viruses. Even simple heating is usually sufficient to destroy harmful microorganisms.

Food contamination can result from any of the following:

- Contamination at the source: Shellfish, for example, may be harvested from polluted water containing hepatitis A virus, *Aeromonas*, *Salmonella*, or cholera bacteria; chicken and beef can be fecally contaminated with *E. coli* during slaughter; lettuce and other uncooked vegetables may be contaminated in the field from contact with fecally contaminated soil and transmit a variety of bacteria and parasites; unpasteurized dairy products, made from milk produced by sick cattle, can transmit brucellosis, listeriosis, and tuberculosis.

- Contamination from handling: This includes foods that require a lot of touching during preparation, such as salads and raw vegetables. Salads may have also been rinsed with contaminated water during preparation.
- Contamination from bacterial growth: Foods that are prepared moist and warm and that are allowed to sit unrefrigerated are risky. Under these conditions, bacteria, such as staphylococci, can rapidly multiply, producing toxins that cause sudden, severe vomiting and diarrhea. The term "food poisoning" describes this type of toxin-related gastrointestinal illness. Reheated foods are particularly dangerous in this regard.
- Contamination from parasitic larvae: Beef, pork, fish, and shellfish may contain parasitic larvae encysted in their flesh. Aquatic plants (watercress, water chestnuts) may have parasitic cysts attached to their shoots. Examples of illness transmitted by encysted parasites include trichinosis, beef and pork tapeworm disease, anisakiasis, and clonorchiasis, paragonimiasis, and fascioliasis (liver fluke and lung fluke diseases).

Guidelines to Reducing Risk

No matter where you decide to eat, if you follow the guidelines below, you'll improve your chances of staying healthy.

- Eat only meat and fish that have been thoroughly and recently cooked, not re-warmed. Beef and pork should be well done without any pink areas.
- CAUTION: Because of uneven heating, microwaving may not completely destroy surface bacteria. Microwave thoroughly.
- Eat only cooked fruits and vegetables or fruits that you can peel.
- Wash the surface of melons before slicing. Bacteria can otherwise be carried onto the cut surface.
- Foods that require little handling are safer.
- Order hard-boiled eggs served in the shell.
  - Choose dairy products from large, commercial dairies. Boiled milk is safe.
  - Milk and dairy products in Canada, Western Europe, Australia, and Japan are considered safe. Canned milk is safe.
  - NOTE: Commercially prepared mayonnaise is safe. The combination of vinegar, lemon juice, and salt in mayonnaise actually helps kill bacteria, such as *Salmonella*.

Foods to Avoid

- Rare or raw meat; raw fish, shellfish, crayfish, and sushi that have not been previously frozen. In the United States, Food and Drug Administration regulations stipulate that fish to be eaten raw—whether as sushi, sashimi, ceviche, or fish tartare—must be frozen first to kill parasites. (Tuna is the only exception.) Other countries have enacted similar laws.
- Raw vegetables, especially leafy salads served in restaurants

- Fruits not peeled by you and fruits with punctured skins. Watermelons, for example, are often injected with tap water to increase their market weight.
- Aquatic plants in Asia (e.g., watercress, water chestnuts)
- Raw eggs, undercooked eggs, unpasteurized milk and cheese. Some cooking techniques (sunny-side up, "soft" scrambled) won't kill *Salmonella* bacteria.
- Street vendor food unless it is hot and well cooked
- All food that has been left out in the sun, especially dairy products
- Buffet food that has been re-warmed or recycled (e.g., the same cheeses that are at each meal)

Street Vendor Guidelines

- Choose food that is cooked, boiled, steamed, or grilled directly in front of you. These items are safe if served fresh and hot.
- Avoid food handled excessively by the vendor after cooking.
- Avoid juices and other drinks unless they are commercially bottled.
- Eat only food that is served in a clean container.

Wash Your Hands

Wash your hands with soap or detergent, or use a hand sanitizer gel, before you eat. Good hand hygiene not only helps prevent travelers' diarrhea, but there's good evidence that it reduces the risks of colds and respiratory viruses. If you already have travelers' diarrhea, or if you are caring for someone with this problem, be sure to wash your hands after using the toilet, or after having personal contact with the patient. Shigellosis, giardiasis, and viral gastroenteritis are some of the diseases that can be spread from person to person.

Contact with Animals and Eating

Outbreaks of *E. coli* O157: H7 gastroenteritis have occurred among visitors to a petting zoo and a farm in the United Kingdom. Visitors to zoos and farms should know that various pathogens such as *E. coli*, *Salmonella*, and *Campylobacter* can be transmitted to humans from animals, and that hand-to-mouth contact, eating, drinking, and smoking should be discouraged during these visits. Hand washing should be encouraged.

"Safe" Restaurants

Appearances can be deceiving. It's not always possible to tell if a particular restaurant serves safe food. Although the big, established restaurants and hotels may have better safety records, even their kitchens can have lapses in sanitation. As for eating in local restaurants, ask for a recommendation from business contacts, hotel managers, tour guides, etc. When in doubt, don't hesitate to eat in a deluxe hotel restaurant. Some travelers say that Chinese restaurants are often the safest. These restaurants use fresher ingredients, cooked at high temperatures (not reheated), which are served immediately. Mexican-style restaurants are riskier because many dishes require more handling to prepare and often contain eggs, lettuce, and uncooked vegetables.

The following checklist will also help you decide which restaurants may be safer than others.

- Are the silverware, tablecloths, glasses, and plates clean?
- Are the toilets clean? Are soap and water provided for hand washing?
- Are there many flies inside? (Flies can carry disease germs.)
- Is there adequate screening to keep out flies and other insects?
- Is there excess/uncovered garbage outside?
- Are the waiters well groomed?
- Is the restaurant recommended by knowledgeable people?

Remember that the enjoyment of eating is partly what travel is all about. Eating well will also help you stay well, provided you use common sense. Getting enough to eat and drink helps avoid fatigue and dehydration. Within reason, you can often eat what the locals eat. For example, if you're traveling in Europe, choose a tasty but well-cooked specialty such as wiener schnitzel and pass up the risky, uncooked, steak tartare. In Asia, enjoy the Peking duck but skip the raw fish.

WATER AND BEVERAGES

All surface water supplies can be expected to be contaminated at one time or another, no matter how pristine the source, and water from most streams, ponds, wells, and irrigated areas should be considered unsafe to drink. Tap water is often contaminated in less developed countries, but many hotels and resorts maintain safe water systems. You need to judge each facility individually. If you are on a typical tourist itinerary, you are probably going to play it safe and stick to commercially bottled water, soft drinks, fruit juices, beer, and wine, etc. If you plan to obtain drinking water from potentially contaminated sources you need to employ methods that lessen your risk of illness.

Remember that water is only one potential source of illness. Harmful microorganisms also can be transmitted by contaminated food, person-to-person contact, and touching contaminated objects, so there is no absolute protection against the acquisition of an infectious disease. The goal is to reduce your risk by methods that are not too inconvenient or too expensive.

Safe Water and Beverages

- Boiled water—The traditional "standard" of water purification
- Chemically treated water—Chlorine dioxide is becoming more widely used as a replacement for iodine and chlorine.
- Filtered water—Filters remove bacteria and parasites, but not viruses (see "Recommendations").
- Hot tea and coffee are generally safe. Even if the water was never actually boiled during preparation, heating water over a period of time is similar to pasteurizing it. Be sure the drinking cup is clean.

Avoid—If Possible

- Untreated tap water by the glass, in mixed drinks, or in the form of ice cubes Commercial ice in blocks should be suspect.
- Locally bottled water: Be suspicious: These bottles are sometimes refilled with local tap water.
- Uncapped bottled water: These bottles may also have been refilled locally and are best avoided.
- Sea water is always unfit to drink because of the salt content, but it can be used for cooking.
- Pristine-looking water in wilderness lakes and streams may be contaminated with *Giardia* or *Cryptosporidium* parasites, or pathogenic bacteria, such as *Campylobacter*.

Planning Your Water Needs

Review your itinerary to determine what your water needs and sources will be. Will you be vagabond traveling, wilderness trekking, living in tropical countries, or touring under-developed countries? All present different problems and require different strategies. You may be faced with preparing quantities of safe drinking water from polluted sources or simply disinfecting small amounts of tap water in your hotel room. If you will be depending on a filter for much of your water, pump speed, ease of pumping, and ease of cleaning are important factors. Can the filter element be cleaned and re-used, or must it be replaced? When planning your water needs, consider the following:

- Will you be in an urban, rural, desert, mountain, or jungle environment?
- For how long will you be there?
- Will you be hiking or trekking? Need to disinfect water en route?
- Will you be staying at a fixed location or base camp?
- Will you be storing drinking water on a boat or vehicle?
- How many people will be in your group?
- How much water (maximum amount) will you need to disinfect at one time?
- How close will you be to rivers, lakes, and streams? Will you be using that water to drink? How safe is that water to drink?
- What illnesses are common at your destination?
- What type of disinfection equipment or chemicals are you planning to take on your trip?
- What type and how many water containers will you carry?

Wilderness hiking and camping in the United States and Canada expose you mainly to *Giardia*, whereas drinking water in less developed countries is potentially more dangerous—especially near population centers where raw sewage may contaminate the drinking water. In less developed countries, additional protection against bacteria and viruses (especially for certain groups) is essential. See "Recommendations" subsequently. Unless you are in resorts, first-class hotels, and cities that properly filter and chlorinate their water, you should disinfect tap water.

Figure 5.1   The Katadyn Drip Filter is useful for treating large quantities of water under field conditions. The ceramic 0.2 micron filter can be cleaned multiple times and a total of 39,000 gallons can be treated before a replacement is needed.

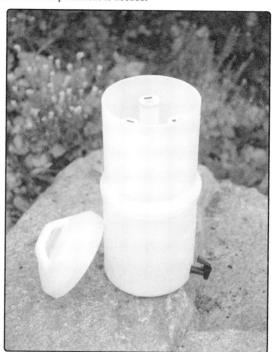

What About Viruses?

You may be advised when traveling in less developed countries, and obtaining water from unsafe sources, not to rely on filters because they do not eliminate viruses. The Wilderness Medical Society states: "Filtration may be used for *Giardia* and . . . bacteria, but for field use, filtration is not practical for viruses (although many are removed by adhering to larger particles)."

But what viral illnesses are we protecting against? And can they be prevented? Should everyone traveling in less developed countries use a water purification device, apply disinfecting chemicals, or boil their water to avoid this threat? Consider the following points:

- Polio is the most dangerous water-borne virus to avoid, but this disease can be prevented by immunization and it has been eradicated from most countries in the world.
- Hepatitis A is spread by contaminated water, but there is an effective vaccine.
- Aside from the common cold, viral gastroenteritis is the most common infectious disease in the world. How preventable is this illness? Recent epidemics on cruise ships illustrate how widespread the problem can be. It is easy to acquire viral gastroenteritis not just by consuming contaminated food or beverages, but also by touching contaminated objects, having close contact with infected people, and not washing your hands. This is usually a self-limited illness, but can be potentially serious for infants

and very young children, the elderly, and people with immune disorders. (These groups are unlikely to be exposed to unsafe water while camping or trekking in a wilderness setting, or traveling off the usual tourist routes.)
- Hepatitis E is the most common form of hepatitis in many countries, and is usually transmitted by contaminated water. There is no vaccine. This disease is much more serious in pregnant women.

Recommendations

Total protection against gastrointestinal illness is not possible, but some groups of travelers are at higher risk than others. These considerations lead the *Health Guide* to recommend the following:
- All travelers should be fully immunized against polio and hepatitis A.
- Pregnant women in regions endemic for the hepatitis E virus should drink only commercially bottled or boiled water, or purified water. Using iodine tablets for longer than 3 weeks is not recommended because of the possibility of thyroid suppression.
- Infants, young children, the elderly, and those with immune disorders should take precautions against exposure to viruses in drinking water.
- All other travelers should be concerned primarily with eliminating bacteria and parasites from their drinking water.

In reality, many travelers may use several methods of water acquisition and treatment as availability, sanitary conditions, itinerary, length of stay, convenience, and personal preference dictate. One method or technology doesn't necessarily exclude the other. Each method has advantages and disadvantages. You may not have your filter or purifier with you at all times. It may clog or break, or you may not have a replacement cartridge. If you are at a base camp you may need large quantities of water for many people and a gravity drip filter plus granular chlorine might be the most convenient and cost-effective method. If on a solo hike, a small water filter or purifier, or disinfecting tablets, may be the most convenient. Whatever the scenario, you often need a backup method of treatment.

Regardless of what system is used to disinfect water, travelers' diarrhea is still a threat because it is also caused by the consumption of contaminated food and spread by person-to-person contact. Treating water—even sterilizing it—reduces, but does not eliminate, the risk of illness.

WATER TREATMENT AND DISINFECTION
Obtaining Clear Water

If you are drawing water from a polluted source, it may be grossly contaminated with organic material. For esthetic reasons alone, you wouldn't want to drink cloudy, scummy water. Furthermore, cloudy water requires more time and bigger doses of chemicals to disinfect, especially if it is cold. Chlorine, in particular, reacts with, and is neutralized by, organic material such as rotting vegetation. Unless you are literally dying of thirst, you should take enough time to clarify your drinking water before it is treated. Here are some techniques:

Sedimentation   Let the turbid water stand undisturbed for several hours, then pour off the upper, clear portion. This works best if the cloudiness is due to sand, silt, or other inorganic material.

Flocculation   Organic impurities may not settle out with gravity alone. Add a pinch of alum (available over the counter in drugstores) to each quart. Flocculation (clumping) of suspended organic impurities will occur, and these clumped particles will settle to the bottom of the container. Pour off the clarified water. To save time, pour the water through a coffee filter, commercial filter paper, fine cloth, or a canvas filter bag to re-move the flocculated sediment more rapidly.

Filtering   Ceramic and glass fiber filters that filter bacteria and parasites also filter out turbidity, but clogging will occur. Ceramic filters can be cleaned many more times than glass fiber filters. Use a pre-filter on the intake hose to eliminate large particles.

Methods of Disinfecting Water

Heating Water   *Cryptosporidium* and *Giardia* cysts (oocysts) are very susceptible to heat. Two minutes at 149° F (65° C) or 20 minutes at 113° F (45° C) (similar to pas-teurization) will inactivate the cysts. Bacteria, such as cholera germs, are killed at 144°F (62°C) for 10 minutes.

Boiling Water   Water that is brought just to a boil and then allowed to cool is safe to consume. Boiling water for 10 to 20 minutes, even at high altitudes, is unnecessary and wastes time and fuel. Some people even question the need to boil water at all—they just "pasteurize" it by heating it for a period of time at a sub-boiling temperature (as men-tioned earlier). NOTE: Boiling water at 10,000 feet raises its temperature to 194° F (90°C)—adequate for killing all microorganisms.

Advantages of Boiling   Boiling water completely eliminates bacteria, cysts of parasites (amoeba, *Giardia*, *Cryptosporidium*), worm larvae that cause schistosomiasis, and viruses (the causes of hepatitis, polio, and viral gastroenteritis). NOTE: Briefly boiling water won't eliminate the spores of certain bacteria; hence, the water can't be considered absolutely sterile. However, bacteria do not cause intestinal illness and can be con-sumed without harm.

Disadvantages of Boiling   It is easier said than done. Heating the water is time-consuming, often inconvenient, and may require you to carry a source of fuel with you. Boiling is usually most easily done at a base camp or other fixed location, not on the trail. Other technologies of water disinfection now make the tedious process of boiling water often unnecessary.

Iodine and Chlorine   Under proper conditions, both iodine and chlorine are excellent water disinfectants for eliminating bacteria and viruses; they are less effective, or even ineffective, against parasites, especially when contact time is brief and/or the water is cloudy and cold.

   Iodine has been used to disinfect water since the turn of the 20th century. U.S. Army studies have demonstrated that under field conditions with dirty, cold water, a

10-minute contact time with iodine kills bacteria, *Giardia*, and viruses; other field studies have shown that at least a 50-minute contact time, and perhaps longer, is necessary to kill *Giardia* under "worst case water" conditions. *Cryptosporidium* cysts are not eliminated by either iodine or chlorine. Boiling, filtering, or using chlorine dioxide are the only ways to eliminate this parasite.

Iodine Tablets   Potable Aqua comes in a small glass bottle that holds 50 tablets and can treat 25 quarts of water. The directions state that it is not for continuous use but for occasional use or emergencies. Potable Aqua is a lightweight, convenient item to carry as a backup purifier. It is not effective against *Cryptosporidium*. Disadvantages are that the need for adequate contact time prevents immediate use. There is a disagreeable taste and odor, but Potable Aqua Plus provides a neutralizer that improves taste and smell. Travelers should avoid prolonged use (more than 3 weeks) of iodine-treated water (as the sole source of drinking water) to avoid potential suppression of thyroid function. This limitation of iodine intake is most important during pregnancy because of the potential adverse effects on fetal thyroid gland development. However, iodine should be used by pregnant women if there is no other short-term alternative to purifying water, especially in areas endemic for hepatitis E.*

Liquid Chlorine Bleach (4% to 6% Clorox)   Household bleach is easily available and cheap, but it doesn't kill *Cryptosporidium* and may not kill *Giardia*. The *Health Guide* does not recommend chlorine as a first-line treatment for water disinfection, but it may have a role when other methods are not available or when the water can also be filtered to remove parasites, if these are a threat. Chlorine is cost effective for treating large quantities of drinking water. The percentage of available chlorine in bleach is usually written on the label. Be sure to use clear water. Mixing directions are as follows: If the strength of the chlorine is unknown, use 10 drops per quart. Double the amount of chlorine if the water is cloudy or cold. Allow the water to stand for 30 minutes. The water should have a slight chlorine odor; if not, repeat the dosage and let stand for an additional 15 minutes.

Table 5.1   Treating Water with Liquid Chlorine Bleach

Available Chloride (%)	Drops per Quart of Clear Water
1	10
4-6	2
7-10	1

*A Peace Corps study published in 1998 in the medical journal *Lancet* described a group of Peace Corps volunteers in Niger who used two-stage iodine-resin filters for more than 24 months as the sole source of potable water. Forty-six percent developed enlarged thyroid glands (goiter) and 34% had abnormalities of thyroid function. The authors recommended not using an iodine-resin filter (or iodine tablets) as the sole source of potable water for more than 3 weeks in any 6-month period.

Granular Calcium Hypochlorite   This method is useful for disinfecting large quantities of water. It uses the granular chlorine often used in swimming pools. Add and dissolve 1 heaping teaspoon of high-test granular calcium hypochlorite for every 2 gallons of water. This will prepare a stock chlorine solution that can be used to disinfect larger quantities of water. Add the chlorine stock solution 1 part to every 100 parts of water. For example, add 1 pint of stock solution to 12.5 gallons of water to be treated.

Chlorine Tablets   Chlorine tablets were once a popular product in the United States, sold under the brand name Halazone. Chlorine tablets are no longer sold in the United States, but are still available in the United Kingdom and elsewhere. Other disinfecting tablets, using iodine or chlorine dioxide, have replaced chlorine tablets in availability and popularity.

Chlorine Dioxide (ClO_2)   Chlorine dioxide is an extremely effective disinfectant, which rapidly kills bacteria, viruses, and *Giardia*, and is also effective against *Cryptosporidium*. ClO_2 also improves taste and odor, destroys sulfides, cyanides, and phenols, controls algae, and neutralizes iron and manganese ions. It is an effective biocide at concentrations as low as 0.1 ppm (parts per million) and over a wide pH range. It is ten times more soluble in water than chlorine, even in cold water. Unlike iodine, chlorine dioxide has no adverse effects on thyroid function. Chlorine dioxide is widely used by municipal water treatment facilities.

The term "chlorine dioxide" is misleading because chlorine is not the active element. Chlorine dioxide is an oxidizing, not a chlorinating agent. ClO_2 penetrates the cell wall and reacts with amino acids in the cytoplasm within the cell, killing the microorganism. The by-product of this reaction is chlorite, which is harmless to humans. Chlorine dioxide is available in both tablet (Micropur MP 1) and liquid (Pristine) preparations.

Micropur MP 1   These tablets are a stabilized form of chlorine dioxide and have a shelf life of 3 years. Each tablet will treat 1 quart of water and they are sold in a 30-tablet blister pack. Effective against *Giardia*, *Cryptosporidium*, bacteria, and viruses, but a 4-hour wait time is required to eliminate *Cryptosporidium* from cloudy, cold water.

Pristine   This is an economical liquid chlorine dioxide product that will purify 30 gallons (120 quarts) of water for about the same price as 30 tablets of Micropur MP 1 (which will

Table 5.2   Chlorine Dioxide Treatment Guidelines

Microorganism Killed	EPA Water No. 1 (Clear, 20° C–68° F)	EPA Water No. 2 (Dirty, 4° C–39.2° F)
Bacteria	15 Minutes	15 Minutes
Virus	15 Minutes	15 Minutes
Cysts	30 Minutes	4 Hours

Figure 5.2 Micropur MP 1 is the only *single-tablet* chemical treatment approved by the Environmental Protection Agency (EPA) to kill bacteria, viruses, and parasites, including *Giardia* and *Cryptosporidium*.

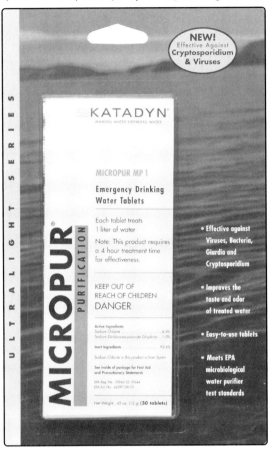

treat 30 quarts). This product is slightly more complex to use than Micropur MP 1 because mixing of two chemicals is required and there is the chance of spillage.

Water Filters and Purifiers

A filter's basic task sounds simple and straightforward: remove microorganisms and other particles larger than a specified size from water. This mission isn't so easy, given the small size and variety of particles, pathogens, and chemical contaminants that may be encountered. Therefore, a variety of devices have evolved: ceramic filters, depth filters, surface filters, etc. These filters all come with a rating of their pore size, which determines what size particles can be physically removed. Pore sizes are measured in microns, and the period at the end of this sentence is about 600 microns across. In practical terms, the most important number is the "absolute" pore size rating, which means the filter element will pass no particle above a certain size.

Figure 5.3 The Katadyn Pocket Filter contains a silver-impregnated ceramic filter and has an 0.2 micron pore size. The filter can be cleaned and has a 13,000 gallon lifetime capacity.

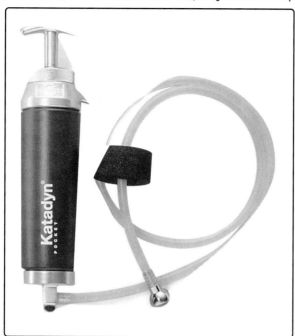

To strain out common parasites (protozoa), such as *Giardia* and *Cryptosporidium*, a pore size of no larger than 4.0 microns absolute is necessary (protozoa range in size from 5 to 15 microns). For bacteria that range in size from 0.2 microns to 10 microns an absolute pore size of 0.2 microns is desirable. A filter this fine is subject to more rapid clogging and will require frequent cleaning. A pre-filter helps reduce clogging.

Water Purifiers   Because viruses can be as small as 0.0004 microns, no field device that relies entirely on filtration will remove them. Water purifiers have both a filter and a de-mand-release iodine-resin element.* A popular model is the Katadyn Exstream. The VirusStat cartridge kills bacteria and viruses and the filter removes parasites. The cartridge needs to be replaced after 100 liters of water have been treated.

NOTE: Choosing a filter/purifier—Aside from removal of microorganisms, consider the following factors when selecting one of these devices:
- Rated output in liters/minute
- Life of filter/purifier element before replacement
- The size and weight of unit with accessories
- Cost, not only of the device, but also of the replacement filter

*How the demand-release iodine system works: iodide ions are bound to an anion exchange resin, creating an electrically charged structure. When negatively charged microorganisms contact the resin, iodine is instantly released, penetrating the microorganism. By this process, bacteria and viruses, and some parasites, are killed. NOTE: the residual iodine in the water may have a concentration of 10 mg/liter, which is significant considering that the RDA (recommended daily allowance) of iodine is only 0.15 mg/day. Some purifiers have a charcoal filter that reduces the iodine content of the treated water.

Figure 5.4   The Katadyn Exstream has a 34-oz. capacity.

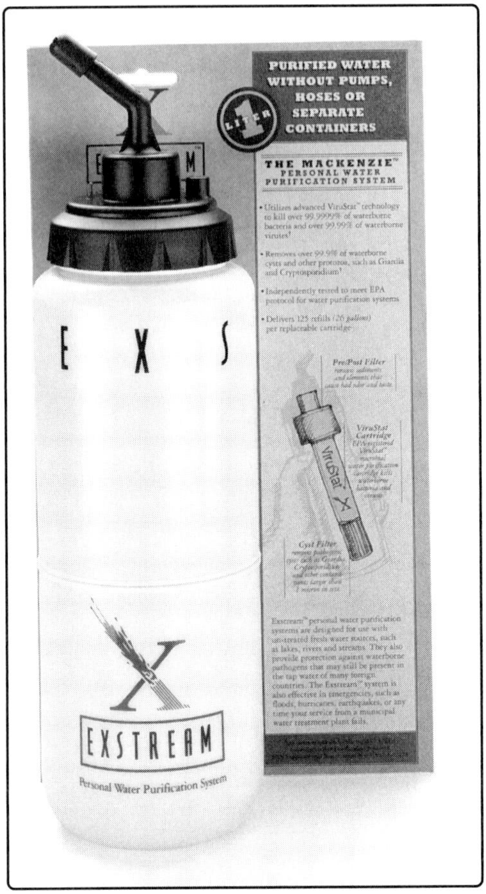

- Whether a carbon cartridge is attached to reduce residual iodine and other chemicals in the filtered water
  Facts about activated carbon filters—What they can and cannot do:
- Carbon filters won't "soften" water.
- Carbon filters will not remove iron, lead, manganese, and copper or chlorides, nitrates, and fluorides.
- Carbon filtration can remove more than 90% of cadmium, chromium, manganese, mercury, silver, and tin.
- Carbon filters are not effective against bacteria, cysts, or viruses; in fact, they may promote bacterial growth when not changed at proper intervals.
- They remove many objectionable tastes and odors.
- Carbon filters are effective for removal of chlorine and iodine taste and smell as well as potentially dangerous and carcinogenic organic compounds.
- If turbidity of the water is the main problem, fiber pre-filters are preferred because they are more cost effective.

CHAPTER 6

Travelers' Diarrhea

KEY POINTS:

▶ Travelers' diarrhea is the most frequent cause of illness among travelers.

▶ Bacterial infections are the most frequent cause of travelers' diarrhea.

▶ Every traveler should carry loperamide (Imodium) and an antibiotic for self-treatment.

▶ Some high-risk travelers may benefit from prophylactic antibiotics.

▶ Food and water precautions may help prevent travelers' diarrhea but are often ineffective because of lack of compliance on the part of the traveler.

▶ Hand washing reduces the incidence of diarrhea.

▶ The oral cholera vaccine (Dukoral) provides up to 60% crossover protection against ETEC diarrhea.

Overview of Travelers' Diarrhea

Diarrhea is by far the most common medical problem among people traveling to less developed tropical and subtropical countries. Travelers' diarrhea, however, is not a specific disease. The term describes the symptoms of an intestinal infection caused by certain bacteria, parasites, or viruses that are transmitted by the consumption of contaminated food or water. The severity and duration of symptoms depend on which microorganism is causing the illness.

Your Risk of Getting Travelers' Diarrhea

Your risk is related to which countries you visit, the month or season of your visit, the duration of your visit, how often you eat in restaurants, and whether or not you eat in local homes or from food vendors. Some studies show that poor restaurant hygiene may be the source of most cases of travelers' diarrhea.

There is little risk (attack rate of about 4%) when visiting North America, northern and central Europe, Australia, and New Zealand. Intermediate attack rates (8% to 20%) are found in travelers to most destinations in the Caribbean, southern Europe, Israel, Japan, and South Africa. High-risk destinations (attack rates of up to 60% during the first 2 weeks) include Mexico, the Dominican Republic and Haiti, and the developing countries of Africa, South and Central America, the Middle East, and Asia. One attack of travelers' diarrhea won't "immunize" you against further episodes. In fact, the attack rate in long-term travelers and expatriates remains unchanged for several years after arrival.

Symptoms of Travelers' Diarrhea

In general, travelers' diarrhea manifests in one of three ways (1) as an acute, watery diarrhea; (2) as dysentery; or (3) as persistent (chronic) diarrhea.

Watery Diarrhea   This is the most common form of travelers' diarrhea, affecting up to 60% of travelers. Most cases of watery diarrhea, worldwide, are caused by a bacterium called enterotoxigenic (toxin-producing) *Escherichia coli*. Other bacterial causes of watery diarrhea include *Salmonella*, *Campylobacter*, and *Vibrio* bacteria. Parasites such as *Giardia*, *Cryptosporidium*, *Cyclospora*, and *Isospora* can also produce watery diarrhea. About 5% to 10% of cases are caused by intestinal viruses.

The symptoms range from several loose or watery stools per day to a more explosive illness with profuse, but nonbloody, diarrhea. Associated symptoms often include nausea, vomiting, abdominal cramps, and a low-grade fever. These symptoms, if untreated, usually last 3 to 5 days. For travelers, this is a major cause of inconvenience and discomfort, potentially ruining a carefully planned vacation or business trip. The main medical danger from profuse diarrhea is dehydration, especially in children and the elderly. Early treatment with fluids, loperamide (Imodium), and antibiotics is usually successful.

Dysentery (bloody diarrhea)   Up to 15% of those with travelers' diarrhea are affected by dysentery. Dysentery results from a more serious intestinal infection caused by certain bacteria (and sometimes parasites) that invade and inflame the wall of the intestine. The most common type of dysentery is bacillary dysentery, also called shigellosis, which is caused by certain species of *Shigella* bacteria. Other bacterial microorganisms that can cause dysentery include *Salmonella*, *Campylobacter jejuni*, *Yersinia*, and *E. coli* serotype 0157:H7. A rare form of dysentery is amebic dysentery (amebiasis), caused when *Entamoeba histolytica* parasites invade the colon wall. Bacterial dysentery is typically recognized by the sudden onset of bloody diarrhea (or bloody, small-volume stools mixed with mucus), high fever, abdominal pain and tenderness, prostration, and the feeling of incomplete evacuation. Blood is visible in only 50% of patients.

If you develop the symptoms of dysentery, you should start antibiotics (as described subsequently), drink sufficient fluids to prevent dehydration, and seek medical attention. If your symptoms are severe, and if you don't improve with antibiotics, you should see a doctor immediately—you may need to be hospitalized.

Chronic Diarrhea   3% to 5% of travelers develop persistent diarrhea, defined as diarrhea lasting more than 1 month. Chronic diarrhea may be accompanied by vague abdominal pain, bloating, nausea, loss of appetite, fatigue, weight loss, and low-grade fever.

If there is an infectious cause, persistent travelers' diarrhea is usually caused by giardiasis, a parasitic disease discussed in Chapter 9. A recent Belgian study reported that *Giardia* and *Campylobacter (C. jejuni)* are the two most commonly found infectious causes of persistent diarrhea. Other unusual causes of chronic diarrhea include amebiasis, cryptosporidiosis, cyclosporiasis, and dientamebiasis.

However, diagnosed infections account for a minority of the causes of persistent travelers' diarrhea. Postinfectious lactose intolerance and irritable bowel syndrome appear to be the most common causes of chronic bowel symptoms in returned travelers. The former results from damage to the cells lining the intestine that contain the enzyme that digests milk, the latter from damage to bowel motility.

If you develop persistent diarrhea, consult your physician or an infectious disease specialist. Testing should be done to establish a precise diagnosis, but in many cases all diagnostic tests are negative, and no definite diagnosis can be made. If medical consultation is not available, assume that you may have giardiasis and self-treat with metronidazole (Flagyl) or tinidazole (Fasigyn). Furazolidone (Furoxone) is effective against both bacterial and parasitic causes of diarrhea. NOTE: Giardiasis, unlike amebiasis, does not cause bloody diarrhea.

Causes and Geographic Variations of Travelers' Diarrhea

The four principal bacterial microorganisms causing travelers' diarrhea in most high-risk areas are *E. coli*, *Shigella* species, *Salmonella* species, and *Campylobacter*.

Temperature; annual rainfall; presence or absence of rivers, lakes, or seacoasts; dry and rainy seasons (monsoons); and other geographic and climatic factors—as well as agricultural, eating, and sanitary practices—will determine which diarrhea-causing bacteria are most common in any particular country, or part of a country. For example, in Thailand, after *E. coli*, *Campylobacter* is most prevalent; in Nepal, after *E. coli*, *Shigella*, and *Campylobacter* are the most common diarrhea-causing bacteria. In Mexico, *E. coli*, *Salmonella*, and *Shigella* predominate in the rainy summer season, whereas *Campylobacter* is more common in the drier winter season. These studies show that globally, the causes of infectious diarrhea are not fixed and that each region has a unique pattern of disease.

TRAVELERS' DIARRHEA FACTS

Bacteria cause about 80% of travelers' diarrhea.

Contaminated food causes more illness than contaminated water.

PREVENTING TRAVELERS' DIARRHEA

Food and Drink Precautions—Are They Effective?

It is commonly believed that your chances of developing a gastrointestinal illness will be reduced considerably by being counseled to "boil it, cook it, peel it, or forget it." Surveys of returning travelers, however, have shown that receiving advice about food and drink safety appears to have no significant effect on rates of diarrhea. In fact, the overwhelming majority of travelers will commit a food and beverage indiscretion within 72 hours after arrival in a developing country, despite pre-departure counseling. Why is this? In some cases, the choice of food may not be under the travelers' control, but it may also be that many people just can't overcome the temptation to sample delicacies in exotic locations. Most travelers find it difficult, impractical, or impossible to resist well-presented, mouth-watering and often prepaid buffets, or to eat only piping-hot foods.

Perhaps then, to the adage quoted above, should be added the words "easy to remember . . . impossible to do!"

Does this mean that travelers should throw caution to the wind and simply forget about prudent dietary habits? No. The medical literature shows a definite correlation between dietary indiscretions and the frequency of travelers' diarrhea. If you can overcome temptation, and stick to safe eating habits, you can reduce your chance of illness. For many, though, this can be a difficult task.

NOTE: An important benefit of prudent eating habits is the prevention of diseases other than travelers' diarrhea. Depending on your itinerary, you could be at risk for acquiring food- and drink-transmitted diseases such as hepatitis A or hepatitis E, typhoid fever, trichinosis, tapeworm and roundworm infestations, and diseases from intestinal, liver, and lung flukes. These are souvenirs you don't want to bring home! The impracticality of following rigid dietary precautions during international travel is a compelling argument for all travelers to carry standby anti-motility drugs (e.g., Imodium) and antibiotics for self-treatment of diarrhea, and for a minority of high-risk travelers, to take prophylactic antibiotics.

Hand Hygiene

Before eating, always wash your hands with soap or detergent. Thirty seconds of washing reduces by 95% the number of bacteria, parasites, and viruses acquired through human contact, or from contaminated surfaces or objects.* Antiseptic towelettes and hand sanitizer gels (e.g., Purell) also do an effective job and are convenient to carry. Hand washing and hand sanitizer gels have also been shown to reduce the spread of colds and respiratory illnesses, including SARS.

Drug Prophylaxis for Travelers' Diarrhea

Self-treatment for travelers' diarrhea has become so predictably effective that most physicians no longer recommend drug prophylaxis against diarrhea except in certain high-risk travelers or when the trip is deemed critical. You might consider prophylaxis with either Pepto-Bismol or antibiotics if you will be traveling short-term (less than 3 weeks) and cannot afford to have your trip interrupted, or travel plans altered, because of illness. You might be, for example, a business person, diplomat, musician, or athlete who can't afford to miss even 1 hour of an important meeting or event.

Or, you might have a medical condition that would be adversely affected by any additional illness. Medical conditions warranting consideration of prophylaxis would include cancer, AIDS, severe inflammatory bowel disease (colitis), kidney failure, and poorly controlled insulin-dependent diabetes. Also, if you have peptic ulcer disease and take a stomach acid-reducing drug (e.g., Zantac, Pepcid, Prilosec, Nexium, Losec, or Protonix), your risk of travelers' diarrhea is increased. Consider taking the anti-ulcer, stomach-coating drug Carafate (sucralfate). This may reduce your risk of diarrhea because Carafate has antibacterial properties.

*In nearly all instances, transmission of acute gastrointestinal illness is caused by organisms that are present transiently on the hands. These organisms are easy to remove by washing. Bacteria that normally live on the hands ("resident flora") are more difficult to remove, but they are not responsible for disease transmission.

Pepto-Bismol   Taking Pepto-Bismol (bismuth subsalicylate) may reduce your chances of getting travelers' diarrhea by about 65% (compared with 90% efficacy for antibiotics). This is a good prophylactic drug for adult travelers and older children, not only because it is effective, but also because there is minimal chance of an allergic or toxic reaction, as sometimes occurs with antibiotic use.

How does it work? Medical studies indicate that Pepto-Bismol actually eliminates harmful bacteria from the stomach. This antibacterial action is due to the bismuth component of the medication. The salicylate in Pepto-Bismol has antisecretory and anti-inflammatory effects on the bowel wall, reducing the output of diarrheal fluid.

Dosage   Two tablets (or 2 oz. of the liquid), 4 times daily. Take with meals and at bedtime. The tablet form of Pepto-Bismol is as effective as the liquid preparation, and the tablets are easier to carry. The downside: taking medication four times a day is very inconvenient for most travelers. Children's dosage: Pepto-Bismol may be used by children older than 3 years. They should use one half the adult dose. For using Pepto-Bismol in a child under age 3, consult your pediatrician. NOTE: 2 tablespoons or tablets of Pepto-Bismol have the salicylate content of about one adult aspirin tablet. Pepto-Bismol is most effective when taken with meals to allow the drug to come into immediate contact with the microorganisms in food.

Contraindications   Pepto-Bismol should be avoided by people who (1) are allergic to, or intolerant of, aspirin; (2) have any type of bleeding disorder; (3) are taking an anticoagulant (warfarin, [Coumadin]); or (4) have a history of peptic ulcer disease or gastrointestinal bleeding.

Side Effects   Pepto-Bismol causes blackening of the tongue and stool, but this is not harmful. Excessive use can cause ringing in the ears (tinnitus) due to salicylate toxicity. Don't take aspirin and Pepto-Bismol simultaneously; the risk of salicylate toxicity (tinnitus, easy bruising) will be increased. If you are on a warfarin anticoagulant (e.g., Coumadin), you should not take Pepto-Bismol because the risk of bleeding will be increased.

Check with your doctor about the safety of Pepto-Bismol if you have any underlying condition for which you are taking medication. Pepto-Bismol should not be taken with doxycycline because it can prevent the absorption of the latter. Pepto-Bismol may also inhibit the absorption of other antibiotics but the extent of this interaction has not been well studied.

Prophylactic Antibiotics   Taking an antibiotic (especially one of the quinolones) can significantly reduce your risk of travelers' diarrhea. However, because all antibiotics have potential side effects, physicians are hesitant to prescribe them routinely to healthy travelers. Also, if diarrhea occurs while taking the antibiotic, then what should you do? Some argue that an antibiotic, such as a quinolone, should not be used for prophylaxis when it is also the treatment of choice, and therefore, should be reserved for the latter. Prophylactic antibiotics are not generally recommended for children, except under rare circumstances.

Rifaximin (Xifaxan)   This is a new, nonabsorbed antibiotic that is effective against non-invasive *E. coli*, the most common cause of travelers' diarrhea. In November 2004, the

Table 6.1   Antibiotics Used to Prevent Travelers' Diarrhea

Ciprofloxacin (Cipro)	250 mg daily
Levofloxacin (Levaquin)	500 mg daily
Ofloxacin (Floxin)	400 mg daily
Moxifloxacin (Avelox)	400 mg daily
Azithromycin (Zithromax)	250 mg daily
Rifaximin (Xifaxin)	200 mg daily

company announced the results of studies that also showed effectiveness in preventing shigellosis (dysentery caused by *Shigella* bacteria).

Pepto-Bismol Combined with Stand-by Antibiotic   Before requesting a prophylactic antibiotic, be aware that the quinolone antibiotics are rapidly effective in the treatment of most cases of diarrhea. In fact, a quinolone usually stops diarrhea within 10 hours or less. Therefore, if you take Pepto-Bismol prophylactically, and carry the antibiotic in reserve, you may significantly reduce your risk of travelers' diarrhea, and at the same time preserve the therapeutic option of an antibiotic. Pepto-Bismol prophylaxis, combined with antibiotic self-treatment, as needed, is a reasonable choice for most travelers requesting prophylaxis. The whole cell/recombinant B subunit oral cholera vaccine (Dukoral) provides crossover protection of up to 60% against ETEC diarrhea.*

TREATMENT OF TRAVELERS' DIARRHEA

The treatment of travelers' diarrhea (depending on the severity) consists of one or more of the following:
- Adequate fluid intake
- Loperamide (Imodium-AD)
- Pepto-Bismol
- Antibiotics

Hospitalization in some cases for treatment of dehydration and toxicity

Fluids

If you are having frequent, copious diarrhea, dehydration is a potential threat and you may need treatment with an oral rehydration solution, as described in the special section, "Oral Rehydration Therapy," starting on page 99. If your diarrhea is not particularly severe, then follow these guidelines:

*ETEC = Enterotoxigenic E. coli, the most common bacterial cause of travelers' diarrhea worldwide.

Mild/moderate diarrhea: Adults—Continue with your regular diet (soup and salted crackers are good additions) and drink at least 2 to 3 liters of fluid (mostly water) daily, or more if you are in a hot climate. Avoid dairy products (milk and cheese) during the acute phase of diarrhea.

Mild diarrhea: Infants—They should continue to receive their regular formula or food and full amounts of whatever liquids they normally consume.

Pepto-Bismol (bismuth subsalicylate)

In addition to its role in prophylaxis, Pepto-Bismol, in conjunction with diet, can also be used for the treatment of travelers' diarrhea. Pepto-Bismol reduces the number of un-formed stools by 50% through its antimicrobial, antisecretory, and anti-inflammatory actions. Bloody diarrhea (dysentery) is not a contraindication to the use of Pepto-Bismol. Pepto-Bismol is more effective in relieving nausea than it is in reducing diarrhea. Pepto-Bismol is not frequently recommended because of its inconvenient dosing and efficacy, which is lower than antibiotics.

Adult Dosage Two tablets or 2 tablespoonfuls (1 dose cup, 30 mL), repeated half hourly, as needed. Do not exceed a total dose of 16 tablets, or 8 oz. of the liquid, in any 24-hour period. Don't take aspirin at the same time you are taking Pepto-Bismol because salicylate toxicity could occur. Use acetaminophen (Tylenol) if you need medication for pain or fever while taking Pepto-Bismol. If your diarrhea is not adequately controlled with Pepto-Bismol in 6 to 8 hours, discontinue the medication and start antibiotics.

Loperamide

Loperamide (Imodium-AD) reduces diarrhea (both the frequency of passage of stools and the duration of illness) by up to 80%. Its action is due to its anti-motility effect (reducing peristalsis) as well as its antisecretory effect (blocking the bowel's output of salt and water).

Adult Dosage Two capsules (4 mg) immediately, then 1 capsule after each loose or watery stool. Don't take more than 8 capsules over any 24-hour period. Don't take loperamide if you have a high fever or are severely ill.

Child Dosage Young infants and children appear to be more susceptible to side effects such as paralytic ileus (distended intestine), vomiting, and drowsiness. If loperamide is used in older children follow label directions carefully. Do not give loperamide to infants and children younger than 2 years old unless you have consulted your pediatrician.

NOTE: A theoretical concern about anti-motility drugs is that they may prolong illness by interfering with the body's natural "flushing" mechanism. In reality, when travelers have used loperamide to treat watery diarrhea, no prolongation of illness has been observed, even when stool cultures have later shown the presence of an invasive microorganism (e.g., *Shigella*). Nevertheless, some medical experts still advise you not to take loperamide if you have bloody diarrhea and/or a fever greater than 101°F. However, the *Health Guide* believes that when a quinolone antibiotic is administered with loperamide, the benefits of combined treatment outweigh any theoretical risk of adverse effects.

Loperamide Plus Antibiotics

The problem with loperamide, used alone, is that it does not treat the cause of the diarrhea—only the symptoms. Recent studies indicate that combining loperamide with an antibiotic is better therapy for diarrhea because it combines the anti-motility action of the former with the curative effects of the latter. Studies in Mexico, for example, showed that a combination of loperamide and a quinolone antibiotic was more effective than loperamide alone.

When to add an antibiotic? If the diarrhea is mild, i.e., does not force a change in your activity, loperamide (and/or Pepto-Bismol) alone is often sufficient. An antibiotic should be added when the diarrheal illness is abrupt, with frequent and/or copious stools, or the diarrhea is bloody or accompanied by fever.

Antibiotics

The quinolone (fluoroquinolone) antibiotics have revolutionized the treatment of travelers' diarrhea. These antibiotics achieve very high fecal drug concentrations, and just one or two doses are often curative. There is, however, increasing evidence that antimicrobial resistance is on the rise as evidenced by a 90% resistance of *Campylobacter* to ciprofloxacin in Thailand (50% in Nepal and 40% in Egypt). The quinolones currently remain the first choice of treatment for all travelers, including pregnant women and children. The best alternative is azithromycin. Other drugs include furazolidone (Furoxone), cefixime (Suprax), trimethoprim/sulfamethoxazole (Bactrim), and rifaximin (Xifaxin).

Quinolones

Single doses are often effective, but a full 3-day course is recommended for individuals who are not well after the first day of illness and in patients with bloody stools, fever, or known *Campylobacter* or *Shigella* infections. Ciprofloxacin is available in liquid form for children. Ciprofloxacin, levofloxacin, and ofloxacin can be given intravenously if vomiting prevents oral administration.

Ciprofloxacin (Cipro)
Dosage: 750 mg once or 500 mg twice daily for 1 to 3 days
Dosage using liquid preparation: 20 to 30 mg/kg/day, divided into two doses per day, for 3 days, if necessary

Levofloxacin (Levaquin)
Dosage: 500 mg once or 500 mg daily for 1 to 3 days

Ofloxacin (Floxin)
Dosage: 400 mg twice the first day or 400 mg daily for 1 to 3 days

Moxifloxacin (Avelox)
Dosage: 400 mg daily for 1 to 3 days

Use of Quinolones for Other Infections
The quinolones are effective in urinary infections and are generally effective for the treatment of typhoid fever. Ofloxacin, moxifloxacin, and levofloxacin are more effective than ciprofloxacin against community acquired pneumonia, acute bacterial bronchitis, skin infections, and uncomplicated pelvic

inflammatory disease (PID) due to gonorrhea and chlamydia. Levofloxacin is effective against methicillin-resistant *Staphylococcus aureus* (MRSA) skin infections.

Alternative Drugs Used to Treat Travelers' Diarrhea

Azithromycin (Zithromax)   This antibiotic is effective against *Shigella*, *Salmonella*, *E. coli*, and *Campylobacter* and it has also shown activity against typhoid fever. In Thailand, azithromycin has shown more effectiveness against *Campylobacter* than ciprofloxacin. The drug is available in both 250-mg and 500-mg tablets.

Adult dosage: 1,000 mg once or 500 mg daily for 3 days
Child dosage: 10 mg/kg/day for 3 days

Cefixime (Suprax)   This is a cephalosporin antibiotic that is effective against most bacteria causing infectious diarrhea, but there have been reports of *Shigella* resistance. Cefixime is also a useful drug for treating ear infections (otitis media), pharyngitis and tonsillitis, acute bacterial bronchitis, urinary tract infections, and gonorrhea. It is available in a liquid form.

Adult dosage: 400 mg once daily for 3 to 5 days
Child dosage: 8 mg/kg once daily for 3 to 5 days

Furazolidone (Furoxone)   This drug is active against most bacterial causes of travelers' diarrhea, as well as *Giardia*, making furazolidone useful as a broad-spectrum treatment when the cause of the diarrhea is not known. Furazolidone is also available in a liquid preparation.

Adult dosage: 100 mg (1 tablet) 4 times daily for 3 days; for giardiasis, treatment is for
    7 to 10 days
Child dosage: 5 years and older—25 to 50 mg (¼ to ½ tablet) 4 times daily
Liquid furazolidone contains 50 mg per tablespoon (15 mL)
5 years and older—½ to 1 tablespoon (7.5 mL to 15 mL) 4 times daily
1 to 4 years—1 teaspoon to 1½ teaspoons (5 mL to 7.5 mL) 4 times daily
1 month to 1 year—½ teaspoon to 1 teaspoon (2.5 mL to 5 mL) 4 times daily

Trimethoprim/Sulfamethoxazole (Bactrim, TMP/SMX, Co-trimoxazole)   TMP/SMX is now considered a last-choice drug, to be used by the traveler who is allergic or intolerant to the other antibiotics mentioned in this section. Worldwide, there is widespread resistance, but it is still effective, to a limited extent, in Mexico.

Adult dosage: One double-strength tablet every 12 hours for 1 to 3 days
Child dosage: 8 mg/kg trimethoprim and 40 mg/kg sulfamethoxazole per 24 hours,
    given in two divided doses every 12 hours
    NOTE: This drug is effective for cyclosporiasis. Adult dosage: One double-strength
tablet every 12 hours for 7 days

Rifaximin (Xifaxin)   This is a new, minimally absorbed antibiotic effective against noninvasive strains of *E. coli* (ETEC), the most frequent cause of travelers' diarrhea in most countries. It may be effective for treating dysentery caused by *Shigella*, *Salmonella*, or

Campylobacter but further studies are required. Rifaximin should be reserved for areas of the world where ETEC is most common, e.g., Latin America. Dosage: 200 mg 3 times daily for 3 days

Metronidazole (Flagyl)   If you have diarrhea that persists longer than 2 weeks, you could be harboring *Giardia* parasites. It is reasonable to start self-treatment for giardiasis if you will be unable to get timely medical consultation.

Adult dosage: 250 mg three times daily for 5 to 7 days; don't drink alcohol when taking metronidazole; severe nausea and vomiting may occur.

Tinidazole (Fasigyn), a derivative of metronidazole, is now the drug of choice for giardiasis; it is administered in a single dose (2 gms). Each tablet is 500 mg.

Treatment of Children and Pregnant Women

Children   The quinolones are currently the most effective treatment for travelers' diarrhea. In some experimental animals, these compounds damage cartilaginous end plates of long bones, but there are no data that show a similar process in humans. Children

SUMMARY OF TREATMENT OF TRAVELERS' DIARRHEA

- Every traveler to the developing world should carry an antibiotic *and* loperamide (Imodium) for self-treatment of traveler's diarrhea.

- Treatment options include loperamide (Imodium), antibiotics, or an antibiotic plus loperamide. If your symptoms are relatively mild, you could start treatment with loperamide. If you are not better after 4 to 6 hours, start antibiotics, preferably a quinolone or azithromycin.

- If you have copious or explosive diarrhea, take an antibiotic and loperamide immediately. Start oral rehydration therapy, as needed. A 1- to 3-day course of an antibiotic combined with loperamide is usually curative.

- Always treat dysentery (bloody diarrhea, high fever) with antibiotics.

- Quinolones are the most effective antibiotics and should not be withheld from pregnant women or children, especially from those who have more severe symptoms.

- Azithromycin is the best alternative drug, particularly for pregnant women and infants or children.

- Diarrhea danger signs include bloody diarrhea, high fever, persistent vomiting, severe abdominal pain, prostration, and dehydration. Seek qualified medical care if your symptoms are not improved after 48 hours of antibiotic treatment, or if you are becoming dehydrated.

- Soup or broth, salted crackers, and extra water will help maintain hydration, and also provide nutrients. Try to eat a normal diet as much as possible, even in the face of diarrhea.

- If you have mostly vomiting—and minimal diarrhea—sipping plenty of slightly salty fluids and taking Pepto-Bismol is a good treatment.

- About 10% of diarrhea is caused by a parasitic disease such as giardiasis or amebiasis. Treat with metronidazole (Flagyl) or tinidazole (Fasigyn).

- Antacids containing magnesium, aluminum, or calcium; sucralfate; iron tablets; or multivitamins containing iron or zinc, or Pepto-Bismol, may interfere with the absorption of quinolone antibiotics. They should not be given with, or within 2 hours, of the administration of a quinolone.

with cystic fibrosis and cancer have been treated with long courses of ciprofloxacin without apparent complications.

Many travel experts now believe that it is unacceptable for a child, who may be more likely to get travelers' diarrhea, may become more dehydrated with it, and may have a more prolonged illness, to receive less effective treatment than an adult. The illness can result in significant suffering for the child and have a major impact on the travel experience for the whole family.

Standby treatment for children should consist of either ciprofloxacin or azithromycin. Ciprofloxacin may be the preferred agent. Because it is not routinely recommended for use in children in the United States or Canada, careful discussion with parents is necessary, weighing the very low risks of giving ciprofloxacin for a very short course against the need for off-label use of an effective, proved therapeutic agent. When using ciprofloxacin for children, give 20 to 30 mg/kg/day, divided into two doses per day, for 3 days. When using azithromycin for children, prescribe 10 mg/kg orally, once daily for 3 days.

Pregnant Women   The same reasoning also justifies the use of quinolones during pregnancy. If antibiotic treatment of diarrhea is indicated, then the most effective drug should be used, especially if the woman could face a prolonged illness with toxicity and dehydration. According to the *Physicians' Desk Reference* (PDR), "quinolones should be used during pregnancy only if the potential benefit justifies the potential risk." In other words, quinolones are not contraindicated during pregnancy (as some would have you believe); they should be administered when untreated maternal illness may result in harm to the mother as well as the fetus.

Standby treatment for pregnant women should consist of a quinolone antibiotic such as ciprofloxacin or azithromycin. Because rifaximin is not absorbed, it should be safe in pregnancy; however, it may have little efficacy against invasive bacteria that cause the most severe illness.

Always follow this principle: The mother's health takes priority. In the case of infectious diarrhea, if her illness is severe, treatment with a quinolone antibiotic should not be withheld because of a theoretical concern about risk to the fetus.

ORAL REHYDRATION THERAPY

The initial treatment of moderate to severe travelers' diarrhea begins by replacing the salt and water lost through your intestinal tract. Severe watery diarrhea (as seen with cholera, for example) can cause life-threatening fluid losses from the intestine of one liter or more per hour. Treating dehydration of this magnitude is an urgent priority, especially in infants, young children, and the elderly. Early, vigorous treatment is even more important in hot, tropical climates where fluid requirements are higher. Hospitalization and intravenous fluid therapy may be required if oral intake cannot keep up with fluid losses. (Additional information on treating dehydration in infants and children is found in Chapter 21).

The first mistake that most people make when treating copious diarrhea is that they don't drink enough fluids. The second mistake they make is using the wrong fluids. They may drink salt-free, high-sugar beverages or a too-salty beverage without the correct glucose concentration necessary to optimize salt and water absorption. Not drinking enough, or using the wrong fluids to treat severe diarrhea, can make matters worse, especially in infants.

Alternatively, you may be in a remote location where you can't get appropriate fluids or the necessary ingredients to prepare a balanced rehydration solution. Under these circumstances, just about any kind of beverage (disinfected tap water, bottled water, tea, coffee, diluted soda pop, etc.) is better than no fluid replacement at all. This will buy enough time (hopefully) to procure the necessary ingredients and prepare a proper solution—or get to a medical treatment facility if you don't improve. First, though, review these basic facts about how the body absorbs salt and water.

Facts About Food, Sugar, Salt, and Water

Your body cannot absorb water by itself. Water absorption only follows the absorption of glucose (or amino acids) and sodium. This fact forms the basis of oral rehydration therapy.

- Glucose (also known as dextrose) rarely occurs by itself in a normal diet. The glucose you consume is mostly in the form of complex carbohydrates (starches) and sugars (disaccharides), such as sucrose, lactose, and maltose. These compounds are broken down by intestinal enzymes to provide free glucose.
- Glucose is transported across the intestinal cell membrane only in conjunction with sodium. Once absorbed through the intestinal wall, glucose and sodium create an osmotic force that pulls in water. The movement of water across cell membranes into the body is entirely passive.
- Table sugar (sucrose) is broken down into one molecule of glucose and one molecule of fructose. Fructose is not co-transported with sodium; it is transported separately and converted to glucose (and fat) in the liver.
- A too-high sugar concentration in the intestine inhibits water absorption. Highly sweetened sugar drinks, especially those with a high fructose content, can actually increase diarrhea by inhibiting water absorption. Apple juice, Gatorade, non-diet cola drinks, and Jell-O have glucose/fructose concentrations of about 6%. Maximum absorption of water occurs when the glucose concentration in your intestine is about 2.5%.
- Starchy foods promote water absorption better than simple sugars. This is because starch solutions in the intestine, before they are broken down to glucose, have less osmotic "back pull" on water.
- Even in the presence of diarrhea, your intestine is still able to absorb glucose, salt, water, and other nutrients. When diarrhea occurs, "resting the intestine" in an attempt to reduce stool output is harmful.
- Rehydration strategies can involve simply the consumption of food plus additional water—or balanced salt/sugar rehydration solutions when diarrhea is more severe.

Oral Rehydration Solutions

Premixed Oral Rehydration Solutions (ORS)   WHO and CeraLyte rehydration salts contain the optimum balance of sodium, potassium, bicarbonate, plus a source of glucose. The WHO formula is glucose-based, whereas Ceralyte uses the advantages of rice carbohydrate as the glucose source. These convenient products are best suited for treating more severe diarrhea and dehydration, especially in infants and children. One packet is added to 1 liter (or 4 cups) of potable water.

Quick ORS formulas   If you don't have packets of ORS formula, you can prepare a basic solution by adding one teaspoon of salt and 2 to 3 tablespoons of sugar or honey to a liter of water. This solution will effectively maintain blood volume and tissue hydration. Another option is to mix one 8-oz. cup of orange juice (or other fruit juice) with three cups of water and add one teaspoon of salt.

Complex Carbohydrate- and Food-Based Rehydration

The glucose-based ORS can keep you hydrated, but they do not decrease stool volume or shorten the duration of acute diarrhea. Cereal- and food-based ORS do both. They also supply up to four times more calories during a time when appetite may be suppressed. With cereal-based ORS, starches (complex carbohydrates) are broken down enzymatically into glucose directly on the intestinal wall with less "osmotic penalty," resulting in better absorption of glucose, salt, and water.

Hydrating Older Children and Adults

This treatment is simple and straightforward, as long as the person is not vomiting:
- Step 1. Drink 2 to 4 liters, or more, of full-strength oral rehydration solution over 2 to 4 hours. Drink enough to restore urine output.

Figure 6.1   WHO rehydration salts

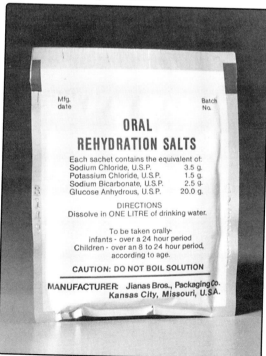

Figure 6.2   Ceralyte

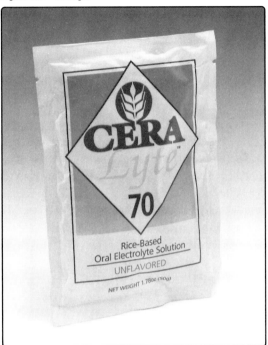

- Step 2. Diet and maintenance fluids—After you are rehydrated and urine output is restored, start to eat (see later) and continue to drink enough fluids to maintain hydration.
- Step 3. If diarrhea continues, continue your diet but drink 8 to 12 oz. of full-strength ORS each time you have a watery stool.

Hydrating Infants and Younger Children

You should know when a child has the potential to become dehydrated. The history is critical: How long has the child had diarrhea, and what are the frequency and volume? Has the child been unable to take oral fluids because of vomiting?

Signs of Dehydration   Observe the child for increased thirst, listlessness or lethargy, decreased urine output, dark urine, and dry mucous membranes. Severe dehydration requires hospitalization and intravenous fluid therapy. Early, vigorous administration of ORS usually keeps a child from reaching that stage.

Children with diarrhea should continue to be fed, but you can interrupt these feedings to administer fluids. Give a dehydrated infant or child 1 to 1-$\frac{1}{2}$ oz. (30-45 mL of

ORS per pound of body weight.) Administer this amount of fluid over 2 to 4 hours. A dehydrated 22-lb. infant, for example, might require as much as 1 quart of ORS during the first 3 to 4 hours of treatment. If the child is not vomiting, give ORS as rapidly as the infant or child will accept it. Use a spoon, dropper, or a baby bottle for infants. Some parents squirt the solution into the child's mouth with a small syringe (ask your doctor for one before leaving or purchase the EZY DOSE syringe, or similar product; these are available in most pharmacies). Watch for the return of urine output and improvements in the child's appearance and behavior.

Vomiting   Don't let it deter you from giving ORS. Even if the child has been vomiting, continue to administer ORS in small amounts. Giving a teaspoon (5 mL) of ORS every 1 to 2 minutes avoids stomach distention, but provides an hourly intake of up to 10 oz. (300 mL). If available, use a feeding syringe (see earlier), an infant bottle, or a medicine cup. This process often requires time and patience, and it may take you 4 to 6 hours to rehydrate the child. Seek medical care if vomiting continues to interfere significantly with oral feedings. Intravenous fluids, or fluids via nasogastric tube, may be required.

Feeding Infants and Children   Early feeding is important. The intestine continues to absorb water and nutrients despite diarrhea. The World Health Organization, in fact, advises parents not to stop giving infants with diarrhea their regular formula or food. Starving an infant to rest the intestine will only make matters worse. Therefore, restore a child's regular diet as soon as possible. Avoid the so-called BRAT diet (bananas, rice, apple sauce, and toast)—it provides insufficient calories and nutrients, and a consensus has developed among pediatricians that this diet is too low in protein, fat, and energy content and may impede the recovery process. Children, like adults, recover more quickly when fed a normal diet.

What Not to Eat and Drink

In moderate to severe diarrhea, avoid fatty foods and also drinks high in simple sugars, including undiluted fruit juices, sport drinks, and soft drinks. These drinks are not appropriate because their carbohydrate concentration is too great and the electrolyte concentration (especially sodium) is too low. Apple and pear juices have greater concentrations of fructose over glucose, and this excess fructose may also aggravate diarrhea. If you do give a child a sugar-containing soft drink, dilute it 2:1 with water and add a teaspoon of salt per liter of diluted drink.

General Dietary Recommendations

Appropriate foods include lean meats, yogurts, fruits and vegetables, as well as complex carbohydrates (starches) such as pasta, rice, potatoes, bread, crackers, and cereals. Cream of Wheat and Gerber Rice Cereal are good choices. It is not clear whether spicy foods (e.g., hot curry) aggravate diarrhea, but these are best avoided unless there is no alternative. Tea is recommended, but alcoholic beverages should be avoided.

CHAPTER 7

Malaria

KEY POINTS:

▶ Malaria, caused by a parasite transmitted by night-biting mosquitoes, is the most important life-threatening infection for travelers and is preventable.

▶ Malaria may be prevented by use of prophylactic drugs. The drug of choice for chloroquine-sensitive malaria is chloroquine. For chloroquine-resistant areas, atovaquone/proguanil (Malarone), mefloquine (Lariam) and doxycycline are the three drugs of choice. Primaquine is an alternative. When primary care providers are not expert in the prevention of malaria, travel medicine advisors should be consulted.

▶ Because no antimalarial drug is 100% effective, mosquito-bite prevention is also important. Methods for prevention include: the use of DEET-based insect repellents; the application of permethrin insecticide on clothing and bed nets; wearing long-sleeved shirts and trousers, weather permitting; and minimizing outdoor exposure between dusk and dawn.

▶ DEET repellents are preferred over non-DEET and biologic repellents when traveling to a malarious region.

▶ Fever in, or after recent return from, the tropics is malaria until proved otherwise, and is a medical emergency. The highest risk of acquiring falciparum malaria (the species that is potentially fatal) is in Oceania and sub-Saharan Africa; illness usually develops within the first 2 months after exposure. Travelers who return with fever should seek medical attention urgently; inform their health-care provider that they have traveled in a malarious area; and request repeated blood films to exclude this infection.

EXTENT AND IMPORTANCE OF MALARIA WORLDWIDE

Malaria is by far the most important insect-borne disease in the world and has been a scourge throughout history, killing more people than all wars and other plagues combined. It remains globally the most important parasitic disease of mankind and claims the lives of more children worldwide than any other infectious disease. In 2005, more than 100 countries were considered malarious, and this disease threatens nearly 40% of the world's population. More than 300 million acute episodes of illness occur every year, and it is estimated that more than 270 million people are chronically infected with malaria parasites. The World Health Organization (WHO) estimates more than 1.5 million people die each year of malaria. The majority of malaria deaths occur among young children in sub-Saharan Africa, especially in rural areas with inadequate or nonexistent health-care services. Along with tuberculosis and HIV infection, malaria forms a disease triad that accounts for almost one half of all infectious disease mortalities worldwide.

Each year, over seven million Americans travel to countries where malaria occurs and in 2000 nearly 1,500 cases of imported malaria were reported to the CDC, an increase of 25% from 1998. Although sub-Saharan Africa is visited by only 2% of U.S. travelers, this region accounts for 83% of malaria cases reported among U.S. civilian travelers.

Malaria is the most important insect-borne disease in many countries, and a delay in diagnosis and treatment may have fatal consequences. If you plan to travel to a malarious region, you must do the following:

- Become informed about your risk of acquiring malaria at your destination.
- Take measures to prevent insect bites, as outlined in Chapter 8. If you prevent mosquito bites, your risk of malaria is decreased considerably. Also, because of increasing drug-resistant strains of malaria, no antimalarial drug is 100% effective. Preventing insect bites gives you backup protection.
- Take a prophylactic drug, if necessary, particularly in countries where there is the risk of *Plasmodium falciparum* malaria, the species most often responsible for fatal malaria. Obtain the most appropriate medication from a health-care provider knowledgeable in travel medicine. To find a travel medicine practitioner in your area, go to www.istm.org, the website of the International Society of Travel Medicine, or www.travmed.com, the website for Travel Medicine, Inc. Both websites maintain travel clinic directories.
- Know the symptoms of malaria.
- Seek immediate medical treatment if symptoms of malaria occur. Be aware that symptoms may be delayed for weeks or months, sometimes years, after exposure and that you may sometimes get malaria even if you took an appropriate prophylactic drug.
- Always consider malaria if you develop a fever after returning from a malarious area, especially within the first 2 months after return.

Your Risk of Getting Malaria

The risk of malaria depends on where you travel and may vary markedly from country to country. The risk of malaria may also vary within a particular destination because the disease may be transmitted only in certain locations within a country, during certain seasons, or below certain altitudes.

Various categories of travelers are also at different risks. Tourists staying in urban, air-conditioned hotels, for example, will usually be at much lower risk than travelers venturing into low-lying rural areas.

Figure 7.1 shows disease rates worldwide.

Travel to Oceania (Papua New Guinea, Irian Jaya, the Solomon Islands, and Vanuatu) and sub-Saharan Africa entails the greatest risk, especially from the potentially

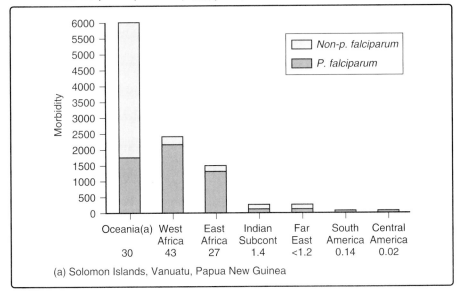

Figure 7.1　Morbidity and Mortality in 100,000 Nonimmune Travelers Exposed for 1 Month Without Chemoprophylaxis* (From Steffen R, DuPont H: Manual of Travel Medicine and Health. Hamilton, Canada, BC Dekker, 1999, p 220.)

(a) Solomon Islands, Vanuatu, Papua New Guinea

fatal *P. falciparum* malaria. There is intermediate risk on the Indian subcontinent and low risk in frequently visited tourist sites in Latin America and Southeast Asia. Tropical Africa is a much higher-risk destination compared with Latin America and Asia for the following reasons:

- Tourists in Africa spend considerable time in rural areas such as game parks, where mosquito activity is high.
- Tourists in Latin America and Asia, however, spend more time in urban or resort areas, where there is little, if any, risk of exposure, and they usually travel to rural areas only during daytime hours when there is little malaria-transmitting mosquito activity.
- In Latin America and Asia, malaria transmission is more seasonal, or focally distributed in rural areas away from the usual tourist routes. For example, 52% of the 1.1 million malaria cases reported from the Americas in 1989 were from Brazil, but 97% of these cases were reported from three gold-mining areas rarely visited by tourists. In Asia (e.g., Thailand), most malaria occurs in remote forested areas—places where few tourists go.
- Malaria is transmitted in both urban and rural areas in sub-Saharan Africa, whereas almost all large cities in Latin America (with the exception of Guayaquil, Ecuador) and Southeast Asia are malaria free. There is no malaria in Hong Kong, Bangkok, Kuala Lumpur, Jakarta, Singapore, Rangoon, Phnom-Penh, Manila, and most other major urban areas. There are some exceptions, such as urban areas of Papua New Guinea and some urban areas in India and Pakistan.

- Mosquitoes in Africa are more apt to be carrying malaria parasites. For example, the proportion of infected anopheles mosquitoes in western Kenya may exceed 20%, whereas in Latin America and Asia less than 1% of anopheles mosquitoes are infected.

> **MALARIA FACT**
>
> In countries where malaria occurs, the highest rates of transmission occur in low-lying rural areas during, and just after, the rainy season. In parts of Africa and Oceania, however, malaria transmission may be high all year, even in urban areas.

The Cause of Malaria

Malaria is caused by a single-cell protozoan parasite of the genus *Plasmodium*. There are four different species of *Plasmodium* parasites that infect humans:

Plasmodium falciparum, which accounts for 40% to 60% of malaria cases worldwide and more than 95% of all malaria deaths

Plasmodium vivax, which causes 30% to 40% of malaria worldwide, but is rarely fatal

Plasmodium ovale, an uncommon parasite found mostly in West Africa

Plasmodium malariae, also uncommon, but distributed worldwide

Worldwide Distribution of Malaria Species

The occurrence of each *Plasmodium* species varies from region to region. *P. falciparum* causes 80% to 95% of malaria in sub-Saharan Africa. It is also the most common species in Haiti and the Dominican Republic, the Amazon Basin, and parts of Oceania (Papua New Guinea, Vanuatu, the Solomon Islands). In South America, outside the Amazon Basin, *P. falciparum* accounts for 10% to 50% of cases. *P. falciparum* is also common on the Indian subcontinent and in Southeast Asia. *P. vivax* causes about 95% of malaria in Mexico and Central America and is also found in South America, North Africa, the Middle East, the Indian subcontinent, China, Asia, and Oceania. Except for Somalia and Ethiopia, *P. vivax* malaria is very rarely encountered in sub-Saharan Africa. *P. malariae* causes as many as 10% to 15% of malaria in sub-Saharan Africa and 1% to 5% of cases elsewhere, worldwide. *P. ovale* is rare. It is found primarily in West Africa where it causes up to 5% of malaria, but it also occurs sporadically in Oceania and Southeast Asia.

Malaria is uncommon at high altitudes because reproduction of the parasites in the mosquito is temperature sensitive. For this reason, *falciparum* malaria rarely occurs over 1,000 meters (3,250 feet) elevation. *P. vivax* parasites, which are hardier, can reproduce at altitudes as high as 2,000 meters (6,500 feet).

How Malaria Is Transmitted

Malaria is transmitted by anopheles mosquitoes. The female mosquitoes require a blood meal every 3 to 4 days to promote the fertilization and growth of their eggs. Anopheles mosquitoes feed from dusk to dawn, so when evening comes you need to take extra measures to prevent bites. Not every mosquito transmits malaria, but it takes just one

Figure 7.2   The Cycle of Malaria Transmission

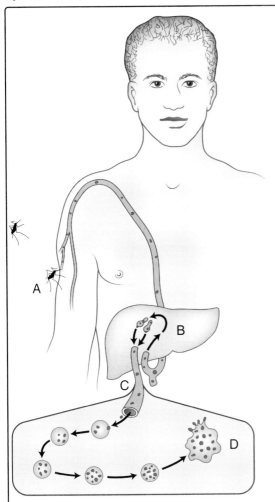

When the anopheles mosquito bites a victim (A) it infects that person with parasites, called sporozoites, which enter the blood stream and travel rapidly (within 30 minutes) to the liver, where they multiply, producing daughter cells, called merozoites (B). Six to 14 days later (approximately), the liver cells burst, releasing large numbers of merozoites that invade red blood cells (C), where they multiply again, rupturing the red cells and releasing even more merozoites (D), triggering an attack of malaria. The merozoite parasites released from the red blood cells then invade new red blood cells, continuing the process. *Plasmodium vivax* and *Plasmodium ovale* parasites have the unique ability to persist in the liver and cause attacks of malaria months, even years, later. Chloroquine, mefloquine, and doxycycline kill malaria parasites only in the blood stage. Atovaquone/proguanil and primaquine destroy *Plasmodium falciparum* in the liver and blood stages; primaquine, but not atovaquone/proguanil, eradicates the dormant forms of *P. vivax* or *P. ovale* from the liver.

bite from an infective insect to give you the infection; therefore, even a brief trip to a malarious area can put you at risk. Malaria may also be transmitted through blood transfusion, or from an infected pregnant woman to her baby at the time of delivery.

How Malaria Causes Illness

After they are injected into the body by a feeding mosquito, malaria parasites first invade the liver, then the red blood cells, where they again multiply. When the parasite-filled red cells rupture, an attack of malaria occurs.

Falciparum malaria is the most serious and sometimes fatal form of malaria. The severity of *P. falciparum* infections is due to the high percentage of red blood cells (RBCs) that are infected by this species. In extreme infections, up to 80% of RBCs may be parasitized and destroyed. This massive red cell destruction has two primary effects (1) severe anemia, and (2) clogging of small blood vessels (capillaries) to vital organs, particularly the brain and kidneys. This circulatory clogging occurs because the infected RBCs produce sticky projections that bind the cells to the walls of the blood vessels and to other RBCs, forming obstructing clumps of cells. Also, chemicals (called cytokines) are released as a result of an immune response to the infection, causing fever, malaise, and other signs of inflammation. In contrast, the other three forms of malaria (*P. vivax*, *P. ovale*, and *P. malariae*) are usually not fatal because fewer than 1% of RBCs become parasitized.

Severe malaria occurs when more than 5% of RBCs are parasitized. Other criteria defining severe malaria include decreased consciousness (indicates cerebral malaria), severe anemia, hypoglycemia (low blood sugar), kidney/liver failure, pulmonary edema (fluid in the lungs), hyperthermia (high fever), and persistent vomiting and diarrhea.

If you are treated appropriately for malaria, you should improve within 48 to 72 hours. Indications of successful treatment include (1) reduction of fever and (2) at least a 75% reduction in the number of red blood cells that are parasitized.

Delayed Attacks of Malaria

If you acquire *P. vivax* or *P. ovale* malaria you may have a delayed attack of malaria because some of the parasites (called hypnozoites) may remain dormant in your liver. In only one third of vivax malaria cases do symptoms develop within 30 days of exposure; about 10% won't develop symptoms for a year or more.

Prophylactic drugs such as chloroquine, mefloquine, and doxycycline work only in the blood (after the liver phase) to eradicate parasites within red blood cells. By taking these drugs during exposure and for 4 weeks after exposure, parasites released from the liver will be killed, and infections without a dormant liver form (*P. falciparum* and *P. malariae*) will be completely eliminated. Primaquine and atovaquone/proguanil act on the liver phase and, therefore, may be discontinued 3 days to 1 week respectively, after exposure. Only primaquine has the ability to eradicate dormant forms of relapsing malarias *P. vivax* and *P. ovale*.

Symptoms of Malaria

Malaria makes you feel like you have "the flu"—only worse. Before an attack of malaria begins, you may have 1 or 2 days of headache, fatigue, muscle aches, loss of appetite, and a low-grade fever. The acute attack starts abruptly with chills, soon followed by a high fever, lasting 2 to 6 hours. During this time you may have a cough and also notice pains in your chest, back, stomach, joints, and muscles. The attack ends with 2 to 3 hours of heavy sweating. If you are not treated promptly, symptoms will recur and complications may develop, especially if the attack is caused by *P. falciparum*. In some cases, malaria fevers recur periodically—every 48 to 72 hours. Death from malaria may occur within only a few days of symptoms. In those U.S. citizens who die from malaria, the most frequent interval from symptom onset to treatment is approximately 4 days.

NOTE: Malaria may occur as soon as seven days after an infective bite, and almost all cases of falciparum malaria occur within 60 days after the bite in people not taking a prophylactic drug or in people using inadequate prophylaxis. Other important causes of fever in the returned traveler include typhoid fever, dengue, gastroenteritis, hepatitis, urinary tract infections, tick typhus, and, rarely, amebic liver abscess.

Although a blood film is required to make the final diagnosis, the most important aspect of diagnosis is always to think of malaria as a possible cause of your illness. This is especially important because not every case of malaria manifests with the typical periodic fever pattern. If you are in a malarious area and you develop fever, and medical care is not available within 24 to 48 hours, it may be advisable for you to start self-treatment before a diagnosis is established. Self-treatment is discussed later, starting on page 127.

Diagnosis

Microscopy of serial blood films to detect the presence of the malaria parasites (plasmodium species) continues to be the standard for diagnosis because it allows estimation of parasite levels, and identification of the four different *Plasmodium* species of malaria. The problem with the malaria blood film is its low sensitivity in light infections, and the need for technical expertise in reading it. Parasites may not be observed unless prolonged, repeated searches are done; also, laboratory technicians—especially in facilities where malaria is rarely seen—may not recognize them. Malaria should not be excluded as a diagnosis until three blood films, obtained 12 to 24 hours apart, have been examined.

Advances in technology have now made the diagnosis of malaria potentially much easier and faster. Sensitive, simple-to-use dipstick assays can now distinguish between *P. falciparum* and *P. vivax*. They have a reported sensitivity of more than 90% and a specificity of 99% for *P. falciparum*. Presently, dipstick tests (e.g., Optimal, PATH Falciparum Malaria IC Strip) have not replaced expert microscopy as a diagnostic standard, but can enhance the speed and accuracy of the diagnosis of malaria, particularly in settings where expertise in microscopy is not immediately available.

NOTE: Although these rapid diagnostic tests for malaria appear promising, various studies have shown that travelers especially when ill, may be unable to perform these tests satisfactorily. In addition, the kits must be stored at temperatures not exceeding 20° C (68° F) to 25° C (77° F). Storing the kits under adverse environmental conditions could invalidate the test results. These tests are not yet licensed for use in the United States but are available in Canada.

MALARIA PREVENTION

Virtually all cases of malaria are preventable. Unfortunately, a significant proportion of travelers who acquire malaria do not receive appropriate information on, or do not adhere to, malaria prevention measures. Failure to take or adhere to appropriate prophylactic medication, and to seek prompt medical attention were significant factors in a recent review of deaths of 185 U.S. travelers who died of malaria between 1963 and 2001.

Chemoprophylaxis

Before departing for a malarious area, you and your health-care provider or travel medicine practitioner should decide if prophylaxis is indicated and which drug, if any, you should take. If the risk of malaria is low, the benefits of prophylaxis must be carefully

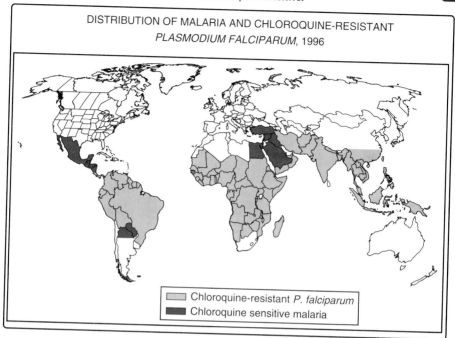

Figure 7.3 Distribution of Malaria and Chloroquine-Resistant Falciparum Malaria–2003*
*Note: Malaria in central China is chloroquine sensitive.

DISTRIBUTION OF MALARIA AND CHLOROQUINE-RESISTANT
PLASMODIUM FALCIPARUM, 1996

Chloroquine-resistant *P. falciparum*
Chloroquine sensitive malaria

assessed. For brief visits to low-risk areas (especially where *P. vivax* malaria predominates) and where prompt medical care is available, it may be acceptable not to take a prophylactic drug, but to rely on insect-bite prevention measures and immediate treatment in the event of illness. However, the issue is controversial; the malaria branch of the CDC recommends prophylaxis in any situation, no matter how low the risk or how long the exposure (even for many years).

Factors determining your need for, and choice of, prophylaxis include (1) your itinerary; (2) the intensity and duration of your exposure to mosquito bites, especially those transmitting *P. falciparum*; (3) your ability to obtain rapid, qualified medical care should symptoms occur; (4) your own knowledge of malaria and its symptoms; (5) your medical history and personal health status; (6) your history of known drug allergies or known ability (or inability) to tolerate certain prophylactic drugs; (7) your use of other medications that may be incompatible with prophylactic drugs; (8) your age; (9) your pregnancy status, if applicable; and unfortunately (10) your financial resources.

The complexity of the situation is one reason why seeing a travel medicine specialist is advisable when exposure to malaria is likely. Remember, though, that the best prophylaxis is still mosquito-bite prevention. If you don't get bitten, you can't get malaria!

NOTE: Recent studies have shown that travelers are being diagnosed with malaria even though they are taking a recommended drug as directed. When these cases were

Table 7.1   Malaria Prophylaxis According to Geographic Area[1]

Chloroquine-Sensitive Areas	First-Line Drug(s)	Alternative Drug(s)
Central America Caribbean Middle East, N. Africa	Chloroquine Chloroquine	Atovaquone/proguanil,[2] doxycycline, mefloquine or primaquine[3]
Chloroquine-Resistant Areas		
South America	Atovaquone/proguanil,[2] doxycycline, or mefloquine	Primaquine[3]
Africa (sub-Saharan)	Atovaquone/proguanil,[2] doxycycline, or mefloquine	Primaquine[3]
Indian subcontinent	Atovaquone/proguanil,[2] doxycycline, or mefloquine	Primaquine[3]
Southeast Asia and Oceania (Papua New Guinea Vanuatu Solomon Islands)	Atovaquone/proguanil,[2] doxycycline, or mefloquine	Primaquine[3]
Thailand[4] (border areas only)	Atovaquone/proguanil[2] or doxycycline	Primaquine[3]

1. In Central and South America and Southeast Asia, travelers are generally at risk only in rural areas during evening and nighttime hours. In sub-Saharan Africa and Oceania, malaria is often transmitted in both urban and rural areas.
2. Atovaquone/proguanil can be carried for use as emergency treatment if malaria is suspected in travelers not using this drug for prophylaxis and who do not have access to medical care within 24-48 hrs.
3. Off-label use. Requires G-6-PD enzyme-screening test.
4. A combination of proguanil and a sulfonamide is an alternative for travelers in Thailand unable to take atovaquone/proguanil, doxycycline, or primaquine. Dosage: proguanil, 200 mg daily, plus either sulfisoxazole, 75 mg/kg daily, or sulfamethoxazole, 1,500 mg daily.

investigated more thoroughly, it was found that the diagnosis of malaria was incorrect due to poor-quality diagnostic facilities. Particularly in Africa, where this problem appears to occur most often, travelers who develop fever while on an appropriate prophylactic agent, and are told that they have malaria, should follow the advice of the local medical practitioner with respect to treatment, but should not discontinue their antimalarial drug. **One important caveat**: those using mefloquine for prophylaxis should not take halofantrine for treatment because of the dangerous interaction of the two drugs.

DRUGS RECOMMENDED IN AREAS OF CHLOROQUINE-RESISTANT MALARIA

Atovaquone/Proguanil (Malarone)

Malarone, a combination of atovaquone (250 mg) and proguanil (100 mg), is the newest drug for the prevention and treatment of malaria. In multiple field trials, atovaquone/proguanil has been shown to be 95% to 100% effective in preventing chloroquine-resistant and multidrug-resistant strains of *P. falciparum* malaria.

Atovaquone/proguanil is active against liver-stage parasites, and requires only a short period of pre-exposure and postexposure dosing. This means the drug may be started 1 day before exposure, continued once daily during exposure, and for 1 week after exposure ceases. The brief postexposure requirement for drug use is ideal for the short-term and frequent traveler, allowing the latter to discontinue medication between trips. In addition, it is an ideal drug for overseas workers who travel into rural malarious areas intermittently, requiring protection for only brief periods. With the exception of primaquine and atovaquone/proguanil, most prophylactic drugs must be taken for 4 weeks after exposure. Mefloquine and chloroquine must be started 1 to 2 weeks before exposure. There is a pediatric formulation of atovaquone/proguanil, making it convenient to prescribe for children, especially those under the age of 8 years who should not take doxycycline.

Atovaquone/proguanil is more expensive than other prophylactic drugs and, therefore, it is less likely to be accepted for long-term prophylaxis. However, because many insurance plans now cover the drug, it is more widely used. Because of its convenient dosing schedule, even in chloroquine-sensitive areas many travelers prefer atovaquone/proguanil to chloroquine.

Adult Dosage One tablet, started the day before travel, taken daily during exposure, and for 7 days after leaving the malarious region.

Child Dosage A pediatric-strength tablet (25 mg proguanil with 62.5 mg atovaquone) is available. The dosage is based on weight: 10 kg to 20 kg = one pediatric-strength tablet, 21 to 30 kg = two pediatric-strength tablets, 31 to 40 kg = three pediatric-strength tablets, and more than 40 kg = one adult-strength tablet. Recent treatment studies showed that atovaquone/proguanil was safe for infants who weighed as little as 5 kg.

Side Effects To date, atovaquone/proguanil (Malarone) has an enviable safety record, with no reports of serious adverse side effects. A recent large-scale trial in travelers from industrialized countries to malarious areas showed that only 1% of users of the drug discontinued it because of side effects—compared with 5% of those using mefloquine (Lariam).

Most complaints include stomach upset, skin rash, mouth ulcers, dizziness, and insomnia in up to 20% of users. Tablets should be taken with food or a milky drink at the same time each day. If vomiting occurs within 1 hour after dosing, a repeat dose should be taken. Atovaquone/proguanil is contraindicated during pregnancy and should not be used by those with severe kidney disease.

Mefloquine (Lariam)

Mefloquine (Lariam) is recommended for both short- and long-term travel to countries where there is chloroquine-resistant *P. falciparum*. The drug is also highly effective against *P. vivax, P. ovale,* and *P. malariae.* In western Cambodia and along the border areas of Thailand, however, the incidence of mefloquine-resistant *P. falciparum* is as high as 50%. Prophylaxis with atovaquone/proguanil (Malarone) or doxycycline is recommended in these areas.

Adult Dosage One tablet, 250 mg once weekly during travel in malarious areas and for 4 weeks after leaving such areas. Mefloquine should be started at least 1 week before departure.

Child Dosage Children: 5 to 14 kg, 1/8 tablet weekly; 15 to 19 kg 1/4 tablet weekly; 20 to 30 kg, 1/2 tablet weekly; 31 to 45 kg, 3/4 tablet weekly; and greater than 45 kg, one tablet weekly. For children weighing less than 5 kg, 5 mg/kg should be given.

Side Effects Mefloquine (Lariam) in prophylactic doses is generally well tolerated, but about 35% of users report mild-to-moderate side effects—sleep disturbances (strange dreams, insomnia), nausea, dizziness, and weakness. Although the gastrointestinal symptoms are the most frequent, it is the neuropsychological side effects (anxiety, dizziness, depression, agitation, nightmares) that cause about 5% of mefloquine users to discontinue the drug. Studies show that men tolerate mefloquine better than women, and infants appear to tolerate the drug well. More severe neuropsychiatric side effects (psychosis, seizures) are extremely rare. Side effects may be reduced by splitting the weekly dose and taking one half tablet twice weekly. Taking the drug with food lessens stomach upset.

Loading Dose of Mefloquine Some travel clinics give a loading dose (one tablet daily for 3 days, then once weekly) to achieve therapeutic levels rapidly and to "screen" for side effects. If there are to be significant side effects, they will usually occur within 1 week instead of 3 to 7 weeks when the drug is initiated on a weekly basis. The loading dose should be taken 2 weeks before travel. If bothersome side effects occur, there will be enough time to switch to another antimalarial, such as atovaquone/proguanil or doxycycline (Vibramycin, Doryx). Alternatively, one may start mefloquine 4 weeks before departure (one tablet weekly) because the majority of side effects will occur within the first three doses.

Travelers with a history of epilepsy, psychosis, recent depression or anxiety disorder, or cardiac conduction disturbances with arrhythmia should not use mefloquine (Lariam). The drug should probably not be given to those on mood-altering drugs such as Prozac, Celexa, Paxil, etc. Mefloquine (Lariam) should be administered cautiously when the traveler is receiving quinine, quinidine, procainamide, or other drugs that affect cardiac conduction. In addition, in countries where halofantrine (Halfan) is used to treat malaria, halofantrine should not be given to those using mefloquine for prophylaxis because of the risk of severe heart rhythm disturbances. Airline pilots, operators of machinery and heavy equipment, scuba divers, and mountain climbers should be informed that mild dizziness is a possible short-term side effect of mefloquine.

Mefloquine has been shown to be safe for prophylaxis during the second half of pregnancy and, by extension, also safe for infants. The drug has not been associated with congenital malformations or adverse postnatal outcomes when used for prophylaxis. There may be a slight trend toward miscarriage when mefloquine is taken during the first trimester, but the data are not firm. Travel medicine physicians will prescribe mefloquine during the first trimester when exposure to chloroquine-resistant falciparum malaria is high and unavoidable. Inadvertent use of mefloquine during the first trimester is not an indication for therapeutic abortion.

Doxycycline (Vibramycin, Doryx)

Doxycycline is an inexpensive tetracycline derivative that also has the advantage of being more than 90% effective in all chloroquine-resistant areas of the world, including along the borders of Thailand. In addition to its effectiveness and low price, prophylactic doxycycline also prevents other serious diseases such as tick typhus, relapsing fever, plague, Lyme disease, and leptospirosis. A disadvantage is that doxycycline must be taken every day. One or two missed doses may put the traveler at risk for malaria.

Adult Dosage   100 mg daily. Doxycycline should be started 1 to 2 days before exposure. It must be continued daily during exposure and for 4 weeks after departure from the malarious area.

Child Dosage (for children older than 8 years of age)   2 mg per kg of body weight per day up to the adult dose of 100 mg daily.

Side Effects   Most travelers tolerate doxycycline well, but nausea, vomiting, and heartburn can occur. Doxycycline should be swallowed in the upright position with sufficient liquid or food to ensure complete passage of the tablet into the stomach. If the tablet or capsule gets stuck in the esophagus it can cause painful mucosal erosions or even esophageal perforation.

Doxycycline may cause phototoxicity, an exaggerated sunburn-type reaction. Avoiding prolonged, direct exposure to the sun, wearing a hat, and using a broad-spectrum sunscreen can reduce the risk, estimated at 2% to 10% of users of the drug. Women taking doxycycline may develop a vaginal yeast infection and are advised to carry a self-treatment dose (one 150 mg tablet) of the antifungal drug fluconazole (Diflucan). Doxycycline is contraindicated for pregnant women and children under the age of 8 unless required for the treatment of a serious infection such as *falciparum* malaria or ehrlichiosis.

Primaquine Phosphate (Primaquine)   This drug has long been used for the treatment of relapsing malaria, but in the last decade it has been re-examined for malaria prevention. Primaquine is considered a *second-line* drug because it is slightly less efficacious than those discussed above, and because a G-6-PD enzyme blood test is required before it is recommended (see later). Field trials in Indonesia, East Africa, and Colombia have shown it to be an effective (albeit off-label) prophylactic agent. When taken by adults in a daily dose of 30 mg (or 0.5 mg/kg per day for children), an effectiveness of 85% to 95% against *P. falciparum* (as well as *P. vivax* and *P. ovale*) has been demonstrated. Primaquine prophylaxis is started 1 day before exposure, taken daily during exposure, and for 3 days after exposure. Primaquine is intermediate in cost between doxycycline and mefloquine. It is an ideal drug for Central America where *P. vivax* malaria is most frequent.

Side Effects Because primaquine is a potent oxidizing agent which is capable of causing severe breakdown of red blood cells (hemolytic anemia), a G-6-PD enzyme screening test is required before using this drug. Primaquine is contraindicated in pregnant women because there is no way to test the fetus for the enzyme deficiency. Taking the drug with food may reduce stomach upset.

DRUGS RECOMMENDED IN AREAS OF CHLOROQUINE-SENSITIVE MALARIA

Chloroquine (Aralen)

For sensitive *P. falciparum* and *P. vivax*, chloroquine remains the drug of choice to prevent malaria. The standard doses are generally well tolerated and are safe for pregnant women and children. Because of widespread resistance, however, the use of chloroquine against *P. falciparum* is limited to persons traveling in Central America, the Caribbean (Haiti and the Dominican Republic), parts of the Middle East, and central China during the malaria transmission season. Although chloroquine remains effective against most strains of *Plasmodium vivax*, *Plasmodium ovale*, and *Plasmodium malariae* as well, *P. vivax* chloroquine resistance is increasing, particularly in the South Pacific, Southeast Asia, and parts of South America (Guyana).

Adult Dosage 500 mg salt (300 mg base) once weekly, beginning 1 week before and continuing 4 weeks after leaving the malarious area. Starting chloroquine before you leave gives you a protective blood level and also lets you know if any unusual side effects will occur.

Child Dosage 8.3 mg/kg salt (5 mg/kg base) once weekly, up to the maximum adult dose of 500 mg salt per week.

Generic chloroquine tablets are sold in the United States in strengths of 250 mg and 500 mg. Only the tablet form of chloroquine is available in the United States. For young children, tablets may be crushed into powder by a compounding pharmacy and the bitter taste masked with syrup. Another strategy is to have a pharmacist pulverize the tablets and prepare gelatin capsules with the proper weekly dose. Mixing the powder from the capsule with food (e.g., chocolate sauce or ice cream) or drink will make the taste more palatable. Liquid chloroquine for pediatric use is available overseas.

Side Effects Chloroquine is generally well tolerated; nausea, however, is not uncommon. Taking chloroquine with meals may usually control gastrointestinal side effects. Dizziness, headache, blurred vision, and itching may also occur, but these symptoms will rarely require you to stop taking the drug. One large European study has shown that seizures and psychosis may occur very rarely with chloroquine. Itching is a frequent occurrence among people of African descent and is not an allergic reaction. Fears about long-term prophylaxis causing degenerative eye (retinal) changes are unfounded. Chloroquine is safe for pregnant women and children, including infants.

WARNING: An overdose of chloroquine (even one tablet in a small child) can be fatal. The drug should be kept in a child-safe container at all times.

NOTE: Chloroquine interferes with the antibody response to rabies vaccine when the vaccine is administered intradermally. If you are taking chloroquine prophylaxis and need rabies vaccination, the vaccine must be given intramuscularly.

Hydroxychloroquine (Plaquenil)

An alternative to chloroquine phosphate is hydroxychloroquine (Plaquenil). It has the same action as chloroquine, but causes fewer gastrointestinal side effects. (Hydroxychloroquine may also be used to treat chloroquine-sensitive malaria.)

Adult Prophylactic Dosage   400 mg salt (310 mg/kg base) weekly.

Child Dosage   6.5 mg/kg salt (5.0 mg base/kg) weekly, up to the adult dosage.

Chloroquine and Proguanil (Paludrine)

In sub-Saharan Africa in particular, proguanil, combined with weekly chloroquine, has been a widely used prophylactic regimen, but it is much less efficacious (<60% efficacy) than mefloquine, doxycycline, and atovaquone/proguanil. This combination should be avoided unless no other regimen can be tolerated. Although the combination is safe for children and in pregnancy, its low efficacy is a reason not to use it in this population that is at greatest risk of severe malaria.

Dosage (adults)   Chloroquine, 500 mg weekly, plus proguanil, 200 mg daily, and continued for 4 weeks after exposure.

Side Effects   The relatively high incidence (about 30%) of gastrointestinal side effects, including mouth ulcers, is reported to cause a significant number of travelers to discontinue prophylaxis with this drug.

Chloroquine-Resistant *Plasmodium Vivax*

Resistance of *P. vivax* to chloroquine has been confirmed in Myanmar (Burma), Papua New Guinea, the island of Nias (Indonesia), Irian Jaya (Indonesian New Guinea) Sabah, Borneo (Malaysia), Colombia, and Guyana. Atovaquone/proguanil, mefloquine, doxycycline, and primaquine are effective prophylactic agents for these strains of malaria.

Other Drugs for Malaria Prevention

Azithromycin (Zithromax)   This is a macrolide antibiotic which has been shown to prevent malaria; one 250 mg dose is taken starting 1 to 2 days before exposure, daily during exposure, and for 4 weeks after exposure. Although safe in pregnancy and in children, the drug has limited efficacy and for this reason is used only as a third-line agent when no other more appropriate drug can be used.

Tafenoquine   This drug is an analog of primaquine that is not only better tolerated but is more potent and long lasting than the parent drug. In one study, a tafenoquine loading dose (one tablet daily for 3 days) protected against *falciparum* malaria for 2 months. Because of its long half-life and its effect on liver-stage parasites, the drug can be discontinued when leaving the endemic area. Like primaquine, a G-6-PD level will be required before usage. This drug is not yet available.

PREVENTION OF RELAPSES (RADICAL CURE)

Most malarious areas of the world (except Haiti) may put you at some risk for having a delayed (relapsing) attack of malaria. Relapsing malaria is caused mostly by *P. vivax* and rarely by *P. ovale*, parasites that reside in your liver, out of reach of standard prophylactic drugs. If you harbor these parasites but are taking a prophylactic drug, the parasites will be suppressed. However, when you discontinue prophylaxis, a delayed attack of malaria can occur, months, even years, later. Your risk of relapsing malaria is proportional to your degree of exposure to infective mosquito bites and the extent of *P. vivax* malaria in the areas where you have traveled. If you were heavily exposed over many months, you have the following three options:

Treat   Take primaquine (see later) when the malaria risk is over to eliminate any possible dormant liver parasites. If you were in a high-risk malarious area for more than 2 to 3 months, then your chance of harboring dormant parasites may be high enough to justify treatment (in sub-Saharan Africa the risk of *P. vivax* is low). Start a 2-week course of primaquine after finishing prophylaxis. Areas of the world with the highest risk of relapsing malaria include Central America, North India, and Oceania.

Adult Dosage   30 mg base daily. The total dose administered should be 6 mg/kg

Child Dosage   0.6 mg base per kg daily for 14 days

A G-6-PD enzyme-screening test is required before using this drug. Primaquine is contraindicated during pregnancy. Pregnant women at risk should continue chloroquine prophylaxis during gestation and receive primaquine after delivery.

OR

Wait and Watch   If your exposure was low to moderate, the chance of infection is less. Be alert for symptoms, especially fever. If *P. vivax* or *P. ovale* malaria occurs, it must be treated with a drug that acts on the blood phase (e.g., chloroquine) followed by primaquine.

OR

Use Primaquine Prophylaxis   Primaquine is the only antimalarial prophylactic agent that acts not only on the liver phase of the malaria life cycle, but also eradicates the dormant liver forms of *P. vivax* and *P. ovale* malaria. When primaquine is used as a prophylactic agent, the likelihood of developing relapsing malaria is very low (except in areas where primaquine resistance occurs—see later). The dose of primaquine starts 1 day before exposure, daily during, and for 3 days after exposure.

Adult Dosage   30 mg (2 tablets) per day for people >60 kg in weight

Child Dosage   15 mg per day (1 tablet) for people <60 kg in weight

Primaquine-Resistant Plasmodium Vivax

Treatment of relapsing malaria may not be 100% effective because primaquine-resistant strains of *Plasmodium vivax* are now reported in scattered areas throughout Southeast Asia, Oceania, and Somalia. For adults who fail the standard treatment, a prolonged dose of primaquine is usually given as 30 mg per day for 28 days. Higher doses of primaquine may be required; however, in such cases, blood counts must be carefully monitored to detect significant hemolysis (breakdown of red blood cells).

MALARIA TREATMENT

Principles of Malaria Treatment

Malaria is a medical emergency and treatment should be initiated as soon as possible. If you develop a fever and there is the possibility it could be caused by malaria, seek medical care immediately, and inform your health-care provider that you have been in a malarious area. If you are carrying standby antimalarial drugs and are still in the tropics, begin self-treatment but seek medical consultation as soon as possible.

Chloroquine (Aralen)

In areas where chloroquine-resistant *P. falciparum* or chloroquine-resistant *P. vivax* is NOT reported, start treatment on the following schedule:

- Day 1. Chloroquine 1 gm (salt) by mouth immediately, then chloroquine, 500 mg (salt), 6 hours later. (500 mg salt = 300 mg base)
- Day 2. Chloroquine, 500 mg orally
- Day 3. Chloroquine, 500 mg orally
  A total of 10 tablets (250 mg each) are required.

Severe chloroquine-sensitive malaria requires an intravenous infusion of chloroquine, 0.83 mg/kg/hr (base), or intramuscular chloroquine, 3.5 mg/kg (base) repeated every 6 hours until parasitemia decreases. Oral chloroquine can then be started: the total dose is 25 mg/kg (base).

NOTE: Because intravenous chloroquine is not readily available in the United States or Canada, intravenous quinidine or quinine may be substituted (see later).

Atovaquone/Proguanil (Malarone)

Atovaquone/proguanil (Malarone) now appears to be the most effective treatment for acute uncomplicated *falciparum* malaria (<5% parasitemia), including multidrug-resistant strains. It has been shown to be effective in regions where high failure rates occur with other anti-malarials including chloroquine, mefloquine, and halofantrine. In Thailand, atovaquone/proguanil cured 100% of cases of *P. falciparum* malaria versus 86% for mefloquine. Elsewhere, an overall success rate of 98.7% has been reported. However, recently, several cases of atovaquone/proguanil treatment failure have been documented.

Adult Dosage   Four tablets once daily for 3 days

Child Dosage   11-20 kg: one adult tablet daily for 3 days; 21-30 kg: two adult tablets once daily for 3 days; 31-40 kg: three adult tablets once daily for 3 days; more than 40 kg: four adult tablets once daily for 3 days

Side Effects   Nausea, vomiting, loss of appetite, abdominal pain, headache, and itching. Dividing the dose and giving it twice daily may reduce the gastrointestinal effects.

Mefloquine (Lariam)
This drug is highly active against all malaria strains, except in Thailand, where cure rates of *P. falciparum* have fallen to 50%-70%.

Dosage   1,250 mg (or a total dose of 15 to 25 mg/kg) is best given as a divided dose of 750 mg (or 15 mg/kg) followed by 500 mg (or 10 mg/kg) 6 to 8 hours later. (25 mg/kg is needed to treat *falciparum* malaria from Thailand and 15 mg/kg elsewhere.)

Unless safer options are not available, mefloquine should not be used for self-treatment because of the frequency and potential severity of neuropsychiatric adverse effects, and is contraindicated (for treatment, not prophylaxis) in pregnancy.

Pyrimethamine/Sulfadoxine (Fansidar)
Fansidar is a combination of pyrimethamine and sulfadoxine, and has been used in the past for self-treatment. Resistance to the drug is widespread in Southeast Asia and South America and is becoming more of a problem in Africa. It is now considered a second-line drug for treatment and should be avoided unless other more effective treatments are not available.

Halofantrine (Halfan)
Halofantrine is chemically similar to mefloquine, with which it shares cross-resistance. It is highly effective against all four plasmodium species. A 3-day course of treatment is 90% curative but side effects, some of which may be potentially fatal, are also increased. Halofantrine is not to be used to treat mefloquine failures (because the combination of the two drugs may cause severe heart rhythm disturbances) and is contraindicated during pregnancy or breastfeeding. The CDC does not recommend halofantrine for treatment because of the potential side effects and the availability of safer alternative drugs. The drug is currently available in many countries in Africa and Europe but is not commercially available in the United States or Canada.

Quinine
Quinine is an ancient drug that originated from the cinchona plant. It is active against all four *Plasmodium* species. Quinine is also one of the most rapidly acting drugs for the

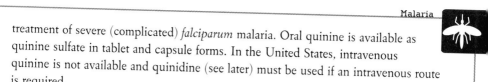

treatment of severe (complicated) *falciparum* malaria. Oral quinine is available as quinine sulfate in tablet and capsule forms. In the United States, intravenous quinine is not available and quinidine (see later) must be used if an intravenous route is required.

NOTE: Quinine by itself may not be adequate for eliminating all parasites permanently from the blood, and recrudescent infections can occur. In addition, resistance to quinine is reported in Thailand and elsewhere, and treatment failures have occurred. Therefore, combination treatment with another drug, such as atovaquone/proguanil, mefloquine, an artemisinin derivative, artemether/lumafantrine or doxycycline, is recommended.

Dosage for Complicated Malaria
Quinine dihydrochloride salt by intravenous infusion, 20 mg/kg loading dose over 4 hours, followed by 10 mg/kg every 8 hours given over 2 to 4 hours. Oral therapy (see later) with quinine sulfate should be started when there has been clinical improvement and the patient is not vomiting.

Oral Dosage for Uncomplicated Malaria
Quinine sulfate, 600 mg (or 10 mg/kg) orally three times daily for 5 to 7 days. Quinine treatment should be combined with one of the following:

- doxycycline, 100 mg twice daily, OR
- clindamycin, 450-900 mg three times daily

Doxycycline or clindamycin should also be administered for 5 to 7 days. The second drug may be administered during or following quinine therapy.

Side Effects (IV and oral routes)
Side effects can be a problem with quinine, especially after several days of treatment. Headache and tinnitus (ringing in the ears) are the most common side effects. Nausea, vomiting, abdominal pain, blurred vision, vertigo, and tremors may also occur. Serious, occasionally fatal side effects (hypotension, convulsions, heart block, ventricular fibrillation) can occur with too rapid intravenous injection of the drug. Slow intravenous administration, or oral administration, is usually safe but can cause minor ECG changes (prolongation of the QT interval and T-wave flattening). Quinine can also cause low blood sugar (hypoglycemia) from stimulation of the insulin producing cells of the pancreas; therefore, the intravenous preparation should be administered with glucose, and blood glucose levels must be measured frequently during therapy. Quinine can be used, if necessary, during pregnancy. On the third day of intravenous therapy (in the pregnant or nonpregnant patient), the dose should be reduced by one half to one third.

Quinidine

Quinidine gluconate (the d-isomer of quinine) is a commonly used cardiac drug that can also be used to treat drug-resistant falciparum malaria. In fact, quinidine has the special status of being the only intravenously administered antimalarial drug available in the United States indicated for use in the treatment of patients with complicated or life-threatening infections.

NOTE: Because newer antiarrhythmic cardiac drugs are replacing quinidine in some hospitals, physicians should check with their hospital pharmacies to ensure the availability

Table 7.2   Summary of Treatment of Malaria (by oral route)

Chloroquine–Sensitive Malaria (*Plasmodium vivax*, *Plasmodium malariae*, and Sensitive Strains of *Plasmodium falciparum*[1])		
	Adult Dose	**Pediatric Dose**
Chloroquine phosphate (Aralen) (250 mg salt = 150 mg base per tablet)	1 g of salt (4 tablets) immediately; then 500 mg (2 tablets) in 6 hr; then 500 mg (2 tablets) once a day for 2 days	10 mg base/kg (max. 600 mg) immediately; then 5 mg/kg in 6 hr; then 5 mg/kg/day for 2 days
P. vivax and *P. ovale* Malaria		
To prevent relapses after chloroquine therapy, add:		
Primaquine (26.5 mg salt = 15 mg base/tablet)	30 mg base/day for 14 days	0.6 mg/kg/day to max. 30 mg base/day for 14 days
Chloroquine-Resistant Malaria		
Atovaquone/Proguanil (Malarone)	4 tablets daily × 3 days	See text
Quinine sulfate 300 mg (salt) = 1 tablet	600 g salt (2 tablets) three times daily × 5-7 days (7 days in SE Asia)	10 mg salt/kg three times daily × 5-7 days (7 days in SE Asia)
Quinine should be taken with the following:		
Doxycycline	100 mg twice daily × 5-7 days	Doxycycline and tetracycline are contraindicated in children younger than 8 years of age, unless the seriousness of the infection warrants their use. The pediatric dose of clindamycin is 10 mg/kg three times daily × 5-7 days.
or		
Tetracycline	250 mg four times daily × 5-7 days	
or		
Clindamycin	900 mg three times daily for 5-7 days	

Alternative treatments

Mefloquine (Lariam)

1-1.5 g (15-25 mg/kg) in a divided dose over 12 hours

Artemether/lumafantrine
(Coartem, Riamet)

4 tablets twice daily × 3 days. The second 4-tablet dose on day 1 should be taken 8 hr, after the initial dose.

Total dose: 24 tablets over 3 days.

Artesunate[2]

100 mg (2 tablets) first dose, then 50 mg twice daily for 3-5 days, plus mefloquine 15 mg/kg once, or doxycycline 100 mg twice daily × 5-7 days

See text

[1]Chloroquine-resistant and primaquine-tolerant *P. vivax* have been described but the management of such cases requires advice of a specialist in travel or tropical medicine.
[2]Quinine-resistant malaria is rare, but it does occur along the border areas of Thailand. Quinine and artesunate should not be used as monotherapy.

of this important agent. If there is difficulty in obtaining the drug locally, physicians should contact the Eli Lilly Company (24 hours) at 800-821-0538, or the CDC's Malaria Branch hotline 770-488-7788; after hours, the on-call person for malaria can be paged.

Dosage   A loading dose of quinidine gluconate, 10 mg/kg (salt), in saline is given intravenously over 1 to 2 hours, followed by a constant infusion at 0.02 mg/kg/minute (1.0 to 1.5 mg/kg/hour). As soon as the parasite density drops below 1% of red cells infected and the patient is not vomiting, intravenous quinidine should be stopped and treatment continued with oral quinine sulfate (as discussed earlier).

Side Effects   Intravenous quinidine therapy should be administered in an intensive care unit. Cardiac effects are similar to those caused by intravenous quinine—dose-related QT interval prolongation and QRS widening.

Artemisinin (Qinghaosu) and Derivatives

Artemisinin and its two derivatives, artesunate and artemether, are the most rapidly acting antimalarial drugs, clearing parasites from the blood faster than quinine, and giving quicker relief of symptoms. Artemisinin is found in the medicinal herb *Artemisia annua* (sweet wormwood), a common plant that the Chinese call Qinghaosu, and used by traditional Chinese practitioners since AD 341 for the treatment of fever. Artemisinin was isolated in 1972 and is chemically unrelated to any other currently used antimalarial drug.

HOW ARTEMISININ WORKS

Artemisinin has a peroxide group in its structure. When it comes into contact with high iron concentrations, the molecule becomes unstable and "explodes" into free radicals. High concentrations of iron are found in red blood cells, which is also where the malaria parasites are found. When the drug enters the red blood cell, it releases the free radicals, which are highly destructive to the malaria parasites.

Artemisinin is effective against *P. vivax* as well as chloroquine-resistant strains of *P. falciparum*, but recrudescence of infection is common when the drug is used as sole therapy. To prevent recrudescent infections, as well as drug resistance, artemisinin and its derivatives should always be given in conjunction with another antimalarial drug, such as doxycycline or mefloquine.

Artemisinin is produced for clinical use in China and Vietnam and is presently available in some other countries in Asia. It is now being used in Africa, often as single-drug therapy, for the treatment of falciparum malaria.[*]

---

[*]When the first signs of drug-resistant malaria appeared in Asia during the Vietnam War, Chinese scientists developed a family of drugs from sweet wormwood, a common shrub that had been used for centuries in traditional medicine. These "artemisinin compounds" are now standard components of malaria treatment in Asia, where they have proved to be the best antimalarial drugs. To circumvent future drug resistance, malaria experts believe the time has come to partner artemisinin with other antimalarial drugs, creating artemisinin combination therapies (ACTs)—the same strategy that underlies the treatment of HIV and tuberculosis. In Africa, deaths from drug-resistant malaria are increasing daily, but the expense of ACT drugs has so far prevented their widespread use on that continent.

Oral Dosage   3 gm (or 50 mg/kg) given over 3 to 5 days. The first dose can be 20 mg/kg.

Intramuscular Dosage   1.0 to 1.2 gm (adult dose) over 3 to 5 days.

Suppositories   2,800 mg total dose given over 3 days.

Side Effects   Nausea, vomiting, rash, fever, transient first-degree heart block.

Use in Pregnancy   Artemisinin and its derivatives appear to be safe in the second and third trimesters; limited studies suggest that these drugs may be safe during the first trimester as well. There are several semi-synthetic derivatives of artemisinin.

- Artesunate is an oral, water-soluble derivative of artemisinin and has been effectively combined with single-dose mefloquine to treat drug-resistant *P. falciparum* in Southeast Asia. Oral dosage—100 mg (two tablets) first dose, then 50 mg every 12 hours for 3 to 6 days.
- Artemether is an oil-soluble compound that is also rapidly effective in severe malaria. Oral artemether, given over 5 days, was found to have a higher cure rate, with fewer side effects, than mefloquine against multidrug-resistant *P. falciparum* in Thailand. In studies done in Malawi, intramuscular artemether acted more rapidly than intravenous quinine in clearing coma and reducing parasite counts in children with cerebral malaria. In Vietnam, intramuscular artemether was as effective as intramuscular quinine in curing severe *falciparum* malaria.

Oral Dosage   700 mg, given over 5 days. (1st day—1.6mg/kg twice. On the 2nd, 3rd, 4th, and 5th days—1.6mg/kg, once daily)

Intramuscular Dosage   3.2 to 4 mg/kg initially, followed by 1.6 to 2 mg/kg once daily for 5 days. A single 300-mg dose of artemether, followed by mefloquine, 1,250 mg, in divided doses, has also been very effective. Artemether in oil is supplied in 1.0-mL ampoules containing 80 mg of the drug for intramuscular injection. The average treatment for adults is six ampoules.

Side Effects   Oral artesunate and artemether appear to be among the safest and best-tolerated antimalarial drugs, but their side-effect profile has not been fully delineated.

Artemether/lumafantrine (Co-artemether, Coartem, Riamet)   This drug combines the fast-acting artemether with the prolonged action of lumafantrine. The drug is currently available in Europe. Unlike halofantrine, lumafantrine is not associated with adverse cardiac effects. A 6-dose regimen over 3 days is reported to cure more than 95% of acute uncomplicated multidrug-resistant falciparum malaria. Because of its rapid onset of action, co-artemether may prevent progression to cerebral malaria. In countries where it is available, the drug is currently recommended as first-line treatment for acute *P. falciparum* malaria. Travelers from North America who are stopping over in Europe on their way to the tropics can obtain this drug for standby emergency treatment.

Oral Dosage   Four tablets, twice daily × 3 days. The second four-tablet dose on day 1 should be taken 8 hours after the initial dose. Total dose: 24 tablets over 3 days.

Table 7.3   Drugs for Self-Treatment in Adults[1]

Drug	Dose
Chloroquine[2] (Aralen)	1,000 mg salt (4 tablets) followed by 500 mg salt (2 tablets) at 6, 24, and 48 hours later. Total dose: 10 tablets of the 250 mg salt
Atovaquone/proguanil (Malarone)	4 tablets once daily for 3 days
Mefloquine (Lariam)	3-5 tablets (750 mg-1,250 mg) in divided doses over 12 hours
Artemether/lumafantrine[3] (Riamet, Co-Artem)	4 tablets twice daily for 3 days
Quinine plus	600 mg every 8 hours for 5-7 days
Doxycycline[4,5]	100 mg twice daily for 5-7 days

[1]The self-treatment drug should not be the same as the prophylactic medication if one is being taken. See text for pediatric dosages.
[2]For Central America, the Caribbean, and parts of the Middle East only.
[3]Artemether/lumafantrine. Not currently available in the United States or Canada.
[4]A second drug should always be added when quinine is used.
[5]Tetracycline, 250 mg, four times daily, or clindamycin, 900 mg three times daily, can be used in place of doxycycline.

Scientists now agree that the most effective treatment against malaria is a combination of drugs using artemisinin derivatives. Artemisinin-based combination therapy (ACT) is the quickest and most reliable way of clearing malaria infection, and it is very well tolerated. Using a combination of drugs shortens the treatment course, and has also been shown to protect each individual drug from resistance. These drugs, however, are not currently available in the United States or Canada. Co-artemether is available in Europe.

In Africa, single, stand-alone treatments for malaria, such as chloroquine, are rapidly losing their effectiveness. In some regions, malaria is resistant to all traditional first-line therapies. As a result, many countries* are moving toward the use of a combination of drugs that include an artemisinin derivative to treat malaria, which helps to slow the development of resistance. To date, no clinical resistance has been documented for ACT therapies, making these drugs the optimal first-line treatment where they are available.

*Twelve countries have already adopted artesunate plus amodiaquine as their national first-line treatment. These countries are (as of 2004) Indonesia, Burundi, Cameroon, Equatorial Guinea, Gabon, Ghana, Liberia, Mali, Sao Tome, Sierra Leone, South Sudan, and Zanzibar. Five countries have adopted first-line artesunate plus mefloquine. These countries are Cambodia, Myanmar, Thailand, Bolivia, and Peru.

SELF-TREATMENT

Standby emergency medication is a part of malaria protection for a very few, carefully selected, travelers and should be prescribed only by a well-trained travel medicine provider. The traveler must know that use of the standby drug must be followed by a medical consultation as quickly as possible to assess efficacy of treatment and to rule out other causes of fever.

The ideal standby drug should have few adverse effects; act rapidly against all species of malaria parasites, especially drug-resistant *P. falciparum*; be safe for children and pregnant women; and be simple and straightforward to use. Currently, no one drug satisfies all of these requirements. In the United States and Canada atovaquone/proguanil (Malarone) is emerging as the self-treatment drug of choice because of its effectiveness and relative lack of adverse side effects. In Europe artemether/lumafantrine (Riamet) is gaining favor. (See Table 7.3 for current self-treatment drug options.) Travelers who are potential candidates for self-treatment include the following:

- Travelers to moderate- and high-transmission endemic areas in countries where they will not have access to medical care within 24 to 48 hours.
- Travelers in chloroquine-resistant areas who are taking a less-than-optimal prophylactic drug such as chloroquine, chloroquine/proguanil, or azithromycin.
- Travelers whose exposure to malaria is likely to be so low or brief (especially if they are taking precautions to prevent insect bites) that chemoprophylaxis is not considered essential. This would include travelers to Central America and parts of Southeast Asia.
- Frequent short-term travelers to endemic countries (e.g., airline personnel).
- Expatriates or other long-term travelers whose compliance with regular intake of a prophylactic drug may be a problem. Some travelers are unable to tolerate, unwilling to take, or even unable to afford an optimal chemoprophylactic regimen for prolonged periods.

Fever, without clear evidence of other causes, after a stay of at least 7 days in a risk area is an indication for using the standby drug. Several studies, however, have shown that travelers who carry a self-treatment drug rarely use it appropriately and often do not seek medical attention as soon as possible as is recommended in all cases.

Advice for the Returning Traveler   Fever in the tropics, or in a traveler returning from the tropics, *is malaria until proved otherwise, and is a medical emergency.* Travelers who develop fever should seek medical attention urgently. If they are at home they should inform their health-care provider of their recent travels and request thick and thin blood films to confirm, or exclude, the diagnosis of malaria. If the first test is negative, examination of the blood should be repeated several more times over the next 12 to 24 hours. Treatment, however, should not be delayed while waiting for the test results if the diagnosis of malaria is strongly suspected.

CHAPTER 8

Insect Bite Prevention

KEY POINTS:

▶ A single bite from an infected insect can result in disease transmission; it is essential to know which repellent products can be relied on to provide predictable and prolonged protection.

▶ Botanical and other non-DEET repellents do not provide protection for durations similar to those of DEET-based repellents and should not be relied on to prevent insect-borne diseases, such as malaria.

▶ Low-concentration (5% to 15%) DEET repellents may be acceptable for preventing nuisance bites but may not provide enough protection in areas of the world where insect-borne diseases are a threat.

▶ The fear of "DEET toxicity" prevents many people from using repellents properly; this fear is unfounded.

▶ Permethrin is an insecticide that is chemically related to natural pyrethrum. It kills mosquitoes and ticks, but is nontoxic for human use.

▶ The combination of a properly applied DEET skin repellent and permethrin-treated clothing can give 99% to 100% protection against insect bites.

Mosquitoes

Mosquitoes are ubiquitous insects. They are found in every region of the world except Antarctica. Mosquitoes breed in standing water in diverse aquatic habitats, including fresh water (even if heavily polluted), saltwater marshes, brackish water, and even water found in discarded containers and old tires.

Both male and female mosquitoes feed on flower or fruit nectar, but only female mosquitoes bite; they require a blood meal every 3 to 4 days for the protein necessary to produce eggs. Mosquitoes can be divided generally into two types: daytime and nighttime biters. Those mosquitoes that transmit malaria and Japanese encephalitis (*Anopheles* and *Culex* mosquitoes) bite mostly at twilight or during the night, whereas Aedes mosquitoes, which transmit dengue and yellow fever, are daytime biters. Mosquitoes also bite indoors, so you need to prevent mosquitoes from gaining entry into living and sleeping quarters and to eliminate those that might already be there. The most common mosquito-transmitted diseases that you need to protect yourself from in tropical and subtropical climates are the following:

- Malaria
- Dengue fever
  Less common mosquito-transmitted diseases include the following:
- Yellow fever
- Filariasis
- Viral encephalitis (e.g., Japanese encephalitis, Venezuelan equine encephalitis)
- Miscellaneous viral illnesses. In addition to Rift Valley fever, West Nile fever, Chikungunya fever, and Sindbis fever, there are about 30 rarely diagnosed viral illnesses, such as epidemic polyarthritis, that are also mosquito transmitted.

NOTE: Mosquitoes cannot transmit HIV. The virus neither survives nor replicates in mosquitoes, and the blood from the last bitten person is not transmitted into the next bitten person.

Ticks and Biting Flies

The same personal protection measures that you use against mosquitoes will also protect you against ticks and biting flies—insects that transmit Lyme disease, tick-borne encephalitis, relapsing fever, typhus, leishmaniasis, onchocerciasis, trypanosomiasis, and several other tropical and infectious diseases. Of these diseases, leishmaniasis, transmitted by sand flies, is the most common.

You will want to avoid mosquitoes and biting flies for another reason—insect bites, even without the risk of disease, can make you miserable. Bites usually cause localized swelling and itching, and certain bites, such as from black flies, are very painful. Bites can also become infected, usually from excessive scratching (excoriation). Rarely, bites can cause systemic reactions, including anaphylaxis, from a person's sensitivity to the insect's salivary antigens. Protecting yourself from insect bites entails more than just applying an insect repellent to your skin. A multi-pronged approach is essential. The combined use of a skin repellent, permethrin-treated clothing, and/or shelters is the best way to avoid insect bites. By using the personal protection methods described in this chapter, you can achieve more than 90% protection against mosquitoes and other biting insects. Not every mosquito or insect carries disease, but just one bite from an infected mosquito or other insect can make you sick.

INSECT REPELLENTS

Insect repellents fall into two categories, (1) chemical and (2) botanical.

Chemical Repellents

Repellents containing DEET (acronym for the chemical diethyltoluamide) are the most effective and widely used. DEET was developed in the 1930s by the U.S. Department of Agriculture and registered for use by the general public in 1957. Over 200 million persons now use DEET-containing repellents annually worldwide. In the past 45 years, people have applied DEET more than 10 billion times. Features of DEET are:

- Repels insects for up to 12 hours
- Effective against more species of biting insects than any other repellent

- The best studied and analyzed of all repellents
- Remains the standard of chemical insect repellents
- Forty years of testing more than 20,000 compounds has not led to a better repellent being brought to market.

How DEET Works   The female mosquito in search of a blood meal is guided by several clues, the most important being heat, moisture, carbon dioxide, and odor. DEET works in part by masking the insect-attracting odor of carbon dioxide and lactic acid given off by the human body. At very close range DEET also appears to work by interfering with an electrophysiological homing mechanism in the mosquito's antennae.

DEET is effective in relatively small amounts provided it is spread evenly and completely over all exposed areas. DEET, however, has little "spatial activity," meaning that nearby, untreated skin is still likely to be bitten. Factors playing roles in any repellent's

Table 8.1   Comparative Protection Times of Insect Repellents

Product	Active Ingredient	Mean Protection Time (Minutes)
Ultrathon*	DEET, 33%	720
MaxiDEET	DEET, 100%	600
Ben's 30	DEET, 30%	480
Off! Deep Woods	DEET, 23.8%	301
Sawyer Controlled Release	DEET, 20%	234
Avon Skin-So-Soft Bug Guard Plus	IR3535	22.9
Repel Lemon Eucalyptus	Oil of Eucalyptus	120
Bite Blocker	Soybean oil	90
Natrapel	Citronella	20
Green Ban	Citronella, peppermint oil	14
Avon Skin-So-Soft Bug Guard	Citronella	10
Avon Skin-So-Soft Bath Oil	Uncertain	9.5
Repello Wristbands	DEET	9.5

*DEET-based repellents protect for the longest duration and this protection increases with higher concentrations of DEET. The exception is Ultrathon. This repellent contains a polymer that prolongs DEET effectiveness. Botanical repellents, with the exceptions of soybean oil and oil of eucalyptus, perform poorly. The IR3535-based Skin-So-Soft Bug Guard Plus (Avon) repellent, also sold in the United Kingdom and Europe as Autan, protects for an average of only 22.9 minutes. (IR3535 is ethyl butylacetylaminopropionate.) Repellent-impregnated wristbands provide minimal protection.

effectiveness include its concentration, the frequency and uniformity of application, and the number and species of insects attempting to bite. Evaporation and absorption from the skin surface, wash-off from rain or sweat, higher temperatures, or a windy environment all reduce effectiveness. Higher concentrations of DEET provide longer-lasting protection, but as the concentration of applied DEET climbs above 50%, each incremental increase provides relatively less additional protection. Extended-release formulations, however, have made it possible to reduce the concentration of DEET without sacrificing duration of action. DEET is most effective against mosquitoes and ticks, less so against gnats, black flies, biting flies, fleas, and mites. It has no effect against bees and wasps.

DEET Toxicity/Safety

It is not known exactly how many adverse reactions might be caused by DEET, but millions of people have used DEET over the last 40+ years without significant problems. The Environmental Protection Agency (EPA) completed a comprehensive re-evaluation of DEET in 1998 and concluded: "As long as consumers follow label directions and take proper precautions, insect repellents containing DEET do not present a health concern." Adverse side effects fall primarily into two categories:

Dermatologic Side Effects   Preparations containing less than 50% DEET are almost free of side effects when applied to the skin of adults. Skin reactions (contact dermatitis) may include itching, hives, blisters, or redness. Contact with the mouth can cause transient burning or stinging of the lips, tongue, and oral mucosa.

Neurologic Side Effects, Including Seizures   Concerns over the potential neurologic toxicity of DEET are based on a very small number of case reports in the medical literature. Between 1961 and 2000, there were only 23 reported cases of seizures and other neurologic symptoms associated with the use of DEET. Six of these cases were deliberate ingestions. Regarding the remaining cases:

- Details were often poorly documented and the symptoms could not be positively attributed to DEET.
- Most cases involved "heavy, frequent, or whole-body" application of DEET.
- There was no correlation seen between the severity of side effects and the concentration of DEET applied.

Given the small numbers of neurologic side effects reported since the 1960s and the 50 to 80 million people using DEET each year in the United States, the risk of serious side effects appears to be very low. If properly applied, DEET-containing repellents can be regarded as safe.

The potential of greater DEET toxicity in children has been a concern because their thinner skin and greater body surface area-to-weight ratio theoretically could enhance DEET absorption. This concern, however, has not been upheld by scientific study, and neurologic toxicity in children has not been substantiated by detailed surveillance. In a 1994 report reviewing 9,086 cases of DEET exposure from 71 poison control centers in the United States, the most severe reactions to DEET were caused by inhalation or eye contact, not skin application. The report also reached the following conclusion: There was no correlation between the severity of symptoms and age, gender, or concentration of applied DEET.

These reports, and others, indicate that side effects from proper DEET use are rare. Despite years of use and millions of applications, no clear pattern of DEET toxicity has emerged. It should be noted in this respect that the EPA does not require a cautionary statement on the label of repellents warning about the possibility of seizures or other neurologic side effects.

Although a direct link between DEET and significant health problems is extremely remote, the EPA recommends you follow these precautions to minimize any possible risks:

- Apply just enough repellent to lightly cover the areas of exposed skin. Do not saturate the skin. DEET may also be applied to clothing.
- Do not get DEET in eyes or mouth and avoid applying repellents to children's hands to prevent contact with these areas.
- Avoid inhaling DEET aerosol or spray.
- Wear long sleeves and long pants, when possible, to reduce the skin surface area that needs to be treated with DEET.
- Don't apply repellents on open cuts, or inflamed or irritated skin.
- Shower or wash repellent-treated skin after coming indoors.

Until recently, manufacturers of 5% to 10% DEET repellents have made label claims that their products are safer for use in children. However, because there is no evidence that DEET toxicity correlates with DEET concentration, the EPA has ruled that manufacturers can no longer place child safety claims on products. One other potential problem with the low-concentration "for children" formulas is that they usually last for shorter periods of time, requiring more frequent application of the repellent, with potentially greater risk of toxicity.

Figure 8.1   Repellents often used for foreign travel include Ultrathon, a controlled-release formula lasting up to 12 hours and Fite Bite 30, a 30% DEET repellent that lasts for 6 to 8 hours. Repellents with lower DEET concentrations may not be sufficiently protective where there is the risk of malaria or other insect-transmitted diseases. Oil of eucalyptus and soybean oil repellents are acceptable alternatives for travelers declining to use a DEET-containing repellent.

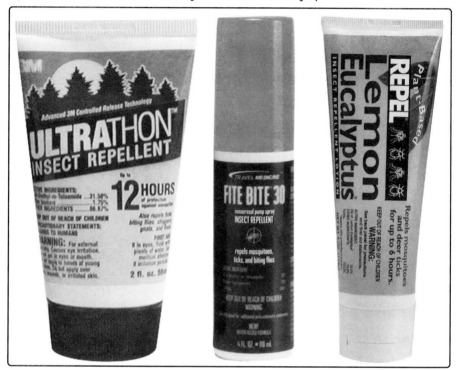

How Low Should You Go?

Despite the lack of scientific evidence showing that higher DEET concentrations are more toxic, manufacturers have responded to consumer fears of "DEET toxicity" by producing repellents with DEET concentrations in the 5% to 10% range. These low-concentration products may be perfectly acceptable for preventing nuisance bites, but may not provide enough protection in areas of the world where insect-borne diseases are a real threat.

What Should the Traveler Do?

The *Health Guide* believes that travelers (including children) who are visiting areas where insect-transmitted infectious and tropical diseases are found should use a repellent with a DEET concentration of 20% to 35%. Repellents in this range are effective for 6 to 8 hours. Under conditions of high temperatures or humidity, which increases loss of repellent from the skin surface, or when there is intense insect-biting activity, higher concentrations of DEET may be justified. Choosing a controlled-release formulation of DEET (e.g., Ultrathon) is another way to prolong the efficacy of a repellent (up to 12 hours) without requiring the use of DEET concentrations over 33%. There is no convincing evidence that infants and children are harmed by DEET if the repellent is used according to the label. If parents choose to use a low-concentration DEET repellent on their children, additional measures of protection, such as permethrin-treated clothing, mosquito nets, and elimination of indoor insects, should be used.

Botanical Repellents

Long before the advent of synthetic chemicals, people used plant-derived substances to repel mosquitoes. Most plant-based insect repellents currently on the market contain essential oils from one of the following plants: citronella, cedar, eucalyptus, peppermint, lemon grass, geranium, and soybeans. Citronella is the most common botanical oil found in natural repellents. When compared with DEET, however, citronella and most other essential oils give only short-lasting protection, lasting anywhere from minutes to less than 2 hours. Exceptions are the soybean oil-based and lemon eucalyptus repellents; they give 90 to 120 minutes of protection.

One reason natural repellents are popular is because some consumers are concerned about "DEET toxicity" and they prefer a "nonchemical" repellent, despite DEET's safety and effectiveness. Others reasons cited include a dislike of the odor and DEET'S adverse effects on synthetic fabrics and plastics. The true safety profile of natural repellents has yet to be determined. Plant-derived repellents are not inherently safe just because they are "natural." Citronella, for example, caused the death of a 21-month-old child after ingestion of only one ounce of the oil. Drinking eucalyptus oil has also caused poisonings and fatalities.

The Bottom Line

Using DEET is an essential step in preventing insect bites. If you are traveling in an area where insect-borne disease is a real threat, the most prudent repellent choice is one that contains DEET. These products are effective and necessary to safeguard your health. Because of their relatively poor efficacy, the *Health Guide* does not recommend that plant-derived repellents be used when either children or adults are traveling to areas where insect-borne diseases may be found.

PROTECTIVE CLOTHING

Clothing provides a physical barrier to biting insects, provided it is sufficiently thick or tightly woven. For increased protection, especially when there is more intense mosquito activity (e.g., in the evening), you should wear, weather permitting, long-sleeved shirts and trousers. Tucking your pant leg into your socks or boots can prevent both mosquito bites and tick attachment.

Chemically Treated Clothing

Clothing protection is dramatically increased when the fabric is sprayed or impregnated with a chemical that will either repel or directly kill any insect that alights on the fabric. Both DEET and permethrin are used as clothing treatments, but DEET has been largely replaced for this purpose by the more-effective permethrin.

PERMETHRIN

Unlike DEET, which is used primarily on the skin, permethrin is applied to fabric, such as clothing or bed nets. Permethrin, however, is not a repellent—it is a powerful, rapidly acting contact insecticide that knocks down, or kills, insects that come in contact with it. Features of permethrin:

- Permethrin kills or stuns insects touching treated fabric.
- Permethrin adheres tightly to fabric and will last through multiple washings. It will not harm or stain fabric, even silk.
- Unlike DEET, permethrin will not soften plastic or synthetic materials.
- It is effective against mosquitoes, ticks, flies, and chiggers. Permethrin is more effective against ticks than DEET.
- Permethrin is biodegradable and does not accumulate in the environment. However, it should not be disposed of in ways that will harm marine life.

Permethrin is a synthetic chemical analog of the naturally occurring insecticide pyrethrum that is found in chrysanthemums. It acts as a neurotoxin. The stunning and direct killing effects of permethrin are caused by its blockage of sodium transport in in-

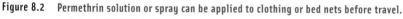

Figure 8.2 Permethrin solution or spray can be applied to clothing or bed nets before travel.

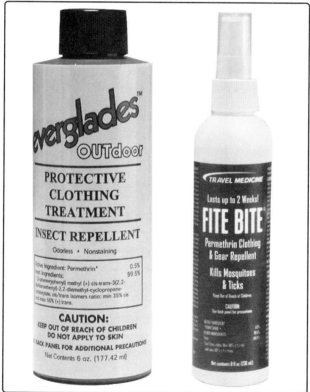

sect nerve fibers. Although highly toxic to insects, permethrin is not hazardous to mammals; skin absorption of the chemical is extremely low, and any absorbed permethrin is rapidly metabolized. To date, no cases of human toxicity, carcinogenicity, or mutagenicity have been reported. In fact, products such as 5% ELIMITE anti-scabies cream contain permethrin, and are safe enough to be applied overnight directly to the scalp and skin for medical purposes.

DEET and Permethrin—The Ideal Combination?

The best way to avoid insect bites—and the diseases that insects transmit—is to apply a DEET repellent to your exposed skin and treat your clothing with permethrin. The effectiveness of this combination is confirmed by many studies. In one study, conducted in Alaska, the use of permethrin-treated clothing and 33% DEET afforded 99.9% protection. In comparison, untreated control subjects sustained more than 1,000 bites per hour!

Preventing Tick Bites

The measures described are also dramatically effective against ticks. Protection against tick attachment is 100% possible when using the combination of DEET and permethrin. **Tip:** also wear a permethrin-treated bandana and treat your socks. This deters ticks from attaching about the head and neck and crawling up your legs from your ankles. If you are not wearing long sleeves and long pants, you need to rely more on a DEET skin repellent and vigilant self-inspection for ticks attached to your skin, especially about the legs, thighs, neck, and waist—the regions where ticks tend to migrate.

Treating Mosquito Bites

Topical corticosteroid creams and ointments can reduce redness, itching, and swelling. Avoid any topical skin preparation containing an anesthetic. Both lidocaine and benzocaine can cause localized and generalized allergic reactions. Oral antihistamines, however, can be effective in reducing the symptoms of mosquito bites. An ammonium solution (AfterBite) applied to the bite can help relieve itching.

BED NETS

Herodotus mentioned bed nets in the 5th century B.C. when he described how fishermen were protected by nets that were naturally impregnated with fish oil. Mosquito nets now play an important role in preventing malaria and other insect-borne illnesses such as leishmaniasis, filariasis, and encephalitis. Nets are less important in preventing dengue because the *Aedes* mosquitoes that transmit it are daytime biters.

Treatment of nets with insecticidal or repellent compounds started in the 1930s in the USSR, using lysol, and in the American and German armies during World War II, using DDT. In 1973, photostable insecticidal pyrethroids, developed as molecular analogs of the natural plant insecticide pyrethrum, were synthesized and found to be highly effective against mosquitoes when applied to fabric. In 1984, field trials of permethrin-impregnated nets were first carried out. These and subsequent trials demonstrated that

Figure 8.3 Technique for Impregnating Clothing or Mosquito Netting with Permethrin Solution.

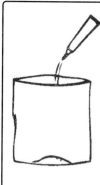

1. Pour contents of one bottle of 0.5% permethrin solution into treatment bag.*

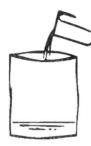

2. Fill bottle with tap water and pour it into the treatment bag.

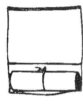

3. Place bed net or rolled-up garments in bag. Close bag tightly.

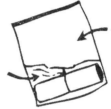

4. Shake bag to get uniform coverage. Let stand for 2-3 hours.

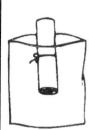

5. Remove items from solution. Wring out excess solution.

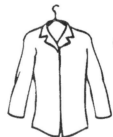

6. Hang up clothing or netting for 2-3 hours to dry. Treatment lasts 4-6 weeks.

*Everglades or Fite Bite permethrin. If more solution is needed to cover garments or net, double or triple the amounts of permethrin and water you mix together.

Directions for Spraying

One pump spray or aerosol will treat 2 sets of clothing (shirt & trousers = 1 set) or 1 net.

1. Place the clothing or mosquito net on a plastic sheet outside.
2. Spray, using a slow, circular motion, holding the can 8"-12" above the fabric. Moisten all areas. Fabric will temporarily darken when moistened.
3. Shirts: Spray each side 30-45 seconds. Trousers: Spray each side 30-45 seconds. Jackets: Spray each side 30-45 seconds.
4. Mosquito nets: Partially unroll the net onto the plastic sheet. Spray 30-45 seconds. Turn net and spray another 30-45 seconds. Keep turning and spraying the net until you've moistened all areas.
5. Hang up, or lay out, clothing or net to dry. Allow 2-3 hours for complete drying. Effective for 2-6 weeks. Fabric, when dry, is odorless. Permethrin is nonstaining.

(1) permethrin binds tightly to nylon, polyester, and cotton; (2) insecticidal fabric levels can be maintained for 6 to 12 months; (3) permethrin-treated nets kill insects that land on it; and (4) treated nets reduce mosquito counts in dwellings. Studies from many countries show that malaria rates are reduced in communities where permethrin-treated nets are used. Many tropical countries now have public health programs that supply permethrin-impregnated nets to villages in malaria-endemic areas.

The use of bed nets and other personal protection measures against bites is increasing among travelers as more are being exposed to multidrug-resistant malaria, for which no prophylactic drug regimen is 100% effective. The prevention of mosquito bites, in fact, is the best defense against malaria and other insect-transmitted illnesses. Bed nets, however, have certain problems. They may not be well fitted and can be torn, allowing insects to enter. This problem can be overcome by using a permethrin-treated net. Insects always stop first on the net before going through an opening. Permethrin kills or knocks down these insects before they have a chance to enter through a hole or feed through the net on a body part touching it. Lack of adequate ventilation in a hot climate can also be a problem, more so with tightly-woven nets. A tightly woven net might have 300 holes per square inch versus a bed net with a mesh size of with 156 holes per square inch. A tighter mesh bed net, however, will keep out tiny sand flies.

Types of Nets

Bed nets come in various shapes and sizes. Conical nets hang from a single attachment point in the ceiling; rectangular nets are slightly more spacious, but require an attachment at each corner. The type of mosquito net you use depends on several factors. If you are traveling solo from location to location, the net should be compact, light, and easy to set up. If there are two of you in a fixed location for an extended period of time, then a larger model is preferable, even though it may be heavier and take more time to install. Some types of bed net used by travelers are

- The Spider—This popular conical net (Fig. 8.4) has a large mesh (156 holes per square inch) for better ventilation, can cover a king-sized bed, but is compact and lightweight (17 oz.).

  Products shown in this chapter are available through Travel Medicine, Inc., 800-TRAVMED.

- SleepScreen—This free-standing net sets up with easy-to-assemble fiberglass poles and is carried in a small stuff sack that fits easily into a pack or carry-on luggage. The small mesh size also keeps out sand flies and no-see-ums. Larger models have nylon floors. This type of net can be set up indoors over a bed or used outdoors.

Insect Proofing Your Sleeping Quarters

According to a large European survey of tourists who have visited east Africa, sleeping in air-conditioned rooms significantly reduces the incidence of malaria. Those travelers not staying in well-screened or air-conditioned rooms should spray living and sleeping quarters in the evening with a pyrethroid-containing insecticide. Brands such as RAID Flying Insect Spray and Green Thumb Flying Insect Killer are commonly available in the United States and Canada but aerosols such as these can't be transported by air so

Figure 8.4 When bed nets are treated with permethrin, malaria rates decrease.

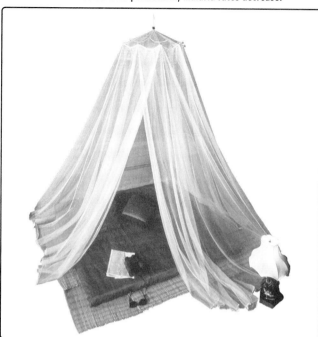

Figure 8.5 Free-standing nets are tightly woven; they also protect against sand flies, gnats, and no-see-ums.

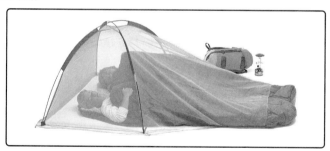

you will have to find their local equivalent. In East Africa, Doom Insect Spray, containing permethrin and pyrethrum, is widely used; similar preparations are available in many other countries. One spraying should last several days because of the residual effect of the insecticide. NOTE: When spraying indoors, vacate the sprayed areas until the product "settles." Don't spray on food or eating surfaces.

CHAPTER 9

Insect-Borne Diseases

KEY POINTS:

▶ Travelers must be aware of how to protect themselves against insect-borne diseases, particularly malaria, yellow fever, dengue fever, Japanese encephalitis, and leishmaniasis.

▶ Yellow fever, found only in Africa and South America and transmitted by a day-biting mosquito, is preventable by immunization. The yellow fever vaccine, however, can cause severe side effects in older individuals and should be administered in this age group only when there is the real risk of exposure.

▶ Dengue is the most common arthropod-borne virus infection globally, a viral infection transmitted by day-biting mosquitoes in the Caribbean, Latin America, and Southeast Asia. There is no vaccine; mosquito-bite prevention measures will significantly reduce the risk of infection.

▶ A night-biting mosquito transmits Japanese encephalitis, a very serious vaccine-preventable viral infection of the brain that is found only in rural South and East Asia. However, because the risk to travelers is low, only those traveling in rural areas for prolonged periods should consider being vaccinated.

▶ Leishmaniasis, found in Mediterranean countries and Latin America eastward to the Middle East and South Asia, is a parasitic infection that causes skin ulcers as well as a severe generalized illness. It is transmitted by a rural, night-biting sandfly.

Overview of Insect-Borne Diseases

This chapter describes a number of important but rather uncommon (at least for the traveler) diseases caused by viruses, parasites, and bacteria. Unlike a common disease such as hepatitis A, these insect-borne diseases often require the diagnostic and treatment expertise of a travel/tropical medicine or infectious disease specialist. This chapter also underscores the importance of insect-bite protection measures because there are no vaccines available for most of these diseases.

YELLOW FEVER

In 1900, Dr. Walter Reed demonstrated that yellow fever is a viral illness transmitted by mosquitoes. The disease is so named because jaundice, the result of liver damage, is a common sign of this illness.

There are two distinct cycles of transmission, but the resulting disease is the same. Urban yellow fever is transmitted by an *Aedes aegypti* mosquito from an infected person to another person. In jungle yellow fever, mosquitoes transmit the infection between nonhuman primates (e.g., monkeys) and humans or vice versa.

Yellow fever occurs in tropical areas of certain countries in Africa and South America. These countries comprise the yellow fever endemic zones. Interestingly, there is no yellow fever in other regions with warm climates and *Aedes* mosquitoes, such as the Middle East, Southeast Asia, and the Pacific. The reason for this has never been clearly understood.

Since the 1980s, yellow fever has re-emerged across Africa and South America. In Africa, both jungle and urban transmission cycles occur. The largest number of cases in Africa has been reported from Nigeria. In 1992, yellow fever reappeared in Kenya after an absence of 50 years, and in 1994 and 1995, Gabon reported its first outbreak ever. Outbreaks have also been reported from Cameroon, Ghana, Liberia, Senegal, and Sierra Leone.

In South America in 1995, Peru experienced the largest yellow fever outbreak from any country in South America since 1950, and in 1998, 45% of the world's cases were documented there. Between 1985 and 1998, yellow fever cases have been reported from Bolivia, Brazil, Colombia, Ecuador, and Peru. In South America, the jungle transmission cycle predominates, and about 80% of yellow fever cases are reported in adult male forest workers. Urban yellow fever has not been reported from South America since 1954, but the *Aedes aegypti* mosquitoes have reinfested many tropical cities and some suburban areas of South America, setting the stage for potential urban outbreaks of this disease.

Yellow fever is underreported; epidemiological investigations have found the true number of cases to be 10 to 500 times higher than the number reported. Among unvaccinated individuals, it is estimated that the risk of yellow fever in endemic areas in South America is approximately 1:25,000 per 2-week stay. However, in Africa, during epidemics, the risk is estimated to be 1:250; between epidemics 1:2,500 per 2-week stay.

Symptoms

Most yellow fever infections are mild and go unrecognized, but severe, life-threatening illness occurs in about 15% of people exposed to the disease. Symptoms of severe illness start with fever, headache, muscle aches, nausea, abdominal pain, and vomiting. These acute symptoms last for 3 to 4 days and are followed by a toxic phase characterized by jaundice, vomiting of blood, bloody stools, coma, and, in 50% of severe cases, death.

The differential diagnosis includes malaria, leptospirosis, viral hepatitis, typhus, dengue fever, and other viral hemorrhagic fevers. The laboratory diagnosis of yellow fever can be made by measuring IgM antibody response.

Treatment

Specific drug treatment is not available. Supportive care is indicated.

Prevention

Vaccination—The best way to prevent yellow fever is by immunization and the current vaccine is highly effective. Most travelers to rural areas of endemic-zone countries should be immunized. To meet international requirements, the vaccine must be administered at least 10 days before arrival when administered for the first time. However, booster doses are effective immediately.

Mosquito Protection Measures   All travelers should take measures to prevent mosquito bites at dawn and dusk when *Aedes* mosquitoes are most likely to bite. These measures include applying a DEET-containing insect repellent, wearing permethrin-treated clothing, eliminating indoor mosquitoes through screening and spraying, and sleeping under a permethrin-treated bed net.

DENGUE FEVER

This viral illness occurs in more than 60 tropical and subtropical countries, with more than one half the population of the globe at risk for infection. The incidence and geographic distribution of the disease have greatly increased in recent years. Dengue (pronounced DENG-ee) is now prevalent in the Caribbean, Central and South America, Mexico, the Pacific Islands, and South Asia and Southeast Asia. In the United States, the majority of dengue fever cases occur in tourists who have returned from Puerto Rico, the Virgin Islands, Mexico, and Thailand. Unless there is an epidemic in progress, the risk of acquiring dengue by the average tourist is low, perhaps 1:15,000 to 30,000 travelers.

Dengue is spread by *Aedes* mosquitoes. These mosquitoes feed during the day, with most biting activity in the morning for several hours after daybreak and in the late afternoon for several hours before dark, but the mosquito may feed at any time during the day, especially indoors, in shady areas, or when it is overcast. Dengue is primarily an urban disease because *Aedes* mosquitoes usually breed in small pools of stagnant water that collect in discarded tires, buckets, bottles, flower vases, barrels, etc. There are four (serotypes) dengue viruses. If you are infected with one type of virus, you will gain life-long immunity against that particular serotype, but not against the other serotypes. In fact, subsequent infection with a different serotype may result in more severe disease including dengue hemorrhagic fever or dengue shock syndrome. Severe infections, however, are very rare among travelers.

Symptoms

Dengue virus infections may be asymptomatic or may lead to a range of symptoms, including death. The vast majority of infections, especially in children younger than 15 years of age, are asymptomatic or minimally symptomatic. More severe illness is seen with increasing age, or with repeat infections with a different serotype, especially in children living in endemic areas.

Dengue Fever (DF)   Typical symptoms include chills and fever ("breakbone fever"); severe headache, especially behind the eyes; muscle and joint pain; nausea and vomiting; flushing of the face, neck, and chest; and a rash. The rash appears in 3 to 4 days and may be confused with measles. Low white blood cell count and low platelet count occur frequently. In uncomplicated cases, acute symptoms resolve in 5 to 7 days, but fatigue may linger for many weeks.

NOTE: Other illnesses that can mimic dengue include malaria, leptospirosis, typhoid, measles, and chikungunya fever. You should be checked immediately for malaria if you develop fever while in or after visiting a malaria-endemic area.

Dengue Hemorrhagic Fever (DHF)   This is a severe, sometimes fatal form of dengue fever that rarely strikes Western tourists. Dengue hemorrhagic fever is diagnosed when there is minor or major bleeding, low platelets, and evidence of plasma leakage from capillaries into the tissues or body cavities. A progressively decreasing platelet count and a rising hematocrit from ongoing plasma loss herald the impending onset of dengue shock syndrome (DSS).

Treatment

Treatment consists of bed rest, fluid replacement, and analgesics. Aspirin and other non-steroidal anti-inflammatory drugs should be avoided because they interfere with platelet function and may promote further bleeding. Antibiotics and steroids are not beneficial. The prognosis in DHF and DSS depends on the prevention or early recognition and

Figure 9.1   World Distribution of Dengue
Source: Division of Vector-Bourne Infectious Diseases, National Center for Infectious Diseases, Centers for Disease Control and Prevention.

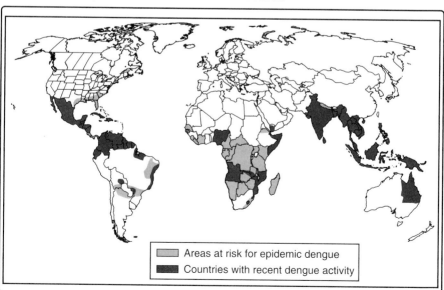

Areas at risk for epidemic dengue
Countries with recent dengue activity

treatment of shock. Early, judicious treatment with intravenous fluids and plasma ex-panders can keep mortality below 1%. Once DSS is established, mortality can exceed 40%.

Prevention

No vaccine is available. Reduce your risk by preventing mosquito bites. Remember, the *Aedes* mosquito is a day biter and found mostly in urban centers. Follow the guidelines in Chapter 7.

JAPANESE ENCEPHALITIS

Japanese encephalitis (JE) is a mosquito-transmitted viral illness and the number one cause of brain infection (encephalitis) in Asia and the Western Pacific. More than 50,000 of cases of JE are reported annually from Southeast Asia, India, China, Japan, and Korea.

Japanese encephalitis (encephalitis = inflammation of the brain) occurs in rural-agricultural areas throughout Asia. In temperate regions such as the People's Republic of China, Japan, and Korea, JE transmission is highest from April to September. In northern India and Nepal, peak transmission is from June to November. In the tropical regions of Asia and Oceania, JE occurs year round.

The virus of Japanese encephalitis is transmitted by *Culex* mosquitoes. These mos-quitoes breed where there is abundant water, such as in rice paddies, and feed primarily on birds and local domestic animals, usually pigs. Visiting a rural-agricultural rice-growing, pig-farming region, therefore, can put you at risk. About 1% to 3% of the *Culex* mosquitoes in endemic areas are infective. Because these mosquitoes are night feeders, there is less risk of JE transmission during the day.

The average tourist is not at risk. If you are a short-term traveler, and if you are visiting only urban areas, your risk of getting JE is very low—approximately one in one million. You will be at greater risk if living in rural agricultural (rice-growing, pig-farming) areas during the season of peak transmission. Your risk then rises to approxi-mately 1 in 5,000 per month of exposure. Of the small number of Americans who have developed this illness in the last 2 decades, most were military personnel or their dependents.

Symptoms

Nausea, vomiting, headache, and fever are the most frequent symptoms. A severe attack may cause seizures, paralysis, confusion, coma, and death. Fortunately, most JE infections are asymptomatic—only 1 in 250 individuals who are infected becomes sick. Unfortunately, if one does develop symptoms, the resulting illness can be severe, with death occurring in up to 25% of patients, and permanent neurologic damage in about 30%.

Treatment

There is no drug treatment for JE. Good nursing care is essential in severe cases.

Figure 9.2   Distribution of Japanese Encephalitis

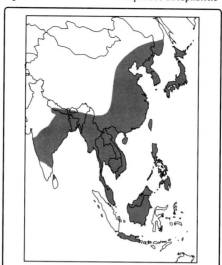

Prevention

Mosquito Protection Measures   All travelers should take measures to prevent mosquito bites, particularly during the evening and nighttime when staying in rural areas.

Vaccination   See Table 3.2, Chapter 3, for JE vaccine schedule, indications, precautions, and contraindications.

AFRICAN TRYPANOSOMIASIS (SLEEPING SICKNESS)

African trypanosomiasis, or sleeping sickness, is transmitted by the bite of a tsetse fly. This disease is endemic in sub-Saharan Africa, and major outbreaks are now occurring in Sudan, Uganda, Congo, and Angola. The number of cases is estimated at 300,000, with about 60 million people at risk. Sleeping sickness, however, almost never occurs in tourists, although occasional cases are reported in travelers, usually those visiting game parks. Long-term travelers or expatriates living in rural endemic areas may be at slightly increased risk.

There are two forms of this disease. Gambian, or West African, trypanosomiasis (caused by *Trypanosoma brucei gambiense*) is a chronic disease that takes several years to reach the advanced stage. It occurs primarily in the forested areas of western and central Africa. Rhodesian, or East African, trypanosomiasis (caused by *Trypanosoma brucei rhodesiense*) manifests more acutely and progresses more rapidly. It occurs primarily in the savannah and woodlands of eastern and southern Africa and is the form seen (rarely) in travelers.

Symptoms

Symptoms start 5 to 15 days after the bite of an infected fly. (NOTE: Tsetse fly bites may be quite common on safari but only a very small percentage of tsetse flies are infected. Tsetse flies are not affected by insect repellents and the bites are not particularly painful). An inflamed nodule (inoculation chancre) develops at the site of the bite and may measure one half inch or more in diameter. Chancres are typically seen only in *T. rhodesiense* infections. Other symptoms include fever, headache, rash, lymph node swelling, enlarged spleen, swelling of the face and joints, and, occasionally, inflammation of the heart. In East African disease, the brain is invaded early, and, unless treated, progresses to lethargy, coma, and, ultimately, death within 6 weeks to 9 months. The onset of West African trypanosomiasis is more insidious. A localized skin lesion is the first symptom. Fever, rash, and lymph node swelling take weeks to months to appear. Brain damage symptoms occur later. The diagnosis of East African sleeping sickness is made by demonstrating trypanosomes in blood, chancre, or spinal fluid.

Treatment

Management of this disease requires the expertise of a specialist. Suramin is the treatment of choice for early-phase East African (Rhodesian) trypanosomiasis. Melarsoprol, an arsenic compound, is indicated for the treatment of second-stage disease, when there is central nervous system involvement. Treatment of the second stage, however, is long and complicated, and can be hampered by severe side effects. In the early stage, Gambian sleeping sickness may be treated with pentamidine and the 2nd stage with eflornithine.

Prevention

The only prevention is to avoid the day-biting tsetse fly.

CHAGAS DISEASE

This is a potentially fatal disease, but one that rarely affects travelers. Chagas disease* is caused by a parasite that is most often transmitted by the reduviid (triatomine) bug, known colloquially as the kissing bug. The insect lives in cracks and holes in poor housing, where it bites people, often on the face, while they sleep. Parasites in bug feces deposited on the skin enter the body through the bite or when the bite is scratched. The disease can also be transmitted through blood

---

*This disease, American trypanosomiasis, is named after Carlos Chagas, a Brazilian physician, who first described it in 1909. The causative organism is *Trypanosoma cruzi*, a single-cell parasite.

transfusions, organ transplants, and from mother to child at birth. Oral transmission may occur with the ingestion of food contaminated by feces of infected Triatominae. In 2005, Brazilian health officials reported a widespread outbreak in which Chagas disease was transmitted through the consumption of contaminated sugar cane juice. This mode of transmission may be particularly frequent among the settlers of Amazonian areas.

Chagas disease occurs in Latin America in rural areas extending north from Chile and Argentina to Mexico. The highest incidence occurs in Bolivia, where 20% of the population is infected; Brazil, with a 1.3% global prevalence rate, has 5 million persons with Chagas disease. Prevalence is estimated to be 5% to 10% in Argentina, Honduras, Paraguay, and El Salvador; 1% to 5% in Chile, Columbia, Ecuador, Uruguay, and Venezuela; and less than 1% in Mexico and Nicaragua.

Symptoms

The parasites may cause an acute illness, but more frequently the symptoms are mild or overlooked. Decades later, in about 30% of infected individuals, damage to the heart and/or the gastrointestinal tract becomes evident.

The initial symptoms of Chagas disease are usually mild or nonexistent; less than one-third of persons develop an acute illness and most of these are children and young adults. One to three weeks after insect-bite exposure there may be a swollen nodule or pimple (chagoma) at the inoculation site, accompanied by fever and localized lymph node swelling. A facial bite (which is common) with entry of parasites through the conjunctiva causes painless swelling of the eyelids and conjunctivitis (Romaña's sign) is considered a reliable diagnostic indicator in suspected cases. Localized symptoms may be accompanied by a flu-like illness with fever, headache, muscle aches, vomiting, and a rash. Some degree of heart muscle inflammation (myocarditis) occurs in 30% of infected people but severe disease, requiring hospitalization, is uncommon.

The chronic phase—After 30-60 days all initial symptoms will have resolved, but the parasites remain active in the body, causing a chronic, but largely silent, infection. By the fourth decade of life, about one-third of chronically infected people will develop symptoms of heart and/or gastrointestinal disease. Cardiac problems include cardiomyopathy, heart block, and heart failure. Chronic enlargement of the esophagus and colon may cause difficulty swallowing, abdominal pain, bloating, and constipation.

Acute Chagas disease may be confused with malaria, mumps, eye infections, sinusitis, and cellulitis of the skin. The diagnosis can be made by identifying T. cruzi parasites under the microscope. Serological testing is useful during the long asymptomatic period or when late-stage disease of the heart or intestine occurs.

Treatment

The acute illness may be treated with either benznidazole (Ragonil®, Roche) or nifurtimox (Lampit®, Bayer). Neither drug is commercially available in the United States or Canada. Although there is no drug that currently provides satisfactory treatment for chronic Chagas disease, there is an increasing trend to treat silent chronic infections before late-stage illness begins.

Prevention

Transmission by insect vector occurs primarly in areas where there is poorly constructed adobe-style mud and thatched roof huts. People staying in tourist accomodations are not at risk. If you are sleeping in a structure that is possibly infested, take the following precautions:

- Spray your living and sleeping quarters with an insecticide. (e.g., RAID Formula II Crack and Crevice Spray).
- Use a residual insecticide on the walls and roofs of houses.
- Sleep under a permethrin-impregnated bed net that is tucked under the mattress.
  Remember that Chagas disease can also be spread by unscreened blood transfusions, so these should be avoided.

FILARIASIS

Filariasis is prevalent throughout the tropics and is a group of diseases caused by thread-like roundworms, called filaria, which are transmitted by various mosquitoes, flies, and biting midges. Varieties of filariasis include (1) lymphatic filariasis—bancroftian and Malayan filariasis (elephantiasis); (2) subcutaneous filariasis-onchocerciasis ("river blindness"); and (3) loiasis.

BANCROFTIAN AND MALAYAN FILARIASIS

These illnesses are transmitted by several different species of mosquitoes found in tropical regions of Central and South America, the Caribbean, Africa, China, India, Southeast Asia, and Oceania. Infective larvae (microfilariae) are injected into the skin by the bite of the mosquito. The larvae migrate through the lymphatic channels of the skin and become trapped in lymph nodes, where the adult worms develop. For the most part, disease results from damage to lymphatic channels caused by the host's immune response to adult worms.

Symptoms

Light infections rarely lead to symptoms. Heavier exposure (many bites over many months) is generally necessary to cause symptomatic disease. Initial symptoms consist of redness of the skin and swelling of lymph nodes of the arms and legs, headache, weakness; in some cases muscle pain, coughing, wheezing, and fever occur. Thousands of mosquito bites are often required before symptoms develop. Continued exposure may result in permanent lymphatic obstruction. Progression of the disease, usually observed only in the indigenous population of the endemic area, can lead to the grotesque swelling of the legs (and scrotum in males) known as elephantiasis.

To check for exposure to filariasis, your doctor may wish to examine your white blood cells for eosinophilia, and your blood at midnight for microfilaria because these larvae enter the blood stream mostly between 10 P.M. and 2 A.M. Antibody tests are more than 95% sensitive but are nonspecific. A negative antibody test virtually rules out an active infection.

Treatment

Treatment of filariasis with diethylcarbamazine (DEC) is effective. The dosage is 6 mg/kg/day for 12 days. Repeated single doses of DEC at monthly intervals for 6 to 12 months appear to increase effectiveness. An effective alternative is albendazole.

Prevention

See measures described subsequently.

ONCHOCERCIASIS

One type of filariasis that is particularly devastating is onchocerciasis, or river blindness, common in equatorial Africa, the Sahara, Yemen, and parts of Latin America (Mexico, Guatemala, Venezuela, Ecuador, Colombia, and Brazil). The disease is transmitted by black flies that breed in vegetation along fast-flowing rivers in these regions. Onchocerciasis is occasionally acquired by long-term travelers such as expatriates and Peace Corps volunteers. In this infection, adult worms are found in nodules under the skin, and microfilaria released from the worms are located in the skin.

Symptoms

Symptoms include a skin rash with intense itching (the most common symptom in infected travelers), skin nodules, swollen lymph glands, inflammation of the eyes, and, in heavy, prolonged infections, blindness.

Symptoms don't occur for several months or more after exposure. By this time, the blood eosinophil count will usually be elevated; therefore, a complete blood count is often a good screening test. Blood tests (antifilarial antibody and antigen assays) can help establish the diagnosis. (The Clinical and Parasitology section of the National Institutes of Health [NIH] can do the serology testing; call 301-496-5398.) To make a definitive diagnosis, skin snips are obtained to identify filarial larvae.

Treatment

Treatment is with ivermectin (Stromectol, Merck), 150 to 220 μg/kg in a single dose every 6 months until symptoms do not recur. (Two 6-mg tablets is the usual adult dose.) Ivermectin does not kill the adult worm, but only suppresses symptoms by temporarily reducing the number of larvae in the skin. The CDC's Parasitology Hot Line (301-496-5398) can answer further questions.

Prevention

There is no prophylactic drug. Take precautions to prevent bites from day-biting black flies.

LOIASIS

This form of subcutaneous (below the skin surface) filariasis is common to the rain forests of West and Central Africa. Loiasis is also the most frequently diagnosed blood filarial infection in travelers returning to North America and the United Kingdom from

Africa, though it is still rare. *Loa loa* larvae (microfilariae) are transmitted by the bite of an infective *Chrysops* fly, also known in Africa as the deer fly. This is a day-biting fly that breeds in rain forests. After the microfilariae enter the body they develop into adult worms in the subcutaneous tissues (under the skin) and larvae are released into the blood stream.

Symptoms

Symptoms of loiasis are caused by migration of the adult *Loa loa* worms just beneath the skin. Symptoms—which take 12 months or more to develop—include fever, itching, and skin swellings (Calabar swelling), usually involving the hands, wrists, forearms, or face. Adult worms can also be observed migrating on the surface of the eye, beneath the conjunctiva.

Diagnosis

A blood test for eosinophilia and microfilariae (which peak in the blood during the day), and an ELISA screening test, can be done to check for exposure.

Treatment

Diethylcarbamazine (DEC) is the treatment of choice for *Loa loa* and consists of a total dose of 75 mg/kg. Although DEC is usually innocuous to humans, serious allergic reactions induced from the destruction of filarial worms may occur. In heavy infections, the full dose of medication should be administered over 2 to 3 weeks. Refractory cases of loiasis have responded to albendazole, 200 mg orally, twice a day, for 21 days.

Prevention of Filariasis and Loiasis

No vaccines are available. You should take measures to prevent insect bites during the day for loiasis and at night for bancroftian filariasis. These measures include applying a Deet-containing skin repellent, wearing permethrin-treated clothing, and sleeping under a mosquito net or in an insect-free room.

Prophylaxis   You can take DEC either weekly or monthly to prevent loiasis or lymphatic (bancroftian or Malayan) filariasis. These regimens are recommended rarely to expatriates living in highly endemic areas. Dosage—300 mg DEC weekly to prevent loiasis and 500 mg DEC 2 days each month to prevent lymphatic filariasis.

NOTE: DEC is available in the U.S. and Canada from the CDC, USA, and Health Protection Branch, Canada, respectively, as an investigational drug for the treatment of filariasis. It is available in many developing countries.

Leishmaniasis

Leishmaniasis is one of the most common parasitic infections in the world, occurring in various forms in 80 countries. The disease is found on all continents except Australia and Antarctica. It is an important public health problem in Mexico, Central and South

America, North Africa, sub-Saharan Africa, the Middle East, central Asia, southern Russia, northern China, and India. Scattered areas of disease activity occur in southern Europe, mainly Portugal, southern France, Italy, the Greek isles, the Costa del Sol, and Majorca. In the United States, cases of the disease have been reported in Texas and Oklahoma.

Leishmania are single-cell organisms (protozoa) smaller than a red blood cell. Infection occurs when these tiny parasites are injected into the body by the bite of an infective sand fly. Which form of leishmaniasis (visceral, cutaneous, mucocutaneous) that develop depends on (1) which species of Leishmania (there are about 20) causes the disease; (2) which organs and cells are predominantly infected; and (3) the host's state of immunity (many cases of leishmaniasis are self-healing). Sand flies are usually found in focal areas on the edge of forested areas or in rodent burrows. They feed from dusk to dawn and have a very limited flight range.

VISCERAL LEISHMANIASIS (KALA-AZAR)

This disease affects primarily the internal organs and bone marrow. About one half a million people are infected annually, with about one half of the cases in northeast India. Visceral leishmaniasis is also found in and around the Mediterranean Basin, southern Russia, China, East Africa (Kenya, Sudan, Uganda), Central America, Brazil, Venezuela, and Paraguay. In India and China it is widespread throughout rural areas.

Symptoms
Hallmarks of the disease are marked enlargements of the liver and spleen, chills and fever, and anemia. Symptoms include fatigue, weight loss, cough, and diarrhea. Many infections are asymptomatic; however, the parasites may remain dormant and cause severe disease at a later date if the immune system is weakened as in patients with AIDS.

Diagnosis
To diagnose visceral leishmaniasis, blood tests and a bone marrow examination and culture may be necessary. An antibody test may be helpful. Diseases that can be confused with visceral leishmaniasis include malaria, typhoid fever, brucellosis, Chagas disease, schistosomiasis, tuberculosis, and amoebic liver abscess. Because massive enlargement of the spleen sometimes occurs, kala-azar can also mimic leukemia or lymphoma.

Treatment
Symptomatic visceral leishmaniasis is usually fatal unless treated. Pentostam, the drug of choice, is given in an intravenous dose of 20 mg/kg daily for 30 to 40 days. Pentostam is available from the Parasitic Disease Drug Service Branch of the Centers for Disease Control in Atlanta, Georgia, and the Special Access Program, Health Protection Branch, Health Canada. Amphotericin B is an alternative where there is Pentostam-resistant dis-

ease. A new oral drug, miltefosine, also appears to be very effective when administered for 28 days.

For further information about drug treatment and the serologic diagnosis of leishmaniasis, physicians should contact the Parasitic Disease Drug Service of the CDC at 770-488-7760 or 770-488-7775.

CUTANEOUS LEISHMANIASIS (OLD WORLD VARIETY)

This infection is characterized by ulcerative skin lesions, and occasionally nodules, caused by one of several species of *Leishmania*. Local names for this disease include *Oriental sore* and *Baghdad boil*. Risk areas include the Mediterranean Basin, the Middle East, Africa (stretching from Senegal to Sudan, Ethiopia, and Kenya), southern Russia, central Asia, and northwestern India.

Symptoms

As the name implies, cutaneous leishmaniasis affects the skin. A variety of lesions can occur: self-healing ulcers, chronic nonhealing sores or ulcers, or nonulcerating and warty skin nodules. Chronic skin ulcers are the most common form of the infection. The skin sites involved are those areas usually not covered by protective clothing, that is, the face, forearms, back of hands, and legs. Symptoms usually occur 2 to 8 weeks after a bite. The lesions may ulcerate and discharge fluid, or they may remain dry. Spontaneous healing tends to occur over a period of several months to 2 years.

CUTANEOUS LEISHMANIASIS (NEW WORLD VARIETY)

Two species complexes of leishmania (*Leishmania mexicana* and *Leishmania braziliensis*) are responsible for most of the cutaneous leishmaniasis occurring in Mexico and in Central and South America.

Symptoms

Skin nodules and/or ulcers are found on exposed skin areas, usually the face and ear. These lesions appear 2 to 8 weeks after exposure. Spontaneous healing may take 6 to 18 months, or longer.

MUCOCUTANEOUS LEISHMANIASIS (ESPUNDIA)

This disease is almost exclusively confined to the Western Hemisphere, occurring mostly in the northern half of South America.

Symptoms

This illness occurs when parasites spread from the skin to the mucous membranes of the mouth, nose, and throat. Espundia is usually preceded by a simple skin ulcer, which may heal. Then 1 month to many years after the initial exposure, destructive ulcerations of the nose and mouth occur. Severe disease with disfigurement (espundia) results if treatment is delayed.

Diagnosis

To diagnose cutaneous leishmaniasis, tissue samples are obtained from the skin for microscopic examination and/or for culture. Antibody tests are of limited use except in espundia and the nodular form of the disease. The Parasitic Disease Branch of the Centers for Disease Control can identify parasites from tissue, carry out appropriate antibody tests, and offer advice on treatment.

Treatment

The treatment of choice for large cutaneous lesions is intravenous sodium stibogluconate (Pentostam) in a dose of 20 mg/kg daily for 30 days. Other drugs are available (dapsone, ketoconazole, pentamidine), but their effectiveness depends on the species of infecting parasite, the geographic location where the infection was acquired, and the form of the disease.

Prevention

This illness in its various forms is transmitted by sand flies. To protect yourself, you must use a DEET-containing insect repellent, treat your clothing with permethrin, and, if necessary, sleep under a mosquito net. There is no vaccine.

RELAPSING FEVER

This is an acute bacterial infection that can be transmitted to humans by ticks or lice. The cause is a spirochete (*Borrelia recurrentis*). Tick-borne relapsing fever is found in Asia, Africa, Europe, and the Americas, including mountainous areas of the western United States. Louse-borne relapsing fever, seen almost exclusively among the poor or those in refugee camps, is found in Asia, Africa, and Europe.

Symptoms include chills, fever, nausea, vomiting, severe headache, and a variety of rashes. The most effective treatment is tetracycline, erythromycin, or penicillin. Without treatment, the attack terminates in 3 to 10 days but may recur in a milder form 1 to 2 weeks later. Prevention consists of tick- or louse-bite prevention.

RIFT VALLEY FEVER

This is a viral disease of animals, but it can be transmitted to humans by mosquitoes. Rift Valley fever occurs primarily in sub-Saharan Africa. The initial symptoms (chills, fever, headache, backache, weakness, and vomiting) are similar to malaria and dengue, but reddening of the eyes helps distinguish Rift Valley fever from malaria. The illness lasts 4 to 7 days and complete recovery is the rule, but 2% of infected people develop hemorrhagic complications, jaundice, or inflammation of the brain and/or the membranes covering the spinal cord. No specific treatment is available, but ribavirin and interferon may offer some benefit. Prevention entails avoiding mosquito bites.

WEST NILE VIRUS

This mosquito-transmitted virus was first isolated from a patient in Uganda in 1937, spread from Africa to parts of Europe and Asia, suddenly appearing in New York City in 1999. The disease was most likely imported to the United States by air travelers from Europe. In 2002, almost 3,000 cases of neuroinvasive disease (encephalitis) were reported in the United States, but in 2004 the total number of cases declined to 741. The disease is now moving from the East Coast across the country to the west. Almost one-third of the cases of neuroinvasive disease in 2004 occurred in Arizona and California; the other cases occurred throughout the rest of the country. About 20% of persons infected with the West Nile virus develop symptoms and of these only 1 in 140 will develop serious neurologic disease or die. No vaccine is currently available.

SAND FLY FEVER

Sand fly fever is a viral disease transmitted by the bite of an infective sand fly and occurs in parts of Europe, Asia, Africa, and Latin America. It occurs primarily in tropical and subtropical areas with hot, dry weather. The vector of the causative virus is the common sand fly, which bites at night.

Symptoms appear 3 to 6 days after the sand fly bite and consist of fever, headache, nausea, weakness, and myalgia. These symptoms may be severe but are rarely, if ever, fatal, and treatment with fluids and analgesics is usually sufficient. Prevention of sand fly fever consists of nighttime protection against insect bites.

SCRUB TYPHUS

This is a mite-transmitted disease found in Asia, the western Pacific, and Australia. Scrub typhus is endemic in a triangular area between northern Japan and southeast Siberia to the north; Queensland, Australia, to the south; and Pakistan to the west. The cause is a rickettsial organism, *Rickettsia tsutsugamushi*. The disease is transmitted in scrub lands and forest clearings where mites abound on the vegetation.

Symptoms
The larval form, called chiggers, can bite humans who come in contact with vegetation infested with mites. One to three weeks after the mite bite, symptoms occur and consist of chills, fever, rash, lymph node swelling adjacent to the bite, and prostration. A blister,

followed by a black scab, or eschar, may occur at the site of the bite. This infection may cause serious illness.

Treatment

Tetracycline or doxycycline is the treatment of choice.

Prevention

Prevention consists of using personal protection measures against mite bites. In particular, permethrin-impregnated clothing should be worn (long-sleeved shirts are suggested) with trousers tucked into boots when walking through grasslands and forests in endemic areas. Prophylaxis with 200 mg of doxycycline weekly is effective.

PLAGUE

Plague is a disease of extreme poverty. The risk of tourists contracting plague is extremely low. Plague is caused by infection with the bacterium *Yersinia pestis*, which is carried by rats, other rodents, and their fleas. Most cases result from the bites of infected fleas, but can also result from handling infected animals or inhaling infectious airborne droplets from persons with plague pneumonia (pneumonic plague), who may spread the disease by coughing. The disease occurs rarely and sporadically in the southwest United States, and in Africa, Asia, Asia Minor, Europe, and South America. Vietnam and Bolivia report the largest number of cases annually.

Symptoms of plague start 2 to 7 days after exposure with rapid onset of fever, chills, headache, generalized aches and pain, and exhaustion. Patients with the bubonic form develop painful swelling of the lymph glands (buboes) in the groin, armpit, or neck; those with the pneumonic form develop a cough and difficulty breathing.

Treatment

Plague is fatal in 50% to 60% of untreated cases. Early treatment with antibiotics is effective, especially if started within a few hours of the onset of symptoms. The preferred drugs are streptomycin, chloramphenicol, and tetracycline.

Prevention

The plague vaccine is of unproved effectiveness; the vaccine is no longer available in the United States. Prophylactic antibiotics can prevent plague; they should be taken by certain individuals (medical personnel, relief workers, etc.) when face-to-face transmission of bacteria has potentially occurred or is anticipated. Adults should take doxycycline, 100 mg daily, or tetracycline, 500 mg twice daily; children 9 years of age, or younger, sulfonamides. The most important measure to prevent bubonic plague is to avoid fleas and rodents such as rats, rabbits, squirrels, and chipmunks in endemic areas. Sick or dead animals should also not be handled. Regular use of flea powders on domestic pets having access to both human and rodent habitats is strongly advised in plague-active areas. The application of DEET-containing repellents on exposed skin and permethrin on clothing will reduce the chance of flea bites. People at high risk of exposure to infected fleas should also consider prophylactic antibiotics.

MEDITERRANEAN SPOTTED FEVER

This tick-borne rickettsial disease is also known as Boutonneuse fever in North Africa, African or Kenyan tick typhus in sub-Saharan Africa, and Indian tick typhus in southern Asia. The disease is caused by *Rickettsia conorii* in the Mediterranean and *Rickettsia africae* in southern Africa and is transmitted by ixodid ticks. Exposure to the ticks usually results from close contact with tick-carrying dogs, rodents, or cattle. Tick typhus is one of the more frequent causes of fever in returned travelers. Symptoms include chills, fever, headache, and a rash. An ulcer with a black crust (eschar) may be noted at the site of the tick bite.

Treatment
Tetracycline and doxycycline are both effective.

Prevention
Take the standard measures (DEET and permethrin) to prevent insect bites, including trousers tucked into your socks, and a skin check for ticks after exposure.

TICK-BORNE ENCEPHALITIS

Tick-borne encephalitis (TBE) viral disease occurs in forested areas of the former Soviet Union, eastern and central Europe, and Scandinavia.* TBE is transmitted by ixodid ticks (the same ticks that transmit Lyme disease) and presents a small risk, primarily campers and hikers engaging in prolonged outdoor activities in endemic areas. The disease can also be spread by the consumption of unpasteurized dairy products from infected cows, goats, or sheep.

The greatest risk of disease occurs during periods of high tick activity, usually March through September. Infective ticks are found in mixed coniferous-deciduous forests, extending into the shrubby forest edge and meadows, as well as along river and stream valleys (including forests bordering large cities).

Symptoms
After an incubation period of 8 days (4 to 28 days) affected individuals develop fever and headache which in about one third of patients may progress to confusion, imbalance, memory changes, decreasing level of consciousness, and limb paralysis. Almost 45% of patients are left with permanent neurologic sequelae. Death occurs in less than 2% of individuals.

*There are two subtypes of TBE: (1) Western subtype (or Central European encephalitis) transmitted by *Ixodes ricinus* ticks. This subtype occurs in the forested areas of Central, Eastern, and Northern Europe, and (2) Eastern subtype (or Russian spring/summer encephalitis) transmitted by *Ixodes persulcatus* ticks. This subtype occurs in the former USSR, east of the Ural Mountains, and also in areas of China, Japan, and Korea.

Treatment

Treatment consists of supportive care only.

Prevention

TBE vaccine is available in Canada and Europe (and also Russia) and is administered in three doses over 12 months. Immunization is recommended only for people who anticipate intense, long-term exposure in endemic areas. It is not recommended for the average tourist. Travelers who expect to have significant exposure should take precautions against tick bites while in endemic areas.

EHRLICHIOSIS

This disease is caused by bacteria (ehrlichia) transmitted by ticks. Five species infect humans. Two types of human ehrlichial infections are recognized in the United States. The infections have the same symptoms and the same treatment but differ in their geographic distribution because of the fact they are transmitted by different species of ticks.

- Human monocytic ehrlichiosis (HME), caused by *Ehrlichia chaffeensis*, is transmitted by Lone Star ticks (*Amblyomma americanum*). These ticks are found predominantly in the Southeast and Mid-Atlantic states.
- Human granulocytic ehrlichiosis (HGE) was first recognized in Minnesota and Wisconsin. HEG is transmitted primarily by deer ticks (*Ixodes scapularis*) and thus, the disease occurs predominantly in the Northeast, upper Midwest, and other areas where deer ticks make their habitat. Overseas, cases of HGE have been documented in many countries in Europe, as well as Argentina, Japan, Malaysia, and Venezuela.

Symptoms

Symptoms of the two infections are practically identical. Most patients have a nonspecific flulike illness with chills, fever, headache, muscle aches, and malaise. In 15% of the cases, however, the disease is more severe and patients can develop kidney failure, pneumonia, and neurologic changes such as seizures and coma. The fatality rate is 2% to 5%.

Diagnosis

Typical laboratory findings include a low white blood cell count (leukopenia), a low platelet count (thrombocytopenia), and abnormal liver function tests. The white blood cells of some patients with HME and HE will have characteristic inclusion bodies in their white blood cells. Antibody tests may be used to establish a diagnosis.

Treatment

When a case of ehrlichiosis is suspected, treatment should be started immediately. A typical candidate for treatment is somebody with a flulike illness who has a low white blood cell count and low platelets, as well as potential exposure to ticks in an endemic area, especially between April and September. The drug of choice is doxycycline, 100 mg twice daily for 10 to 14 days.

Prevention

This is a tick-borne illness that can be prevented by insect bite prevention measures, as outlined in Chapter 8.

OTHER TICK-BORNE DISEASES IN THE UNITED STATES

Lyme disease (Chapter 11) and ehrlichiosis are not the only illnesses transmitted by ticks in the United States. Rocky Mountain spotted fever, Colorado tick fever, tick paralysis, tularemia, babesiosis, and relapsing fever are some of the other diseases of importance. A summary of the tick vectors that spread these diseases and their geographic distribution follows subsequently.

IMPORTANT TICKS AND TICK-BORNE DISEASES IN THE UNITED STATES

The deer tick (*Ixodes scapularis*) is found in great abundance from Virginia to Maine, as well as in Wisconsin and Minnesota, whereas its first cousin, the western deer tick (*Ixodes pacificus*, the black-legged tick) is active along the West Coast. The deer tick is a very small tick, much smaller than the dog tick or wood tick. Deer ticks, both adults and nymphs, are dark reddish brown and have black legs and a pear-shaped body. All stages, especially nymphs and adults, feed on people. The deer tick is the most important carrier of Lyme disease and is the only known carrier of babesiosis. It is also the primary transmitter of human granulocytic ehrlichiosis.

The Lone Star tick (*Amblyomma americanum*) is found throughout the south and southeastern United States, with a high density in the Ozarks. Adults are about one-quarter inch long; nymphs, which are the most aggressive biters, are pinhead sized. The ticks are reddish brown, and the female has a white mark on the middle of her back. The smaller male has lacy white markings on the rear edge of his back. Lone Star ticks transmit monocytic ehrlichiosis, tularemia, and a variant form of Lyme disease, Southern tick-associated rash illness (STARI).

The American dog tick (*Dermacentor variabilis*) is widely distributed in the eastern half of the United States and is also found on the West Coast. It resembles the wood tick in appearance. The unfed female has silvery-gray markings on the shield on her back; the rest of the body is reddish brown. It is bigger than other ticks—approximately one-eighth inch to one-quarter inch long—and although it prefers dogs, it does bite people. The dog tick is the most important transmitter of Rocky Mountain spotted fever. It also transmits tularemia and probably transmits human granulocytic ehrlichiosis. The dog tick can cause tick paralysis.

The Rocky Mountain wood tick (*Dermacentor andersoni*) is a hard tick that resembles the American dog tick and the Pacific coast tick. The female has silvery-gray markings on the shield on her back; the rest is reddish brown. This tick is the prime carrier of Rocky Mountain spotted fever in the West, and it also transmits tularemia and Colorado tick fever (mountain fever). It is the most important cause of tick paralysis in the United States.

Relapsing fever ticks (*Ornithodoros hermsi, O. parkeri, O. talaje, O. turicata*) are soft ticks that transmit relapsing fever, a spirochetal disease. Their bites can be painful. Relapsing fever ticks are widely scattered west of the Mississippi River. Adults are oval-shaped and colored gray to pale blue. Larvae and nymphs are gray.

The brown dog tick (*Rhipicephalus sanguineus*) is found throughout the United States wherever you find dogs. Although suspected of carrying ehrlichiosis, these ticks are probably not disease transmitters. The male is uniformly dark brown. The female is brown but the shield on her back is darker than the rest of her body.

GIARDIASIS

The parasite that causes giardiasis (*Giardia lamblia*) is found in contaminated water (and less frequently in food) and water as a result of fecal contamination from humans or animals (mostly dogs, beaver, and cattle). Giardiasis occurs worldwide, but a higher incidence has been reported in travelers returning from the Indian sub-Continent, Southeast Asia, and Indonesia. Although travelers to Mexico and Latin America and the countries in Asia and Africa may also acquire infection, fewer than 3% of travelers returning from these areas have been found to harbor *Giardia* parasites. *Giardia* cysts can be spread easily from person-to-person in households and in day care centers. Poor personal hygiene, lack of hand-washing, and close physical contact, especially oral-anal sexual contact, promotes transmission.

Giardiasis is also known as backpacker's diarrhea because the parasites may be found in ponds, lakes, and streams in rural or mountainous areas, even in the U.S. and Canada, and pose a potential risk to campers and hikers drinking from these sources. NOTE: Published reports of confirmed giardiasis among outdoor recreationists in North America clearly demonstrate a high incidence among this population. However, the evidence for an association between drinking backcountry water and acquiring giardiasis is minimal. Person-to-person spread appears to be a more significant factor in acquiring backpacker's diarrhea, and perhaps more emphasis should be placed on hand washing, personal hygiene, and other behavior modifications during backcountry travel, rather than simply on water purification.

Symptoms can be sudden and severe or occur gradually. Some travelers may have no complaints except one large, loose bowel movement daily. Nausea, fatigue, weight loss, abdominal cramps, non-bloody diarrhea, excessive gas, abdominal rumblings (borborygmi) and bloating can also occur to varying degrees. A taste of "rotten eggs" is common. Fever is very rare in giardiasis. When the illness is persistent, symptoms may last for weeks or months and be passed off as indigestion, or irritable bowel syndrome. Some cases of chronic fatigue syndrome may be caused by giardiasis. Fatigue, out of proportion to the degree of diarrhea is frequent. In severe cases, malabsorption of food may lead to severe weight loss and malnutrition.

If you have diarrhea lasting more than 2 to 3 weeks, you should be tested for intestinal parasites. Most likely, your doctor will ask you to submit several stool samples for microscopic examination. Detecting *Giardia* parasites can be difficult because organisms are not constantly present in stool; therefore, if the microscopic examination is negative, a more invasive method, such as a small bowel biopsy, may be required. A very sensitive and specific noninvasive screening test of stool, the enzyme immunoassay, is also available. (GiardEIA *Giardia lamblia* Testing Kit; Antibodies Incorporated, Davis, California; 800-824-8540 or 530-758-4400; http://www.antibodiesinc.com). If the immunoassay test is negative, then giardiasis is unlikely. Less common intestinal parasites that can also cause chronic diarrhea include *Dientamoeba fragilis, Isospora belli, Cryptosporidium, Cyclospora cayetanensis,* and *Entamoeba histolytica* (the cause of amebiasis).

Treatment

The drug of choice, tinidazole (Tindamax), has recently been released in the United States for the treatment of giardiasis. The dose in adults is 2 grams once daily. For children older than 3 years up to 40 kg in weight, the dose is 50mg/kg once daily. Another new product, Nitazoxanide (Alinia), is now available as a liquid preparation for children 1 to 11 years of age. Under 4 years of age the dose is 1 teaspoon twice daily for 3 days and 2 teaspoons twice daily in those older than 4 years. Single-dose metronidazole (2 gm in adults) administered with food at bedtime once daily for 3 days is as effective as the standard 5-day course of 250 mg three times daily. The single dose regimen for children less than 25 kg is 35 mg/kg (in a single dose daily for 3 days). For children who weigh 25 kg to 40 kg, the daily dose is 50 mg/kg for 3 days. Alternative treatments include tinidazole (2 gm once), furazolidone, albendazole, and bacitracin zinc. Furazolidone (Furoxone), 100 mg four times daily for 7 to 10 days, is a good, but very expensive, alternative for several reasons: (1) it is available in a liquid preparation (useful for children), and (2) the drug is also effective against most bacterial causes of travelers' diarrhea, making furazolidone useful as broad-spectrum treatment when the cause of the diarrhea is not known. Albendazole, 400 mg twice daily for 7 days (3 days is usually insufficient), is a safe alternative drug with a varying cure rate.

If you are in a remote area with symptoms compatible with giardiasis, and testing is not available, start treatment with one of the drugs above on the assumption that giardiasis is the probable cause of your diarrhea. If no improvement occurs, seek medical consultation as soon as possible. NOTE: Lactose intolerance frequently accompanies giardiasis and may persist for weeks or months following parasite eradication.

Prevention

There is no prophylactic drug or vaccine to prevent giardiasis. Follow the food, drink, and water disinfection guidelines as outlined in Chapter 5, but note that chlorine and iodine may not be effective against parasites. Hand washing and good personal hygiene are important measures.

AMEBIASIS

This potentially serious illness is caused by *Entamoeba histolytica* parasites, a single-celled parasite that invades the wall of the large intestine, causing either acute dysentery or chronic diarrhea of varying severity. These parasites can also infect the liver, causing inflammation and liver abscess. In the carrier state, which is common, parasites live in the intestine without causing symptoms. Recent studies show that 90% of those with *E. histolytica* are actually infected with a microscopically identical but harmless nonpathogenic protozoan parasite now called *Entamoeba dispar*, for which no treatment is necessary.

Transmission occurs through the ingestion of fecally contaminated food or water. Flies can serve as carriers of the amebic cysts. Infected food handlers and houseflies can also spread the disease. Person-to-person contact is important in transmission; household members and sexual partners, especially men who have sex with men, can easily become infected. High-risk areas (where up to one half of the population carries the parasite) are Mexico, South America, India, and West and southern Africa.

Amebiasis is distinctly rare in travelers and is frequently over-diagnosed in developing countries. Most cases of gastrointestinal infection are not caused by *E. histolytica*, but the presence of the harmless *E. dispar* can confuse the diagnosis. An amebic antibody test can differentiate these two identically appearing parasites. If the serology (blood) antibody test for amebiasis is negative, you can presume that you may be infected with *E. dispar*, or that some other organism is causing the illness. *E. histolytica* antigen or DNA can be also be detected by a stool test (TechLab *E. histolytica* II test kit. TECHLABS Inc., Blacksburg, VA; 540-953-1664; www.techlabinc.com).

The symptoms of amebiasis are variable. Most infected persons carry the parasite and have no symptoms whatsoever. Mild illness causes abdominal cramps, little or no fever, and semi-formed stools. Mucus may be present but usually without blood. Soft stools or diarrhea may alternate with constipation. You may experience fatigue, loss of appetite, and some weight loss. The symptoms at this stage are similar to those of giardiasis, except that the abdominal discomfort is in the lower abdomen and the diarrhea is of smaller volume. More severe illness (amebic dysentery) causes high fever, bloody diarrhea, generalized abdominal tenderness, vomiting, and much greater toxicity. Illness at this stage requires urgent care.

Travelers who develop an amebic liver abscess usually don't have diarrhea or other intestinal symptoms. Instead, they may note fever, right upper abdominal pain, and have an enlarged, tender liver. Sweating, chills, weight loss, and fatigue are usually present. NOTE: Amebic abscess is rare, even in long-term travelers.

A microscopic stool examination to identify trophozoites or amebic cysts will point toward the diagnosis, especially if red cells are detected in the parasites. Antibody tests are usually diagnostic, especially if an amebic liver abscess or colitis is suspected. Amebic dysentery must be distinguished from other infections causing bloody diarrhea (e.g., enterocolitis caused by shigella, campylobacter, salmonella, yersinia, or *Clostridium difficile*). Crohn disease and ulcerative colitis can mimic amebiasis and must be considered in the younger patient. In older persons, diverticulitis or malignancy should be suspected.

Treatment

The ideal treatment of invasive amebiasis (colitis or abscess) in the United States is now tinidazole (Tindamax), 2 grams once daily for 3 days. Metronidazole, 750 mg, three times daily for 5 days or 2.5 grams once daily for 3 days, is equally effective. Both regimens must be followed by a drug that acts in the lumen of the bowel such as iodoquinol, 650 mg, three times daily for 20 days. This regimen cures 100% of those with amebic liver abscess and 93% of those with amebic colitis. Even a single dose of metronidazole (2.5 grams) is usually effective in curing an uncomplicated liver abscess. Asymptomatic cyst passers and those without documented invasive disease require iodoquinol alone.

CHOLERA

This disease is caused by *Vibrio cholerae* bacteria, that are commonly transmitted by contaminated food and water or by person-to-person contact. Cholera is often asymptomatic, but in heavy infections it sometimes causes life-threatening diarrhea, particularly among the indigenous people in developing countries. Severe diarrhea from cholera requires the ingestion of large numbers of bacteria, hence the severe form of the disease is rarely seen in healthy tourists who follow prudent dietary habits.

Cholera occurs both sporadically and in worldwide epidemics. Sub-Saharan Africa has the highest reported cholera incidence and mortality rates in the world. By the end of 1999, 61 countries reported cases, but the disease is much more widespread than officially recognized.

Cholera is basically a disease of poverty, and most illness occurs among those people in lesser-developed countries who are exposed to heavily contaminated water or food. Therefore, most travelers on a tourist itinerary need not worry about this disease. In fact, cholera is officially reported in only 1 in 500,000 returning travelers. The healthy people at risk of acquiring cholera disease usually work in high-risk environments, such as refugee camps or relief centers.

Unlike some microbes, cholera bacteria are readily killed by stomach acid. However, if you do ingest a large dose of bacteria from heavily contaminated water—or if you are taking antacids or antiulcer drugs—bacteria can get past the stomach and enter your small intestine. Cholera enterotoxin then acts on the intestinal wall to cause outpourings of water and salt into the gut.

The clinical picture of cholera varies widely. Seventy-five percent of infections are mild or without any symptoms. Only 2% to 5% of infections cause severe symptoms. Cholera in its most severe form is characterized by massive watery diarrhea, vomiting, and muscle cramps. Vomiting is common and may be severe. The frequent, watery stools soon lose all fecal appearance ("rice water stools") and practically all odor. Loss of fluids and electrolytes can cause shock and death in hours if fluids are not replaced.

Milder cases of cholera can mimic travelers' diarrhea caused by toxigenic *Escherichia coli*, salmonella, intestinal viruses, and parasites. The absence of blood or pus in the stools, and the lack of fever, are distinguishing features of cholera.

Treatment

Cholera kills solely by dehydration. If you develop severe watery diarrhea, you should immediately start rehydration treatment.

Fluids Drinking an oral rehydration solution (ORS) is essential and its prompt use has saved many lives. ORS can be prepared from water, sugar, and salt or more conveniently, using packets of ready-mixed salts, e.g., CeraLyte (Chapter 6). After rehydration, you should drink 8 to 12 ounces, or more, of full-strength rehydration solution after every loose stool. If your diarrhea is very profuse and exceeds the amount of fluids you can drink, or if you are vomiting and can't retain enough fluids, you may need to be hospitalized and treated with intravenous fluids. NOTE: Don't underestimate fluid requirements—some patients with severe watery diarrhea may require as much as 10 to 12 liters of fluid replacement daily.

Antibiotics Antibiotics will shorten the duration of illness and are an important adjunct to fluid therapy. The best antibiotics for treating cholera are the quinolones, such as ciprofloxacin (Cipro), ofloxacin (Floxin), or levofloxacin (Levaquin). These antibiotics are effective even when given as single-dose therapy (ciprofloxacin, 1 gm; ofloxacin, 800 mg; or levofloxacin, 500 mg). The greater effectiveness of the quinolones versus other antibiotics is because of their higher concentration in the stool. Alternative antibiotics are doxycycline, tetracycline, trimethoprim/sulfamethoxazole (Bactrim), furazolidone (Furoxone), and azithromycin (Zithromax). NOTE: Globally, resistance of cholera to tetracyclines and trimethoprim/sulfamethoxazole is increasingly common.

Treatment of children: Although the quinolones are generally contraindicated in children, single-dose therapy with these drugs is not harmful. Furazolidone and azithromycin are safe for children of all ages.

Prevention

Food and Drink Precautions The best prevention against cholera is to pay careful attention to what you eat and drink (Chapter 5). It is particularly important (1) to avoid raw or undercooked food and seafood (e.g., ceviche), and (2) to drink only commercially bottled, boiled, filtered, or chemically disinfected water without ice.

Vaccination The manufacture and availability of the injectable cholera vaccine in the United States ceased in June 2000. Newer vaccines are now available: a live attenuated oral vaccine (Mutachol and Orachol) and a killed whole-cell bacterial oral vaccine (Dukoral). Because the risk of cholera is extremely low for the average traveler, vaccination is recommended only for those going to high-risk endemic or epidemic areas where they will be living under unsanitary conditions. The oral vaccines are yet not available in the United States.

TYPHOID FEVER

Typhoid fever (sometimes called enteric fever) is a serious, sometimes life-threatening disease caused by one particular species of *Salmonella* bacteria (*Salmonella typhi*) and is contracted by the consumption of contaminated food or water, or by contact with an infected person. Untreated, typhoid lasts 2 to 6 weeks with a mortality rate of up to 30%. However, with treatment mortality is less than 1%.

Although typhoid fever is found in all countries in the developing world, the highest disease rates are reported from Peru, Chile, Haiti, Nigeria, India, Pakistan, Southeast Asia, and Indonesia. Most cases of typhoid reported in American travelers originate in the Indian subcontinent or South America.

The early symptoms of typhoid fever usually consist of chills and fever, headache, weakness, loss of appetite, abdominal pain, body aches (myalgia), cough, and constipation. A rash, with pink spots measuring 2 to 4 mm, may appear on the chest and abdomen. There is a 50% occurrence of diarrhea, which is sometimes bloody in the second to third week of illness. Diarrhea occurs most often in children and in the second to third week of illness. In fact, if your doctor considers diarrhea a prerequisite for the diagnosis of this disease, the diagnosis may be missed. The usual method for diagnosing typhoid fever is a blood culture combined with a stool culture (40% to 80% positive). Although a bone marrow aspirate is more sensitive (80% to 95% positive), it is a more painful and invasive procedure.

Treatment

Strains of *Salmonella typhi*—resistant to ampicillin, trimethoprim/sulfamethoxazole, and chloramphenicol—have become increasingly prevalent, especially outside Latin America (where these drugs may still be effective). The fluoroquinolones (ciprofloxacin, ofloxacin, levofloxacin) are currently the drugs of choice, although there are reports from India, Nepal, and Vietnam of quinolone resistance. Oral administration of a quinolone results in (1) very high fecal drug concentrations; (2) rapid control of diarrhea and elimination of *Salmonella* from stool; (3) reductions in rate of relapse and carrier rates; and (4) prevention of blood stream infection (bacteremia) and other complications. A distinct advantage of the quinolones in uncomplicated typhoid is their efficacy with treatment courses as short as 3 days. Cure rates with ofloxacin given for 3 days (15 mg/kg daily) have been as high as 96% to 100%, but most experts, because of the increase in drug resistance, now recommend a full 10- to 14-day course of treatment to reduce relapses. The longer course of treatment is recommended primarily for travelers who acquire the illness in Asia or Southeast Asia. Third-generation cephalosporins (for example, ceftriaxone) are also effective, but patients may remain ill for more than 1 week, whereas the average time to fever clearance with the quinolones is about 4 days. Another advantage: The quinolones can be self administered by a traveler, whereas most cephalosporins must be given by intravenous or intramuscular injection.

The quinolones are very effective in children with multidrug-resistant typhoid fever or other systemic salmonelloses. Quinolones, however, should not be used to treat *Salmonella* meningitis; a third-generation cephalosporin is preferred.

Azithromycin (Zithromax) is also an effective drug. One thousand milligrams (1,000 mg) taken on the first day, followed by 500 mg daily for 6 additional days, was 100% effective in one study. In children, a dose of 10 mg/kg/day for 7 days was more than 90% effective with few adverse effects.

Prevention

Human carriers transmit *Salmonella typhi* bacteria, and in all countries where there is substandard sanitation there is the risk of typhoid transmission. Pay close attention to dietary safety. Especially avoid raw vegetables and salads because these items are often grown in contaminated irrigation water. All food should be well cooked. You should drink only commercially bottled, boiled, or treated water, or commercial beverages. Flavored ices sold by street vendors are especially risky.

Vaccination See Chapter 3 for typhoid vaccine schedules, indications, precautions, and contraindications. Currently available vaccines are about 70% effective. Travelers, therefore, can still acquire typhoid, or paratyphoid (a similar illness), if exposed to a heavy dose of bacteria, or if the vaccine had not been properly administered or handled, as can happen with the oral vaccine. In 1994, eight Dutch travelers in a tour group to Indonesia were diagnosed with typhoid fever, despite having received the oral Typhim 21a vaccine. Therefore, dietary discretion remains an important factor in disease prevention. Don't rely entirely on the vaccine for protection.

SALMONELLA ENTERITIS (SALMONELLOSIS)

Other species of salmonella bacteria (*Salmonella enteritidis, Salmonella cholerae-suis*) cause primarily diarrhea, an intestinal illness termed salmonella enteritis. Typical symptoms include fever, nausea, vomiting, abdominal cramps, and diarrhea. Occasionally, salmonella bacteria enter the blood stream and cause a severe, life-threatening illness termed salmonella bacteremia, characterized by chills, high fever, and prostration. Fatalities from bacteremia occur most often in infants, the elderly, the chronically ill, and those with immune system deficiencies.

Unlike *Salmonella typhi* bacteria, which are harbored only by humans, other salmonella species are found in a variety of animals including poultry (especially chickens), turkeys, ducks, livestock (pigs, horses, sheep), dogs, cats, rodents, and reptiles (snakes, lizards, turtles). Be aware that purchasing a pet anywhere in the world carries the risk of salmonella infection. Up to 60% of turtles, snakes, iguanas, and lizards in pet stores may harbor bacteria.

Infection is usually transmitted by direct contact with the flesh of an infected animal (e.g., during butchering or food preparation) or by the consumption of undercooked, contaminated food. Undercooked chicken eggs and unpasteurized dairy products are also common sources of illness. Poultry products account for more than one half the cases of salmonellosis.

Treatment
Salmonellosis is best treated with a quinolone antibiotic. A third-generation cephalosporin (ceftriaxone or cefixime) is an alternative drug.

Prevention
There is no vaccine. The typhoid fever vaccine is not effective against the other salmonella bacteria that cause salmonellosis. Prevention is entirely dependent on eating well-cooked food (especially dairy products) and avoiding disease-carrying pets such as turtles and lizards.

SHIGELLOSIS (BACILLARY DYSENTERY)

The most common cause of bacterial dysentery is shigellosis, an infection with *Shigella* species bacteria. This disease accounts for 10% to 40% of diarrhea worldwide. Because very small numbers of bacteria are needed to transmit this disease, the infection can be easily acquired, either from contaminated food or from person-to-person contact with carriers of the bacteria. Flies can also carry and transmit shigella.

Bacillary dysentery is characterized by an abrupt onset of high fever, abdominal cramps, small-volume bloody diarrhea, and the repeated feeling of incomplete bowel evacuation. Voluminous, watery diarrhea may precede the onset of bloody diarrhea. In contrast, amebic dysentery manifests with a gradual onset of diarrhea, associated with low-grade fever. Fulminating colitis with shigellosis is uncommon.

Although a stool culture is needed for exact diagnosis, shigellosis should be suspected on the basis of the symptoms. Other bacteria that can cause similar symptoms include *Campylobacter, Salmonella, Vibrio parahaemolyticus, Yersinia*, and enteroinvasive *E. coli*. Because these microorganisms, like *Shigella*, can all be treated with a quinolone antibiotic, it is not necessary to know the exact bacterial diagnosis before starting treatment.

Treatment
Because bacterial resistance to tetracycline, trimethoprim/sulfamethoxazole, and furazolidone has increased worldwide, shigellosis is best treated with a quinolone antibiotic. The oral cephalosporins do not appear to be effective. If your initial symptoms are severe with high fever and dehydration, hospitalization may be necessary. One species of *Shigella* (*Shigella dysenteriae*) is often more resistant to antibiotics and causes more severe illness and 5 to 10 days of quinolone treatment are usually required.

Azithromycin (Zithromax) is also an effective drug. Take 500 mg on the first day, then 250 mg for an additional 4 to 5 days. The cure rate is approximately 80%, which is similar to the quinolones. (The cure rate with ciprofloxacin is about 90%.)

MENINGOCOCCAL MENINGITIS

This illness is caused by bacteria (*Neisseria meningitidis*) that infect the membranes lining the brain and spinal cord. Unless treated immediately, meningococcal meningitis can be rapidly fatal.

The *Neisseria* bacteria are normally carried harmlessly in the nasal passages of a small percentage of healthy people. This carriage of bacteria tends to be seasonal and increases during the dry season. Coughing and sneezing spread the bacteria person-to-person. Crowded living conditions increase the number of carriers and the transmission of disease. Travelers are usually exposed to infection only through close contact with the local population in endemic areas. It is not entirely clear, however, what triggers the infection in people carrying the bacteria. In some cases, it may be that an upper respiratory infection has damaged the immune defenses of the mucous membranes of their nose and throat; climatic conditions, as well as temperature and humidity, may also play roles.

Disease is caused by one of five bacterial serogroups: A, B, C, Y, and W-135. Group A is the most common cause of epidemics in the world, particularly in the African "meningitis belt." W-135 has emerged as a significant cause in Africa and the Middle East, particularly among pilgrims during the Hajj and Umra in Saudi Arabia. Group B

Figure 10.1   Distribution of Meningitis, Central Africa

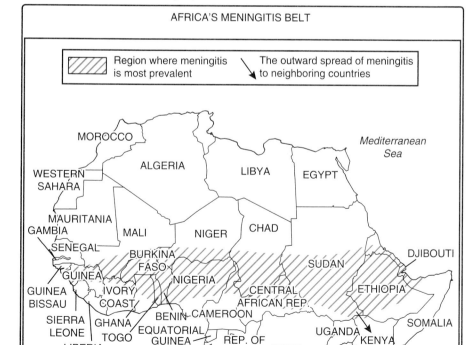

is responsible for most outbreaks in industrialized countries. In the United States, groups B, C, and Y each account for about one-third of cases. Group C causes many cluster outbreaks among college students and military recruits.

Symptoms and Treatment

Fever, vomiting, headache, neck pain and stiffness, and confusion or lethargy are the most common symptoms, but early illness can also mimic "the flu." Neck and back pain and stiffness are the hallmarks of any form of meningitis but are not necessarily present. Effective antibiotics for treating meningococcal meningitis include ceftriaxone (Rocephin) and cefotaxime (Claforan). Vancomycin is usually added while cultures are pending. Chloramphenicol can be used in penicillin-allergic patients, although resistant strains have been reported. Quinolones also appear to be effective. Patients treated with penicillin G may take longer to recover because of the occurrence of relatively resistant strains of *N. meningitidis*.

Prevention

Don't Smoke Cigarette smoking damages the mucous membranes of the airway and has been shown to be a risk factor for contracting meningitis.

Vaccination The quadrivalent polysaccharide vaccine Menomune (Aventis Pasteur) is protective for 3 years against serogroups A, C, Y, and W-135. In January 2005, the U.S. Food and Drug Administration licensed Menactra (Aventis Pasteur), a quadrivalent vaccine also effective against the same four serogroups and approved for adolescents and adults ages 11 to 55 years. Menactra is a conjugate vaccine that protects for 8 years; it also reduces nasal carriage of *Neisseria* bacteria, which limits disease spread during outbreaks. Menactra was developed primarily to prevent meningitis in adolescents, especially college students living in dormitories, but it is likely to become the preferred vaccine for travelers, even those outside the 11- to 55-year age range.

Vaccination is appropriate for travelers going to countries in the meningitis belt of sub-Saharan Africa during the dry season, November through June, who will have close contact with the local population. Travelers at higher risk include those visiting friends and relatives, adventure travelers, health-care workers, missionaries, and volunteer or relief workers. Those who travel on a tourist itinerary, have limited contact with the local population, and stay in tourist accommodations probably don't need to be vaccinated.

Meningococcal vaccine is usually not recommended for children younger than 2 years of age but under special circumstances may be administered to infants as young as 3 months of age. NOTE: The polysaccharide vaccine does not work well in very young children; the new conjugate vaccine (Menactra) is more immunogenic and probably more effective in infants and young children. The CDC no longer recommends meningococcal vaccine for travel to Nepal, India, Mongolia, Kenya, Burundi, or Tanzania. Vaccination, however, is required for entry into Saudi Arabia for those embarking on the annual Hajj pilgrimage to Mecca.

The occurrence of meningitis outbreaks worldwide can be checked on the CDC website at www.cdc.gov/travel.

SCHISTOSOMIASIS

Schistosomiasis (called *bilharzia* in Africa) is a parasitic disease caused by schistosomes, or blood flukes. The disease affects more than 200 million people in 75 countries. The disease is endemic in Africa (most countries), South America (Brazil, Venezuela, Suriname), and parts of the Middle East and Asia. In the Caribbean, schistosomiasis has been reported to occur sporadically in Puerto Rico, Antigua, Dominica, Guadeloupe, Martinique, Montserrat, and Saint Lucia.

The three most common schistosome species are *Schistosoma mansoni* (the cause of intestinal schistosomiasis), *Schistosoma hematobium* (the cause of urinary schistosomiasis), and *Schistosoma japonicum* (Far Eastern schistosomiasis). Other species, such as *Schistosoma mekongi*, found in Southeast Asia, and *Schistosoma intercalatum*, found in Africa, are less common. Infection takes place when schistosome larvae cercariae (larvae), shed into fresh water by snail-intermediate hosts, penetrate within a few minutes the unbroken skin of an individual who is washing, bathing, wading or swimming in ponds, lakes, or slow moving rivers, streams, or irrigation ditches in endemic areas. After skin penetration, there follows a 4- to 6-week incubation period during which time the young schistosome worms migrate to the liver and to the veins draining the intestine or the bladder. The fully grown worms live in the veins of the urinary bladder or the wall of the intestine where they produce large numbers of eggs that cause inflammation and progressive tissue damage. The adult worms can persist for decades, producing various, often puzzling, symptoms.

Light infections are usually asymptomatic. If you are exposed, you should towel off vigorously and wash your skin with rubbing alcohol. This may prevent penetration of the cercariae. When schistosome larvae penetrate the skin, there may be brief tingling

Figure 10.2 Worldwide Distribution of Schistosomiasis

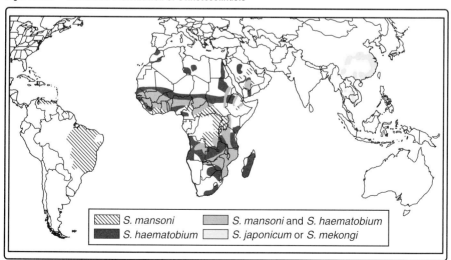

and a rash, called swimmer's itch. Corticosteroid creams and antihistamines can help control symptoms.

Acute schistosomiasis (Katayama fever) Four to 6 weeks after a heavy exposure, you may develop an acute illness called *Katayama fever*. Symptoms include fever, headache, cough, a rash (hives), fatigue, abdominal pain, tender enlargements of the liver and spleen, weight loss, and muscle aches. These symptoms are believed to represent an allergic reaction to the egg deposition. Katayama fever can be confused with malaria or typhoid fever but a white blood count will usually show marked eosinophilia. NOTE: Most persons will not develop Katayama fever during the acute infection; sometimes just a feeling of fatigue or ill health occurs.

Central Nervous System (CNS) Schistosomiasis Rarely, migrating eggs or adult worms can invade the central nervous system. Symptoms of cerebral schistosomiasis include headaches, visual loss, and seizures, if the infection is in the brain. Symptoms of spinal cord schistosomiasis include urinary incontinence, leg pain, and paralysis.

Chronic Schistosomiasis Heavy infections (seen mainly in the indigenous populations) can last for years and can damage the liver, bladder, bowel, and/or nervous system. *S. mansoni, S. japonicum,* and *S. mekongi* parasites primarily affect the bowel and liver; chronic infections can lead to enlargements of the liver and spleen, followed by scarring of the liver and gastrointestinal bleeding from dilated esophageal veins. Bowel involvement may lead to chronic diarrhea and abdominal pain, suggestive of inflammatory bowel disease. *S. hematobium* primarily affects the genitourinary tract. Chronic infections can lead to persistent cystitis, frequency of urination, blood in the urine, obstructive kidney disease, and an increased incidence of bladder cancer; most travelers, however, with

Table 10.1   Schistosomiasis Facts

Always assume that bodies of fresh water in endemic areas are infested with schistosomes. Even deep water, far offshore, may be infective, but is usually safer than the shoreline. Salt and brackish waters are safe.
Water sports are risky because of the degree of exposure.
A history of exposure to infested water is one of the most important elements in the diagnosis of schistosomiasis. A schistosome antibody assay should be done when stool or urine tests are negative for eggs.
High-risk areas for schistosomiasis include the Nile River, the Omo River in Ethiopia, Lake Victoria, Lake Malawi, Lake Kariba in Zimbabwe, Lake Volta in Ghana, and the Tigris and Euphrates rivers.
CDC Schistosomiasis Information http://www.cdc.gov/ncidod/dpd/parasites/schistosomiasis/factsht_schistosomiasis.htm

schistosomiasis are asymptomatic. Symptoms usually occur only when there is a heavy worm burden as a result of repeated or prolonged exposure to infested fresh water.

One of the most important elements in diagnosing schistosomiasis is obtaining a history of freshwater exposure in an endemic area. A white blood cell count may show eosinophilia, but this finding is not specific for schistosomiasis. (About 20% to 30% of patients will have eosinophilia.) The standard diagnostic test is an examination of stool and urine for schistosome eggs. In some cases, a rectal or bladder biopsy will demonstrate eggs; schistosome eggs, however, do not appear for at least 40 days following the initial exposure. In suspected schistosomiasis, a highly accurate serology antibody test using an enzyme-linked immunosorbent assay (ELISA) will usually be diagnostic 6 weeks or more after exposure. This test is far more sensitive than stool or urine examination. The CDC's **Parasitic Disease Branch (404-488-4050)** can provide information about the ELISA assay. A positive test indicates present or past infection, but does not distinguish between the two.

Schistosomiasis of the nervous system, which is extremely rare, causes varying neurological symptoms. The blood eosinophil count may be normal, and the stool and urine egg examination may be negative. Diagnosis is made with the ELISA assay combined with an MRI examination of the central nervous system.

Treatment

For *S. mansoni* and *S. hematobium*, praziquantel is curative in a single dose of 40 mg/kg. For the treatment of *S. japonicum* and *S. mekongi*, praziquantel, 60 mg/kg, is given in three divided doses 6 hours apart.

Prevention

There is no vaccine; therefore, avoiding contact with infested water is the most important preventive measure. Do not swim in slow-moving fresh water unless a reliable source assures you that it is safe. (Chlorinated swimming pools and seawater are safe.) Water for bathing is considered safe if it has been heated to above 50° C (122° F) for more than 5 minutes, if it has stood for more than 48 hours in a tub or container, or if it has been chemically treated (e.g., chlorinated) as for drinking water. If you cannot avoid freshwater exposure, swim or bathe in a rapidly flowing river or stream and stay away from the shoreline of a lake. Researchers have suggested that applying controlled-release DEET may prevent skin penetration by the larvae, but data are preliminary.

LIVER FLUKE DISEASES

These other flukes, unlike the blood flukes (which cause schistosomiasis), are acquired by eating raw or undercooked fish, shellfish, or raw water vegetables.

Clonorchiasis Infection with *Clonorchis sinensis* occurs after the consumption of raw, undercooked, pickled, or smoked freshwater fish that contain parasitic larvae. Clonorchiasis is common in Laos, Cambodia, Thailand, southern China, Hong Kong,

Korea, Japan, and far eastern Russia. Travelers can avoid this disease by eating only well-cooked fish. Symptoms relate to obstruction of the bile ducts and include abdominal pain and jaundice. Most infected individuals, however, are asymptomatic. Clonorchiasis is treated with praziquantel, 75 mg/kg in three divided doses in 1 day. Albendazole has also been shown to be an effective alternative. Untreated clonorchiasis has been associated with bile duct cancer and gallstones.

Opisthorchiasis This disease is caused by *Opisthorchis* species of flukes. It is acquired in the same way as clonorchiasis, and the symptoms and treatment are also the same.

Fascioliasis Human infection is quite widespread, occurring in 66 countries in Africa, China, Latin America, and Europe. *Fasciola hepatica* parasites are acquired by ingesting parasitic larvae attached to aquatic plants, usually watercress. Symptoms include fever, upper abdominal pain, weight loss, and marked elevation of blood eosinophils. Hypodense cystic lesions are frequently found in the liver on imaging studies. Treatment is with triclabendazole, 11 mg/kg in a single dose.

LUNG FLUKE DISEASE

Paragonimiasis Humans develop paragonimiasis after consuming raw, salted, or wine-soaked crustacea (freshwater crabs, crayfish, and shrimp). The species *Paragonimus westermani* is prevalent in parts of China, Korea, Japan, the Philippines, and Taiwan. Other *Paragonimus* species infect humans in West Africa and Central and South America. Symptoms include coughing up blood and chest pain. It is treated with praziquantel, 75 mg/kg in three divided doses on 2 consecutive days. Triclabendazole has also been shown to be effective. Travelers can avoid lung fluke disease by not eating raw or undercooked freshwater shellfish.

INTESTINAL FLUKE DISEASE

Fasciolopsiasis Giant intestinal fluke disease is common in the Far East and is acquired through the ingestion of parasitic larvae attached to aquatic plants such as water chestnuts, which have been contaminated by sewage from mammals (pigs, humans). The causative parasite is *Fasciolopsis buski*. Symptoms of heavy infection include abdominal pain, chronic diarrhea, loss of appetite, and weight loss. Treatment is with praziquantel.

OTHER PARASITIC INTESTINAL INFECTIONS

The rat lung worm, *Angiostrongylus costaricensis*, is the cause of abdominal angiostrongyliasis, and its cousin, *Angiostrongylus cantonensis*, as well as the most common cause of eosinophilic meningitis (inflammation of the spinal cord coverings) in humans. It occurs in Costa Rica and other Central American countries, as well as Southeast Asia, and the Pacific basin and the Caribbean. Human infection occurs through ingestion of larvae present in snails or slugs; or transport hosts, such as freshwater prawns, frogs, or fish; or vegetable produce contaminated by either. The ingested larvae penetrate the abdominal wall and travel to intestinal lymph nodes, causing inflammation that can mimic appendicitis. Larvae that travel to the brain can cause meningoencephalitis (inflammation of the brain). Treatment is with albendazole and corticosteroids.

INTESTINAL ROUNDWORM DISEASES

Whipworm Disease (trichuriasis) *Trichuris trichiura* is one of the most prevalent worm (helminth) infections in the world. The adult worms can live up to 7 years in the intestinal tract, producing thousands of eggs that are passed in the stool. Heavy infections can cause abdominal pain, chronic diarrhea, rectal prolapse, and stunting of growth in children. However, most infections are asymptomatic. Treatment with mebendazole, 100 mg twice daily for 3 days, or albendazole, 400 mg daily for 3 days, is recommended. Travelers can prevent infection by eating only cooked food and rinsing vegetables in hot water (65° C [149° F] or above), an iodine solution, or bleach.

Intestinal capillariasis—This is a serious infection that occurs in the Philippines, in Thailand, and occasionally in other countries in Southeast Asia. The infection is acquired by the ingestion of raw freshwater fish that harbor infective worm larvae. The parasitic worms, *Capillaria philippinensis*, invade the small intestine and can cause chronic diarrhea, malnutrition, and wasting. The disease may be fatal.

The diagnosis of capillariasis is made by finding characteristic eggs in the stool or by examining tissue obtained from a biopsy of the small intestine. A blood serology (ELISA) test is available in certain research laboratories. Eosinophilia occurs but is a nonspecific finding. Treatment with mebendazole, 200 mg twice daily for 20 days, is curative. Albendazole is also effective. Avoiding raw fish prevents this (rare) infection.

Ascariasis This is the most common helminth infection in the world. The roundworm, *Ascaris lumbricoides*, lives in the intestine and produces eggs that are passed in human feces; eggs then incubate in soil for 2 to 3 months before becoming infective to humans. When these eggs are ingested through fecally contaminated food or water, they enter the intestinal tract and hatch into larvae that penetrate the gut wall and are carried to the lung, coughed up, and swallowed. Then larvae develop into adult worms and produce eggs, and the life cycle is completed.

Symptoms of ascariasis are produced by migration of larvae through lung tissue during early migration and also by the presence of adult worms in the intestinal tract. Symptoms of ascariasis include cough, wheezing, fever, and chest pain. There may be eosinophilic inflammation of lung tissue. Intestinal symptoms from heavy infection include nausea, loss of appetite, and abdominal pain. Migrating worms can cause intestinal perforation, bile duct obstruction, appendicitis, and pancreatitis. In children in the developing world, ascariasis is the most common cause of bowel obstruction. Most infections are asymptomatic. Occasionally, the 8-inch adult worm (it looks like an earthworm) will pass spontaneously in the stool or out the mouth or nose. Treatment with a single 400-mg dose of albendazole cures 100% of infections. Mebendazole, 100 mg twice daily for 3 days, or pyrantel pamoate (Antiminth, Reese's Pinworm), 11 mg/kg in one dose, is also effective.

Hookworm Disease (ancylostomiasis) This disease is acquired by walking barefoot in areas where there is fecal contamination of the soil harboring hookworm larvae. The larvae enter the body by penetrating the unbroken skin of the foot, pass through the lungs, and end up in the intestine, where they develop into adult worms. Symptoms of hookworm disease may include coughing and wheezing, peptic ulcer-like pain, and fatigue from anemia. Most infections are asymptomatic. Treatment with mebendazole, 100 mg twice daily for 3 days, albendazole, 400 mg (single dose), or pyrantel pamoate, 11 mg/kg daily for 3 days, is effective.

Strongyloidiasis Like hookworm, *Strongyloides* larvae also enter the body through skin penetration, pass through the lungs, and enter the intestine. In travelers, strongyloidiasis is one of the most important intestinal worms because it is a potentially fatal disease in those whose immune system is compromised by conditions such as cancer, AIDS, radiation therapy, and medication (especially corticosteroids). Symptoms include hives and peptic ulcer-like abdominal pain. Diarrhea and a cough are early symptoms in heavily infected individuals. However, most infected people are asymptomatic. Because this is one of the only worms capable of multiplying in humans, it will often live indefinitely in the body unless it is treated.

Strongyloidiasis and hookworm disease are common causes of undiagnosed eosinophilia in travelers. *Strongyloides* infection is often missed even after multiple stools have been examined. Serology testing through the CDC is 95% sensitive and should be carried out when the diagnosis is suspected and laboratory examination of the stool are negative. Treatment is with ivermectin, 200 μg/kg daily for 2 days, or albendazole, 400 mg twice daily for 7 days.

Anisakiasis This is a parasitic disease transmitted by eating raw, undercooked, or lightly pickled saltwater fish, especially salmon, herring, mackerel, whitefish, cod, pollock, bonito, and sole. The parasite is the larval form of a marine roundworm, which may be present in the muscles and organs of the fish just mentioned. The worm attaches to the lining of the stomach or intestine. Symptoms include nausea and vomiting, or abdominal pain that mimics appendicitis. All good sushi chefs prepare raw fish so as to virtually eliminate the risk of anisakiasis. Freezing fish also kills the parasite. The treatment is surgical excision of the worm from the intestinal tract.

INTESTINAL TAPEWORM DISEASES

Diphyllobothriasis (fish tapeworm disease) This is an infection caused by a fish tapeworm called *Diphyllobothrium latum* and occurs among people who eat raw, smoked, pickled, or undercooked freshwater fish. These include Eskimos, fishermen, devotees of sushi bars (salmon), and people who taste raw fish (such as whitefish) while cooking. Symptoms are uncommon but may include primarily abdominal cramps and diarrhea, but fatigue and, rarely, anemia from vitamin B_{12} deficiency can also occur because fish tapeworms consume this important vitamin. Treatment (adults and children) is with a single dose of praziquantel, 10 mg/kg.

Beef Tapeworm Disease This is an infection acquired by eating raw or undercooked beef and is caused by the beef tapeworm *Taenia saginata*. Many infections are asymptomatic. Classically, people with this infection may notice a small worm segment, or longer piece of the worm, passed in their stool during a bowel movement or crawling out of their anus between bowel movements. Symptoms may include nausea and abdominal cramps. Treatment (adults and children) is with a single dose of praziquantel, 10 mg/kg.

Pork Tapeworm Disease This intestinal infection, similar to beef tapeworm disease, is caused by the pork tapeworm *Taenia solium* and is acquired through eating under-cooked pork that contains the encysted larvae of the tapeworm.

Cysticercosis This is a more serious infection than pork tapeworm disease because it involves organs outside the intestine. Cysticercosis occurs when a person ingests pork tapeworm eggs (not the larvae), usually by eating fecally contaminated food. The eggs hatch in the intestine and develop into larvae that penetrate the intestinal wall and in-vade various organs and tissues of the body. The most serious illness that results, neurocysticercosis, occurs when tapeworm larvae invade the brain and form cysts, causing seizures and other neurological symptoms. Cysticercosis is common in Mexico, Central and South America, Africa, India, China, Eastern Europe, and Indonesia. Infection is very rare in travelers but not uncommon in immigrants from developing countries.

Both praziquantel and albendazole are effective drugs for treating cysticercosis, but the latter is preferred (15 mg/kg/day for 10 to 30 days, or up to 400 mg twice daily for 10 to 30 days). The dose of praziquantel is 50 to 75 mg/day for 15 days. Corticosteroids are often prescribed as adjunctive treatment to prevent serious allergic reactions to dying larvae.

Trichinosis This disease (also called trichinellosis) occurs worldwide, except in Australia, and is most often acquired when people eat raw or undercooked pork con-taining the larval cysts of the parasite *Trichinella spiralis*. Trichinosis, however, can also be acquired by the ingestion of undercooked meat of other carnivorous animals and wild game such as black bear, polar bear, walrus, wild boar, bush pigs, and wart hogs.

During the first week after ingestion, the larvae in the intestine develop into adult worms, causing abdominal pain, diarrhea, nausea, vomiting, and prostration. Next, there is tissue invasion by newly produced larvae, bringing fever, headache, swelling of the eyelids and face, conjunctivitis, muscle pain, weakness, and hives. Symptoms caused by larval invasion of the heart and central nervous system include heart rhythm disturbances and seizures.

Treatment with prednisone (60 mg/day) is used in acute trichinosis to reduce inflam-mation and alleviate symptoms. Albendazole, 400 mg twice daily for 14 days, is the treatment of choice. An alternative treatment is mebendazole, 400 mg, three times daily for 4 days, then 400 to 500 mg/day for 10 days. Adequate cooking will prevent this in-fection. Freezing, smoking, or pickling is as effective.

BRUCELLOSIS

This is a bacterial disease contracted through (1) the consumption of contaminated dairy products, particularly unpasteurized soft cheeses and milk, or (2) by exposure to the flesh of infected animals, particularly that of cattle, hogs, or goats. In this regard, farmers, herdsmen, veterinarians, and slaughterhouse workers are at particular risk.

The highest incidence of brucellosis occurs in Middle Eastern countries such as Saudi Arabia, Kuwait, and Lebanon, but the incidence is also high in Central and South America, sub-Saharan Africa, India, Greece, France, and Spain. Brucellosis should be suspected in travelers who have visited these areas and later develop a prolonged illness with fever.

The brucella bacteria may incubate in the body for a month or more before causing symptoms, and the diagnosis, initially, may not be suspected. The most common symptoms include fever, chills, sweating, muscle and joint aches, abdominal pain, weakness, weight loss, and headache. Backache and testicular pain are not uncommon. The physical examination often demonstrates enlargements of the spleen and liver and swelling of the lymph nodes. Other diseases that mimic brucellosis include typhoid, mononucleosis, leishmaniasis, and tuberculosis.

Early diagnosis of brucellosis depends on a high degree of suspicion for the illness; knowing the travel history and possible exposure to the disease is very important. A positive serology test and positive blood or bone marrow cultures confirm the diagnosis.

Treatment

Brucellosis bacteria often persist inside white blood cells despite antibiotics. Treatment with two antibiotics for at least 6 weeks is, therefore, required. Doxycycline, 100 mg twice daily, is administered for 6 weeks, while a second agent (rifampicin, streptomycin, or gentamicin) is given in conjunction for at least several weeks. The quinolones and co-trimoxazole are also effective.

Prevention The destruction of infected dairy animals, immunization of susceptible animals, and pasteurization of milk and milk products can prevent brucellosis. Travelers should not consume unpasteurized milk and other dairy products and should avoid contact with animal carcasses in risk countries.

LEPTOSPIROSIS

Leptospirosis is the most common zoonosis in the world. (A zoonosis is any disease that humans may acquire from animals.) Distribution is worldwide (except in polar regions), but the disease is most prevalent in the tropics. The causative spirochete *Leptospira interrogans* is transmitted by contact with contaminated fresh water or moist soil, including jungle swamps and mud. (Contamination is usually from the urine of infected animals, such as rats, mice, pigs, cattle, and dogs.) Contact with the tissue of infected animals can also spread disease. Leptospires enter through cuts or abrasions on the skin or exposed mucous membranes (nose, mouth, eyes). Traditionally recognized as an occupational disease (e.g., farmers, sewage workers, butchers) leptospirosis is becoming more frequently associated with recreational exposure (e.g., hiking, swimming, rafting) and following heavy flooding; major outbreaks have recently occurred among eco-challenge racers in Costa Rica and Borneo, in Nicaragua, Honduras, and Guatemala following heavy flooding. Recreational and wilderness travelers to the tropics should be aware of the risk for infection.

Many cases are asymptomatic or mild. More severe cases manifest with high fever, headache, conjunctival suffusion (eye redness and edema without secretions), severe muscle pain (myalgia), and stiff neck (from aseptic meningitis). Weil disease, the most severe and sometimes fatal form of leptospirosis, is associated with liver dysfunction and jaundice, but death is almost always the result of kidney (renal) failure, not liver failure. Other findings in severe leptospirosis include bleeding from hemorrhagic coagulopathy and capillary damage, marked leukocytosis, and hemorrhagic pneumonitis. Differential diagnosis includes hepatitis, malaria, typhoid fever, dengue fever, scrub typhus, and hemorrhagic fever with renal syndrome.

Treatment and Prevention

The incubation period is usually 7 to 14 days (range 2 to 21 days). You should seek prompt medical advice if symptoms suggestive of leptospirosis develop within the incubation period after freshwater exposure.

Effective antibiotics include penicillin, amoxicillin, erythromycin, doxycycline, and ceftriaxone. Dialysis is indicated for acute renal failure. Prevention consists of avoiding potentially contaminated fresh water (rivers, lakes, streams) and soil. Drinking water should be filtered, boiled, or treated with iodine. Chemoprophylaxis with doxycycline, 200 mg weekly, is effective and safe for short-term, high-risk exposure.

RABIES

Rabies is one of the most ancient and feared diseases. It is estimated that as many as 50,000 people worldwide die each year from rabies, mostly in the developing countries of Africa, Asia, and Latin America. Travelers to these countries (especially those visiting small villages and rural areas) need to assess their potential risk of exposure, especially to dogs, which transmit most cases of human rabies in less developed countries.

The highest risk of rabies occurs in El Salvador, Guatemala, Mexico, Colombia, Ecuador, Peru, Nepal, India, Pakistan, Bangladesh, Sri Lanka, Thailand, Vietnam, and the Philippines. More than 50 countries reportedly have no rabies cases.*

All mammals are susceptible to rabies and can transmit the virus, but true reservoirs, which maintain the virus in nature, persist only among carnivorous mammals and bats. Unvaccinated domestic animals and humans can become rabid after exposure to such

---

*These countries include Australia, New Zealand, Papua New Guinea, most islands of the Pacific Ocean, most Caribbean islands (except the island of Hispaniola), the United Kingdom, Cyprus, Finland, Iceland, Norway, Portugal, Spain, Sweden, Japan, Korea, Malaysia, Singapore, and Taiwan.

reservoirs. Infected livestock will die of the disease before transmitting it; cats (usually infected by dogs or wild animals) can transmit the disease, but are not reservoirs of infection.

In North America, raccoons, skunks, bats, and foxes are the primary reservoirs capable of transmitting infection. Because most dogs are now vaccinated, fewer than 100 rabid dogs were reported in the United States in 2002. In fact, more cases of cat rabies were reported, because these animals are less supervised and are vaccinated less often. The mongoose is an important vector in Puerto Rico, the fox in Europe, the jackal in much of Africa, the wolf in Iran and neighboring countries, and the vampire bat in certain Latin American countries. Therefore, at the very least, travelers should not approach or pet stray dogs, cats, monkeys, or feral animals.

Pre-Departure Vaccination Adventure travelers and long-term expatriates often underestimate the risk of rabies. If you plan to stay for more than 30 days in a country where rabies is a constant threat, especially if you travel to remote areas, you should strongly consider pre-departure rabies vaccination. This is particularly important for children who are often attracted to animals and who may not report a bite, and for long-stay travelers and expatriates. In case of a bite from a potentially rabid animal, the advantages to pre-departure vaccination include the following:

- You won't need to receive rabies immune globulin (RIG), which is often not available in developing countries.
- You will need only 2, not 5, doses of rabies vaccine after exposure. Although three pre-exposure doses of vaccine provide lifetime protection, postexposure booster doses are always required.
- A delay in treatment will be less critical because you already have some immunity. If rabies vaccine is not locally available you will need to travel to where the vaccine is available, but there is a bit less urgency.

There are three equally effective rabies vaccines commercially available in the United States: (1) Imovax (human diploid cell vaccine-HDCV); (2) RabAvert (purified chick embryo cell culture-PCEC); and (3) Rabies Vaccine Adsorbed (RVA from fetal rhesus lung cells).

Pre-Departure Vaccination Schedule Rabies vaccine is given as three doses on days 0, 7, and either 21 or 28. RabAvert and RVA should be injected into the deltoid or quadricep (anterior thigh) muscle. The gluteal region should be avoided. Imovax can be administered intramuscularly (IM) or intradermally (ID). NOTE: Intradermal rabies vaccination must be completed before starting chloroquine or mefloquine. If this is not feasible, then the vaccine must be given IM.

Accelerated Schedule Two doses, 1 week apart (intramuscular route only) when time does not allow three doses to be administered over 21 to 28 days.

Postexposure Treatment Following exposure to an animal known or suspected of being rabid, the most important first step is to clean the bite site thoroughly with soap and water or an antiseptic solution. Unvaccinated individuals should receive rabies immune globulin (RIG) *and* rabies vaccine. People already vaccinated should receive rabies vaccine *only*. NOTE: Exposure consists of a bite or a scratch, or the licking of a minor wound or abrasion, by the animal. Coming into contact with a bat, even without an observed bite, may constitute exposure. The rabies virus is contained in the saliva and certain body tissues (e.g., the brain and spinal fluid) of the infected animal. Therefore, contact with the blood, urine, or feces of the animal does *not* constitute exposure and does not require vaccination.

If you completed a pre-departure rabies vaccination series, you will need two additional doses of intramuscular vaccine (given on days 0 and 3). If not vaccinated, you must receive RIG followed by five doses of rabies vaccine (given on days 0, 3, 7, 14, and 28). Treatment is best started within the first 24 hours after exposure. *If anatomically feasible, the entire calculated dose of rabies immune globulin (either human or equine) should be injected directly into the bite(s) and the tissue around the bite(s).* If there are large or multiple bites, RIG can be diluted with normal saline if more volume is needed to infiltrate all wound areas. If it is not anatomically feasible to inject the entire volume of RIG into the wound(s), any remaining volume should be injected intramuscularly at a remote site, usually into the deltoid or anterolateral thigh muscles. NOTE: Injecting into the gluteus muscle risks injury to the sciatic nerve. There is also a greater chance of depositing the injection into fat tissue, resulting in less absorption. RIG dosage: 20 IU/kg (human RIG) or 40 IU/kg (equine RIG). NOTE: Theoretically, chloroquine may interfere with the immune response, and this drug should be discontinued during post-exposure rabies prophylaxis. The patient, of course, should be monitored for malaria symptoms if chloroquine has been discontinued.

Treatment failures can occur, but these failures are usually preventable and caused by (1) bite wounds not having been immediately and thoroughly cleaned with soap and water; (2) delayed (over 24 hours) treatment; (3) RIG not given with the vaccine; or (4) RIG not infiltrated directly into and around the wound(s). The wounds with the highest risk involve bites of the head, neck, and hands. NOTE: Prophylaxis should be initiated whenever exposure occurs or is strongly suspected, regardless of the time interval. The incubation period of rabies is 1 to 3 months, but cases have occurred within 2 weeks of exposure, and as long as 1 year later.

Vaccines Overseas In less developed countries, the vaccines used in the United States and Canada are often not available. The same is true for human rabies immune globulin (Imogam, BayRab), also a very expensive product. In the event of rabies exposure abroad, you would likely be given a Vero cell vaccine, a chick cell-derived vaccine, or a purified duck embryo-derived vaccine. These products are effective and safe and have few side effects. Instead of human RIG, you might get purified equine RIG, which has the potential to cause significant side effects unless the newer preparations (from Europe) are used. If you return to the United States or Canada after starting postexposure treatment abroad, the vaccination schedule can be completed using intramuscular Imovax (HDCV), RabAvert (PCEC), or RVA. In many developing countries, neural-tissue vaccines (Semple, Fermi, suckling mouse) are still in common use.

These vaccines are cheap but are less effective and potentially very dangerous. They should be avoided, if possible. In the event of a possible rabies exposure, contact the nearest U.S. or Canadian embassy to obtain the location of the nearest reliable medical facility. You should be prepared to evacuate to another country for appropriate medical care (with rabies immune globulin and tissue culture vaccines) if necessary. However, if you begin treatment overseas with a neural-tissue (Semple, Fermi, suckling mouse brain) vaccine, you should try, as soon as possible, to get to a facility (even if it means returning to Europe or North America) that can re-initiate vaccination with one of the newer cell-culture vaccines.

SEAFOOD TOXINS

Poisonous toxins in seafood can be an important and often overlooked cause of illness in travelers. Unfortunately, the toxins are often difficult or impossible to detect because they do not usually affect the appearance, smell, or taste of the fish or shellfish. In addition, freezing, drying, smoking, or cooking does not usually destroy them.

Fish Poisoning

Scombroid Poisoning This occurs after eating fish that has been inadequately chilled after capture. It occurs most commonly in tuna and related species and also in mahi-mahi. Affected fish contains histamine and may have a sharp, bitter, or peppery taste. Often, however, the fish looks, smells, and tastes normal. Symptoms of scombroid poisoning resemble an allergic reaction and include flushing, headache, nausea, vomiting, abdominal cramps, and diarrhea. In addition, there may be hives and wheezing. Treatment with antihistamines is very effective.

Ciguatera Poisoning This occurs after eating coral reef fish containing potent toxins that originate in algae found in coral reefs, especially after storms, which may cause an increase in algae. The toxin is passed up the food chain through herbivorous fish to carnivorous fish and eventually to humans. Any part of the fish may contain toxins but the highest concentrations are found in the head, gut, roe, and liver. Almost any reef fish can cause ciguatera poisoning, but it is most common in barracuda, moray eel, grouper, snapper, jack, and sea bass. Large carnivorous fish weighing more than 6 pounds are the most dangerous. Symptoms include diarrhea, nausea, vomiting, and abdominal cramps followed by neurological symptoms such as numbness and tingling involving the arms and legs and the area around the mouth. There may be temperature reversal where cold objects feel hot. For example, ice cream may cause a burning sensation in the mouth. Another bizarre symptom is that the teeth often feel numb or loose. In addition, there may be muscle aches, fatigue, itchiness of the skin, and depression. Some of the symptoms may last weeks or several months. After an episode, travelers should avoid, for several months, alcohol, fish of any kind, and nuts. These substances may exacerbate symptoms. Treatment is directed to relieving the symptoms, but mannitol, given intravenously within 72 hours of onset, may occasionally produce a dramatic improvement. A commercial test (Cigna-check, Oceanit Test) has recently become available to test fish for ciguatoxin (http://www.cigua.com). This test is very sensitive and easy to perform, but it is relatively expensive and probably of limited value for travelers.

Pufferfish or Fugu Poisoning This occurs after eating pufferfish (a bad idea) and less commonly porcupine fish or ocean sunfish, which contain a highly potent toxin known as tetrodotoxin. It is 50 times more potent than strychnine and is usually concentrated in the ovaries, liver, gut, and skin of affected fish. Most cases of pufferfish poisoning occur in Japan where pufferfish or fugu is eaten as a very expensive and prized delicacy. The fugu experience is a feeling of euphoria and exhilaration and is the result of ingesting minute amounts of toxin. Unfortunately, larger quantities of toxins can be rapidly fatal. Symptoms of poisoning include nausea, sweating, dizziness, and neurological symptoms such as numbness, tingling, and weakness. In severe cases, there is widespread paralysis often involving the respiratory muscles. Mortality rates of up to 60% have been reported. Unfortunately, there is no specific antidote, and treatment is directed at relieving the symptoms and providing supportive care.

Shellfish Poisoning

There are two important types of shellfish: crustaceans (e.g., crabs, shrimp, and lobster) and bivalve mollusks (e.g., oysters, mussels, clams, and scallops). Most cases of toxic shellfish poisoning occur after eating bivalve mollusks. The toxins originate in algae, and outbreaks of shellfish poisoning are particularly common after algal blooms or "red tides." There is no specific treatment or effective antidote for any of the shellfish poisonings, and treatment is directed at relieving symptoms and providing supportive care.

Paralytic Shellfish Poisoning This is the most common and most serious form of shellfish poisoning. Typical symptoms include numbness, tingling, and a sensation of floating. In severe cases, there may be paralysis of respiratory muscles. Deaths are most common in children, and mortality rates of over 40% have been reported.

Neurotoxic Shellfish Poisoning This causes nausea, vomiting, diarrhea, and neurological symptoms such as numbness, tingling, weakness, and dizziness. When the aerosolized toxin is breathed in rough surf, coughing, wheezing, and eye irritation may occur in exposed individuals.

Diarrheic Shellfish Poisoning This causes gastroenteritis with symptoms such as diarrhea, nausea, vomiting, abdominal cramps, weakness, and chills. No deaths have been reported.

Amnesic Shellfish Poisoning This is rare but can cause gastroenteritis and neurological features such as headaches, memory loss, seizures, and long-term dementia. It may be fatal in elderly patients.

GUIDELINES FOR THE PREVENTION OF SEAFOOD POISONING

- Avoid fish that has not been promptly chilled after capture (risk of scombroid).
- Avoid fish that has an ammonia smell or sharp, peppery taste (risk of scombroid).
- Avoid reef fish, especially large carnivorous fish such as barracuda, moray eel, grouper, snapper, jack, and sea bass (risk of ciguatera).
  The maxim is: "Eat no carnivorous fish larger than your plate."
- Never eat shellfish associated with algal blooms or "red tides."
- Avoid consumption of bivalve mollusks (oysters, clams, scallops, and mussels) in developing countries.
- Some researchers suggest that ciguatoxin-laden fish can be detected by rubbing a piece of the fish along the gums (before ingestion) to see if a tingling feeling occurs.

CHAPTER 11

Lyme Disease

KEY POINTS:

▶ Lyme disease is the most common vector-borne disease in the United States, with cases reported from every state except Montana, Hawaii, and Oklahoma.

▶ Most cases of Lyme disease are transmitted by deer ticks; in the south, however, a slightly different "Lyme disease" may be transmitted by the Lone Star tick.

▶ It takes more than 24 hours for a feeding tick to transmit infection, and 3 to 5 days for the typical expanding bull's-eye rash to develop after the bite.

▶ A single 200-mg dose of doxycycline, taken at the time of the bite, can prevent infection.

▶ The diagnosis of Lyme disease is based primarily on the characteristic rash and other symptoms, not blood tests.

▶ Treatment may require 2 to 3 weeks, or more, of antibiotics

▶ Signs and symptoms of Lyme disease may be mistaken for another illness. Untreated illness may result in chronic, disabling health problems.

THE PATTERN OF LYME DISEASE

Lyme disease is a potentially serious illness that occurs worldwide. The disease was first recognized in the United States in 1975, following an investigation of a group of children with arthritis in Lyme, Connecticut. Lyme disease is now the most common vector-borne illness in the United States. In 2002, nearly 24,000 cases were reported, but the true number is probably higher. In the United States, 90% of cases are reported from nine states—Connecticut, Delaware, Maryland, New Jersey, New York, Pennsylvania, Rhode Island, Wisconsin, and Minnesota. In Canada, the disease is concentrated in Ontario and Manitoba.

Overseas Most cases are reported from Europe (especially Germany's Black Forest region, southern Sweden, southern and eastern Austria, and the northern Swiss plateau), the former Soviet Union (from the Baltics to the Pacific), China, Japan, and Australia. The incidence of Lyme disease in Latin America appears to be very low. In Africa, cases have been reported from Nigeria, Angola, Kenya, Tanzania, and Zambia. Antarctica is apparently free of the disease.

Different Types of Lyme Disease in the United States

Lyme disease occurring in the Northeast, the upper Midwest, and the Pacific states is caused primarily by the spirochete *Borrelia burgdorferi*, and is transmitted by deer ticks. Southern tick-associated rash illness (STARI) is a Lyme disease—like infection described in patients in the southeastern and south-central United States, whereas classic Lyme disease is relatively rare. STARI develops following the bite of a Lone Star tick (*Amblyomma americanum*) and is believed to be caused by infection with a spirochete tentatively named *Borrelia lonestari*. Some cases of STARI have been reported in New Jersey and Maryland.

How Ticks Develop

Larval ticks feed in the late summer, nymphs feed during spring and early summer, and adults feed predominantly in the fall. The tiny nymphs are your chief threat because they are the most active feeders, and their small size (Figure 11.1) makes casual detection very difficult. In fact, three-quarters of the people who get the disease never spot the tiny ticks which tend to hide in the hair, groin, and armpits and at the back of the knees. Not all ticks, however, are infected with the Lyme spirochete. In some areas, only 1% of ticks carry the spirochete; in other areas the percentage can be much higher.

Ticks primarily inhabit grassy or wooded areas. They are not found on sand dunes, where there is no grass. Ticks don't fly, jump up from the ground, or drop from trees. Instead, they climb to the tips of vegetation and wait for you to brush by. Because the ticks are so small, and their bite is painless, you will probably be unaware when a tick attaches itself to your clothing or skin.

People Most at Risk People most at risk are those engaged in outdoor activities—campers, hikers, hunters, farmers, gardeners, telephone line workers, foresters, and military personnel on training maneuvers.

Symptoms

Because you may not have noticed the tick bite and because the symptoms of Lyme disease are sometimes passed off as "the flu," illness can be overlooked or misdiagnosed. Ten to 20% of infected people may not even develop early symptoms. Up to 40% of victims may not develop or recall having the typical rash.

Stage 1 (early localized infection) A spreading, circular, pink or red rash (erythema migrans) is the hallmark of early Lyme disease. This rash, which originates at the site of

Figure 11.1   Text Actual Size of Deer Ticks in Five Stages. From left to right: larva, nymph, adult male, adult female, and engorged (fed) female tick.

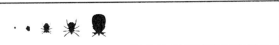

the tick bite, is caused by the *Borrelia burgdorferi* spirochetes migrating in an expanding fashion from the central point of inoculation. The rash can become quite large—5 to 10 inches, or more, in diameter. The appearance of the rash is somewhat varied. In some cases it is halo shaped with an almost clear central area surrounded by a pink or red outer ring (bull's-eye rash). Other rashes have a deep red center with secondary rings and a red outer border. The red areas may be slightly raised and warm to the touch. You may also notice localized lymph node swelling and fatigue. There's a 15% to 40% chance you won't have the characteristic rash. Absence of the typical rash makes early diagnosis more difficult.

Stage 2 (early disseminated infection) After stage 1, the spirochetes spread throughout the body, causing flulike symptoms: fever, headache, muscle and joint aches, swollen glands, increased fatigue, nausea, and loss of appetite. Other symptoms include multiple skin rashes; pains in the muscles, joints, and tendons (fibromyalgia); meningitis; encephalitis; and facial nerve paralysis (Bell's palsy). Cardiac problems include conduction abnormalities with varying degrees of heart block, myopericarditis, and cardiomyopathy. Stage 2 symptoms can occur while the primary erythema migrans rash is still visible or can be delayed by weeks or months.

Stage 3 (late infection) If untreated, you can develop prolonged arthritis attacks in one or multiple joints (often the knees), chronic fatigue, and disorders of the nervous system (polyneuritis, paralysis, encephalopathy). Neuritis symptoms include backache with shooting pains and lack of feeling in the hands and feet.

Symptoms of encephalopathy include mental changes such as forgetting names, misplacing objects, or missing appointments. There may be problems speaking and trouble finding words. A variety of rashes with inflammation and thinning of the skin may also occur.

Prevention

The primary defense against Lyme disease and other tick-borne diseases remains avoidance of tick-infested habitats, use of personal protection measures, and checking for and removing ticks.

Tick Bite Prevention The best way to prevent tick bites is to combine protective clothing with "chemical warfare." Cover as much exposed skin areas as weather conditions allow. Tucking long pants into socks is highly effective. Treat outer clothing with the insecticide permethrin (Chapter 8). Apply a DEET-containing insect repellent to exposed skin. Inspect your body daily for attached ticks.

Prophylactic Antibiotics Finding a tick attached to you doesn't automatically mean you will get Lyme disease because (1) the tick may not be infective, or (2) the tick may not have been attached long enough to transmit spirochetes. (Transmission of spirochetes takes 24 to 36 hours.) Nevertheless, a tick bite signifies potential risk if the tick has fed (it will be engorged with blood). A *single* 200-mg dose of doxycycline is effective for prevention. Don't let a doctor prescribe 2 to 3 weeks of antibiotics just for a bite. That much antibiotic is used for *treatment*.

Vaccination The Lyme vaccine (Lymerix—GSK) was taken off the market in 2002 and is no longer available. Lack of a vaccine makes tick-bite prevention measures more important.

Diagnosis

The diagnosis of early Lyme disease should be based primarily on a history of possible exposure in an endemic area and on the presence of typical symptoms. To make a diagnosis of Lyme disease, you need to have either (1) the typical rash, or (2) symptoms consistent with Lyme disease, in combination with a positive blood test.

NOTE: The most available laboratory test, the ELISA, is both insensitive in the early stages of infection and lacks sufficient specificity to be used as a reliable diagnostic test. Immunoblotting, although it improves the specificity for the diagnosis during the later stages of infection, also lacks both specificity and sensitivity in cases of early infection. A combination of both antibody capture enzyme immunoassay (EIA) and immunoblotting, with proper interpretations, provides the best information.

LYME DISEASE FACT

Tests for Lyme disease may not be diagnostic during stage 1. Therefore, prompt, aggressive antibiotic treatment of early Lyme disease can be started solely on the basis of symptoms, especially a typical "bull's-eye" rash. The absence of the rash, however, should not eliminate Lyme disease from consideration if the symptoms also suggest other features of the infection.

Treatment

If the diagnosis seems clear cut on the basis of your exposure and symptoms (especially the rash), you should receive immediate antibiotic treatment. The treatment of choice for early Lyme disease is doxycycline. Don't let your doctor withhold treatment just to see if your blood test will turn positive.

Treatment recommendations are based on limited data. The duration of treatment is not well established for any stage of the disease and relapses are possible despite a full course of a recommended antibiotic. A second course of antibiotic treatment may, therefore, be required. Table 11.1 summarizes current treatment recommendations.

Treatment of Children and Pregnant Women Amoxicillin is the drug of choice for pregnant women and children younger than 8 years of age. Women who are allergic to penicillin should receive erythromycin base, 250 mg to 500 mg, four times daily for 4 weeks.

Tick Removal

- Grasp the head of the tick with tweezers as near to the skin as possible and gently pull upward and backward until the head of the tick is completely removed. Try not to crush or puncture the tick. Don't try to twist or jerk it out. If the body of the tick tears off and the mouth parts remain embedded in the skin, see your doctor, or go to an emergency department or ambulatory care center to have the mouth parts removed. (They may need to be scraped out under local anesthesia.)

Table 11.1   Treatment of Lyme Disease

	Drug	Adult Dosage	Pediatric Dosage[2]
ERYTHEMA MIGRANS	Doxycycline[3]	100 mg PO bid × 14-21 days	
	OR Amoxicillin	500 mg PO bid × 14-21 days	25-50 mg/kg/day divided tid
	OR Cefuroxime axetil (Ceftin)	500 mg PO bid × 14-21 days	250 mg bid
NEUROLOGICAL DISEASE			
Facial nerve palsy	Doxycycline[3]	100 mg bid × 14-21 days	Contraindicated for children <8 years of age
	OR Amoxicillin	500 mg PO tid × 21-28 days	25-50 mg/kg/day divided tid
More serious CNS disease	Ceftriaxone (Rocephin)	2 g/day IV × 14-28 days	75-100 mg/kg/day IV
	OR Cefotaxime (Claforan)	2 g q8h × 14-28 days	90-180 mg/kg/day in three doses
	OR Penicillin G	20-24 million units/day IV × 14-28 days	300,000 units/kg/day IV
CARDIAC DISEASE			
Mild	Doxycycline[3]	100 mg PO bid × 21 days	
	OR Amoxicillin	250-500 mg PO tid × 21 days	25-50 mg/kg/day divided tid
More serious[4]	Ceftriaxone	2 g/day IV × 14-21 days	50-75 mg/kg/day IV
	OR Penicillin G	20-24 million units/day IV × 14-21 days	300,000 units/kg/day IV

Table 11.1　Treatment of Lyme Disease—cont'd

	Drug	Adult Dosage	Pediatric Dosage[2]
ARTHRITIS[5]			
Oral	Doxycycline[3]	100 mg PO bid × 28 days	
	OR Amoxicillin	500 mg PO qid × 28 days	50 mg/kg/ day divided tid
Parenteral	Ceftriaxone	2 g/day IV × 14-28 days	50-75 mg/kg/day IV
	OR Penicillin G	20-24 million units/day IV × 14-28 days	300,000 units/kg/ day IV

[1] Recommendations are based on limited data and should be considered tentative. The duration of treatment is not well established for any indication. Relapse has occurred with all of these regimens; patients who relapse may need a second course of treatment. There is no evidence, however, that either repeated or prolonged treatment benefits subjective symptoms attributed to Lyme disease.
[2] Should not exceed adult dosage.
[3] Neither doxycycline nor any other tetracycline should be used for children under the age of 8 or for pregnant or lactating women.
[4] A temporary pacemaker may be necessary.
[5] In late disease, the response to treatment may be delayed for several weeks or months.
Abbreviations: bid, twice daily; IV, intravenously; PO, by mouth; qid, four times daily; tid, three times daily.
From The Medical Letter, Vol. 39, 1997. Reprinted with permission.

- If the tick won't release with the above technique, apply a small amount of permethrin spray to the tick. Wait 10 minutes and try the removal technique again.
- Don't use petroleum jelly or a hot object to remove the tick.
- Never use bare fingers to remove a tick. The infection could be passed to you.
- After removing the tick with tweezers, wipe off the attachment site with alcohol or Betadine.
- Dispose of the tick in a safe manner, or cremate it with a match. However, if you want the tick examined or tested, put it in a capped container for later examination (see later).
- When finished, wash your hands thoroughly with soap and water—or use a hand sanitizer gel, such as Purell.

After removing the tick, observe the bite area for any sign of a rash. The typical Lyme disease rash, if it's going to occur, appears from 3 to 30 days after the bite. If you get a rash immediately, or within 24 hours after being bitten, it is not a Lyme disease rash—it is an allergic (hypersensitivity) reaction to the bite. (These allergic rashes are usually itchy.)

IS THE TICK INFECTED?

Once you have removed a tick, you can have it tested for Lyme disease by polymerase chain reaction (PCR), a technique that detects the DNA of the Lyme disease spirochetes in the tick. Without knowing if the tick is infected, the medical profession is divided on whether to treat on the basis of a tick bite alone. A positive PCR test is a strong indication that you should take antibiotics after a tick bite. The PCR test can be done on live or dead ticks sent through the mail. A doctor's order is not necessary to have testing done.

Procedure: Place the tick (dead or alive) in a clean, covered prescription vial that has been thoroughly washed and rinsed with tap water. Refrigerate the vial until it can be sent. Mail the vial with a check or money order for $35 to Imugen, Inc., 220 Norwood Park South, Norwood, MA 02062. Tel: 781-255-0770. Specify that you want Lyme disease testing done because other PCR tests are also performed at this laboratory.

Hepatitis

KEY POINTS:

▶ Hepatitis A is one of the most common vaccine-preventable diseases in the world.

▶ Vaccination against hepatitis A should be routine for all travelers.

▶ Hepatitis B is spread by infected blood, contaminated needles, and unprotected sex.

▶ Hepatitis B vaccine is recommended for long-stay travelers; those who are at occupational or social risk; anybody desiring maximum protection.

▶ The combination vaccine TwinRix (GSK) prevents both hepatitis A and B and is convenient to administer.

▶ Hepatitis E is the most common form of hepatitis on the Indian subcontinent. It is fatal in up to 20% of women in late pregnancy. There is no vaccine for hepatitis E, which is usually transmitted by contaminated drinking water.

Four Distinct Types

Hepatitis is a generic term for inflammations of the liver. It is caused by a number of viruses, other infectious agents, and toxins. There are four hepatitis viruses of which all travelers should be particularly aware: A, B, C, and E.* The means of transmission and long-term effects vary, depending on which virus causes the disease. For the traveler, viral hepatitis is a major concern—not only because of the potential health risks, but because many cases can be prevented by immunization.

Hepatitis A and E are transmitted primarily by contaminated food and water. High-risk areas are less developed countries where poor sanitation results in contamination of groundwater, tap water, and well water. Outbreaks of hepatitis A are also caused by food that has been contaminated by an infected food handler. Hepatitis B and C are spread by sexual contact, exchange of body fluids, injections from contaminated needles and syringes, and unscreened blood transfusions.

Symptoms of Hepatitis

The symptoms can vary. Most cases of hepatitis, in fact, go completely unnoticed. In a textbook case, however, you would develop fever, fatigue, loss of appetite, jaundice (yellow skin), dark urine, abdominal pain, and aching joints.

*A fifth virus, hepatitis D, is an incomplete virus that requires the presence of hepatitis B virus and is of little concern to the average traveler. It can occur in people who are chronically infected with hepatitis B, or occasionally as a combined acute infection with hepatitis B. It is contracted primarily through intravenous drug use or sexual contact with a carrier. Most hepatitis D is found in southern Italy, parts of North Africa adjacent to the Mediterranean, and the upper reaches of the Amazon Basin.

Symptoms of acute hepatitis may occur weeks to months after exposure and typically last from 2 to 6 weeks. The likelihood of complete recovery depends on the particular viral infection and your underlying health. Complete recovery occurs in most cases of types A and E hepatitis, but 5% to 80% of types B and C may progress, causing chronic, sometimes fatal, liver disease.

HEPATITIS A

This is one of the most common vaccine-preventable viral illnesses in the world and the most frequently diagnosed form of hepatitis in travelers returning from developing countries. Hepatitis A is very widespread and close to 100% of people in less developed countries are infected with the hepatitis A virus (HAV) by 10 years of age. In some industrialized countries, however, no more than 10% of the population has been infected. In the United States, about 33% of the population has serologic evidence of previous HAV infection.

Risk to Travelers The risk to a nonimmune traveler of acquiring hepatitis A is estimated at 1 per 1,000 per month of exposure in resort areas, and 5 per 1,000 per month in remote areas of developing countries. Although the risk of hepatitis A is certainly higher in countries with substandard sanitation and hygiene, travel to developed or industrialized countries still carries some risk.

Symptoms usually appear 2 to 6 weeks after exposure. HAV infection is often mild or asymptomatic in children, but there are increased morbidity and mortality in adults. About 0.15% to 0.5% of infected adults develop fulminant liver failure, fatal in one half of these cases. In those older than age 50, mortality in the acute infection may reach 3%. In individuals with chronic hepatitis C or other forms of chronic liver disease, a superimposed HAV infection may carry even higher risks of severe disease and death.

Treatment

Treatment consists of supportive care. Eat a nutritious diet and avoid alcohol. Be aware that the combination of alcohol and acetaminophen (also called paracetamol in some countries) can cause direct hepatic toxicity. There is no specific treatment that will shorten your illness. Limiting exercise has no effect on the rate of recovery. Hospitalization is unnecessary unless you suffer more severe signs of acute liver failure or refractory nausea, vomiting, and dehydration. Close contacts such as family members or companion(s) who have not previously been infected or vaccinated should immediately receive immune globulin (if available) or hepatitis A vaccine.

Prevention

Hepatitis A vaccine—Several effective vaccines are available. These include: VAQTA (Merck), Havrix (GlaxoSmithKline), Avaxim (Aventis Pasteur MSD) and Apaxal (Berna). There is also TwinRix (GlaxoSmithKline)—a combination of hepatitis A and B vaccines. These vaccines give rise to measurable serum antibody levels within 2 weeks after a single injection; a booster dose, recommended at 6 to 12 months, dramatically boosts antibody levels and provides virtually 100% immunity for at least 10 to 20 years, and probably for life. Hepatitis A vaccine is now recommended for all nonimmune travelers older than age two, (age one in Canada and Europe), especially those going to less developed countries.

Immune Globulin When nonimmune travelers are departing imminently for hepatitis A endemic areas, it has previously been recommended that the traveler receive either (1) immune globulin (IG) alone, for brief visits; or (2) hepatitis A vaccine, plus immune globulin. The rationale for giving IG with the vaccine is to provide immediate protection until vaccine-derived immunity takes effect. Most travel medicine physicians, however, now believe that giving immune globulin is unnecessary. The reason is that it takes the hepatitis A virus 2 to 6 weeks to cause clinical infection; vaccine-derived immunity develops in sufficient time to prevent illness—therefore supplemental IG is really not needed. Already in an increasing number of travel clinics, IG (which is often in short supply anyway) is no longer used to protect travelers against hepatitis A.

Vaccination of Children Extensive safety and efficacy studies have not been done on the use of the vaccine in children younger than two years of age; therefore, it is not FDA-approved for this group in the United States. Nevertheless, the vaccine does appear to be effective in infants once they no longer are protected by maternal antibodies against HAV. In cases where the mother has transmitted HAV antibody to the child, this passive immunity wears off in several months, so vaccination of the child is likely to be effective.*

Children still officially too young for HAV are usually given immune globulin (IG), the dose determined by the weight of the child and the length of exposure to hepatitis A. The disadvantage of IG is that it protects for no longer than 6 months. It also interferes with live attenuated virus vaccines such as measles, mumps, rubella, and varicella.

Safe Food and Drink Even if you have been immunized against hepatitis A, follow these rules to reduce your risks of acquiring other infections transmitted by contaminated food and water. This is especially important for pregnant women who may be exposed to hepatitis E:

- Drink only boiled, commercially bottled, carbonated, or chemically treated water, soft drinks, fruit juices, beer, or wine.
- Don't put ice cubes in your drinks unless they have been made from safe water.
- Eat only well-cooked foods. Avoid raw or undercooked meat, fish and shellfish, and raw fruits and vegetables, unless you peel them yourself. Stick to piping hot foods, if possible.
- Avoid salads

Hand hygiene is also very important and effective. Hand washing before meals, or using a hand sanitizer gel such as Purell, not only reduces gastrointestinal disease, but also reduces the transmission of respiratory viruses.

---

*Hepatitis A vaccine is safe in infants younger than 1 year of age, but is effective only after the disappearance of maternal antibodies. Infants vaccinated at 2, 4, and 6 months of age have shown 100% seroconversion, indicating that hepatitis A vaccine (Havrix 360 ELISA Units) is highly immunogenic in seronegative infants and could be included in the routine harmonized infant immunization schedule.

HEPATITIS B

Hepatitis B is important because of its potential severity and widespread occurrence worldwide. Although the hepatitis B virus is not as lethal as the AIDS virus, it is 100 times more infectious and is more easily spread by person-to-person contact.

Acute hepatitis B occurs from 6 weeks to 6 months after exposure, with an average of 75 days. The most common response to the virus is asymptomatic infection, so you may not even be aware of the illness. (Your chance of developing jaundice during the infection is less than 50%.) Whether you are symptomatic or not, your illness may last for several weeks, or even months, but if you are an adult you have a 90% to 95% chance of recovering completely and having lifelong immunity against any further attacks. Hepatitis B, though, differs in an important respect from hepatitis A: there is a 0.1% to 1% risk of death with the acute infection and an overall fatality rate of 1% to 3%. Five percent, or less, of infected adults (but up to 90% of infected newborns) become chronic carriers of the virus. Seniors who become infected also are at greater risk of becoming chronic carriers of the virus. If you do become a carrier of the virus, you can infect others, and you are also at risk for the development of chronic hepatitis, cirrhosis, and liver cancer. In fact, 10% of chronic carriers develop liver cancer.

High-Risk Countries and Exposure to the Virus

Areas where up to 5% to 20% of the population are carriers of the hepatitis B virus include all of sub-Saharan Africa, the Balkans, the Middle East, China, Southeast Asia, including Korea and Indonesia, the South Pacific Islands (Oceania), the interior Amazon Basin, Haiti, and the Dominican Republic. Travelers to these areas are at increased risk if they are exposed to the blood or body fluids of infected people. Sexual contact appears to be the most frequent mode of disease transmission, especially among expatriates staying long term in a risk area. The risk of hepatitis B in expatriates is 1:1,000 per month of stay abroad. Virus transmission also occurs from intravenous drug use, medical injections or vaccinations with contaminated needles and/or syringes, receipt of unscreened blood transfusions, or skin-to-skin contact with carriers of the virus who have open sores caused by tropical ulcers, impetigo, scabies, or infected insect bites. Fluid from these open sores can transmit the virus, and children especially may be at risk from playmates who have these open skin sores.

Diagnosis of Acute and Chronic Hepatitis B Virus (HBV) Infection

Table 12.1 gives a summary of the serologic tests used to evaluate the status of a traveler who may be (1) acutely infected with HBV, (2) chronically infected and a carrier of HBV, or (3) nonimmune and susceptible to infection.

Treatment

The treatment of hepatitis B is summarized subsequently.

Table 12.1 Summary of Serologic Tests for Hepatitis B

Tests	Results	Interpretation
HBsAg	Negative	
Anti-HBc	Negative	Susceptible
Anti-HBs	Negative	
HBsAg	Negative	
Anti-HBc	Negative or positive	Immune
Anti-HBs	Positive	
HBsAg	Positive	
Anti-HBc	Positive	
IgM anti-HBc	Positive	Acutely infected
Anti-HBs	Negative	
HBsAg	Positive	
Anti-HBc	Positive	
IgM anti-HBc	Negative	Chronically infected
Anti-HBs	Negative	
HBsAg	Negative	
Anti-HBc	Positive	Four interpretations possible*
Anti-HBs	Negative	

*Possible interpretations:
1. May be recovering from acute HBV infection
2. May be distantly immune and test not sensitive enough to detect very low level of anti-HBs in serum
3. May be susceptible with a false positive anti-HBc
4. May be undetectable level of HBsAg present in the serum and the person is actually a carrier. HBsAg: If positive, obtain IgM anti-HBc to differentiate acute hepatitis B from chronic hepatitis B. Chronic hepatitis B is also defined by two HbsAg-positive tests separated by at least 6 months.

Prevention

Both hepatitis B immune globulin and vaccination will protect you against hepatitis B. The vaccines available in the United States, Recombivax-HB, Engerix-B, and TwinRix are genetically engineered vaccines derived from yeast. These vaccines are completely safe and virtually 100% effective in those who develop an antibody response after three doses have been administered. About 10% of recipients do not develop measurable antibody levels. Some recipients will develop measurable antibodies from additional, or increased, doses of vaccine.

If you have not been immunized, your risk of getting hepatitis B can also be reduced or eliminated by practicing safe sex or avoiding sexual contact. You should avoid medical injections or surgical procedures in less developed countries, if possible, because the equipment may not be sterile. Consider carrying a sterile needle and syringe kit.

Accelerated Immunization Because most travelers leave within a month after their first travel clinic visit, they may not have enough time to be fully immunized against hepatitis B if it is administered according to the standard schedule (0, 1, and 6 months). Studies have shown, however, that an accelerated vaccination schedule (0, 1, and 2 months or 0, 7, and 21 days) produces measurable antibodies in 80% of recipients by day 28 and more than 90% protection at 3 months. If you are departing on short notice the clinic can administer the vaccine on the accelerated schedule. NOTE: Even a single dose of hepatitis B vaccine may possibly "prime" your immune system and afford some protection. If you have time for only one injection of vaccine before departure, it seems worthwhile to receive it.

Immunization should be considered for the following groups: Frequent short-term travelers or any short-term traveler who engages in risk-taking activity; persons living for prolonged periods (more than 3 months) in endemic areas; adventure travelers; travelers with chronic diseases, especially chronic liver disease; older travelers; people who will have close, prolonged contact with the local population, such as health-care workers, missionaries, and relief workers; travelers who might have sexual contact with the local population; any risk-averse traveler desiring maximum preparation, especially if they are traveling in a country where the sterility of needles and syringes for medical injections cannot be guaranteed and there is the possibility of receiving a dental or medical injection.

Booster Doses Booster doses of vaccine are routinely not recommended for people with healthy immune systems. Studies suggest that about one third of those vaccinated against hepatitis B will no longer have measurable antibodies after 5 years, yet they are still considered to be protected against infection because of the body's "immune memory." For this reason the measurement of hepatitis B neutralizing antibody is not routinely recommended, except in people who are in high-risk occupations, such as health care, who are accidentally exposed to the virus.*

Prevention After Exposure If you are unvaccinated and have blood or body fluid exposure, you should receive hepatitis B immune globulin (HBIG), as well as the vaccine. This should be given within 24 to 48 hours following exposure to blood. If you have sexual exposure, you should receive HBIG plus the vaccine within 14 days of unsafe sexual contact.

---

*Some travelers who were vaccinated in the remote past and who expect possible exposure to HBV (such as a nurse or doctor going to work with refugees) might be given a booster dose without first measuring antibody levels.

HEPATITIS C

Hepatitis C typically does not cause noticeable symptoms when initially acquired. It is usually diagnosed, often by chance years or even decades later. In 80% of those exposed, the infection becomes permanent, these people being "chronic carriers." The carrier state is a persistent, active viral infection (chronic hepatitis C) that damages the liver, progressing over decades in 20% to 50% of carriers to cirrhosis (fibrous scarring of the liver) or, more rarely, liver cancer.

The number of new cases of hepatitis C in developed countries has decreased more than fivefold since the discovery of the hepatitis C virus (HCV). In the 1960s and 1970s, when there was a lot of experimentation with drugs, HCV got into the population that donated blood. Today, when all blood in developed countries is screened for HCV, the most common means of transmission is the sharing of needles by drug users.

In developed countries, HCV is acquired by:

- Intravenous drug use (50% to 60% of cases)
- Sexual contact (10% to 15%). HCV is not spread by sexual contact as efficiently as is HBV or HIV.
- Miscellaneous or unknown causes: Some people are believed to have been exposed while working in a hospital, while receiving hemodialysis, during birth, or by sharing a toothbrush or razor or being exposed in some other way to infected blood. For 10% of people, there is simply no explanation for the infection. One possibility: intranasal cocaine use has recently been associated with HCV infection in persons without other risk factors.

Comparable information on trends of HCV incidence in less developed countries is unavailable. Some less developed countries don't screen blood for HCV, so transfusions in these countries must be avoided, unless the situation is a dire emergency. Needles and syringes may also be contaminated, and you should avoid unnecessary medical injections or other forms of skin puncturing, e.g., acupuncture or tattooing, in these areas.

Treatment of Hepatitis B and C

With either hepatitis B or C, supportive treatment is indicated, but bed rest is neither necessary nor helpful. Your diet should be nutritious, but otherwise can be unrestricted. However, alcohol, the most important factor in disease progression, must be eliminated. Even more damaging is the combination of alcohol and acetaminophen. Even healthy persons who drink moderate amounts of alcohol, perhaps as little as three to four beers or mixed drinks per day for at least several weeks, and who take normally recommended doses of acetaminophen (6 to 8 extra-strength tablets) per day, are at risk for acute toxic hepatitis.

Interferon At this time, interferon α-2b (Intron A, Schering) as well as pegylated interferons are the FDA-approved drugs for the treatment of hepatitis B. About 40% of patients who are HBeAg(+) become HBeAg(−) after 6 months of treatment. Recently, the drug lamivudine has been associated with substantial histologic improvement in many patients with chronic hepatitis B.

Interferon and Ribavirin Three interferons have been approved for treatment of chronic hepatitis C: interferon α-2b (Intron-A, Schering-Plough); interferon α-2a (Roferon, Roche); alfacon-1 (Infergen, Amgen) as well as pegylated interferons (Pegasys and PegIntron). The combination of ribavirin and interferon α-2b (Rebetron, Schering-Plough) has been demonstrated to be superior to interferon α-2b alone. The genotype of hepatitis C determines the duration and response rates with combination treatment. Thirty percent of persons with genotype 1, which accounts for 70% to 80% of persons with HCV infection, remain virus free 6 months after completion of a 12-month course of treatment, whereas more than two thirds of persons with genotype 2 or 3 clear HCV after 6 months of therapy. Liver transplantation is the treatment of last resort for either disease.

Prevention of Hepatitis C

You should avoid unscreened blood transfusions in less developed countries. If a blood transfusion is required, locate a family member or colleague who would be a compatible donor. If a donor is not available, consider medical evacuation to a country with more advanced facilities. Also avoid unsafe sex and the use of potentially contaminated needles and syringes. Persons with hepatitis C should not share toothbrushes or grooming implements, should cover cuts and open sores, and should not donate blood or tissue.

There is no vaccine to prevent hepatitis C and immune globulin is not recommended after exposure. However, HCV carriers should be vaccinated against hepatitis A and hepatitis B because a superimposed infection with either virus can cause further liver damage.

HEPATITIS E

Hepatitis E has many features in common with hepatitis A. They are transmitted by the same route, and in most cases the infection they cause is acute and self-limiting. The hepatitis E virus can be transmitted from person to person, but such secondary transmission is much less common, the incidence being 5% in hepatitis E compared with 50% for hepatitis A. This is probably because larger doses of virus are needed to transmit this disease. Hepatitis E is endemic in many tropical and subtropical countries, with outbreaks being reported in India, Southeast Asia, China, and Russia. No outbreaks have been described in developed countries presumably because water supply and sanitary systems are satisfactory.

Most cases of hepatitis E are reported in young adults, who usually experience mild symptoms, followed by complete recovery. Chronic liver disease does not develop. However, fulminant liver failure, with a mortality rate of 20%, can occur in pregnant women, especially in the third trimester. Infected mothers can also transmit the hepatitis E virus to the fetus with significant consequences.

The risk to the average tourist is quite low, but the data are scarce. The risk to long-term expatriates appears to be higher. A recent study found an overall seroprevalence of 5.2% in development aid workers who lived in various underdeveloped countries for 9 years. The Indian subcontinent showed the highest incidence (10%) of infection.

Infection rates for Latin America, East Africa, West and Central Africa, and Asia ranged between 6% and 9%. The Middle East had a prevalence of 2.1%. Individual countries with the highest risk of acquiring hepatitis E include Burma, Nepal, Pakistan, Sudan, China, and India.

Diagnosis

Hepatitis E should be considered in returned travelers with fever and hepatitis. If tests for other forms of hepatitis are negative, serologic testing for HEV should be done. Information regarding serologic testing can be obtained from the CDC's Hepatitis Branch in Decatur, Georgia (404-371-5910).

Treatment

No specific treatment is available. Follow the same advice as given in this chapter for hepatitis A.

Prevention

A vaccine is not available. If you are in an endemic area, especially a rural area, strictly adhere to food and water precautions, especially if you are pregnant. Avoid untreated tap water, well water, or surface water. If you are treating potentially contaminated water, remember to use a method that eliminates viruses, such as boiling, chemical disinfection, or purification with a water purifier, not a filter. Purifiers, unlike filters, eliminate viruses. Immune globulin is not protective against hepatitis E because the product in this country is not made from donors carrying sufficient antibodies to this virus.

CHAPTER 13

Diabetes

KEY POINTS:

▶ Pre-departure planning is very important for people with diabetes, especially those on insulin.

▶ Crossing more than five time zones may require adjustments in dosages of medications.

▶ When an insulin-dependent diabetic traveler has unpredictable food intake or eating habits, insulin lispro (Humalog) and insulin aspart (Novolog) offer flexibility in that these ultra–short-acting insulins can be timed with meals.

▶ Long-acting insulin glargine, combined with ultra–short-acting insulin lispro or insulin aspart, may provide the best, most convenient control of blood sugar on long-haul flights.

▶ Frequent blood glucose monitoring is the key to good diabetes control.

The thought of traveling with diabetes can discourage the most confident of travelers. Diabetes may not be the ideal travel companion, but with adequate preparation and common sense, the two are very compatible. Anticipating and avoiding common health problems in both tropical and temperate climates, and being able to manage them on your own, will ensure a more pleasurable, healthier journey. Being cavalier and leaving home without the necessary preparation can be fraught with danger, whereas excess caution might lead you to avoid adventurous travel altogether; the appropriate balance is somewhere in between.

Pre-departure Consultation In addition to contacting your primary care provider, it may be advisable to visit a travel medicine specialist 6 to 8 weeks before departure. You may need itinerary-specific advice, and one or more immunizations. Also obtain a summary of your medical history, including allergies. Ask for a signed and dated letter on your physician's letterhead outlining your diabetes care and the need for you to carry medications and injection supplies. This letter will help avoid problems from overly zealous or suspicious customs and security officials. FAA guidelines allow you to board aircraft with insulin pens/needles/syringes if these items are identified with their original pharmaceutical company labels; it is recommended also to bring the packaging with the affixed pharmacy label.

Time Zone Changes If you will be crossing more than five time zones, you may need to modify your insulin or oral medication dosing. Your doctor or diabetes educator can help you plan the dose and timing of the injections. Eastward travel means a shorter day, and less insulin may be needed. Westward travel means a longer day, and more insulin may be needed.

Medications Review Chapter 2 to see which medications are recommended for such illnesses as travelers' diarrhea. Put all medications and glucose-monitoring equipment in your carry-on luggage. Checked bags may be exposed to extremes of temperature, and, most importantly, your luggage may get lost. Although insulin can be stored for 30 days at room temperature, in warm climates you may wish to request a room with a refrigerator or air conditioning. Before using insulin, check vials for signs of damage (crystals, clumps, discoloration, etc.) and discard frozen or damaged vials. Insulin travels well, except above 86° F and below 32° F, so never keep insulin in direct sunlight or on ice. Where temperatures might be an issue, consider carrying an insulated medication kit. These are available from B & A Products: 918-696-5998 and www.baproducts.com. Bring snacks and bottled water in your carry-on luggage in the event of unanticipated delays or a sudden change in plans.

Medical Care Abroad Identification cards and useful phrases in foreign languages (such as "sugar, please") are available from the American Diabetes Association (www.diabetes.com). Information on health-care providers abroad can be obtained from the International Diabetes Federation (www.idf.org) and from the following commercial organizations, which charge a fee or request a donation: The International Association for the Medical Assistance of Travelers (IAMAT: 417 Center Street, Lewiston, NY 14092; 716-754-4883), the International SOS (www.internationalsos.com), and Medex Assistance Corporation (www.medexassist.com).

TRAVEL CHECKLIST

The supplies below are in addition to those basic supplies listed in Chapter 2. NOTE: a small first-aid kit is essential. Be sure to bring blister pads. An infected blister could put your health at risk and possibly spoil some planned activities.

Oral diabetes medication
Other prescription medications
Copies of prescriptions with both brand and generic names
Bottles of each kind of insulin
Syringes
Insulin pen and cartridges
Lancing device or lancets
Blood glucose testing strips
Urine ketone testing strips
Blood glucose meter
Insulin pump supplies
Extra batteries for each device
Alcohol wipes, tissues, cotton balls
Glucagon for injection

Carbohydrate sources (e.g., snacks, glucose gel, Glutose)
Diabetes medical identification/wrist bracelet
Doctor's/clinic telephone number and e-mail address
Pharmacy telephone number
Diabetes travel letter signed by your physician or health-care provider

Further trip preparation checklist guidelines can be found on the website of the American Diabetes Association: www.diabetes.org/pre-diabetes/travel/when-you-travel.jsp

Going Through Airport Security

Notify the screener that you have diabetes and are carrying your supplies with you. The following diabetes-related supplies and equipment are allowed through the checkpoint once they have been screened:

- Insulin and insulin-loaded dispensing products (vials or box of individual vials, jet injectors, pens, infusers, and preloaded syringes) that are clearly identified and labeled
- Unlimited number of unused syringes when accompanied by insulin or other injectable medication
- Lancets, blood glucose meters, blood glucose meter test strips, alcohol swabs, meter-testing solutions
- Insulin pump and insulin pump supplies (cleaning agents, batteries, plastic tubing, infusion kit, catheter, and needle)
- Glucagon emergency kit clearly identified and labeled
- Urine ketone test strips
- Unlimited number of used syringes when transported in sharps disposal container or other similar hard-surface container

Pump Wearers Although insulin pump manufacturers indicate that pumps can safely go through airport security systems, pump wearers may request a visual inspection rather than walking through the metal detector or being hand wanded. Note that this may subject you to closer scrutiny or a "pat-down."

- Advise the screener that the insulin pump cannot be removed because it is connected to a catheter inserted under your skin.
- Insulin pumps and supplies must be accompanied by insulin with a label clearly identifying the medication.

During the Flight

Keep your carry-on bags within easy reach. Show your travel companion, or tour group leader, where your glucose meter and medications for the treatment of hypoglycemia are located. When traveling at altitudes above 8,000 feet, pressure in insulin vials needs to be equalized; be sure to re-equalize the pressures once you are back at sea level. Insert the syringe without the plunger into the vial. Then, withdraw the syringe, replace the plunger, and withdraw insulin as usual. It is not necessary to inject air into the vial at high altitude.

Two health tips to consider during a flight: (1) drink fluids liberally, and (2) exercise frequently to improve lower limb circulation and glucose control. Take a walk around the cabin for at least 10 minutes every two hours, and do isometric exercises such as pressing your toes against the seat in front of you to tighten calf muscles.

Meal Options During Flight Diabetic diets on air flights are quite low in carbohydrates and are designed more for type 2 diabetics. These diets may predispose to hypoglycemia. It is better to order a regular meal and make up for it with insulin rather than run the risk of hypoglycemia from a too-low carbohydrate meal.

Adjusting Insulin Dose and Meal Times Across Time Zones*

One of the more challenging aspects of diabetes management is the problem of travel across many time zones. No alteration in your dose is needed if you are crossing fewer than five times zones, nor does north-south travel require insulin-dosing adjustment.

The goal of control during travel is to avoid extremes—tight control is not the objective. Better to let your glucose level run a bit higher than usual than to suffer a bout of hypoglycemia in a strange land with strange people speaking a strange language. At the risk of being redundant, "monitor, monitor, monitor your blood glucose level!" Even if you don't test frequently at home, you should test your blood every 4 to 6 hours while traveling. This is the only way to determine how travel is affecting you and what adjustments you need to make in diet or insulin dosing. Be aware that glucose meters may be affected by high altitude. Check the manual or contact the customer service toll-free hotline before departure, and be sure to carry an extra battery.

Ultra–short-acting insulin lispro (Humalog) and insulin aspart (Novolog) and long-acting insulin glargine (Lantus) add flexibility to diabetic management. You administer Lantus (insulin glargine) once daily at bedtime, to get a 24-hour basal insulin activity; then, simply administer an ultra–short-acting insulin (either Humalog or Novolog) within 15 minutes before each major meal, or immediately afterward. Figure 13.1 illustrates the more rapid activity of insulin lispro (Humalog) compared with regular insulin.

Complex tables have been published advising diabetics how to administer insulin during a trip, but insulin pumps and the recent availability of ultra–long-acting insulin glargine (Lantus) and the ultra–short-acting insulins—Humalog and Novolog—have simplified matters. You get long-acting baseline control with Lantus and on-the-spot mealtime control with one of the others. Here's how it can work on an eastbound flight lasting about 11 hours. For example, if you fly from San Francisco to Paris (9-hour time difference), departing in the evening, you would

- Take your full 24-hour dose of insulin glargine (Lantus) at 10.00 P.M. (while on the plane).
- The next day, cover your meals with a short-acting insulin, the amount depending on meal size and carbohydrate content.

*See Appendix A for further details on insulin doses and pump management across time zones.

Figure 13.1 Serum Humalog and Insulin Levels After Injection of Human Regular Insulin or Humalog Immediately Before a High-Carbohydrate Meal in a Patient with Type 1 Diabetes

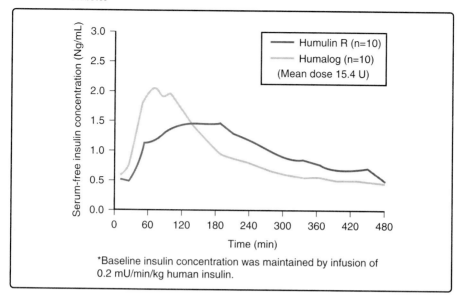

*Baseline insulin concentration was maintained by infusion of 0.2 mU/min/kg human insulin.

- Twenty-four hours later (it is now 7.00 A.M. in Paris), take one half of the insulin glargine dose, and the other one half that evening at 10.00 P.M., thus keeping the 24-hour insulin glargine dose the same.
- The next evening at 10:00 p.m. (the third night), take the full insulin glargine dose.

NOTE: It is best to keep your watch on home time during travel to determine when your meal/insulin doses should be taken. Set your watch on local time the morning after arrival to get in step with meal activities of the destination country. During the flight, administer ultra–short-acting insulin with meals.

An example of a westward-bound flight would be from New Jersey to Honolulu, Hawaii. The flight departs New Jersey at 11:40 A.M., which is 6:40 A.M. in Honolulu (5-hour time difference). It arrives in Honolulu at 10:40 P.M. New Jersey time, which is 5:40 P.M. Honolulu time. Total flight time is 11 hours.

- Take your daily dose of long-acting insulin glargine (Lantus) at 10.00 P.M. the night before departure.
- Adjust for meals with rapid-acting insulin.
- Twenty-four hours later, just before landing in Honolulu at 10.40 P.M. New Jersey time, take one half of your usual dose of insulin glargine
- That night at 10.00 P.M. Honolulu time, take the remaining one half dose of insulin glargine.

Pre-meal coverage with rapid-acting insulin would remain the same, unless you consume extra food during the flight, the amount based on the carbohydrate content of the food and your blood glucose levels.

Oral Medications for Type 2 Diabetes The timing of oral medications for diabetes is not as crucial as that for insulin. If you are on twice-daily metformin (Glucophage), a thiazolidinedione (Actos, Avandia), or a sulfonylurea (e.g., glipizide, Glucotrol) it might be easier to skip a dose if you are on twice-daily dosing; if you are in once-a-day dosing, reduce the dose by one half. It is better to have slight hyperglycemia for 1 to 2 days than to risk low blood sugar. Patients on carbohydrate absorption inhibitors or one of the newer nonsulfonylurea drugs, such as Prandin or Starlix, can continue these drugs as usual.

If you take both insulin and oral diabetes medications, discuss your medications with your health-care provider. Remember that hypoglycemia is what you want to avoid, and that frequent monitoring of blood sugar is key. Hypoglycemia can occur if you do not eat enough or you take too much medication.

After Arrival

Your blood glucose meter is your best travel guide to continued good health, and it is a must because your eating pattern and activity level are likely to be different during travel. You must test your blood glucose level more often to make appropriate adjustments after arrival.

Insulin Abroad Insulin produced in other countries may have reduced purity, and hence reduced activity. Outside of North America, insulin is often dispensed as U80 or U40 concentration, instead of the standard U100. Syringes corresponding to these concentrations may be the only ones available. Read labels carefully to avoid dosing disasters. It is not recommended to use a U100 syringe to draw up U40 or U80 insulin because a very serious dosing error could occur. Also, cartridges and/or pen needles may not be available worldwide. The best safeguard is to bring extra medication and supplies from home.

When going on an outing, always take vital supplies with you regardless of the proposed duration and type of outing. Don't forget bottled water. Try to eat as close to your usual meal plan as possible. Counting carbohydrates and the plate method of meal planning can be especially useful.

Travelers' Diarrhea Although the standard food rules for the prevention of travelers' diarrhea are often impractical, make an effort to avoid the following: raw, undercooked foods (e.g., salads); roadside stands; unpurified water and ice cubes; buffets; and unpasteurized milk products. Every traveler with diabetes should carry an antibiotic (preferably a quinolone) for self treatment of travelers' diarrhea.

Sun Exposure Travel to hot climates brings the risk of sunburn, a particular concern for those with diabetes, because healing is slower and secondary infection is more likely to occur. Wear light colored, cotton clothing and a hat, and use sunscreen (minimum 15 SPF); postpone strenuous activity soon after arrival and drink enough sugar-free fluids to promote urination, whether or not you are thirsty; moderate intake of alcohol and caffeine is acceptable.

Altitude Sickness At high altitudes, hypothermia may be mistaken for hypoglycemia, and vice versa. At about 16,000 feet, retinal hemorrhages may occur, a particular concern for those with preexisting diabetic retinopathy. Altitude sickness, characterized by headache and fatigue, can usually be prevented by slow ascent and dosing with acetazolamide (Diamox).

Foot Care Foot problems can ruin your trip. Never travel with a new pair of shoes that has not been broken in. Take one or more pairs of worn-in walking shoes, slippers for your hotel room, and beach shoes. Avoid pressure points by changing socks and shoes frequently. Inspect feet daily for blisters, redness, and skin breakdown. Never delay treatment of injuries. Never walk barefoot, even on a beach.

Don't forget to review the potential risks of travel medications with your pharmacist or health-care provider: glyburide and doxycycline increase sun sensitivity; chloroquine, quinine, and Pepto-Bismol may increase hypoglycemia; acetazolamide (Diamox) may aggravate hyperglycemia; and antibiotics predispose to vaginal yeast infections. Keep in mind that not taking medication, such as antimalarial medication, may increase your risk of illness, which in turn can cause loss of blood sugar control. In this regard, protection with DEET repellents, permethrin fabric spray, a mosquito bed net, and protective clothing is crucial to the prevention of malaria (transmitted by night-biting mosquitoes) and dengue fever (transmitted by day-biting mosquitoes).

Accidents It is worthwhile to keep in mind that the major cause of preventable death during travel is not an infectious disease such as malaria, cholera, or Ebola virus. A motor vehicle accident is a much more likely cause. Your risk of an accident is increased overseas (especially in less developed countries) because of poor road conditions, poorly maintained vehicles (often without seat belts), inexperienced and/or reckless drivers, and a general disregard for rules of the road. Here are three important safety tips to remember: don't ride on motorcycles; don't travel in overcrowded public vehicles; and never travel by road at night in rural areas.

The vast majority of diabetic travelers return safe and sound from their trips. Remember that healthy, comfortable travel is enhanced by adherence to common sense precautions with respect to food, water, insect bites, safe sex, and road travel, as well as close attention to diabetic control.

CHAPTER 14

HIV/AIDS and Sexually Transmitted Diseases (STDs)

KEY POINTS:

▶ AIDS and HIV infections occur worldwide and the true number of cases is likely far greater than officially reported.

▶ The risk for a traveler of acquiring HIV, however, is statistically very low.

▶ The chances for acquiring HIV is determined primarily by a traveler's lifestyle.

▶ Unprotected sex with a high-risk partner and injecting drug use account for most cases of AIDS.

▶ Unscreened blood transfusions and medical injections with nonsterile equipment can also transmit HIV, but these are largely avoidable.

▶ Mosquitoes cannot transmit HIV.

▶ Some countries require an HIV test for entry, but these tests are usually reserved for long-stay travelers and immigrants.

▶ India, Russia, eastern Europe, and the Caribbean have the fastest growing incidences of AIDS and HIV.

Overview of HIV and AIDS

The development of AIDS should not be a primary concern for the traveler. However, there may be a concern for a subset of travelers who may be exposed to HIV, the virus that causes AIDS, through contact with another person's body fluids or blood. Although travel has contributed in a general way to the global spread of AIDS, fear of traveling because of this disease is not warranted.

What are HIV and AIDS?

The acquired immunodeficiency syndrome (AIDS) was first recognized in 1981 and has since become a major worldwide epidemic. AIDS is caused by infection with HIV—the human immunodeficiency virus. This virus causes the destruction and/or impairment of the body's immune system. It takes months to years before HIV impairs the immune system sufficiently to cause the symptoms of AIDS.*

The HIV virus is commonly transmitted by:

- Having unprotected vaginal or anal sex with an infected person. (There is less risk from oral sex.) The virus can enter the body through the breakage of any mucous membrane of the vagina, vulva, penis, rectum, or mouth. This is the most common pathway through which at-risk travelers acquire HIV, and they may not be aware of the risk.
- Sharing needles or syringes for injecting drugs with an infected person
- Less commonly, HIV is transmitted by
  - Accidental contact with infected blood. This is often an occupational exposure in a medical worker, such as a splash on an open cut or wound, or an accidental needle stick.†
  - Transfusion of contaminated blood or blood products. Some blood banks in less developed countries do not screen blood for the AIDS virus.
  - An unsafe medical injection or surgical/dental procedure using nonsterile equipment. Many less developed countries recycle needles and syringes, which may be contaminated with HIV (as well as hepatitis viruses).
  - Acupuncture, tattoos, or body piercing with nonsterile needles

AN OVERVIEW OF HIV/AIDS WORLDWIDE

HIV/AIDS in the United States, Canada, Western Europe, Australia, and New Zealand

In these countries, AIDS is still largely a disease of men who have sex with men (MSM) and urban drug users, with the rates of HIV and AIDS increasing in the female partners of bisexuals and injecting drug users. In the United States, the epidemic is growing most rapidly among minority populations and is a leading killer of African-American males.

HIV/AIDS in Latin America and the Caribbean

AIDS is spreading rapidly in Latin America, the Bahamas, and the Caribbean. HIV is spilling over to women from infected bisexuals and intravenous drug abusers, and through drug-related commercial sex.

HIV/AIDS in the Middle East and North Africa

Only small numbers of cases are reported in the Middle East, and these are mostly in people returning from areas with higher infection rates. In these countries, the generally conservative social and political attitudes tend to make it difficult to address risk behavior directly, or discuss it.

---

*AIDS is the end result of HIV infection. It generally occurs when the concentration of immune T cells (CD4+ T cells) falls below 200 per cubic milliliter of blood, and is characterized by the appearance of unusual infections and certain cancers. These include: *Pneumocystis jiroveci* pneumonia; toxoplasmosis; tuberculosis; extreme weight loss and wasting, often exacerbated by diarrhea; fungal infections, including meningitis; syphilis; malignancies such as lymphoma, cervical cancer, and Kaposi's sarcoma, which affects the skin and mouth, and may spread elsewhere—it can occur in earlier stages of HIV as well.
†Compared with the hepatitis B and C viruses, the human immunodeficiency virus is much less infectious. For example, the chance of getting hepatitis B from a contaminated needle stick is about 1 in 3, from hepatitis C, 1 in 10, and from HIV, 1 in 200 to 300.

HIV/AIDS in Russia, Eastern Europe, and Central Asia

The countries most affected are the Russian Federation, Ukraine, and the Baltic states (Estonia, Latvia, and Lithuania), but HIV continues to spread in Belarus, Moldova, and Kazakhstan, whereas more recent epidemics are now evident in Kyrgyzstan and Uzbekistan. Driving these epidemics is a widespread change in behaviors—increasing injecting drug use and unsafe sex—especially among young people. Drug abuse is rampant, especially in Russia, and is still the main route of HIV transmission, but the spread of the disease has now reached a critical point: the virus is moving from high-risk groups such as drug users, sex workers, and prisoners to a bridge population—the wives of convicts and the partners of drug abusers, and into the general population. The forecast is that the epidemic will then progress by the same pattern as in Africa, where HIV is contracted primarily through heterosexual sex.

HIV/AIDS in Sub-Saharan Africa

In sub-Saharan Africa, AIDS is a devastating problem. In the "AIDS-belt"—countries of central and east Africa—the infection is spread primarily through heterosexual intercourse, and men and women are infected almost equally. In many urban areas, 30% or more of sexually active people carry HIV and up to 90% of commercial sex workers are infected. Four out of five HIV-positive women in the world live in Africa. The factors behind the epidemic in Africa include:

- Multiple sexual partners—There is widespread, culturally tolerated male promiscuity in many countries.
- Commercial sex—As many as 90% of commercial sex workers in the larger cities in sub-Saharan Africa are HIV infected.
- Widespread incidence of sexually transmitted diseases—These diseases greatly enhance the transmission of the HIV virus.
- Social resistance to the use of condoms and lack of effective public health programs directed against HIV/AIDS and other sexually transmitted diseases thwart containment.
- Contaminated needles and syringes—Few countries can afford sterile, disposable supplies for safe injections. Needles and syringes are often reused, a problem common to almost all less developed countries.
- Blood transfusions—Some countries do not have the means to screen blood for HIV (as well as hepatitis B and C viruses).

  The social implications of the AIDS epidemic in Africa are profound and affect other countries as well. The shrinkage of the adult population in sub-Saharan Africa presents increasing social and security problems. The absence of adults in communities, including the parents, police, teachers, laborers, doctors, nurses, and many others of the middle class, invites economic chaos, social disorder, the rise of demagogues, and increased regional instability. Many of these conditions already exist in some pockets in Africa. AIDS orphans, or children without their parents who have died from AIDS, are a growing problem in these areas.

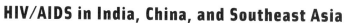

HIV/AIDS in India, China, and Southeast Asia

The AIDS epidemic in India is expanding rapidly. It is estimated that more than four million people are living with HIV, which makes India the country with the largest number of HIV-infected people in the world. HIV has spread beyond high-risk groups and is now firmly embedded in the Indian population and is fast spreading into rural areas. Between 30% and 60% of commercial sex workers and 15% of truck drivers are infected with HIV or have AIDS. Sex workers continue to play a critical part in the heterosexual spread of HIV, which is the dominant mode of transmission in India, except in two regions (Nagaland and Manipur) where intravenous drug use is widespread. Another mode of transmission is through contaminated blood and blood products and nonsterile needles and syringes. Children sold into prostitution are yet another avenue for the transmission of the HIV virus.

Figure 14.1   AIDS Belt Countries in sub-Saharan Africa

AFRICA'S AIDS BELT

Region where AIDS is most prevalent → The outward spread of AIDS to neighboring countries

NIGER
CHAD
SUDAN
NIGERIA
SOMALIA
CENTRAL AFRICAN REPUBLIC
ETHIOPIA
CAMEROON
EQUATORIAL GUINEA
UGANDA
GABON
CONGO
KENYA
RWANDA
ZAIRE
BURUNDI
TANZANIA
ANGOLA
MALAWI
ZAMBIA
MOZAMBIQUE
ZIMBABWE
NAMIBIA
BOTSWANA

No AIDS cases were reported in China until 1988, when an outbreak was reported among the tribesmen of the Yunnan Province in the western part of the country, bordering the "Golden Triangle." The government of China estimated that at the end of 1996 as many as 200,000 people were living with HIV/AIDS. It is estimated that this figure had doubled by the beginning of 1998. The increase in injecting drug use, particularly in the Southwest, and the increase in commercial sex on the eastern seaboard are primarily responsible.

In Thailand infection rates among drug users increased from 1% to 43% between 1987 and 1998. Up to 70% of rural commercial sex workers in Thailand are now infected, and spillover into the heterosexual population is occurring, causing a serious public health problem. The Thai government has begun to formally address these issues in ways in which it has not been addressed in many other countries.

HIV/AIDS in the Philippines, Korea, Indonesia, Japan, and Oceania

At present, the incidence of AIDS in these regions is still low, although spread into the heterosexual population is a threat wherever commercial sex is widespread.

PREVENTING HIV TRANSMISSION

Travelers can virtually eliminate the possibility of becoming infected with HIV if they are not sexually active, or are in a monogamous relationship with an uninfected partner or spouse, and are not injecting drug users. Many travelers, however, do have sex with new acquaintances, even strangers. What is their risk of acquiring HIV? As shown earlier, some countries have a much higher incidence of HIV/AIDS than others; so being in certain geographic areas may automatically put them at a higher risk. But what other factors are involved? Just how risky is sex?

As a starting point, one may ask: What is the estimated risk in the United States for acquiring HIV by vaginal intercourse? The actual risk throughout the general population is statistically low. Researchers estimate that the odds are 5 million to 1 against acquiring HIV after a single act of unprotected vaginal sex with a "low-risk" partner. The per-event, male-to-female HIV transmission rate is about 1 in 1,000 with a "high-risk partner" and 1 in 500 if the partner is HIV-positive. Condoms will reduce transmission tenfold. These statistics are reassuring because they demonstrate that it is relatively difficult to acquire HIV from random sex with people in populations deemed to be "low-risk." But there is a significant flaw in these numbers—statistics can mislead. It is still possible to transmit HIV from a single act of unprotected intercourse. And the traveler may be among a "high-risk" population. Indeed, studies have shown that frequent travelers do represent a higher risk group. In some cases, travelers had rates of HIV that were 50 to 500 times the rate in their home countries. Travelers may engage in behaviors while traveling that they would not engage in at home. In addition, although travelers may not engage in casual and unprotected sex with a commercial sex worker, they may do so with a new acquaintance who they deem is from a similar socioeconomic and educational background. Unfortunately, this is poor judgment. Therefore, the only way to really protect oneself is to take preventive measures, which include:

- Avoid sex with high-risk partners.
- Use a condom, or insist on condom use.

What is a high-risk partner? In general, it is someone who is sexually active with many people (i.e., promiscuous), or is an injecting drug user, or is someone who is, or has been, a partner of a high-risk individual. In addition, anyone with an STD (later) should be considered high risk, as well as uncircumcised males; they have a greater chance of being infected with HIV. Also, some people with HIV may be much more infectious than others with this disease. For example, if your partner has a newly-acquired HIV infection, there is much more HIV virus in his/her blood and body fluids than during a later phase of infection; and if you happen to have an open sore in your mouth or on your genitals, you are much more susceptible to getting infected.

If you do have unprotected sex, having a low-risk partner is safer, but it is rare that you can feel certain about the safety of a casual acquaintance. When you met, were you under the influence of alcohol? Or drugs? Many people, whether heterosexual, homosexual, or bisexual, don't practice safe sex, may not tell the truth about it, and don't reveal their sexual orientation. Your intuitive sense about the safety of the relationship may be misleading. Asking a new acquaintance about his or her past sexual habits or drug use may not be adequate. In fact, the *Archives of Internal Medicine* (1998) reports that of 203 consecutive HIV-positive patients at two U.S. hospitals, 40% had not told their partners, and nearly two thirds of them had not always used a condom. People with multiple partners, homosexual and heterosexual, were three times less likely to reveal their HIV status than those with one partner.

Condoms You should always use a condom, or insist one be used, for anal, oral, and vaginal intercourse. But how effective are they? Simply put, very effective, but not 100% effective. A study published in 1994 in *The New England Journal of Medicine* looked at 256 heterosexual HIV-discordant couples (i.e., one partner is HIV negative and the other is HIV positive). Of the 124 couples that consistently used condoms, none of the HIV-negative partners in the study became infected. Among the 121 couples that did not consistently use condoms, 12 (about 10 percent) of the HIV-negative partners became infected. This is not to say that a condom cannot break or slip off, but considering that semen (and pre-ejaculatory fluid) has the greatest concentration of HIV of any body fluid, the use of condoms is highly logical.

There are many ways in which HIV can be spread, but first you should realize that HIV is not spread by

- Casual contact at work or school
- Touching or hugging
- Handshakes
- Coughs or sneezes
- Insect or mosquito bites
- Food or water
- Eating utensils, cups, plates
- Toilets
- Swimming pools or baths

Spermicides and Diaphragms A female should also use a diaphragm along with a spermicidal jelly; this further protects the cervix and uterus from HIV (but not the vaginal walls). Condoms, diaphragms (or cervical caps), and spermicidal jellies, used together, also help prevent other sexually transmitted diseases, as well as pregnancy. NOTE: Used by *themselves*, contraceptive jellies *may not prevent pregnancy* and probably are not effective in preventing HIV transmission. Diaphragms and spermicidal jelly, used together, somewhat reduce the risk of a sexually transmitted infection, but not as effectively as condoms.

NOTE: Women taking oral contraceptives have a lower risk of HIV transmission. Women who have unprotected sex, who are using IUDs, have a higher risk of HIV transmission. Men who are circumcised have a lower risk of acquiring HIV.

> With HIV, a single act of unprotected vaginal or rectal intercourse *may* be sufficient for transmission. It is believed, however, that in the majority of cases, repeated exposure to the virus through multiple acts of intercourse is necessary for transmission to take place.

Emergency Prevention

Postexposure Prophylaxis for HIV People exposed to the AIDS virus through a lapse in safe sex or drug-use behavior, or are exposed through sexual assault or accidents, or who experience condom slippage with a partner who is HIV positive can receive emergency prophylaxis with a combination of three antiretroviral drugs. This complex "morning-after pill" regimen must be started within 72 hours of exposure and taken for 28 days. It should not be considered a substitute for abstinence, safe sex, mutual monogamy, consistent condom use, or sterile needles. Choices of drugs include the three-drug combinations of antiretroviral medications recommended by the U.S. Department of Health and Human Services, except those containing nevirapine, which has been associated with severe reactions and liver damage. Medical attention should be sought immediately should postexposure prevention be required.

HIV TESTING AND FOREIGN TRAVEL

In most countries, tourists staying less than 1 month do not need to show evidence of an HIV test. But dozens of countries—including the United States—do require an HIV test for those coming to study, work, reside for long periods, or apply for immigrant status.* Under these rules, those who test HIV positive usually are denied entry, although sometimes a waiver may be issued. Countries that screen immigrants for HIV include Argentina, China, Colombia, Costa Rica, Cuba, Hungary, Iraq, Israel, Mongolia, Myanmar (Burma), the Philippines, Russia, South Africa, South Korea, Syria, Thailand, and the United Kingdom. Furthermore, several countries have policies of rejecting or expelling all foreigners with AIDS. Among those countries are Indonesia, Malaysia, Sri Lanka, and Thailand. Policies tend to change; seeking information from the United States Department of State website (see later) is useful.

*According to the U.S. Department of State "Travelers to the United States who are HIV positive are not eligible, under current United States visa law, to travel visa free under the Visa Waiver Program. They are required to apply for a visa and a waiver of the ineligibility before traveling."

Sometimes visa forms ask whether a visitor has any infectious or communicable diseases, so if you are HIV positive, be prepared for this question—and rejection of the application if you answer truthfully. The World Health Organization regards HIV screening as discriminatory and unnecessary from a public health perspective.

For the most current HIV testing requirements for foreign travel, go to the Bureau of Consular Affairs website at www.travel.state.gov. Click on "International Travel" then on the side bar, open "Travel Brochures." Scroll down to "Human Immunodeficiency Testing Requirements for Entry into Foreign Countries." This information may also be found at www.thebody.com/state_dept/entry.html. To confirm requirements, telephone the country's consulate in the United States because these requirements may change. Some of the countries requiring testing will accept a test done in the United States. If you need a test, contact the country's nearest consulate to find out which laboratories in the United States can perform the test and how the results are authenticated and certified. You want to avoid, if possible, having your blood drawn overseas. Consider carrying sterile, disposable needles and syringes with you if you anticipate overseas testing. If you will be tested overseas, call the U.S. embassy in the country of your destination to inquire about the safety of a test done locally and if sterile needles are used.

Be aware that a country's announced policy and what actually happens may differ. Random testing may also be performed. Also, travelers found carrying an anti-HIV drug, such as AZT, may be turned away.

SEXUALLY TRANSMITTED DISEASES (STDs)

In addition to HIV, other STDs may be acquired from unsafe sex. Risky behavior relates to the number of sexual exposures, number of different partners and/or anonymous partners (e.g., commercial sex workers), anal intercourse (especially MSM—men having sex with men), and use (or nonuse) of condoms. Having another sexually transmitted disease greatly increases the risk of HIV transmission.

Causes of STDs

Sexually transmitted diseases can be caused by bacteria, fungi, parasites, and viruses. Some STDs can be spread by kissing and mouth-to-genital contact (e.g., herpes and genital warts).

Bacteria-Caused STDs

- Gonorrhea; syphilis; chancroid
- Chlamydia infections (urethritis, lymphogranuloma venereum)
- *Shigella, Salmonella*, or other bacteria transmitted, often transmitted by MSM

Virus-Caused STDs

- AIDS; hepatitis B; hepatitis C
- Hepatitis A (oral-anal contact)
- Genital herpes; genital warts

Parasite (protozoa)-Caused STDs

- *Giardia, Isospora, Cryptosporidium, Entamoeba histolytica,* or other parasites, especially in MSM
- Vaginal or urethral infections caused by *Trichomonas*

Symptoms of STDs

The most common STDs infections in the United States are caused by gonococcus and chlamydia, and by the herpes virus, but statistics are lacking about the extent and type of STDs occurring in travelers. In those with gonorrhea or genital herpes, symptoms usually occur 4 to 10 days after exposure, and the association with travel would be obvious. Diseases that have much longer incubation periods, such as hepatitis, may not be recognized as being travel related because their symptoms may occur well after the traveler has returned home.

Pelvic Inflammatory Disease Women who develop lower abdominal pain, vaginal discharge, and fever should be examined for the possibility of pelvic inflammatory disease (PID), which is an infection of the uterus and/or fallopian tubes. This is often a mixed infection, usually caused by gonococci and/or chlamydia, along with other bacteria. Bear in mind that appendicitis; an ovarian cyst; and even an ectopic pregnancy can mimic PID, so a precise diagnosis is important.

If you notice any ulcers or sores on your genitals—herpes, syphilis, or chancroid may be the cause. A painless ulcer may indicate syphilis, whereas herpetic ulcers are usually shallow and quite painful. These lesions require a specific diagnosis for appropriate treatment. Be sure to seek qualified medical care.

Several regimens are available for the treatment of uncomplicated PID:

- A 250-mg injection of ceftriaxone (Rocephin) plus a 14-day course of doxycycline, 100 mg twice daily (or tetracycline, 500 mg four times daily), plus metronidazole (Flagyl), 500 mg twice daily for 14 days.
- Ofloxacin (Floxin) 400 mg twice daily for 14 days (or levofloxacin 500 mg daily), plus metronidazole 500 mg twice daily for 14 days.

Gonorrhea in Men For the treatment of gonorrhea in men, a coinfection with chlamydia must be considered. Use either of the above treatments, but without metronidazole. Oral therapy for 7 days is sufficient.

A single 1-gm oral dose of azithromycin is effective against both gonorrhea and chlamydia. It is easier to administer and there are fewer problems with compliance.

Quinolone-Resistant Gonorrhea Quinolones are no longer recommended for gonorrhea in Hawaii or California, or for patients who may have acquired their infections in Asia or the Pacific. In other areas, a regimen of levofloxacin, 500 mg daily for 7 days is effective.

Treatment During Pregnancy If you are pregnant and have PID, you can safely be treated with ceftriaxone or procaine penicillin plus Benemid. These are often administered with azithromycin, 500 mg daily for 3 days, to eliminate chlamydia. Avoid the quinolones when alternative drugs (as earlier) are available.

Post-Treatment Follow-Up If you were treated for gonorrhea or PID while traveling, you should contact your physician when you return home. Women should have follow-up cultures of the cervix to see if they are still carrying gonorrhea and/or chlamydia. Both men and women should have blood tests to check for syphilis and should be screened for HIV infection (as well as hepatitis B and perhaps other infections as well). HIV screening tests may not be positive for 12 weeks or longer after exposure. Early diagnosis of HIV infection is important because early, aggressive anti-HIV therapy with antiretroviral drugs may preserve crucial components of the immune system. NOTE: There is also an FDA-approved home HIV test, made by Home Access, which is similar to the test done in hospitals. It is sold in most drug stores and can be ordered by phone (800-HIV-TEST) or online (www.homeaccess.com).

Prevention of STDs

Follow the same prevention guidelines as for HIV (pages 210-212).

CHAPTER 15

Altitude Illness

▶ Acute mountain sickness (AMS) is common, affecting up to 40% of travelers at moderate altitudes (up to 10,000 feet).

▶ Headache is the most common symptom of AMS.

▶ Acute pulmonary edema is the most common cause of death from altitude illness.

▶ Travelers should never continue ascending if they have any symptoms of altitude illness.

▶ Descent is the most reliable treatment for any type of altitude illness.

▶ Ascending to moderate altitude appears to entail little risk for people with stable coronary artery disease.

The term "altitude illness" describes disorders affecting the brain and the lung that can occur after a climber ascends to altitudes over 8,000 feet (2,500 meters).

The most common altitude-related disorder is acute mountain sickness (AMS), which affects the brain. The hallmark of AMS is headache and the AMS syndrome has been defined as the presence of headache in an unacclimatized person who has recently arrived at an altitude above 2,500 meters plus the presence of one or more of the following symptoms: loss of appetite, nausea, vomiting, fatigue, dizziness, or insomnia. The headache is dull and throbbing, worse during the night and in the morning, and increased by straining or bending over. AMS symptoms typically develop within 6 to 10 hours (but sometimes as soon as 1 hour); attain maximum severity within 1 to 2 days, and begin to decrease about the third day—provided additional ascent does not occur. AMS represents one end of the spectrum of altitude illness affecting the brain: it can progress to high-altitude cerebral edema (HACE), a life-threatening form of altitude illness.

High-altitude pulmonary edema (HAPE) affects the lung. It is less common than AMS, but accounts for most deaths from high-altitude illness. HAPE often occurs in someone already suffering from AMS. In fact, 50% of climbers with high-altitude pulmonary edema have acute mountain sickness and 14% have high-altitude cerebral edema.

Incidence of AMS

The incidence of altitude illness depends on the altitude reached, the rate of ascent, and individual susceptibility. AMS occurs in 22% of adults ascending to 7,000 to 9,000 feet; 42% going to 10,000 feet, and approximately three fourths going to 15,000 feet. One study in Nepal showed an attack rate of 58% among trekkers who were ascending to 16,000 feet and also sleeping at high altitudes. A special cohort of potential victims are climbers ascending to, and often staying at, very high (12,000 to 18,000 feet) and extremely high altitudes (18,000+ feet). About 8% of the climbers who develop AMS at higher than 15,000 feet go on to develop cerebral and/or pulmonary edema.

Factors That Increase Your Chance of Getting AMS

Susceptibility to AMS can vary over time. Previous ability to ascend to high altitudes without getting AMS is no guarantee you won't become afflicted in the future, but if you have been to a certain altitude before with no problems, you probably can return to that altitude without developing symptoms as long as you acclimatize properly. Risk factors for AMS include the following:

- Fast ascent (more than 3,000 feet/day)
- Altitude reached, especially a sleeping altitude over 10,000 feet
- Strenuous exertion at high altitudes
- Age younger than 50 years
- Time spent at high altitudes
- History of high-altitude illness (the most important risk factor)
- Not becoming sufficiently acclimatized

Factors NOT Associated with—or Not Protective Against—AMS

- Previous high-altitude experience
- Smoking
- Younger age
- Gender
- Pre-ascent training
- Good physical condition

It may seem surprising that good physical condition does not prevent AMS, but young, fit persons often go higher and faster than others and they also engage in more strenuous activity at high altitudes. Although smoking is not a risk factor for AMS, smokers may have less physical endurance than nonsmokers. Common conditions such as hypertension, coronary artery disease, mild, chronic obstructive pulmonary disease (COPD), diabetes, and pregnancy do not appear to affect susceptibility to high-altitude illness.

Normal Symptoms at High Altitude

Shortness of Breath on Exertion Shortness of breath (dyspnea) on exertion is normal for anyone exercising at high altitudes. If dyspnea occurs at rest, however, high altitude pulmonary edema should be considered.

Frequent Nocturnal Awakening This often occurs because of periodic breathing (see later) or the need to urinate.

Edema of Altitude Edema of the extremities and face because of fluid retention can occur as an isolated finding without symptoms of AMS. It responds to diuretics, dexamethasone, and descent.

Periodic Breathing Periodic breathing during sleep occurs normally at high altitudes. It is characterized by periods of rapid, deep breathing followed by slowing of respiration, then complete cessation of respiration (apnea). The period of apnea may last 10 to 15 seconds before breathing resumes and the cycle starts over. This can be quite startling to observe because the person really does (briefly) stop breathing. It occurs in everyone above their personal altitude "threshold." The degree (severity) of periodic breathing is genetically determined. Acetazolamide (see page 220) reduces periodic breathing, which improves oxygenation and reduces the risk of AMS.

Hypoxic Ventilatory Response (HVR)

What is HVR? Simply put, it is the increase in breathing that occurs when you're not getting enough oxygen. A person with a lower hypoxic ventilatory response is more likely to suffer AMS, HACE, and HAPE than those with a high HVR. The HVR is controlled by a receptor (the carotid body) located in the carotid artery in your neck, and it signals the respiratory center in your brain to increase ventilation when it detects hypoxia. The increased rate and depth of respiration blow off carbon dioxide from your blood, allowing for a corresponding increase in arterial oxygen. Persons who have a sluggish HVR and who under-ventilate remain more hypoxic, especially during sleep. Adverse effects of hypoxia include increased cerebral blood flow triggering cerebral edema, pulmonary vasoconstriction and increased pulmonary artery pressure, and increased water retention by the kidney.

Causes of AMS

The physiologic changes that occur during ascent to high altitudes are complex, and there is considerable variation in how each individual responds. Perhaps the most important change that occurs is the increase in blood flow to the brain. The resulting rise in cerebral artery capillary pressure, in association with hypoxia, results in fluid leakage across the blood-brain barrier, and the resulting increase in brain water is termed vasogenic cerebral edema. This process appears to be the critical step in the genesis of AMS and the syndrome of HACE.

Facts About AMS

- Of all the organs, the brain seems to be most vulnerable to the hypoxia of high altitudes, particularly extreme altitudes.
- The dilation of the cerebral arteries caused by hypoxia is lessened by the constricting effect on the arteries caused by hypocapnea (low arterial carbon dioxide). Overall oxygen delivery to the brain is a result of the balance between vasodilation and vasoconstriction. In general, vasodilation overrides vasoconstriction.
- The combination of increased cerebral blood flow and hypoxia can lead to vasogenic cerebral edema (as described).
- Increased cerebral blood flow can also cause brain swelling from engorgement of the brain with blood.
- All brains swell on ascent to high altitudes—either as a result of cerebral edema and/or engorgement with blood, but not all climbers develop AMS.

218

- According to the "tight fit" hypothesis, cranial anatomy determines who might develop AMS. In climbers who remain relatively asymptomatic, the brain volume increase and corresponding rise in intracranial pressure are "buffered" by decreased intracranial blood flow (from vasoconstriction) as well as increased displacement of cerebral spinal fluid out of the skull.
- If buffering is unsuccessful, cerebral edema and intracranial pressure continue to rise, resulting in the symptoms of AMS.
- AMS can evolve into high HACE. HACE strikes only a minority of climbers, usually those at extreme altitudes.
- Cases of mild AMS are probably caused by early cerebral edema.
- There is a hazy line between moderate-to-severe AMS and HACE. Symptoms of more severe AMS include unrelieved headache, decreased urine output, vomiting, and lethargy—but not the loss of balance (ataxia) and the mental confusion or coma that define HACE.

High-Altitude Cerebral Edema

This is the most severe form of AMS. At this stage, significant brain edema and increased intracranial pressure have developed. HACE can be preceded by symptoms of AMS or occur suddenly. Symptoms include confusion, disorientation, irrational behavior, lethargy, and especially, ataxia. Nausea and vomiting may be severe. The progression from initial symptoms to coma may take as little as 12 hours. Death follows if early treatment is not administered.

High-Altitude Pulmonary Edema

The second organ of the body most affected by hypoxia is the lung, but the cause of high-altitude pulmonary edema is completely different from AMS and HACE. Basically, in HAPE, a high-pressure fluid leak occurs in the lung. Here's the mechanism: Hypoxia causes pulmonary artery vasoconstriction and an elevation of pulmonary artery pressure. The vasoconstriction, however, is unevenly distributed throughout the lung, and those regions of lung tissue less constricted become overperfused with blood, resulting in regional elevations of pulmonary capillary pressure. The increased capillary pressure forces water and proteins through the capillary walls into the pulmonary air spaces, resulting in pulmonary edema (high-pressure overperfusion edema). The flooding of these patchy areas of lung tissue further reduces oxygen delivery to the blood, further increasing hypoxia.

Persons who have a low hypoxic ventilatory response (HVR) have more pulmonary hypertension and are more susceptible to HAPE. More importantly, a low HVR may permit extreme hypoxemia during sleep, explaining why HAPE often strikes in the middle of the night. In addition, persons susceptible to HAPE have other genetic differences; for example, their production of nitric oxide (a chemical that dilates arteries) in the lung is diminished.

HAPE usually occurs after a rapid, strenuous ascent to high or very high altitudes and staying there. The early symptoms of HAPE are breathlessness on exertion and reduced exercise tolerance, greater than expected for the altitude. Untreated, there is progression to breathlessness at rest, especially at night, and persistent cough. The cough can be dry or progress to produce white, watery, or frothy fluid. Severe fatigue or exercise intolerance is nearly universal and may be the most reliable hallmark of HAPE. The most reliable combination of diagnostic signs and symptoms is dry cough and fatigue plus lung crackles and oxygen desaturation (measured with a pulse oximeter and more pronounced than calculated for the altitude) or tachycardia and increased oxygen desaturation.

HAPE strikes 1% to 2% of those who travel above 12,000 feet. (Fatal cases, however, have occurred as low as 8,000 feet.) HAPE kills more travelers each year than any other altitude-related condition but is reversible if recognized early and treated properly. At increased risk are those who have previously experienced HAPE; they have a 60% chance of recurrence during another exposure to high altitudes.

Reducing the Risks of AMS and HAPE

Reduce Activity If you travel rapidly to an elevation higher than 8,000 feet (2,500 meters), you can reduce your chance of illness by not engaging in strenuous activity for the first 2 days.

Acclimatize The major cause of altitude sickness is going too high too fast. You can avoid or lessen AMS by making a slow, gradual ascent. Slow ascent means not increasing your sleeping altitude by over 2,000 to 3,000 feet (600 to 900 meters) on successive nights, especially when climbing above 10,000 feet. An alternate strategy, called staging, is to spend 2 to 3 days at an intermediate altitude (e.g., 8,000 to 10,000 feet) before resuming ascent. Every 3,000 to 4,000 feet thereafter, you should stop for a day to acclimatize further. In addition, no matter how high you are climbing during the day, try to sleep at a lower altitude, if this is an option.

Unfortunately, cautious guidelines on the rate of ascent are impractical for most climbers. For example, if you were to climb Mt. Kilimanjaro on a guided tour, you would find yourself ascending on a schedule that forces you to sleep at much higher altitudes each successive night. You begin the climb at 5,000 feet. The huts where you sleep are at 9,000, 12,000, and 14,500 feet. Only a single rest day is spent (sometimes) at the highest hut before the final ascent to the 19,000-foot summit the following morning. Needless to say, AMS is a frequent occurrence among those climbing Mt. Kilimanjaro.

Take a Prophylactic Drug In situations where you are going rapidly to altitudes above 8,000 feet, or arriving by airplane at a high destination (Table 15.1), there are two drugs that can help: (1) acetazolamide, which accelerates acclimatization; and (2) dexamethasone, which reduces symptoms, but has no effect on acclimatization itself. Prophylaxis is especially important if you have previously experienced altitude sickness, but drug prophylaxis isn't uniformly recommended by some experts for those who plan a reasonably slow ascent schedule to moderate altitudes. The problem here is: How many people actually practice *slow ascent*?

Acetazolamide (Diamox)—Acetazolamide has been shown to reduce susceptibility to AMS and the incidences of HAPE and HACE. This is the drug of choice for preventing AMS. Acetazolamide works through several mechanisms: (1) It forces the

Table 15.1   AMS Treatment Options

Descent
Pro   Rapid recovery patients generally improve during descent; recover totally within several hours.
Con   Loss of progress toward summit or trek goal; descent may be difficult in bad weather or at night; personnel need to accompany patient.
Rest at same elevation
Pro   Acclimatization to current altitude; no loss of forward progress
Con   It may take 24-48 hours to become symptom free; condition of climber may deteriorate.
Rest plus acetazolamide
Pro   Benefits of rest alone, plus acclimatization is accelerated; recovery is likely within 12-24 hours.
Con   Recovery may take 12-24 hours.
Rest plus dexamethasone
Pro   Benefits of rest alone, plus recovery of moderate AMS in 2-6 hours. This protocol is essentially as rapid as descent, without the walk.
Con   Potential for steroid side effects (unlikely)
Rest plus acetazolamide plus dexamethasone
Pro   Benefits of rest alone, plus acceleration of acclimatization and resolution of pathology
Con   Probably treatment of choice for most cases of AMS if immediate descent is not indicated
Oxygen and/or hyperbaric treatment
Pro   Oxygen at 2-4 L/m, or simulated descent in a hyperbaric bag works as well as descent in the short term, without the walk.
Con   Not generally used because oxygen tanks are heavy, and hyperbaric bags are very expensive and labor intensive; these are usually reserved for more serious illness and are usually found only on more elaborately equipped, very high-altitude expeditions. Treatment for 2 hours with either will resolve symptoms in most patients, but rebound symptoms can occur.

kidneys to excrete bicarbonate, acidifying the blood. The resulting metabolic acidosis acts as a respiratory stimulant, increasing ventilation and improving arterial oxygenation. The drug is especially effective in preventing extreme hypoxia during sleep—a situation that can also trigger HAPE, especially in persons with a history of this disorder; (2) It reduces cerebrospinal fluid (CSF) formation and possibly CSF pressure; and (3) It causes a diuresis, counteracting the fluid retention that occurs in AMS.

Standard dosage: 125 to 250 mg every 12 hours, or 500 mg daily of the slow-release preparation (Diamox-SR). Start acetazolamide 24 hours before starting your ascent and continue it for 3 days at the higher altitude. Side effects include frequent urination (polyuria) and a tingling sensation of the face and lips (paresthesia).

Dexamethasone (Decadron)—Although effective in treating cerebral symptoms of AMS, dexamethasone is not routinely recommended as a prophylactic agent. It may be a useful drug, however, for those who need to ascend abruptly to very high altitudes—for example, those going on a mountain rescue mission—or for those allergic to acetazolamide. The drug is usually used for the treatment of AMS (see the Treatment Section).

Prophylaxis dosage: 2 mg every 6 hours, begun the day of ascent, continued for 3 days at the higher altitude, then tapered over 5 days. Side effects: weaning from dexamethasone may increase risk of depression.

Nifedipine—In someone with a history of HAPE who desires prophylaxis, use either the 20-mg slow-release capsule (available in Europe and Asia under various brand names) every 8 hours, or the 30-mg slow-release (available as Adalat-CC or Procardia-XL in North America) every 12 hours. All climbers above 10,000 feet should also carry standby treatment doses of the rapid-acting 10-mg capsules.

Aspirin—Pretreatment with aspirin before travel to high altitudes appears to decrease the incidence and severity of headaches, the main symptom of mild AMS. Take one aspirin tablet every 4 hours for three doses before arrival. After arrival, take two tablets three times daily for 3 days. (Ibuprofen also works.)

Ginkgo biloba—This herb has shown mixed results in preventing AMS.

DIAGNOSING ALTITUDE SICKNESS

When diagnosing and treating AMS, HACE, or HAPE keep in mind other diagnoses that can mimic altitude sickness. Consider:

- Dehydration (can cause nausea, weakness, headache)
- Hypothermia (can cause loss of balance, staggering gait)
- Exhaustion (can cause lethargy, loss of balance, staggering gait)
- Respiratory infection (symptoms include coughing, shortness of breath)
- Carbon monoxide poisoning (can result from cooking in enclosed spaces such as tents, snow caves; causes rapid breathing, headache, mental changes, coma.)
- Hyperventilation (rapid breathing from anxiety; may simulate pulmonary edema)
- Psychiatric problems with psychosis can cause irrational behavior mimicking some aspects of HACE.

- The combination of high altitudes, hypoxia, and dehydration can predispose to venous thrombosis—cerebral, retinal, and pulmonary. Women on birth control pills who smoke may be at higher risk for a pulmonary embolus.
- Altitude—unrelated illness, e.g., diabetes, a seizure disorder, symptoms of an undiagnosed brain tumor, viral or bacterial infection

Although the valuable aphorism "any illness at altitude should be considered AMS until proved otherwise" is usually true, it is sometimes impossible, perhaps even unnecessary, to make an immediate diagnosis. Symptomatic treatment, such as oxygen, quickly followed by descent, should be the first priority. An exact diagnosis can often wait until after the climber has descended.

TREATMENT

Mild AMS by itself is a benign illness but you must watch for progression to more severe AMS, HACE, or HAPE. In general, management depends on the acuity and severity of symptoms. The principles of treatment are as follows:

- Stop further ascent and rest. Administer adjunctive treatment, as indicated.
- Descend if there is no improvement or if symptoms worsen.
- Descend immediately if there are symptoms or signs of cerebral or pulmonary edema.

Mild AMS

The first rule applies: Stop your ascent and rest. Symptoms should improve in 8 to 12 hours; if not, descend. To help the headache, take aspirin, acetaminophen, or ibuprofen. Acetazolamide (Diamox), 125 mg to 250 mg twice daily may reduce symptoms within 12 hours. Dexamethasone (4 mg orally or intramuscularly every 6 hours) works within 6 hours and is possibly more effective than acetazolamide. Combining dexamethasone and acetazolamide may be even more effective but no studies have yet proved this. No further ascent should be attempted until symptoms have cleared. Continue to take acetazolamide for several days as prophylaxis. Drinking extra fluids doesn't help AMS, but if you are dehydrated you will feel better.

More Severe AMS

Treatment of more severe AMS (which is essentially a pre-HACE condition) is directed at reducing brain volume and intracranial pressure and stopping the formation of vasogenic cerebral edema. A descent of 1,500 to 3,000 feet is the best initial treatment. Adjunctive measures include oxygen, steroids, acetazolamide, rest, and keeping the climber warm. Start oxygen, if available, at a flow rate of 2 to 4 liters/minute, and administer dexamethasone, 8 mg immediately, then 4 mg every 6 hours, plus acetazolamide, 250 mg every 12 hours. Plan for descent as soon as possible.

High-Altitude Cerebral Edema (HACE)

The hallmarks of HACE are confusion and ataxia. To test for ataxia, have the climber attempt to walk a straight line, one foot in front of the other, heel to toe. A climber who struggles to stay on the line, falls off to one side, or falls down should be considered to have HACE. At the first sign of ataxia, if not before, descent should be started. Adjunctive treatments are listed in the preceding paragraph. A portable hyperbaric chamber, such as the Gamow bag (see later), will improve oxygenation, give temporary relief, and will facilitate descent; but use of the Gamow bag should not unduly delay descent. NOTE: HACE and high-altitude pulmonary edema (HAPE) often occur simultaneously, but HACE can also occur as a single entity without pulmonary symptoms.

High-Altitude Pulmonary Edema (HAPE)

Treatment depends on the severity of the illness and the environment. If oxygen and medical expertise are not available, immediate descent is indicated. If diagnosed early, a descent of 1,500 to 3,000 feet usually gives rapid improvement within 2 or 3 days of rest at the lower elevation usually adequate for complete recovery. Once the symptoms have resolved, cautious re-ascent may be attempted. NOTE: Some authorities state, however, that once a diagnosis of HAPE is made, the individual should be evacuated to a medical facility for proper follow-up treatment. This is probably indicated only in more severe cases. If re-ascent is attempted, prophylactic acetazolamide and nifedipine should be considered.

Adjunctive treatment measures include the following:

- Oxygen, at an initial flow rate of 2 to 4 liters/minute, can be lifesaving. Reduce flow to 1 to 2 liters to keep SaO_2 >90%.
- Administer nifedipine. Although oxygen and descent are the best treatments for HAPE, nifedipine is an effective adjunct, especially when oxygen is not available. If conscious, have the patient swallow one 10-mg capsule for the first dose. If comatose, pierce the capsule and squirt it under the tongue. Continue treatment with the slow-release form, 20 to 30 mg every 12 hours. Nifedipine rapidly reduces pulmonary vasoconstriction, thus reducing pulmonary hypertension and over-perfusion edema. The reduction in vasoconstriction also makes pulmonary blood flow more homogeneous, which improves oxygenation. Sublingual administration of nifedipine results in a 10% rise in arterial oxygen saturation within 10 to 15 minutes. Nifedipine can sometimes be used alone with strict bed rest in a person with only very mild HAPE, otherwise it is used only in combination with the other treatments: descent, oxygen, and hyperbaric therapy.
- NOTE: Sildenafil (Viagra) has recently been shown to be effective for treating HAPE. The dose is 50 mg every 8 hours. It has the advantage of not reducing systemic blood pressure.
- Administering hyperbaric treatment in the Gamow bag (see next) for a total of 2 to 4 hours usually results in dramatic improvement, facilitating descent.
- Keep the patient warm. Not only will the patient be more comfortable, cold stress increases pulmonary artery pressure.

The Portable Hyperbaric Chamber (Gamow Bag)

This device is an airtight, 7-foot cylindrical bag made of coated nylon weighing about 18 lbs. with a pump and/or rebreathing unit. It is used for the treatment of more severe AMS or HACE, especially when a person is too ill to descend immediately.

The stricken climber is placed inside the bag, which is then pressurized with a foot or hand pump. This pressurization simulates a decrease of 1,500 to 2,500 meters in altitude and, depending on the starting altitude, is usually sufficient to raise arterial oxygen saturation to more than 90%. A 1-hour treatment provides rapid relief from most symptoms of AMS, but the effect is temporary, lasting only 10 to 11 hours. This may buy enough time to walk the stricken climber to a lower altitude. By contrast, climbers receiving dexamethasone will improve more slowly but with sustained, longer-lasting effects. Although the administration of dexamethasone is simple, the same can't be said for the mobile hyperbaric chamber. Maintaining therapeutic pressure and air flow in often extreme weather can be a daunting task. In addition, access to the victim is restricted.

The main advantages of the Gamow-type bag are its rapid action and independence from consumable oxygen. The device is best suited for alpine expeditions and search and rescue teams that don't carry bottled oxygen. Gamow bags can be purchased or rented form Chinook Medical Gear, Inc., 120 Rock Point Drive, Unit C, Durango, CO 81301; 970-375-1241; 800-766-1365.

Oxygen

This is usually supplied by "E" type cylinders that weigh about 18 lbs. One full tank will last about 4 hours at a flow rate of 2 liters/minute. Supplemental oxygen is slightly more effective than the Gamow bag in raising arterial oxygen saturation and its use does not restrict access to the victim.

Sleeping Pills

It is usually recommended that high-altitude travelers not take sleeping pills because they might depress respiration, increase oxygen desaturation and hypoxia, and increase the incidence or severity of AMS. However, a recent study (conducted at an elevation of 5,300 meters) among members of the British Mount Everest Expedition found that small doses (10 mg) of the short-acting benzodiazepine, temazepam (Restoril), improved the subjective quality of sleep without adversely affecting respiration. Better sleep, defined as longer periods without arousal, resulted in less daytime drowsiness and improved endurance. In 1996, French researchers found that a 10-mg dose of zolpidem (Ambien) taken at a simulated altitude of 4,000 meters was associated with fewer sleep arousals and no increase in period breathing. From these studies, it appears that the short-acting hypnotics may actually be safe adjuncts for improving comfort and rest as well as high-altitude performance.

Acute Altitude Sickness in Children

The incidence of AMS in children is about the same as in adults, but diagnosing the condition can be problematic because the symptoms—cough, headache, irritability, and loss of appetite—are often mistaken for a viral illness. If a child does become sick at altitude, the parents should assume that AMS is a possibility, descend, and seek prompt medical consultation. Drug prophylaxis/treatment for AMS could be considered as for adults, but with appropriate pediatric doses. These medications have not been specifically studied for treating children with AMS.

THE HEART AT HIGH ALTITUDES

Ascent to moderate altitude appears to entail little risk for travelers with coronary artery disease who are ordinarily asymptomatic or who have moderate exercise tolerance. They may develop angina at a lower level of exertion, but generally have no impairment of their ability to acclimatize. They should rest for a few days after arrival at altitude, and ascend slowly thereafter. If the traveler is on treatment for angina, atrial fibrillation, hypertension, or mild compensated congestive heart failure their medications should be carefully adjusted, especially to keep the blood pressure and pulse well controlled.

However, the question that many people (and their doctors) ask about high-altitude travel is "will it trigger a heart attack?" or "Is there a risk of sudden death?" Younger people need not worry about this, but what if you're a 50-year-old man in relatively poor physical condition, perhaps with several cardiovascular risk factors? Is trekking a good idea? Reports in the medical literature demonstrate an increased incidence of sudden cardiac death associated with abrupt exercise in sedentary people, but there are little data about the risk during participation in mountain sports.

In a report of sudden deaths among high mountain hikers and skiers in Austria, hikers were more than twice as likely to die as skiers. Among the hikers, the risk of death was highly associated with an age of more than 40 years and lack of prior physical activity. In contrast, a study of medical evacuations of climbers and trekkers in Nepal showed that cardiac disease accounted for only 5% of the evacuations, and none of the deaths. One reason for this difference could be that the climbers that went to Nepal were in much better physical condition.

The possibility of an acute cardiac event has prompted efforts to screen asymptomatic travelers in an effort to identify the presence of coronary disease before the occurrence of a serious problem. A stress test is often recommended. Unfortunately, exercise stress tests have limited effectiveness because they don't show the anatomy of the coronary arteries. They miss plaques that are not large enough to obstruct blood flow, but that have the potential to destabilize and rupture, causing new-onset angina, heart attack, or cardiac arrest. More sensitive tests are needed to detect these asymptomatic plaques, and if found, to stabilize them.

- Coronary artery disease (CAD) is a disease where there is build-up of atherosclerotic "plaques" within the arterial wall.
- Plaques consist of a lipid-rich core, inflammatory cells, calcium, and a fibrous cap.
- Your risk of heart attack is related not only to the existence and extent of coronary artery plaques, but to their biochemical *stability*.
- Unstable plaques can fissure or rupture, triggering thrombosis and blockage of the coronary artery.
- Larger plaques are more likely to rupture than small plaques, but smaller plaques are more numerous, and present the greater risk for a heart attack.
- Stabilizing plaque is a key goal in reducing risk.
- Statin drugs can stabilize plaques. Regular exercise reduces the risk of plaque rupture.

- Reducing cardiac risk factors reduces plaque formation.
  Exercise stress tests are probably most useful for evaluating the functional capacity of the hearts of people who already have diagnosed coronary artery disease. The results can also help their physician adjust their medication for maximum benefit. If you are planning a trip to moderate-to-high altitudes, here are some guidelines:
- If you are younger than age 50, without symptoms of heart disease, and in good physical condition, and you have no cardiac risk factors, especially no family history of early heart disease, you don't need a cardiac evaluation before your trip. Standard pre-travel counseling (Chapter 2) is sufficient. Follow the guidelines in this chapter for preventing altitude illness.
- If you have one or more risk factors (including male older than age 50), but have no cardiac symptoms, consult your physician. Depending on the nature of your planned excursion, the number of risk factors, your overall medical and physical condition, plus whatever anxiety you might have about your heart—pre-ascent treadmill exercise testing may be recommended. However, there can be drawbacks to testing asymptomatic people. The exercise test can be normal even when there is significant underlying coronary artery disease. And if the test is equivocal, or mildly abnormal, it could open a diagnostic Pandora's box. Next you'll need a nuclear perfusion scan;

Table 15.2   Some Cities at Elevations of More Than 7,500 Feet Above Sea Level

Location	Altitude (feet)
Addis Ababa, Ethiopia	7,900
Thimphu, Bhutan	7,700
Bogota, Colombia	8,653
Cuzco, Peru	11,152
Arequipa, Peru	7,559
La Paz, Bolivia	12,001
Darjeeling, India	7,431
Toluca, Mexico	8,793
Sucre, Bolivia	8,530
Lhasa, Tibet	11,830
Quito, Ecuador	9,300
Mexico City	7,546

you may even get an angiogram. Angiograms are invasive, and not without risk. A newer technology, the multidetector CT scanner, can show your coronary arteries in enough detail to diagnose coronary artery disease and the extent of any plaque formation. The test is noninvasive and takes only 15 minutes.

- If you have a history of heart attack, coronary artery bypass grafting (CABG) surgery or angioplasty, climbing or travel to high altitudes is certainly possible, but the indications for ascent should be examined carefully. If you have a normal exercise stress test you are probably at low risk. If you are in a higher risk category, as shown by your stress test and/or symptoms, precautionary measures should be more rigorous.
- If you have symptoms or established CAD, and your exercise test is abnormal, your activity level should be related to the test results. If the test is mildly abnormal and you are able to perform the test at a high exercise level, almost no limits should be imposed on your physical activities, except those that evoke symptoms. If you have symptoms or an abnormality at a low exercise level, it is best to exercise below that level.

Pearls About Heart Disease and High Altitudes

- Judicious exercise at altitude usually causes few problems in the traveler with stable cardiac disease.
- High altitude increases cardiac work during the first 3 or 4 days at altitude. Overly strenuous activity should be avoided during this time. Activity should be limited to that tolerated at lower altitudes.
- At least a moderate degree of physical conditioning is desirable before commencing any strenuous activity in the mountains. Physical conditioning is especially important for those ages 40 and older.
- Heart attack (myocardial infarction) can be triggered by heavy physical exertion in habitually sedentary people. Regular exercise protects against it.
- Gradual, rather than abrupt ascent is always better.
- Blood pressure should be kept under good control.
- Travelers with a history of congestive heart failure often decompensate at high altitudes because of fluid retention.
- When angina drugs are prescribed, calcium channel blockers may be preferable to beta blockers.
- Cardiac arrhythmia, such as atrial fibrillation, may worsen after rapid ascent to altitude, even without underlying coronary artery disease.
- Trekkers who have had cardiac bypass surgery have climbed as high as 19,000 feet without problems, but the risks for them from mountaineering and trekking at extreme altitudes are simply not known. Every traveler must be evaluated individually.
- Your maximal physical exertion at high altitudes is usually limited more by your lung function than by your heart.
- The guidelines for travel to higher altitudes by people with heart disease are somewhat elusive and not well standardized.
- Taking a cholesterol-lowering statin drug, such as atorvastatin (Lipitor), may reduce the risk of a cardiac event. Atorvastatin, in higher doses, stabilizes coronary artery

plaques, reducing the risk of plaque rupture and acute coronary syndrome (new-onset angina, heart attack).

- Aspirin and clopidogrel (Plavix) reduce the risks of heart attack and stroke, but bleeding can be a side effect.

The decision to travel should be based on your physician's advice, plus your own desire to go. Bear in mind that if problems occur, you could be far away from a hospital. However, many intelligent, well-informed people, knowing the risks, as well as their own capabilities and limitations, want to live life to the fullest. This is a human desire that should not unnecessarily be restricted.

How Two Physicians Advise Their Patients Who Climb

Dr. Drummond Rennie, an internist and experienced trekker/climber advises, "My own practice is to take a careful history from people who ask if they can go trekking at high altitudes. I explain that if they are able to carry out strenuous, long, continued exercise at sea level, they can probably expect to do so at high altitude. I suggest also that, if possible, they should give themselves a trial at moderate altitude, say 8,000 feet. If they have any symptoms, say angina, they should ascend even more slowly than usual so that they can acclimatize." And Dr. Charles Houston, who is a world-renowned expert on altitude sickness, says, "Coronary artery disease, per se, is not an absolute contraindication to trekking at higher altitudes. If reserve circulation is sufficient, if the patient is wise in recognizing symptoms and accepting limits, if the anticipated stresses of hiking and climbing do not produce signs and symptoms at sea level, then a person may go ahead, properly warned and prepared, because the emotional and psychological benefits are large."

CHAPTER 16

Medical Care Abroad

H

KEY POINTS:

▶ Good trip preparation helps reduce the need for medical care abroad.

▶ Short-term travelers are most concerned about emergency medical care; expatriates and long-stay travelers may have different health-care needs.

▶ Travelers with an acute medical or surgical emergency should seek the nearest facility for immediate care. Most of the time this care will be adequate.

▶ Most travelers should purchase a travel insurance policy that includes assistance benefits.

▶ An assistance company can provide referrals to English-speaking physicians, monitor health care, and arrange emergency medical evacuation, if those become necessary.

▶ Medical care abroad varies widely, and in many countries is of high quality. This high-quality care, however, may be available to only a small segment of the general population. Travelers should find out how to locate this care.

▶ All travelers should carry at least a basic medical kit. They should have their own supply of pain medication, antibiotics, drugs for diarrhea, heartburn, etc. This can help avert a trip to a doctor or hospital.

▶ Travelers should consider carrying a mobile phone that can make international calls. They should bring with them their personal physician's office telephone, mobile phone, and fax numbers and e-mail address so the traveler, or his family, and/or the physician overseas will be better able to assess the medical problem.

What do you do if you are suddenly taken ill or have a serious accident in a foreign country? How do you find an English-speaking physician? Or locate a reputable hospital? Where do you turn for help and advice? The first step in avoiding disaster is prevention. This means careful pre-trip planning as outlined in this *Health Guide*. But what if an unexpected illness or accident occurs? Statistics show that 25% of travelers develop some type of medical problem over a 2-week period. Most accidents and cases of medical illness are relatively minor. The problem may be self-evident. Most conditions resolve by themselves or can be treated with simple first-aid measures or with the medication you have on hand.

But what if you need a physician's treatment or hospitalization? When an emergency happens far from home, even a seasoned traveler may have trouble coping, especially if medical care is urgently needed. What starts out as a routine vacation or business trip could end up as a real nightmare.

How to Cope When Illness or Injury Suddenly Strikes

Stay Calm You may be able to solve the problem yourself. You may already have medicine with you to treat a minor infection, a rash, a cut, a bruise, or a sprain. If diarrhea should occur, follow the treatment guidelines for travelers' diarrhea in Chapter 6. Check to see what's in your medical kit. Home health-care guides and first-aid manuals are sources of useful advice, so you may wish to bring one of these with you.

Serious Accidents or Illness Demand Immediate Attention If you sustain a more serious injury, such as a deep laceration or a fracture, or have bleeding, unremitting chest or abdominal pain, or trouble breathing, don't waste your time trying to find a local physician. Go immediately to the nearest hospital. If you are in a large city, go to a hospital associated with a medical school if possible (these hospitals usually have English-speaking doctors as well as qualified specialists on staff). You can ask for directions or assistance from your hotel, your tour guide, a taxi driver, or the police. A taxi or private car may be faster than waiting for an ambulance. Remember, in an emergency, minutes count. Don't delay!

NOTE: If you think you are having a heart attack, early diagnosis and treatment are critical. Administration of a thrombolytic (clot dissolving) drug, or angioplasty, will greatly improve your chance of survival.

Less Urgent Illness This can usually be treated during a daytime visit to a doctor's office, but some doctors will make an after hours hotel "house call." Your hotel can usually provide the names of one or more English-speaking physicians. Better yet, if you have friends, relatives, or business associates who are residents of the area, ask them for a referral to a doctor they know is qualified.

Colds, sore throats, ear aches, bronchitis, diarrhea, most urinary infections, and the flu are some of the conditions that usually don't require emergency attention, but do require monitoring and possible physician follow-up. You won't find overseas the widespread availability of over-the-counter drugs there is in the United States and Canada; so bring your own supply of antibiotics, pain medication, diarrhea pills, etc. The medication you bring may cure or sufficiently ameliorate the problem or make you feel better while waiting to see a physician. You can take levofloxacin (a standby antibiotic for travelers' diarrhea) for painful, frequent urination (urinary tract infection?) or a cough with fever (pneumonia?) pending further medical evaluation. Self treatment with an antimalarial drug is a good example of how self medicating can be potentially life saving. However, if you do have a fever that might be from malaria, be sure you are examined within 24 hours.

Request that all medications you receive from the doctor be identified or labeled with the generic as well as the trade name. This is important if you have drug allergies and must avoid certain medications or if you develop a drug-related reaction or have to see another doctor for ongoing care. That doctor will need to know what drugs you have been taking. NOTE: Familiar drugs will have different brand names in other countries, but generic names may also vary. For example, acetaminophen (Tylenol) has another generic name, paracetamol, in some countries; and meperidine (Demerol), is sometimes generically identified as pethedine.

Bring a Medical Kit and First-Aid Manual You can often save yourself a trip to the doctor if you are able treat cuts, abrasions, and other minor injuries yourself. Be sure your routine immunizations are up-to-date so you don't have to go to a hospital for a tetanus booster.

Carry a Phrase Book A phrase booklet or pamphlet that provides medical words and phrases in various foreign languages, or the KwikPoint medical visual language translator (www.kwikpoint.com), can be invaluable when a language barrier prevents the adequate communication of immediate medical needs. Find an interpreter as soon as possible.

Contact Your Doctor in the United States Bring a mobile telephone with you on your trip. If you are hospitalized, a consultation with your own physician back home can be invaluable. Hopefully your doctor, or an associate, will be available at the time you call. (Leave your number, or another call back number, if necessary.) Describe the history of your illness, your symptoms, what the diagnosis is, and what treatment you are receiving. Let your doctor know if you are in a country where there are tropical diseases. Have your own doctor discuss your case with the local doctor caring for you. Obviously, for certain conditions, treatment is standard and straightforward—surgery for appendicitis, casting for fractures, etc.—and your treatment may have already been rendered. However, for more serious or life-threatening problems, this consultation can be important. Your diagnosis may be in doubt, and the hospital and physician may not have the expertise to provide adequate care. Your physician can help assess the situation and reassure you that you are receiving proper care and that there's no need to worry, or your physician may feel that a second opinion is warranted or even that transfer to another facility is advisable.

FACTORS DETERMINING EMERGENCY MEDICAL EVACUATION

- Qualified medical consultation has determined that local medical care is not adequate.
- Another facility, one that can provide a higher level of care, is available and accessible, and has accepted the patient in transfer.
- The patient's condition has been sufficiently stabilized before transport.
- The patient can pay the cost of the transport.

Locating Physicians Abroad

In many cases, finding good medical care abroad is not a problem—maybe even less of a problem than back home where you may have to wait for hours in an ER! You have many options when it comes to finding a physician to care for you. The American and

Canadian embassies and consulates maintain referral lists from which you can choose. The embassy or consulate, however, won't officially recommend individual doctors on the list. Other options to consider include the following:

Travel Insurance/Assistance Companies If you have purchased a travel health policy, call the 24-hour hotline number and you'll be connected with an assistance center that can give a physician referral. Companies such as International SOS Assistance and Shoreland, Inc. (publisher of *Travax EnCompass*), provide corporate and travel physicians, for a fee, with a list of worldwide medical facilities and contact information.

International Medical Clinics Because of globalization, there is a growing market for Western-style medicine* to serve the medical needs of the employees of multi-national corporations, visitors, expatriates, and insured travelers. These clinics, usually part of a chain, are found in large cities and may provide the best first contact for any medical problem. One such provider is the American Medical Centers that maintains clinics in Moscow, St. Petersburg, and Kiev. International SOS and MEDEX run clinics in Beijing and many other locations throughout the world.

IAMAT The International Association for Assistance to Travelers (IAMAT) is a Canadian foundation that publishes a booklet listing hospitals and English-speaking physicians who have agreed to adhere to a standard schedule of fees. Physicians are not listed by specialty. Contact IAMAT (www.iamat.org), 417 Center Street, Lewiston, NY 14092; 716-754-4883; in Canada, 40 Regal Road, Guelph, Ontario, N1K 1B5; 519-836-0102; no charge, but a donation is encouraged.

Cardholder Assistance Credit-card companies provide 24-hour emergency medical hotlines available to many of their cardholders, usually those in the "gold card" or "platinum card" category. Typically, the hotlines can refer you to English-speaking doctors and dentists and to hospitals with English-speaking staff members, arrange for replacement of prescription medicines, and help you charter an air ambulance. If you are an American Express cardholder, call the Global Assist hotline at 800-554-AMEX (301-214-8228 collect from overseas). If you are an American Express Platinum cardholder, call your special assistance number, 800-345-2639 (202-331-1688 collect from overseas). Visa Gold and Classic cardholders can call 800-332-2484 (410-581-9994 collect from overseas). MasterCard cardholders can call 303-278-8000 (collect from overseas).

Hotel and Resort Doctors Most large hotels will refer you to a local doctor or to a doctor who will come to your room to render treatment. Be warned, however, that the main qualification some of these doctors have is a payback arrangement with the hotel management. They may be helpful in providing referrals.

The Telephone Book You may find many doctors and clinics listed in the "yellow pages" of the local telephone book. These physicians often mention their qualifications and

---

*Western-style medicine has three main components: (1) evidence-based medicine; (2) quality assurance; and (3) patient-centered delivery of care. Evidence-based medicine means practicing medicine using diagnostic and treatment protocols that have been developed through research, not handed down from generation to generation.

some may indicate that they have received specialty training in the United States, Canada, the United Kingdom, or other medically advanced country.

Personal Recommendation A time-tested method of locating a qualified physician (assuming time allows it) is to find a satisfied patient. Ask locals for personal recommendation. Contact employees of multi-national corporations or expatriates such as schoolteachers, relief workers, or missionaries who may have received medical care in-country. They are often familiar with high-quality private general hospitals or specialty clinics.

FOREIGN PHYSICIANS

Because of cultural differences, the attitude of physicians toward their patients in foreign countries is often different than in the United States or Canada. Physicians abroad are often perceived as being more autocratic and authoritarian. This can make patient-doctor communication difficult. The doctor caring for you may not want you to question his or her care and may not be available to answer your questions (to be fair, this can sometimes be said of American physicians also). This does not mean that your care is substandard. In fact, the doctor caring for you may have more knowledge of local diseases than your own physician and be perfectly well qualified to diagnose and treat your illness. Nevertheless, you should seek a second opinion if you have doubts about the quality of your care.

FOREIGN HOSPITALS

Foreign hospitals can range from basic to the most advanced, but the quality of your medical care shouldn't necessarily be judged by your surroundings. If you're hospitalized in a less developed country, you might wonder if you should be moved to a "more modern" facility. This question faces hospitalized patients everywhere, not just travelers overseas. An analogy to being hospitalized in the United States might be appropriate. In the United States, the smaller community hospitals are adequate for almost all medical care. Occasionally, however, a patient requires transport to a specialty center for advanced, sometimes life-saving treatment. The same is true overseas. You may be in a small, seemingly inadequate facility that may, in fact, be perfectly adequate for your medical needs. Having someone available, in serious situations, to assess your diagnosis and treatment will help you or your family know when transfer or medical evacuation may be indicated.

Assessing Foreign Hospitals

If you need emergency care and minutes count, go to the closest facility. However, if the situation is not immediately critical—and there's more than one hospital nearby—use the following checklist to get a basic idea of what level of care is available to you. The checklist will also help you tell your doctor at home, if the occasion arises, what services are being provided.

- Does the hospital have a coronary care unit, ICU, recovery room, and advanced resuscitation and diagnostic equipment?

- What medical and surgical procedures can be performed? Are orthopedic surgeons, neurosurgeons, and other specialists on staff? If not, where is the closest referral facility?
- Can they treat heart attacks with thrombolytics (clot-dissolving drugs), angioplasty, stenting, or cardiac bypass surgery (CABG)?
- Can the hospital render qualified obstetric and postpartum care? Do they have a renal dialysis service?
- Are computed tomography (CT), MRI, and ultrasound available?
- Does the hospital or clinic stock disposable supplies, especially needles and syringes?
- Does the blood bank screen for HIV, hepatitis B antigen, and hepatitis C antibody?
- What vaccines are available (e.g., tetanus, rabies, rabies immune globulin, hepatitis B, hepatitis B immune globulin)?
- Is the hospital air-conditioned? Are there private rooms? What types of meals are served?
- Are private duty nurses available?
- Does the hospital have 24-hour admitting capability?
- Does the hospital have an emergency room, receive ambulances, and treat major trauma?
- Do most of the doctors speak English?
- What are the room rates and the charges for various medical and surgical procedures?
- How will you pay the hospital? Do they accept major credit cards? Do they demand guarantee of payment from you or your travel insurance/assistance company "up-front?"

CHAPTER 17

Travel Insurance

KEY POINTS:

▶ Foreign hospitals and doctors won't accept your regular health insurance and usually require payment with cash or a credit card at the time of treatment. Your insurance company may reimburse you later (for approved treatment only) after your claim has been processed and the trip long over.

▶ Travelers can avoid this problem with a travel health insurance/assistance policy. These policies guarantee on-site payment of medical bills abroad.

▶ These policies also include another essential benefit—medical evacuation, by air ambulance if necessary, to a higher level, or more appropriate, medical facility. Assistance companies can also help with other matters—obtaining prescription drugs, legal matters, lost documents, and more.

▶ There are many different policies available that cover different types of overseas travel, including: short-term, frequent, long-term, study abroad, and living abroad. There are also many medical assistance companies. They vary in size from having one small office to having offices or representatives in many countries. Generally, it is wise to choose a policy associated with a larger assistance company with offices in many countries.

WHY TRAVELERS NEED TRIP INSURANCE

Health insurance in the United States is characterized by its diversity. There are a multitude of plans with different costs, benefits, deductibles, exclusions, and restrictions. However, many insured travelers lack adequate travel protection. Government sponsored health programs such as Medicare almost never cover treatment received in a foreign country.* Employer-sponsored plans usually limit overseas coverage to emergency care only (and the burden will be on you to prove it's an emergency). Emergency medical evacuation is almost never covered. Even if you're traveling on business, you may have significant gaps in your coverage.

Before you travel, check your existing health insurance policy to see what it pays for. It will probably reimburse you for 100% of the cost of emergency treatment abroad, ex-

---

*Medicare does not cover health-care costs outside the United States and its territories, except under limited circumstances in Canada and Mexico. For this coverage, you will need a Medigap policy, but not all Medigap policies cover foreign travel, and the policies vary from state to state. For example, in Massachusetts, three out of the four available Medigap plans do provide coverage for travel abroad. (These are Core Policy with Rider, Supplement 1 and Supplement 2).

cluding any deductible or co-payment. You normally will have to pay the doctor or hospital at the time of treatment, or before hospital admission—perhaps thousands of dollars. Of course, for this to work the hospital must accept your credit card and your card must have a sufficient credit limit. You then hope your insurance company will reimburse you later. This, however, can get complicated: did you notify your insurance carrier within the 24-hour time period required for hospital admission, or other treatment? (This requirement may be waived for emergencies.) Do you have copies of your treatment record and medical bills in English, or are they all in a foreign language? The insurer may not accept incomplete records or bills that are not itemized.

The same dilemma occurs if you need emergency medical evacuation, perhaps by air ambulance. Once again, you will have to pay up front, but air ambulance transport can be much more expensive—sometimes tens of thousands of dollars.

Travel Insurance with Assistance

Imagine the following scenario: You find yourself hospitalized with a serious illness in a foreign country and the doctor caring for you speaks hardly any English. You're being treated with an unfamiliar drug, and you are worried about an allergic reaction or a serious side effect. The doctor then says you may need surgery, but you're not sure of the diagnosis, or the surgeon's qualifications. The situation is becoming more and more like a nightmare. Where do you turn for help and advice? If you find yourself in this situation, then having *travel insurance with assistance* can be a godsend. Following are some of the reasons:

Medical Monitoring Travel insurance with assistance gives you a 24-hour telephone number of an assistance center where multi-lingual personnel, backed up by physician specialists, are available around the clock to evaluate your treatment and to monitor your medical care.

Emergency Medical Transport/Repatriation If it is determined that you need to be transported immediately by air ambulance, or another form of emergency medical transportation, to a higher level or more appropriate medical facility, the assistance center will arrange for it and pay the costs, up to the policy limit. (Some policies have an unlimited evacuation benefit.) And if you're unable to return home unassisted after your condition has stabilized, the insurer, working through the assistance center, will arrange and pay for transport (with a qualified medical attendant) so that you can recover closer to home and family.

Emergency Medical Payments The assistance center will also guarantee payment to those providing your medical care or, when necessary, can advance money for on-site payment. This means that, aside from possibly paying a small deductible, you will not have to make cash payments yourself, provided the policy covers the illness and the doctor and/or hospital will accept the travel insurance (which they often will).

Traveler's Assistance Assistance centers can also help with a variety of other problems, including replacement of lost prescriptions, physician referral, or finding you a local dentist. Non-medical assistance includes travel document and ticket replacement, emergency cash transfer, emergency message center, legal assistance (e.g., lending you bail money, locating a lawyer), and assistance in replacing a lost prescription or lost passport or other document. (Some of these services are also provided by the Bureau of Consular Affairs in the U.S. Department of State, but the assistance companies often have a faster, more complete response.)

Travel Safety Assistance This is a growing service area because of geopolitical turmoil and terrorist threats. Some assistance companies have the capability to locate travelers and provide them with updated health and security e-mail alerts. The recent tsunami in Indonesia has made many travelers, as well as their employers, aware of the need for communication when a disaster strikes.

What Else Can These Policies Cover?

Accidental death and disability—For additional fees most policies will cover accidental death and disability (AD&D), lost luggage, collision damage waiver, and trip interruption or cancellation insurance. Consider whether you really need this extra coverage. If you already have your own life insurance, the small AD&D benefit is probably not worth the cost; and lost luggage may be covered by your homeowner's policy.

Trip Interruption Insurance This can be an important money saver if illness or other problems force you to miss your scheduled flight. Some medical emergency policies offer this benefit in the basic package or as an optional benefit available for an additional fee. A trip interruption policy should cover the following:

- Interruption because of sickness, injury, or death to you, members of your immediate family, your traveling companion, or your business partner
- Accidents or emergencies that cause you to miss a scheduled departure (or connection) when you're traveling to the departure point
- Travel delays caused by an unannounced strike, bad weather, or a hijacking
- Terrorist-caused incident at destination that results in trip cancellation

How Much Travel Insurance Do I Need?

Some policies let you buy up to $100,000 of medical coverage, but if you are a tourist or short-term traveler it is unlikely you would ever need this much insurance to pay medical bills abroad because (1) travel policies pay only for emergency medical care; (2) if sick or injured, you most likely will be repatriated home once your condition has stabilized; and (3) medical care abroad (at least in less developed countries) is usually less expensive than in the United States.

Be sure, however, that the policy's evacuation benefit is adequate. A long-range chartered air ambulance can cost $75,000, or more. For trips to the Caribbean or Europe, an evacuation benefit of $30,000 is probably sufficient, but if you are going on a trip halfway around the world, you want a policy that pays unlimited evacuation costs, or a high dollar amount, for example, $100,000.

Types of Policies

You can purchase coverage for a single trip, or buy an annual subscription or membership that covers multiple trips throughout the year. The cost of shorter trips is about $4 to $8/day per person, depending on age. An individual annual membership typically costs $450 to $475 for a $25,000 medical benefit and unlimited evacuation payments. There are also various policies for corporate travelers, students abroad, and people living abroad.

Exclusions—Read Carefully!

Read the policy carefully to see what is not covered. Exclusions and restrictions vary among the policies. For example, most policies pay for complications of pregnancy, but some will not. Sports activities such as scuba diving, sky diving, and mountain climbing are usually not covered, but separate scuba coverage is available from Divers Alert Network (DAN).

Probably the exclusion of greatest significance to many travelers—particularly the elderly—is the exclusion for preexisting medical conditions. This exclusion could prove financially burdensome if a condition becomes active during travel and requires emergency treatment or medical evacuation. An exclusion may state that coverage is excluded for "any injury or sickness (or complications arising therefrom) which manifests itself, or for which treatment or medication was prescribed or taken in the 180 days immediately prior to the period of insurance." However, other policies may be less restrictive, excluding only "any condition that has required treatment in the past 60 days, unless the condition is controlled through the taking of prescription drugs or medication and remains controlled throughout the 60-day period." In some cases, there are no exclusions for preexisting conditions provided you purchase the insurance within 7 days of making a deposit on your trip.

Travel Insurance with Assistance

There is a very large number of policies available, covering almost every travel situation. Each company's website offers the best overview of their products.

International SOS Assistance, Inc.
3600 Horizon Boulevard, Suite 300
Trevose, PA USA 19053
800-523-8930 or 1-215-942 8000
http://www.internationalsos.com/

Membership provides assistance (e.g., medical monitoring) as well as worldwide emergency medical transport. There is no cost limit on the evacuation benefit and no preexisting condition exclusion for medical care, if not treated within 60 days. SOS maintains offices in 50 countries and alarm centers in 24 countries, and staffs their own medical clinics in China.

Worldwide Assistance Services, Inc.
1133 15th Street, N.W., Suite 400
Washington, DC 20005
800-821-2828 or 1-202-331-1609
www.worldwideassistance.com

Comprehensive emergency medical evacuation and medical coverage available on a per-trip or annual basis. Individual, student abroad, and corporate programs. Their

Travel Assistance International Plan A provides up to $60,000 in medical benefits plus $1,000,000 for emergency medical evacuation. There are 36 assistance centers worldwide and coordinators in 200 countries. Policy covers medical complications of pregnancy through the third trimester. $100 deductible. Preexisting conditions: 60 days.

MEDEX Assistance Corporation
8501 LaSalle Road
Suite 200
Towson, MD 21286
800-732-5309 or 410-453-6300
www.medexassist.com
  $100,000 medical and air ambulance coverage for $4 a day. Age 71 and older, $5 a day. $25 deductible. SCUBA coverage, $1.00 a day extra. Preexisting conditions: 6 months.

International Medical Group (IMG)
407 N. Fulton Street
Indianapolis, IN 46202
800-628-4664 or 309-296-0600
www.imglobal.com
  IMG offers a variety of plans, including coverage for extreme sports, long-term major medical coverage for people residing abroad. Coverage up to $5 million is available. Plans include emergency evacuation, in-patient and out-patient coverage, and choice of deductibles.

Wallach & Company
107 West Federal Street
Middleburg, VA 20118
800-237-6616 or 540-687-3172
www.wallach.com
  The HealthCare Abroad policy pays $250,000 in benefits, and will cover downhill skiing and SCUBA up to $10,000. Coverage is available up to age 85.

Credit-Card Assistance

American Express will pay all costs for emergency medical evacuation to the nearest adequate medical facility for holders of the American Express Platinum and Centurion cards. American Express will also assist *any* cardholder with a medical problem overseas. For example, American Express can help cardholders arrange air ambulance transport, or find a doctor overseas, but they won't pay the cost.
  American Express Global Assist hotline: 800-345-2639 or 202-331-1688 collect from overseas.

Scuba Diving Insurance

Divers Alert Network
800-446-2671 or 919-684-2948

DAN scuba diving insurance is secondary coverage, available to DAN members. The scuba diving insurance policies listed below are in addition to DAN members' automatic $100,000 DAN TravelAssist medical air evacuation benefits.

DAN Standard Plan

$45,000 (maximum lifetime benefit) coverage for decompression illness incurred within the 130-foot depth limit.

DAN Plus Plan

$50,000 (maximum lifetime benefit) coverage for decompression illness plus up to $10,000 in accidental death/dismemberment benefits resulting from a covered diving illness or injury, plus up to $10,000 in total disability benefits.

DAN Master Plan

$125,000 (maximum lifetime benefit) coverage for decompression illness and ALL covered in-water injuries, plus up to $15,000 in accidental death and dismemberment benefits resulting from a covered diving illness or injury, plus up to $15,000 in permanent total disability, plus the policy pays up to $1,500 for accommodations, $1,000 for airline tickets, and $2,500 for lost dive equipment.

CHAPTER 18

Medical Transport

KEY POINTS:

▶ Companies that provide emergency medical transport require prepayment or guarantee of payment

▶ Travelers, especially those going to remote or medically underserved locations, should be covered by insurance that pays for emergency medical transport

▶ Stretcher transport on a commercial airliner is much less expensive than a chartered air ambulance

▶ Flight clearances into many countries may be difficult to obtain in short notice. The larger, more experienced air ambulance and assistance companies are generally better able to arrange flights to countries in Africa, the Middle East, and Asia.

What is Medical Evacuation?

Medical evacuation is required when a medical condition cannot be adequately treated in the current location. It involves moving a patient to another location with a higher standard of care. Medical evacuation may not involve moving the patient to their home country; it may be more appropriate to bring the patient to a location with quality medical care within the same region.

Medical evacuation can be as simple as a ground ambulance ride or as complicated as an air ambulance moving an unconscious patient from one country to another. Air ambulances are basically flying intensive care units with specially trained medical staff.

Arranging Medical Transport

Medical evacuations are complex to organize, especially if you are the patient! Even for family or friends, the logistics and cost can be daunting. If you are covered by a travel insurance policy, the insurance company will work with a medical assistance company to make all the arrangements (Chapter 17) and hopefully pay the costs through the insurance policy.

If you are uninsured, you can make the arrangements yourself or contact a medical assistance company directly and pay their fees. Either way, you will have to pay up front and hope your medical plan or HMO back home will reimburse you. Before you are reimbursed, your plan will want to see documentation verifying why the transport was medically necessary and also see copies of all invoices. They could very well delay or deny your claim. So, unless the situation is extremely urgent, try to contact your primary care provider or health plan from overseas to obtain authorization for the transport. This will help prevent problems later over reimbursement. If you are making the arrangements yourself, here is some information that will assist you.

Transport by Commercial Airliner This can range from transporting a wheelchair-bound traveler who only requires assistance with boarding, to transporting a bed-ridden patient. In cases where the patient must lie down, the airline curtains off a section of seats and installs a stretcher unit and oxygen (if needed). Seats are allotted for a medical attendant and sometimes a family member.

Stretcher transport is offered by some, but not all, airlines. The arrangements are more complex if the travel involves a change of aircraft or airline. Commercial airlines will not accept patients with unstable medical conditions. This is because if the patient's medical condition deteriorates in flight, the aircraft (and it's passengers and crew) may need to be diverted to the nearest location that can treat the patient. This is very expensive for the airline and inconvenient for the other passengers. Unstable patients can only be evacuated by air ambulance.

To arrange medical transportation by commercial aircraft, your first step is to call the airline/s and ask for their medical department, special services department, or "stretcher desk." (If you are the patient, have a friend or relative make the arrangements.) Explain the problem and the airline will tell you if and how they can assist. The airline's medical director must authorize the transport, and a medical attendant, either a nurse or a doctor, must accompany the patient. Sometimes a family member can be the attendant when medical treatment or monitoring will not be needed en route.

Ground ambulance pick up must be arranged at either end and coordinated with departure and arrival. Often the stretcher will not fit down the jetway and through the aircraft door. In these cases, a lift truck (the same as is used to load food and supplies onto the plane) is used to lift the stretcher up to a larger rear aircraft door. All these arrangements must flow smoothly, and making these arrangements can be quite a feat, especially when you may be dealing with non-English-speaking people halfway around the world and many time zones away.

The cost of stretcher transport on a commercial airliner is usually nine to ten times the cost of a one-way economy seat (or four times the cost of a first-class seat). Oxygen, nurse or doctor's fees, and ground transport will be extra. Scheduling normally takes 48 to 72 hours, or more, and is dependent on seat availability as well as the airline's acceptance of the case.

Most U.S. airlines do not perform stretcher transportation. If you are arranging stretcher transport of a sick or injured relative back to the U.S., the patient will first arrive at a major U.S. international airport and then you will have to arrange further transport to their hometown—this can only be done by ground or air ambulance.

Some air ambulance and assistance companies can also make stretcher arrangements on a commercial airliner on your behalf. This can be very helpful, especially in complex cases where there is considerable leg work involved. They will provide medical attendants for the flight, obtain medical clearances and have their physician consultant speak with the doctors caring for the patient, arrange ground ambulance pick up, and arrange, as necessary, ongoing air ambulance transport in the United States after arrival from overseas. The fees charged will vary from company to company, so it's best to get several price quotations.

Transport by Air Ambulance If the medical condition requires immediate air ambulance evacuation, you must contact an air ambulance company that can provide a medically equipped and staffed aircraft—often a small jet or turboprop. Air ambulance companies vary in their capabilities, especially outside developed countries, and it may be difficult to determine if the company provides quality medical care and safe aviation. Also, air ambulances are expensive, usually three times the cost of a comparable stretcher-equipped commercial flight. You will be required to prepay the total cost of the flight—or arrange guarantee of payment if you have insurance coverage.

Because of their geographic proximity, it is best to use a U.S.-based air ambulance company for evacuations from Mexico, the Caribbean, Canada, and/or South America. U.S. companies can usually arrange transport from Europe or the Pacific Basin to the United States, but when dealing with medical evacuation from other parts of the world, it may be better to deal with European- or Asian-based companies. This is especially true when charter aircraft must be flown into Africa, Asia, the Middle East, the former Soviet Union, or Eastern Europe. American companies, unless they have overseas affiliates, are too remote to provide this service, and they may have difficulty obtaining the necessary flight clearances to enter countries in these regions.

An air ambulance is often required to provide urgent evacuation from a remote or medically under-served area to a more suitable, higher-level medical facility. For example, an injured patient might be flown from North Africa to Switzerland. After further treatment and stabilization, the patient might be returned home by stretcher-equipped commercial airliner for ongoing treatment or convalescence. This last leg of the trip is called repatriation.

Companies Providing Air Ambulance Services

If you look in the Yellow Pages of any metropolitan telephone book, you'll find listed numerous air ambulance companies. What you can't be sure of is their quality. The companies listed in this chapter are well established and have a record of quality care and reliability. Some of these companies are hospital-based and provide local helicopter "life flights," as well as staffing fixed-wing aircraft with their medical teams for overseas evacuations.

A listing of air ambulance companies and assistance companies is also found on the State Department's website: Medical Information for Americans Traveling Abroad (http://travel.state.gov/travel/tips/health/health_1185.html).

U.S.- and Canada-Based Companies (Also serving the Caribbean/Mexico/ Latin America)

National Air Ambulance
Fort Lauderdale, FL
800-327-3710
www.nationalairambulance.com

Life Flight
Hermann Hospital
Houston, TX
800-231-4357

Skyservice Lifeguard
Montreal and Ft. Lauderdale
800-463-3482

INTERNATIONAL SOS
Philadelphia, PA
800-468-5232 (U.S. and Canada) or
1-215-245-4707 (from overseas)
www.internationalsos.com

MEDEX ASSISTANCE CORP.
Baltimore, MD
1-800-537-2029
1-800-527-0218
1-410-453-6330 (overseas collect)

United Kingdom/Europe

Heathrow Air Ambulance Services
London, England
[44] 208-897-6185 or 800-513-5192
   (toll-free U.S. access)
http://www.heathrowairambulance.com
Connecting Europe, the Middle East,
   North Africa, and West Africa

Swiss Air Ambulance
Zurich, Switzerland
[41] (1)-383-1111
http://www.rega.ch
Extensive operations in Europe, Russia,
   Africa, and the Middle East

Austrian Air Ambulance
Vienna, Austria [43] 1-40-1-44
ambulance@oafa.com
http://www.oafa.com

German Air Rescue
Stuttgart, West Germany
[49] 711-701-070
alertcenter@drf.de
http://www.german-air-rescue.de

MEDIC'AIR International
Paris, France
[33] 1-41-72-1414
http://www.medic-air.com/

Turkey

Redstar/MARM Assistance
Sabiha Gokcen International Airport
Kurtkoy
redstar@redstar-aviation.com
www.redstar-aviation.com
[90] (216)-588-0216
Turkey's primary air ambulance and
   rescue company

Israel

HMC MEDEVAC
   INTERNATIONAL
Herzliya Medical Center
Herzliya
[972] (9)-959-2444 or 972-9-959-2433
aj@hmc-ims.com

East Africa

AMREF Flying Doctors Service
Nairobi, Kenya
Evacuation services for East Africa and
   surrounding countries.
[254] (0)-20 315 454 or
   [254] (0) 20 605 093

Botswana/Zimbabwe/ Zambia/Mozambique

Medical Air Rescue Service, Ltd.
Belgravia, Harare, and Zimbabwe
[263] (0)-73-45-13/14/15

South Africa

Medical Rescue International
Johannesburg
[27] (0) 11-403-7080
Extensive assistance network in sub-
Saharan Africa. Mobile decompression
chamber for diver emergencies.

EuropAssistance (Headquarters in
Europe)
Johannesburg
[27] (0) 11-315-3999

India

East West Rescue
New Delhi, India
[91] (11)-698-865/623-738/698-554
www.eastwestrescue.com
India's largest assistance company. Serves
India, and Bangladesh,
Bhutan, Sri Lanka, Nepal, Maldives, and
Pakistan

Southeast Asia

International SOS
800-468-5232 (U.S. and Canada)
1-215-245-4707 (overseas)
www.internationalsos.com
Evacuations from China, SE Asia,
Pacific Rim, and the western-most Pacific
islands

Medical Transport of the Overseas Employee

If you are an overseas employee and are sick or injured, your company can help arrange medical transportation to a local hospital. If the local hospital is not adequate, you may need to be flown to another hospital, perhaps in the United States. The following check-list will help your company arrange this type of transportation. They can do the following:

- Assess availability of local ground ambulance and rescue services
- Establish ground ambulance access protocols. Determine if you will need a language interpreter in emergency situations. Suggestion: Contact the consular section of the U.S. Embassy, a United States consulate, or a corporate neighbor. Because they have already arranged emergency protocols for their own personnel, they can identify reliable English-speaking doctors and also relate their experience with local hospitals, pharmacies, and ambulance services.
- Formulate medical evacuation protocols for emergencies that can't be handled locally, including planning for disasters as well as individual medical evacuation cases.
- Check availability of stretcher transport on commercial airlines for nonemergency cases.
- Establish access and credit arrangements with an international air ambulance com-pany such as International SOS Assistance, Swiss Air Rescue, EuropAssistance, or one of the other companies listed in this chapter. Commercial airliners will not trans-port emergency cases.
- Determine if exit visas or other formalities are required.
- Provide on-site employees with 24-hour telephone or telex number(s) of an assis-tance company, and/or the home office, in case of a medical emergency.

CHAPTER 19

Business Travel and Health

KEY POINTS:

▶ Corporations have the responsibility to ensure that employee travel is as safe and secure as possible.

▶ This responsibility also extends to an employee's family when they accompany the employee abroad.

▶ Trip preparation must take into account the stress factors not usually encountered by the traveling tourist.

▶ Business travelers should have 24-hour access to an assistance center that can provide emergency medical evacuation or deal with any security/safety issues that may arise.

Business travel is increasingly international in scope, and more companies are taking steps to protect the health and safety of their employees who are traveling or living abroad. The reason? Business travelers may be at significant risks for travel-related health and safety problems.

Business travel is different from tourism. In addition to the multitude of tropical and infectious diseases that the business or corporate traveler may be exposed to, these travelers are often under higher stress because of job performance requirements, tight schedules, sudden departures, separation from home and family—plus the increased fear of kidnapping or a terrorist incident. If you are on a long-term assignment overseas, not only you but also your spouse must deal with culture shock and must adapt to living abroad.

TRIP PREPARATION

As a corporate or business traveler, you need to maintain a high degree of personal health at home, know your medical history, and have access to your medical records. Maintain a close relationship with your corporate medical department. If your company does not have a medical department, contact a travelers' clinic for advice, shots, and medications.

Routine Immunizations These immunizations should be kept up to date and include the following:

- Tetanus/diphtheria (Td)
- Polio
- Measles/mumps/rubella (MMR)

- Varicella (chickenpox)
- Pneumococcal influenza
  - Temperate southern hemisphere: important from April to September
  - Temperate northern hemisphere: important from November to March
  - Tropics: important year round

Trip-Specific Immunizations More and more business trips occur at short notice, so many travelers barely have time to book their tickets and pack their suitcases, let alone time to arrange a visit to their travel clinic. Also, many travelers are unaware that certain immunizations (such as hepatitis B) require up to three injections spanning 6 months.

Many travel-health professionals now practice "proactive" vaccination management so that the traveler is "ready to travel" at any time. The traveler is given the appropriate vaccinations for the most likely destinations and these are kept up to date. These vaccinations may include: hepatitis A, hepatitis B, typhoid, cholera, meningococcal vaccine, rabies, Japanese encephalitis, and/or yellow fever. A baseline PPD/Mantoux skin test for tuberculosis may also be appropriate.

Yellow fever vaccine can be administered only in certified clinics, or at a health department. The vaccination is recorded in the WHO "International Certificate of Vaccination" booklet (often called the "yellow booklet" because of its color) and this must be produced when entering a country that requires proof of yellow fever vaccination. Note that the certificate is not valid until 10 days after receiving the vaccination. Not having a valid vaccination certificate could mean being quarantined, denied entry to a country, or, even worse, being vaccinated on the spot, possibly with a non-sterile needle/syringe.

Hepatitis A Hepatitis A is the most common vaccine-preventable disease in the world and is very common in all developing and even some developed countries. The first dose of the two-shot series gives good protection, even if administered just before departure. The second dose, usually given 6 to 18 months later, essentially gives you life-long immunity to this disease. The hepatitis A vaccine is now considered practically routine for foreign travel.

Hepatitis B Certain travel-health professionals recommend hepatitis B vaccination for all international travelers. However, vaccination is certainly recommended for all health-care workers and expatriates and frequent visitors to developing countries. It is important if there is a possibility of receiving medical or dental injections abroad or the possibility of new sexual partner(s) during the stay. Counseling on body fluid and blood precautions—as well as safe sex—is strongly recommended before departure.

Sexually acquired hepatitis B may be a significant threat to the health of corporate travelers. A study in the British Medical Journal reported a 50% exposure to the hepatitis B virus over a 5-year period in expatriate male company employees in Southeast Asia. Sexual contact with the local populace was the apparent mode of transmission. Males, especially those traveling to Asia or sub-Saharan Africa, where there is a high incidence of hepatitis B, and who want maximum protection against hepatitis B, should be immunized.

- **Medication**—Talk to your travel-health advisor about the need for medication for the prevention or treatment of travel-related problems such as motion sickness, travelers' diarrhea, jet lag (short-acting sleeping pill?), altitude sickness, and malaria.
- **Start medication**—If you're going to a country where there is the risk of *falciparum* malaria and your doctor has prescribed the prophylactic drug mefloquine, start this medication 2 weeks before departure. This time period will ensure protective blood levels of the drug and alert you to possible side effects.

Under special circumstances, your health-care provider may start you on a short-term course (2 weeks maximum) of prophylactic antibiotics to prevent travelers' diarrhea. This may be justified if your project demands your complete availability and physical well-being and you will be at high risk for illness.

Other Medications Carry enough of any medication that you might regularly use for the treatment of any chronic medical condition, such as for high blood pressure or diabetes.

Medical Kit/Travel Supplies Obtain a travel kit that contains basic first-aid supplies, plus analgesics, antacids, a quinolone antibiotic for treating travelers' diarrhea, loperamide (Imodium), antimalarial drugs (if needed), and perhaps a short-acting sleeping pill for jet lag. Mosquito repellents and permethrin clothing spray are very important when traveling to a country where there is the risk of malaria or other insect-transmitted diseases. A permethrin-treated mosquito net is often useful. (See checklist in Chapter 2)

Avoid Unsafe Sex and Unsafe Injections It's virtually impossible to get infected with HIV or hepatitis B if you avoid casual sexual relations (or at least practice safe sex), and avoid unsafe injections and unscreened blood transfusions. Although getting an unsafe injection overseas is unlikely, it can occur when travelers receive emergency medical or dental treatment in hospitals or clinics in developing countries. Some health-care facilities abroad can't afford disposable needles and syringes, so these items are sometimes recycled, usually without sterilization. Because of this situation, some travelers now carry kits stocked with sterile needles and syringes, suture supplies, and, in some cases, in case they need injections, wound repair, or intravenous fluids.

HIV Testing See if this applies to you. Test results are required by about 50 countries for long-stay travelers as a condition for granting certain types of visas. Country-specific testing requirements are available online (http://travel.state.gov) *but* you should contact that country's embassy or consulate before departure to verify the requirement.

Medical Care Abroad Your company may have a contract with a medical assistance or insurance company to look after its international travelers. Know who to call and how to access this system. If no such arrangement exists, make sure that you know how to find, or arrange for, medical care (and medications) abroad (see Chapter 16).

Travel Insurance If your company does not have a program, you should purchase travel health insurance to (1) pay your hospital bills on the spot or (2) evacuate you in event of serious illness or injury. The best travel policies also provide telephone access to an emergency assistance center through a 24-hour hotline. At the assistance center, medically trained multi-lingual personnel refer you to appropriate medical care, monitor your condition and, if necessary, arrange emergency evacuation if the standard of care in the local hospital is inadequate to treat your medical condition. In Chapter 17, you'll find a list of other companies that offer travel health insurance.

Medical Assistance An alternative method of protecting a traveling employee is for a company to purchase travel assistance directly. Your firm sets up a credit account with an assistance company. The assistance company will monitor your medical care, provide direct payments to overseas doctors and hospitals, and arrange evacuation, if necessary. Contact International SOS (215 942 8000), Medex Assistance Corporation (410-453-6300), or AXA Assistance (800-756-5900).

KIDNAPPING AND TERRORISM

Not only should you be concerned about your health, but you should also consider your physical safety. What are the risks of being kidnapped, hijacked, or taken hostage? What's the best way to reduce these risks? How should you react in a terrorist incident? When traveling to a hostile or unstable country, what rules should you follow to maintain a low profile? These and many other questions increasingly concern today's business traveler, especially after 9/11 and the escalating conflicts in the Middle East. Multinational corporations and their employees are often the targets of insurgent or dissident groups who are trying to make a political statement, take hostages, or extort money.

Preparing for a Safe Trip

A large industry has developed in the field of corporate travel safety and security. If your company has a corporate security division, contact that office for a briefing. You also need to start some essential background reading. Suggested titles include *The Safe Travel Book—A Guide for the International Traveler* by Peter Savage (Lexington Books: 800-462-6420) and *The Security Minute: How to Be Safe in the Streets, at Home, and Abroad So You Can Save Your Life!* by Robert L. Siciliano (Safety Zone Press: 800-438-6223).

Safe Travel Tips

Don't
- Dress like a high-profile business person
- Carry expensive luggage
- Display tickets from U.S. airlines
- Wear shirts or hats with logos of U.S. corporations
- Carry English-language publications in plain view

Do
- Take a nonstop flight
- Send sensitive documents separately
- Leave a detailed itinerary at the office
- Carry medical evacuation insurance
- Check Department of State travel warnings and advisories

Risk Management

Risk management firms, usually run by former employees of the State Department or CIA, have sprung up to meet the security needs of multi-national corporations and certain high-risk travelers. These firms do more than just arrange kidnap insurance. They can do the following:

- Train employees to reduce their risk of being taken hostage
- Conduct counter-terrorism-training seminars
- Provide personal security training
- Prepare a crisis management plan
- Negotiate hostage release
- Provide anti-kidnapping equipment (for example, armored vehicles)
- Alert you to which airlines are under increased terrorist threat (and advise appropriate travel alternatives)
- Provide detailed security advisory before travel to a high-risk country

Some well-known firms are listed below. Kidnap insurance is arranged through their affiliated underwriter:

The Ackerman Group, Inc.
1666 Kennedy Causeway
Miami Beach, FL 33141
(305-865-0072)
www.ackermangroup.com

Control Risks Group, LLC
1600 K Street, NW
Suite 450
Washington, DC 20006
1-202-449-3330
www.control-risks.com

iJET Travel Risk Management
910F Bestgate Road
Annapolis, MD 21401
1-410-573-3860
www.iJet.com

Parvus International/Armor Group
1401 K Street, NW, 10th floor
Washington, DC 20005
202-289-5600
www.armorgroup.com

International SOS Assistance, Inc.
3600 Horizon Boulevard, Suite 300
Trevose, PA USA 19053
215-942 8000 or 1-800-523-8930
http://www.internationalsos.com

BUSINESS TRAVEL AND STRESS

Your Health May Be at Risk

Business travel can be stimulating and rewarding, but it also can be stressful to the point of jeopardizing your health. In fact, a study by the Hyatt Hotels Corporation found that business travel lasting more than 5.2 days interfered significantly with a traveler's personal life.

The problem is more than just chronic jet lag. Frequent departures on short notice, high-pressure work schedules, job-performance anxiety, living in hotels and motels, traveling alone and feeling isolated, eating calorie-dense restaurant and airline foods, and not exercising all take their tolls. Add to this being separated from your home, your family, and your usual routines. No wonder you feel depressed and lonely—even disoriented at times. You may start to smoke and drink too much or overeat. You need a sleeping pill at night and then a tranquilizer in the morning. Fatigue mounts and performance suffers. Things spiral downward. The possible outcome? Burnout or worse. You need a plan.

- Start with physical fitness. A regular exercise program promotes physical and mental health. Exercising also helps control your weight and combats insomnia. Not being fit can lower your self-esteem. What's the best exercise? It's the one you like doing, but experts often recommend either walking or jogging. You can do them almost anywhere, without charge, and they build aerobic stamina.
- Plan the exercise activities you want to pursue during your trip and pack the necessary equipment: footwear, gym gear, bathing suit, tennis racquet, etc. Take into account the climate (how hot?) and the geography (seashore? mountains?) at your destination.
- Stay in hotels that cater to travelers interested in fitness. Ask about the facilities when you make your reservation. Most major hotels and resorts now have fitness rooms and health clubs. Is there also a swimming pool? Tennis courts? The Hyatt, Hilton, and Marriott hotels even provide guests with information on dealing with all types of stress.
- Use a guidebook to plan walking tours of local tourist attractions, museums, scenic areas, etc. If possible, walk to your business appointments. Wear walking shoes made by companies such as Rockport; many models are also formal enough for business dress.

Emotional needs of travelers—In addition to exercise and diet, you need to care for your emotional and psychological needs.

- Keep in close touch with your office and family. Carry some photos of your spouse and children, or close friend. Write postcards and letters. Keep a diary. Take pictures. Buy gifts and souvenirs to bring home.
- Carry playing cards, a board game, a walkman with your favorite cassettes (or foreign language tapes), and a short-wave radio to listen to music and news on the Voice of America or the BBC. The Grundig short-wave radio from Magellan's (800-962-4943) is a good choice.
- If you are a recovering alcoholic, find out if there is a local AA chapter or other self-help group in the area. For a directory of AA chapters overseas, contact: AA World Services, P.O. Box 459, Grand Central Station, New York, NY 10163; or call 212-686-1100.

- Research your destination. Find out as much as possible about the country you're in, its history, and its culture. Make it a project to learn something specific about some aspect of the culture. If you can speak some of the language, do this as much as possible.
- Turn your trip into a psychic adventure. Stripped of your ordinary surroundings, your friends and family, and your usual routine, you may be forced into a more direct experience with your new surroundings and yourself. This can be painful, but don't retreat. View your new surroundings not only in terms of work but also as an opportunity to learn and grow.

Long-Term Assignments and Stress

If you are being assigned to an overseas post, and will be living abroad for many months, or even years, you and your family will encounter additional stresses. If your spouse and children are traveling with you, how will they adjust? Studies show that spouses (usually the wife of a busy executive) bear the greatest burden adapting to overseas living. Today, most companies anticipate these stresses and provide appropriate counseling. Pre-departure orientation and counseling can have dramatic effects on your psychological well-being and the success of your trip.

To better prepare for your trip also consider the following:

- *Survival Kit for Overseas Living: For Americans Planning to Live and Work Abroad* by L. Robert Kohls. Widely used guide for adapting to living abroad. Paperback $16.95. Discounted pricing from Amazon.com.
- *Culture Shock!* Country Guides. These individual guides explore the psychological consequences of exposure to unfamiliar environments. They claim to "take you beyond the stereotypes and misinformation that often precede a visit to a foreign country." Available from Amazon.com and other online booksellers.

For further resources, contact the Intercultural Press, Inc., P.O. Box 700, Yarmouth, ME 04096 for their catalog or to order directly, 207-846-5168.

Stages of Adjustment What happens when you are uprooted and sent overseas to live and work? Research has delved into the lives of people stationed abroad to analyze their psychological reactions to their new environment. These studies show that adaptation will typically occur in three phases.

- Phase 1. You experience an initial period of excitement and well being, usually lasting about a month. You then start to "come down" as the reality of life in a foreign country sets in.
- Phase 2. This is a period of disillusionment, usually lasting several months. The disillusionment may be with your host country, your work, or both. Instead of acknowledging your feelings, you may instead experience physical symptoms such as fatigue, headaches, and stomach problems and pass these off as simple stress. You, or your spouse, may even become overtly depressed. In this case, you should seek psychological counseling. (Some employees, or their spouses, don't get over this phase. They can't adapt to their new environment and consequently reconsider their decision to remain abroad.)

- Phase 3. After about six months, you will have adjusted to your new life in a foreign country. You will also have picked up some of the language, your children will have adjusted to school, your home will be established, and social connections will have been made.

OVERVIEW OF STRESS FACTORS AND BUSINESS TRAVEL

The number of international business travelers continues to increase rapidly, perhaps doubling every decade or so, an increase that is likely to continue.

One study reports that the bank's employees who travel frequently see physicians and other health-care professionals about three times as often as a matched group of employees who do not travel. Traveling males are 80% more likely to see a health-care professional than matched nontraveling males; whereas for women, those who travel are 18% more likely to see a health-care professional than matched females who don't travel. Although many of the complaints deal with known travel-related health hazards (e.g., infectious diseases), there is a striking number of psychological complaints. The number of psychological complaints increases as the number of trips per year increases, and the increase is steeper for female travelers than for male travelers.

Employees on business trips tend to feel a strong sense of social and emotional concern for their families and a sense of isolation. These traveling employees believe that there is a strong association between such stresses and their physical and emotional health, making frequent international business travel an important, previously overlooked occupational medical concern. Moreover, it is reasonable to assume that the countless business travelers who work for small companies, or who are self-employed, experience similar stress-related problems. Previous studies, performed among both travelers and nontravelers, have shown that an accumulation of work-related psychological stress is associated with physical illness, including a general perception of poor health, cardiovascular disease, and mental health problems.

Many factors are *not* important determinants of stress, including geographic areas of the world visited, number of time zones crossed, having children at home under the age of 18, satisfaction with work, days off overseas, and length of the mission.

In spite of the frequent complaints raised by business travelers, few missions end in total failure, meaning that it is very rare for a business traveler to return home prematurely because of stress-related problems. But stress does seem to cause many hard-to-quantify, less-than-optimum work performances. Failures are far more common among employees posted overseas (i.e., away for more than 6 months), and in most cases such failures are because of coping problems experienced overseas by accompanying dependents, rather than employees. In financial terms, each such failure costs employers tens of thousands of dollars in actual costs (less employee training and relocation expenses), and additional lost revenue from disruption of business.

Causes of Stress

International business travelers experience the following stressors:

- The routine discomforts and annoyances that all long-distance travelers encounter, such as planning the trip, hassles of getting to and through airports, altered eating and sleeping patterns, changes in climate, safety concerns
- Challenges unique to frequent, long-distance business travelers. These fall into three general categories (two already discussed):
  - Concerns about the effects of frequent and extended travel on one's physical and psychological well being, the effects of jetlag, loneliness, and fear of dangerous ground transportation in many developing countries;
  - The effects on one's family of repeatedly being away from home, which is by far the most frequently cited cause of travel-related stress in self-assessment question-naires, with the number of missions per year an important determinant;
  - The workload that business travelers are expected to accomplish on each mission and the amount of work awaiting them on their return to the office—workloads frequently perceived as "unreasonable." During the mission, stressful activities may include having to make decisions away from the office without the usual office support system, communicating in foreign languages, operating in an unfamiliar business culture, and spending long hours in negotiations.
- The spouse at home often feels abandoned, worries about the traveler's safety, and is sometimes concerned about infidelity. Spouses without children tend to experience stress either before or after the mission; spouses with children primarily experience stress during the mission.

Strategies for Dealing with Stress

Here are some realistic strategies recommended by symposium participants for alleviating stresses when traveling overseas on business.

Better Selection of Employees for Travel Because about one third of business travelers do not complain of travel-related stress, there are clearly differences in people regarding this issue, but little is known about these differences. Perhaps psychological tests could be developed to better screen job applicants for positions that involve extensive travel.

Employers should be more candid with job applicants about how much travel a position requires, which is not always the case today. Job descriptions sometimes change and nontravel positions can suddenly become travel intensive. Promotions within an organization can also change travel requirements. Job applicants should be apprised of the fact that in many organizations experience gained in missions is an important consideration in a promotion. Moreover, overseas travel is often appealing to young (perhaps, unmarried) job seekers, but it becomes tedious and stressful after time.

- **Flexible scheduling of travel to allow more time at home**—Corporate travel budgets are often "penny wise and pound foolish." Cost considerations sometimes force travelers to be away on a Saturday night or to use an airline with limited scheduling flexibility. Ideally, business travelers should be able to return home before weekends and leave home after weekends. When possible, employees should be consulted about the timing of their missions. There should also be realistic limits to the amount of time an employee can spend away from home per year. In fact, many organizations have such limits, but they are rarely followed. In many organizations, immediate supervisors look down on the official policy of reduced travel assignments.

- **Travel schedules and work assignments reviewed by senior staff members who have "been there, done that"**—Realistic scheduling from a human resource point of view may require days off from work before a mission and again on return to take care of both family chores and office matters. Family chores may involve seemingly mundane tasks such as paying bills, servicing the car, and other tasks that, ideally, should not be left for the stay-at-home spouse. Female business travelers seem to have a tougher time preparing for their absences than do males, perhaps because females are generally more involved with arranging for child care and carpools, for example.

- **Office workload tends to increase just before a mission**—Doing routine work plus preparing for the mission—and immediately on return. Optimal office scheduling may dictate that several days be devoted exclusively to the mission before departure, with no other work assignments, a day or two of "debriefing" on return, and another day or so to be spent handling desk work and computer work that has piled up.

- **Minimize trip cancellations and date changing**—It is extremely disruptive to frequent business travelers' personal lives to experience repeated changes in travel schedules, which happens quite frequently, albeit often unavoidably. Having to reschedule missions often requires rescheduling family obligations that have already been changed. Employees should be given the option to decline missions if this happens frequently.

- **Counselors to help with the "nuts and bolts" of overseas travel**—Experts can help travelers cope with many of the basic travel issues (e.g., health and safety concerns). In fact, many corporations already have in-house medical departments, sometimes even travel clinics, and some organizations even maintain extensive websites to help business travelers better plan trips; however, many travelers do not use these available resources.

Preparing to Leave

The effects of a parent's frequent absence from home on children are not well understood, but presumably they have a negative impact on children; sometimes children show anger, especially when a parent is away for an important event. (However, according to one boy who was interviewed, "My father being away on a trip makes little difference. When he is home he spends so much time at the office that he is never home anyway.") The impact can, perhaps, be minimized by scheduling special family events before departure (e.g., a day in the park, a day trip, or a visit to a favorite restaurant). It may also be beneficial to have young children accompany the departing parent to the airport, discuss the itinerary and look at maps, and be provided with books and videotapes about the countries the parent will be visiting.

Coping Overseas and Staying in Touch with Home

Travelers should stay in close touch with spouses and children back home, using regular mail, the telephone, and e-mail, even if the traveler has to bear the costs, which may be high. Some organizations cover the costs of daily e-mail and telephone; those organizations that do not cover such costs should be encouraged to do so. Children like to receive regular mail, even though the parents may call or e-mail daily. E-mail appears to be a very effective way for a parent to stay in touch with a child old enough to use a computer. Sending audiocassettes and videos from overseas may help smaller children. According to some experts, adolescents are the most difficult age group with which to maintain a long distance relationship. Some can be interested in the purpose of the mission and kept informed of day-to-day developments, but most adolescents don't care about that either.

Children and Spouses at Home Children appear to require more personal attention while one parent is away traveling. They appear more comfortable with familiar routines rather than additional changes (e.g., staying at home rather than being shuttled off to a grandparent). Some children seem to find comfort in marking off the days on a calendar until the parent returns home. Support groups with other families of business travelers working for the same organization and living in one neighborhood appear to be very helpful for spouses at home.

Returning Home

Nearly 100% of spouses describe their returning mates as being irritable and withdrawn when they return home, probably the effects of fatigue and stress. Awareness of such behavior helps families deal with it. It's best to postpone any coming-home celebrations for a few days. Travelers should try to return home before a weekend, if possible.

Taking children on work trips is no longer the sole prerogative of Hollywood stars with a legion of nannies, or the last recourse of desperate single parents. Surprisingly, it is a commonplace choice around the world and is often encouraged or at least tolerated by the employer; some of them are even willing to foot the bill. In the United States last year, more than 23 million trips were made with one or more children in tow, about 11% of all business trips. Parents who take children along say it is educational and entertaining and helps build family togetherness. Most parents interviewed believe travel is worth missing a few days of school. Frequent flyer miles often help pay the bill if the company won't.

There are no figures for how frequently children accompany parents on international business trips, but the percentage is probably far smaller than it is for domestic travel. The obvious reason is the cost. Trips are generally longer and may interfere excessively with children's school and spouses' work schedules, and most destinations are not exactly to London, Hawaii, or Hong Kong, but rather to dull, uncomfortable, and, occasionally, dangerous locations.

CHAPTER 20

Travel and Pregnancy

KEY POINTS:

▶ Pregnant women should not travel to areas where adequate health care is not readily available.

▶ Travel to areas of the world with malaria is not advised.

▶ Travel after the 28th week should be limited to a 100-mile radius.

▶ Pregnant travelers should be fully immunized, with the exception of live virus vaccines, excluding yellow fever.

▶ Drugs commonly used for travelers' diarrhea can be safely used during pregnancy.

If you are a healthy woman with an uncomplicated pregnancy, you do not necessarily need to curtail reasonable travel. According to the American College of Obstetricians and Gynecologists, the best time for travel is during the second trimester when your body has adjusted to the pregnancy but is not so bulky that moving about is difficult. The second trimester is also safer because the probability of miscarriage is lower. After the sixth month, the risks of premature labor and other complications increase.

When to Limit Travel

A brief trip to major European cities during the second trimester represents a far safer scenario than an extended trip to a developing country where you might have potential exposure to exotic illnesses, as well as limited access to medical care. If you will be far away from expert medical and obstetric care, and/or have increased exposure to travel-related diseases, such as malaria, then you should consider deferring travel until after delivery.

After the 28th Week—Most obstetricians advise their patients not to travel beyond a 100-mile radius after the 28th week. Problems after this time include increased risk of premature labor, preterm rupture of membranes, development of hypertension, phlebitis, and increased risk of uterine and placental injury should you be involved in a motor vehicle accident.

Pre-Travel Checklist

A careful assessment of your medical and obstetric history, and your current state of health, is mandatory before departure. It should include the following:

- Obstetric history—Have you had any of the following conditions?
- Spontaneous abortion (miscarriage)
  - Ectopic pregnancy
  - Pre-eclampsia or eclampsia
  - Premature labor
  - Incompetent cervix
  - Prolonged labor
  - Cesarean section
  - Premature rupture of membranes
  - Uterine or placental abnormalities
  - Hypertension
  - Pelvic inflammatory disease
  - Phlebitis or pulmonary embolism
  - D (Rho) negative blood group
  - Severe morning sickness
  - Twin births
- Medical history—Do you
  - Have diabetes? Take insulin?
  - Take medication for any other illness?
  - Have symptomatic congenital or acquired heart disease?
  - Have anemia, asthma, epilepsy, phlebitis, or any other significant medical illnesses?
  - Get severe motion sickness?
  - Have significant allergies?
- The current pregnancy—Do you have any immediate obstetric complications (e.g., mild pre-eclampsia)?
- Personal comfort—Will it be manageable and acceptable during your trip?
- The duration of your trip—Will it be more than a few days? Will travel require prolonged sitting?
- The destination—Is it more than 100 miles from home?
- The quality and availability of medical and obstetric care in the countries on your itinerary—Is it available and adequate?

Medical Clearance for Travel—After reviewing the above checklists, your doctor will be able to discuss with you the relative safety of your travel plans and offer appropriate advice.

Prenatal Checkups

You should have your first prenatal appointment at 10 weeks' gestation. The fetal heart tones are usually heard by this time, and their presence is reassuring that your pregnancy is probably proceeding normally. Once fetal heart tones are heard, the chance of spontaneous miscarriage is small. You then should have checkups every 4 weeks until week 30, then every 2 weeks until week 36, then weekly until delivery. Travel plans should not interfere with these important checkups.

Pelvic Ultrasound—Before leaving, discuss with your obstetrician the advisability of having an ultrasound examination to check for tubal pregnancy, multi-fetal pregnancy, or placental abnormalities.

Medical Care Abroad

All travelers should ask: What will I do if an emergency arises? Before leaving home, learn as much as possible about the availability and quality of obstetric and medical care in the countries on your itinerary. Unfortunately, most doctors won't be of much help because few physicians or obstetricians are familiar with foreign doctors and hospitals. A travelers' clinic is better able to assist you. U.S. embassies and consulates overseas usually have lists of local English-speaking physicians and can give you a referral. (Ask which physicians the embassy staff personally would use.)

IAMAT—Travelers can obtain a listing of English-speaking doctors overseas by contacting IAMAT (the International Association for Medical Assistance to Travelers) at 519-836-0102. The list is free but a membership donation to this tax-free foundation is encouraged.

Travel Insurance—Travelers going to a less developed country should purchase a supplemental travel health insurance policy that provides a worldwide 24-hour medical assistance hotline number. This type of policy puts you in telephone contact with medical personnel who can help arrange emergency medical consultation and treatment, monitor care, and provide emergency evacuation to a more advanced medical facility, if necessary.

NOTE: Travel insurance policies won't cover medical expenses associated with a normal pregnancy (e.g., delivery). Some policies don't cover complications in the third trimester. Other policies don't cover miscarriage, which is usually a first trimester problem. Check if the policy covers the neonate. You should compare the various policies and read their exclusions before buying one. The policies of the following companies cover complications of pregnancy through the third trimester:

International SOS Assistance, Inc.
3600 Horizon Boulevard, Suite 300
Trevose, PA 19053
800-523-8930 or 1-215-942 8000
http://www.internationalsos.com/

Worldwide Assistance Services, Inc.
1133 15th Street, N.W., Suite 400
Washington, DC 20005
800-821-2828 or 1-202-331-1609
www.worldwideassistance.com

Calling Home—Travelers should always carry their doctor's telephone number or e-mail address with them. It's usually possible to call the United States or Canada when problems arise and the traveler wants direct advice from the physician who knows her best. In addition, providing the personal physician's telephone number to overseas physicians may be extremely helpful during an emergency.

Obstetric Emergencies

Review with your doctor those signs and symptoms that indicate a possible obstetric emergency and seek immediate, qualified obstetric care if you have any of the following:

- Vaginal bleeding
- Passing of tissue or blood clots
- Abdominal pain, cramps, or contractions
- Gush of watery fluid from the vagina
- Headaches, blurred vision, upper abdominal pain, nausea, and vomiting may be symptoms of severe pre-eclampsia

Other causes of illness should not be overlooked. Abdominal pain, for example, does not necessarily indicate that you have an obstetric emergency. You could have appendicitis, a urinary tract infection, or merely simple indigestion. Diagnosing the cause of abdominal pain is usually more difficult during pregnancy. Readily available, high-quality medical care is essential if you develop worrisome symptoms.

Symptoms that may be no cause for concern (but if persistent should be evaluated) include the following:

- Increased urination
- Fatigue, insomnia
- Heartburn
- Indigestion
- Constipation
- Slight increase in vaginal discharge
- Sore, bleeding gums
- Leg cramps
- Occasional mild dizziness
- Mild swelling around the ankles
- Hemorrhoids

TRAUMA DURING PREGNANCY

Motor Vehicle Accidents—Accidents are the leading cause of death in travelers younger than age 55, and motor vehicle accidents are responsible for most cases of blunt trauma to pregnant women. Maternal mortality is increased sixfold and fetal mortality fivefold when the woman is ejected from the vehicle. Consequently, the use of seat belts is recommended to decrease maternal and fetal trauma. Use of a lap belt alone, however, has been implicated in placental injury and fetal injury. The best protection is provided by the diagonal shoulder strap with a lap belt. The straps should be above and below the abdominal bulge, thus distributing the energy of impact over the anterior chest and pelvis.

Falls—Women in their third trimester tend to have more falls. Eighty percent of these falls occur after the 32nd week and are mostly caused by fatigue, a fainting spell, a protuberant abdomen, a loss of balance and coordination, and increased joint mobility, especially looseness of the pelvic joints. Most of these third trimester falls are usually minor but some might require you to undergo a brief period of observation or fetal monitoring.

Abruptio Placentae (Placental Separation)—A direct blow to your abdomen is more apt to injure the placenta than the fetus. Mild abdominal trauma may cause placental separation in 1% to 5% of cases. Major blunt abdominal trauma causes separation in 20% to 50% of cases. Symptoms of abruptio placentae include abdominal pain and vaginal bleeding; severe pain without bleeding can also occur.

Fetal Monitoring—Early detection and treatment of abruptio placentae are critical to prevent fetal death and preserve the mother's health. Fetal monitoring as early as the 20th week of pregnancy can be diagnostic. Studies show that there is frequent uterine activity—more than eight uterine contractions per hour—during the first few hours of monitoring after trauma in virtually all patients in whom abruption eventually occurs. Monitoring is advised, however, only after the stage of fetal viability (approximately 24 weeks) because no therapy exists for the treatment of fetal distress before this developmental stage. Concern for maternal health is the only indication for hospitalization before the stage of fetal viability.

Ultrasound—Ultrasound may be unreliable for the diagnosis of abruption. Fetal monitoring (cardiotocographic monitoring) is superior. Ultrasound is useful to (1) determine fetal well being if monitoring is equivocal; (2) measure fetal heart rate and verify lack of fetal cardiac activity if fetal death is suspected; and (3) estimate the volume of amniotic fluid if there is a question of ruptured membranes.

When to Monitor—If you sustain a direct abdominal blow or a motor vehicle accident (with or without direct abdominal trauma), then you should have continuous monitoring for at least 4 hours, provided the monitoring is begun promptly after the injury.

If you sustain minor trauma, a short period of monitoring or observation is usually indicated. If fetal monitoring is not immediately possible, you should contact a physician immediately if you have any of the following warning symptoms: vaginal bleeding, leak of fluid from the vagina, decrease in or lack of fetal motion, severe abdominal pain around the uterus, rhythmic contractions, dizziness, or fainting.

VACCINATIONS DURING PREGNANCY

If you are pregnant (or think you may be pregnant or anticipate you may become pregnant while traveling), an immunization strategy for international travel may present special problems. The problem is weighing the peril and benefit of the vaccine against the risk of contracting a serious, possibly life-threatening infection. For many vaccines there are simply no studies documenting their safety in pregnancy, but they are considered safe, on a theoretical basis if indicated by the perceived risk. If possible, your immunizations should be given after the first trimester.

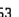

Immunizations Routinely Given During Pregnancy

- **Influenza:** The CDC now states that the flu vaccine is safe in all three trimesters and during breastfeeding. Therefore, all pregnant women should be immunized (using the injectable vaccine, not the live virus FluMist vaccine). Unfortunately, some physicians won't vaccinate during the first trimester, fearing that some women who have a miscarriage will "blame" the vaccine, despite the fact that there is no evidence that flu vaccine causes miscarriages.

    Be aware that the flu season in the Southern Hemisphere is during our summer.

- **Tetanus-Diphtheria (Td):** This vaccine is routinely indicated for susceptible pregnant women.

Immunizations That May Be Administered During Pregnancy, But Only If Indicated by a Definite Increased Risk of Exposure

- **Cholera:** This vaccine is no longer available in the United States and is not recommended for travel. There are no data regarding its safety in pregnancy.
- **Hepatitis A:** The safety of hepatitis A vaccine during pregnancy has not been determined, but the theoretical risk to the fetus is very low. This vaccine is recommended if you are not immune to hepatitis A and plan to travel to a developing country.
- **Hepatitis B:** Hepatitis B vaccine is considered safe and may be administered during pregnancy.
- **Japanese encephalitis:** Significant side effects are possible, including fever, angioedema, and hypotension. There are no data regarding safety in pregnancy. You should receive this vaccine only if travel to an endemic area is unavoidable and your risk of exposure will be significant.
- **Meningococcal:** This vaccine may be given during pregnancy if you have a substantial risk of exposure.
- **Pneumococcal (polysaccharide or conjugated):** If you are a candidate for this vaccine, usually because of a chronic infectious or metabolic state, every attempt should be made to administer it before you become pregnant. The vaccine may be given during pregnancy if you have a substantial risk of exposure.
- **Polio:** A one-time booster with IPV (inactivated polio vaccine) is indicated before international travel.
- **Rabies:** This vaccine, by either the intramuscular or intradermal route, may be given if there is potential risk of exposure.
- **Typhoid:** The Typhim Vi injectable vaccine is indicated for travelers at risk. It is safe and requires only a single dose. The oral Ty21a vaccine (Vivotif-Berna) is not routinely recommended because it is a live (bacterial) vaccine.
- **Yellow Fever:** Although this is a live-virus vaccine, you should receive it if you will be at significant risk in a yellow fever endemic area. Ideally, travel to areas requiring yellow fever vaccination should be delayed until after delivery.

    Yellow fever vaccine may be given after the sixth month of pregnancy if there is substantial risk of exposure according to the World Health Organization. Get a waiver letter from your physician if vaccine is required solely to comply with international travel requirements.

Immunizations Contraindicated During Pregnancy

- **Measles, Mumps, Rubella (MMR):** These are live-virus vaccines and should never be given alone, or in combination, in pregnancy. If you are not sure about your immunization status, you can be tested for immunity to these diseases. Do not become pregnant for at least 3 months after receiving this vaccine.
- **Varicella (Chickenpox):** This is a live-virus vaccine and should never be given in pregnancy. If you are not sure about your immunization status, you can be tested for immunity. Chickenpox is a particularly serious disease in pregnancy and every attempt should be made to give this vaccine before any pregnancy. Avoid becoming pregnant for at least 1 month after receiving this vaccine.

MALARIA

Malaria is the most important insect-transmitted disease you need to avoid, especially the falciparum variety. The disease is more severe in pregnancy, due in part to a decrease in immunity that allows a higher percentage of red blood cells to be infected by parasites, as well as the fact that the placenta is a preferential site of sequestration of parasitized red blood cells.

Maternal complications of falciparum malaria include profound hypoglycemia (low blood sugar), increased anemia, kidney failure, adult respiratory distress syndrome, shock, and coma. Maternal mortality rates of up to 10% can occur. Obstetric complications of malaria include spontaneous miscarriage, premature delivery, stillbirth, and neonatal deaths. Vivax malaria is associated with greater anemia and lower birth weight, but not with miscarriage or stillbirth.

You are best advised to avoid elective travel to malarious areas, especially areas where chloroquine-resistant malaria is endemic (e.g., sub-Saharan Africa, Oceania). If you must travel, it is imperative to (1) prevent mosquito bites and (2) take an effective prophylactic drug.

Prevention

Mosquito Bites—Protection against insect bites is important in the tropics. Malaria, dengue fever, Lyme disease, and other insect-transmitted diseases can seriously affect both you and the fetus. The first line of defense against malaria—and the best—is to prevent bites by mosquitoes. You should apply an insect repellent containing 30% DEET to exposed skin and treat your clothing with permethrin. This combination is 99% to 100% effective in preventing mosquito bites. You should spray residential living areas and sleeping quarters with an insecticide (e.g., RAID Flying Insect Spray). Mosquito nets, especially if sprayed or impregnated with permethrin, have been shown to reduce markedly the incidence of malaria in endemic areas. Vigorous insect-bite prevention measures will not only help prevent malaria but also reduce your risk of other insect-transmitted diseases such as dengue and leishmaniasis.

Drug Prophylaxis—Chloroquine is the drug of choice when traveling to areas endemic for Vivax malaria and chloroquine-sensitive falciparum malaria. Mefloquine (Lariam) is the drug of choice for travel to areas with chloroquine-resistant falciparum malaria. Atovaquone/proguanil (Malarone), doxycycline, and primaquine are not safe to take during pregnancy.

Mefloquine has not been associated with an increase in spontaneous miscarriage, congenital malformations, or adverse postnatal outcomes. It is considered safe for use during the second and third trimesters by the Centers for Disease Control and Prevention (CDC) as well as the World Health Organization. Mefloquine is only 50% effective against *Plasmodium falciparum* along the borders of Thailand with Cambodia and Myanmar, and travel to these border areas should be avoided.

Doxycycline should not be used to *prevent* malaria during pregnancy, but doxycycline can be used during pregnancy to *treat* serious or life-threatening infections such as chloroquine-resistant falciparum malaria and ehrlichiosis when there are no other options.

Treatment of Malaria

Uncomplicated chloroquine-sensitive *Plasmodium vivax* and chloroquine-sensitive *P. falciparum* should be treated with a 3-day course of chloroquine. Uncomplicated chloroquine-resistant *P. falciparum* can be treated with mefloquine or oral quinine plus pyrimethamine/sulfadoxine (P/S) or clindamycin. A recent study has suggested that high-dose mefloquine treatment is associated with an increased risk of fetal death. In the Amazon Basin and Southeast Asia, P/S may not be effective. Falciparum malaria contracted in Thailand can be treated with quinine and clindamycin, but quinine-resistant malaria is increasing in this region.

Atovaquone/proguanil (Malarone) is rated Category C for use in pregnancy, and should be used only if the potential benefits outweigh the possible risks.

Complicated falciparum malaria requires parenteral therapy with quinidine plus doxycycline or clindamycin. Appropriate treatment to save the mother takes precedence over concerns about drug-related fetal toxicity, and individual circumstances will dictate what regimen is best in a given situation. When possible, malaria in pregnancy is best treated by an expert in this area.

Radical Cure

Primaquine should not be used during pregnancy because it may precipitate glucose-6-PD-induced hemolytic anemia in the fetus. If you have been treated for *P. vivax* or *Plasmodium ovale* malaria, you should continue chloroquine prophylaxis until after delivery when you can be treated with primaquine.

DRUG USE GUIDELINES

In general, drugs should be taken only if the severity of the symptoms, or the threat to the mother's health, outweighs the possible risk of fetal damage. As with management of illnesses at home, you should employ nondrug remedies when possible. For example, you can use warm compresses for muscle aches instead of an analgesic. However, if you develop a serious or life-threatening illness, such as an infection, appropriate drugs should not be withheld because of concerns about fetal toxicity.

Drugs for Pain

Acetaminophen (Tylenol)—Safe, in moderation. Analgesic of choice for mild-to-moderate pain.

Acetaminophen with codeine—Safe

Aspirin—Avoid, especially in the last trimester. May increase incidence of bleeding, especially maternal and neonatal blood loss following delivery. Aspirin is a potent prostaglandin synthetase inhibitor, and it has been associated with premature closure of the ductus arteriosus.

Low-dose aspirin—60 to 100 mg daily reduces incidence of pregnancy-induced hypertension; may be indicated for women at risk of developing pre-eclampsia. Should be used only on the recommendation of your obstetrician.

Nonsteroidal anti-inflammatoy drugs (NSAIDs, e.g., ibuprofen)—Avoid NSAIDs do not appear to increase the risk of adverse birth outcomes but are strongly associated with miscarriage. NSAIDs may also increase bleeding potential. Theoretically, any NSAID can cause premature ductal closure.

Opioids—Considered safe

Drugs for Diarrhea and Vomiting

Azithromycin (Zithromax)—Considered safe, although studies are lacking. In Thailand, azithromycin was superior to ciprofloxacin in the treatment of *Campylobacter* enteritis. Other studies have demonstrated some effectiveness against shigella as well as salmonella and *Escherichia coli.*

Bismuth subsalicylate (Pepto-Bismol)—Avoid (contains salicylate)

Furazolidone—Furazolidone is a broad-spectrum antibiotic effective against many diarrhea-causing pathogens (*E. coli, Salmonella, Shigella, Vibrio cholerae*). Furazolidone is 80% effective against *Giardia lamblia.* There are no reports of teratogenicity, carcinogenicity, or other adverse fetal effects.

Lomotil—Avoid. Contains atropine. More potential side effects than loperamide.

Loperamide (Imodium)—Acceptable for watery diarrhea. Avoid with diarrhea associated with a high fever and/or bloody stools.

Metronidazole (Flagyl)—Acceptable for the treatment of giardiasis or invasive amebiasis. Although there is some concern about the use of metronidazole because it is carcinogenic in rodents and mutagenic in certain bacteria, a recent analysis of seven studies suggested that there is no increase in birth defects among infants exposed to metronidazole during the first trimester.

Paromomycin—This is an oral aminoglycoside that is non-absorbed from the intestinal tract and considered to be safe during pregnancy for the treatment of intraluminal, noninvasive amebiasis. As an alternative to metronidazole, it is 60% to 70% effective. Paromomycin can also be used for the treatment of giardiasis.

Piperazines and phenothiazines (Antivert, Compazine)—Acceptable. No reported increased risk of congenital anomalies.

Quinolones—Quinolones are not contraindicated during pregnancy, but they are Category C drugs. According to the *Physicians' Desk Reference* (PDR) "There are no adequate or well-controlled studies in pregnant women. Quinolone antibiotics should be used during pregnancy only if the potential benefit justifies the potential risk to the fetus." Quinolone antibiotics should not be withheld in the presence of serious illness.

Trimethoprim/sulfamethoxazole (e.g., Bactrim, Septra)—In studies of infants exposed to trimethoprim/sulfamethoxazole during early pregnancy, the frequency of congenital abnormalities was not increased. Sulfonamides, however, should be avoided at term due to the risk of hyperbilirubinemia.

Drugs for Altitude Sickness

Acetazolamide (Diamox)—Avoid in the first trimester. Acetazolamide is associated with limb abnormalities in animals. This is a sulfa analog.

Calcium channel blockers (e.g., nifedipine)—No increased risk of fetal anomalies, but decrease in fetal blood flow is possible.

Dexamethasone (Decadron)—Considered safe. No association with congenital anomalies has been reported.

Sleeping Pills and Tranquilizers

Alcohol—Teratogenic; avoid, even in small amounts.

Benzodiazepines—Avoid. One study associated diazepam with cleft lip.

Drugs for Motion Sickness, Coughs, and Colds

Dramamine, meclizine—Considered safe. Use if motion sickness is a significant problem.

Antihistamines—Probably safe, but Benadryl is in Category C.

Cough medicines with iodine—Avoid. Excess iodine may affect fetal thyroid development. Cough preparations with guaifenesin and dextromethorphan are acceptable.

Decongestants—Pseudoephedrine (Sudafed) and oxymetazoline (Afrin) are considered safe.

Drugs for Malaria and Other Infections

Atovaquone/proguanil (Malarone)—Do not use for prophylaxis; safety in pregnancy has not been established.

Cephalosporins—Safe.

Chloroquine—Considered to be safe.

Clindamycin—No studies of adverse embryo-fetal effects. This drug is a good alternative to doxycycline for the treatment of falciparum malaria when used in combination with quinine or quinidine.

Diloxanide—Avoid.

Doxycycline—Avoid. This drug should be used only for the treatment of a life-threatening infection.

Erythromycin—Considered safe. If used to treat maternal syphilis, however, adequate fetal blood levels may not be achieved because little drug passes the placenta.

Halofantrine—Avoid. Halofantrine is embryotoxic.

Iodoquinol—Avoid.

Mefloquine—Drug of choice to prevent chloroquine-resistant malaria.

Nitrofurantoin—Selected by many obstetricians as the initial choice for most urinary tract infections. Congenital anomalies have not been reported.

Penicillin, ampicillin, amoxicillin—Considered safe. This includes the newer penicillins such as piperacillin, as well as those combined with beta-lactamase inhibitors, clavulanic acid (Augmentin), and sulbactam.

Praziquantel—Probably safe. Use only if clearly indicated.

Primaquine—Avoid until after delivery. May cause hemolytic anemia in G-6-PD-deficient fetus.

Proguanil—Probably safe.

Pyrimethamine/sulfadoxine (Fansidar)—Safe as single-dose (three-tablet) presumptive treatment of malaria. This drug is no longer recommended for prophylaxis.

Quinine and quinidine—Indicated for treatment of chloroquine-resistant falciparum malaria. A study in Thailand found no deleterious effect of quinine on the fetus or increased incidence of drug-induced abortion. Quinine may increase the incidence of hypoglycemia in the pregnant patient with malaria.

Sulfisoxazole (Gantrisin)—Acceptable. Avoid at term.

Tetracycline, doxycycline—Avoid unless needed for adjunctive treatment of chloroquine-resistant falciparum malaria or other life-threatening infectious diseases (e.g., ehrlichiosis).

Other Drugs

Iodine tablets and iodine-resin water purifiers—Do not use for more than 3 weeks in any 6-month period as the sole source of purified water. Excess iodine can theoretically cause fetal goiter, but little or no data are available in pregnant travelers using iodine for water purification. Boiling water remains the mechanism of choice for longer-term water purification. NOTE: Prolonged use (more than 2 years) of demand-release iodine-resin filters by Peace Corps workers in Africa resulted in a fourfold increased risk of goiter and thyroid dysfunction (*Lancet*, 1998). Attaching a carbon cartridge to an iodine-resin filter device will reduce iodine concentration in the treated water.

DEET—Considered safe when used according to the directions on the label. There are no reports of teratogenicity nor are there any EPA warnings about the use of DEET during pregnancy.

EXERCISE AND PREGNANCY

Labor is aptly named. Childbearing takes a lot of stamina, and it's no surprise that exercise is appropriate for a healthy pregnant woman. Today, more and more women are active and sports minded, and many obstetricians say that strenuous exercise, even running or jogging, is not harmful to the fetus and may even help build stamina for labor and recovery afterward. But how much exercise is too much? And who should avoid exercise? Guidelines set forth by the American College of Obstetricians and Gynecologists (ACOG) recommend the following:

- Maternal heart rates during exercise should not exceed 150 beats per minute.
- Strenuous activities should not exceed 15 minutes in duration.
- Hyperthermia should be avoided. Body temperature should not exceed 38° C (101.4° F).
- No exercise should be performed in the supine position after the fourth month.

Some authorities believe, however, that the 15-minute limitation may be too restrictive for a woman used to vigorous exercise and advocate the following:

- Pregnant women should tailor exercise to their needs and abilities. For a sedentary person who has never exercised vigorously, low intensity workouts that involve walking, stationary cycling, and swimming are best.
- Exercise should be done within a comfort zone. Special caution should be taken when exercising in a hot, humid climate. (It usually takes about 2 weeks for the body to become acclimated to heat.) Hyperthermia should be avoided, especially during the first trimester when the nervous system of the fetus is developing.
- If the woman is healthy and accustomed to very vigorous exercise, there's probably no reason she can't exceed the ACOG guidelines as long as she does not become hyperthermic, hypoglycemic, or significantly dehydrated.
- The possible effect of low caloric intake on high endurance athletes also warrants caution—this may represent more of a risk than the actual exercise itself.
- Water-skiing is not advised because of the possibility of hydrostatic injury to the vagina, cervix, or uterus. Downhill skiing and horseback riding after the first trimester should be avoided. Cross-country skiing or hiking on uneven terrain should be avoided in the third trimester because of the increased risk of falls.
- Pregnant women should not scuba dive. The fetus is at risk for decompression sickness. No safe depth/time profiles have been established for pregnancy. Snorkeling is safe.
- Relative contraindications to vigorous exercise (or stressful travel for that matter) include hypertension, anemia, thyroid disease, diabetes, cardiac arrhythmia, history of precipitous labor, history of intrauterine growth retardation, any bleeding during current pregnancy, breech presentation during the last trimester, excessive obesity, or leading an extremely sedentary lifestyle.
- Absolute contraindications against exercising include a history of the following conditions: three or more spontaneous miscarriages, ruptured membranes, premature labor, multi-fetal pregnancy, incompetent cervix, bleeding or a diagnosis of placenta previa, or a diagnosis of heart disease.

HIGH ALTITUDES, TREKKING, AND PREGNANCY

There is no known fetal risk if you go to high altitudes for a few days. Some authorities, however, advise against trekking in remote areas above 8,000 feet. Not only may you develop acute altitude sickness, but emergency medical and obstetric care will also be far away.

Women who remain at high altitudes during their pregnancies have altitude-associated increases in fetal growth retardation, high blood pressure, and premature delivery. You should consult your doctor if you will be traveling to, or plan to live at, altitudes greater than 6,000 feet.

COMMERCIAL FLYING

Domestic airlines ordinarily won't allow travel after the 36th week of gestation; the cutoff for foreign airlines is 35 weeks.

After 24 weeks—You should get a letter from your doctor specifying details of your pregnancy and giving you permission to travel. This letter is mandatory for travel after week 35. You should call the particular airline you will be using to verify specific requirements.

Unless you have severe anemia (hemoglobin of less than 8.5 gm%) or sickle cell disease/trait, the reduced cabin oxygen pressure will not cause harm to you or your fetus. If your blood count is reduced more than 25% to 30%, however, you may require pre-travel treatment of the anemia and/or supplemental oxygen en route.

Cosmic radiation is increased at the flight altitudes of commercial jets. Studies suggest that an exposure of 50 millirems of radiation per month (about 80 hours of flight time) will not harm a fetus. This is the permissible monthly exposure allowed pregnant flight attendants. NOTE: Airport metal detectors will not harm the fetus.

Varicose veins and leg edema can be a problem, especially during the third trimester. You should request an aisle seat so that you can get up and walk around every 20 to 30 minutes. If you are in the third trimester, request a bulkhead seat so that you can extend and elevate your legs. These measures will increase comfort, help relieve swelling, and reduce the risk of deep vein thrombosis.

FOOD AND WATER

You should drink only water that has been boiled, bottled (especially carbonated), or chemically treated to remove bacteria, parasites, and viruses. This is especially important if you are traveling in geographic areas where sanitation is poor, hepatitis E is most prevalent (southern and western China, Nepal, northern India, Indonesia, Myanmar, Pakistan, Algeria, Kenya, Sudan, Ethiopia, and Mexico). The hepatitis E fatality rate can be as high as 25% during the second and third trimesters of pregnancy. If necessary, you can use iodine tablets on a short-term basis (2 to 3 weeks) to treat water of questionable purity. Don't use a water filter alone—it won't remove viruses. Use a water purifier instead. Water purifiers contain an iodine-resin matrix that will eliminate hepatitis E and other viruses. NOTE: It is also recommended that an iodine-resin purifier should not be used as the sole source of drinking water for longer than 3 weeks in any 6-month period because of high levels of residual iodine in the treated water (see Chapter 5). All foods should be well cooked and served hot to avoid a variety of infectious illnesses.

TRAVELERS' DIARRHEA

The treatment of travelers' diarrhea can be problematic. You don't want to risk causing a drug-related fetal injury (even though this may be highly unlikely), but not treating diarrhea may result in symptoms ranging from extreme personal discomfort and inconvenience to (rarely) life-threatening illness. Some authorities, worried primarily about the safety of the fetus, focus on fluid replacement and shy away from recommending practically any drug treatment. Others take a different view: they believe that the severity of the symptoms and the circumstances of the particular illness should dictate treatment—not arbitrary guidelines.

Basic treatment—Drink extra fluids to prevent dehydration. If you have mild or moderate watery diarrhea, you can safely take loperamide (Imodium). This drug is especially useful if toilet facilities are not close by and uncontrolled symptoms would cause undue inconvenience, discomfort, or embarrassment.

Antibiotic treatment—Refer to Chapter 5 for antibiotic dosage recommendations. The use of an antibiotic depends on the severity of symptoms: volume and frequency of stools, abdominal pain, general feelings of illness, and degree of inconvenience. The *Health Guide* believes that if you do use an antibiotic, the first choice should be a quinolone, such as ciprofloxacin or levofloxacin. Quinolones are the best drugs for treating infectious diarrhea, and if antibiotic treatment is indicated, then the most effective agent should be used. Alternative drugs, in order of preference, are azithromycin, cefixime, and furazolidone.

- Azithromycin (Zithromax) is emerging as an important drug for treating travelers' diarrhea. It is presumed safe in pregnancy. In one study performed in Thailand, azithromycin was superior to ciprofloxacin in the treatment of *Campylobacter* enteritis. Other studies have demonstrated effectiveness against multi-drug–resistant *Shigella* as well as *Salmonella, E. coli,* and *V. cholerae.*
- Cefixime (Suprax), a cephalosporin, is effective against most pathogens causing infectious diarrhea and is considered safe in pregnancy. There are reports, however, of its lack of effectiveness in the treatment of shigellosis.
- Furazolidone (Furoxone) has activity against a wide range of gastrointestinal pathogens, including *E. coli, Salmonella, Shigella, Campylobacter,* and the *Vibrio* species (which cause cholera). It is also effective against *Giardia.*

Treating more severe diarrhea/dysentery—If you have severe or incapacitating diarrhea, diarrhea causing dehydration, or diarrhea with dysentery, start treatment with a quinolone antibiotic. Institute aggressive fluid replacement therapy. Seek medical consultation if you are not better in 24 hours. Although fluids are very important, antibiotics are also essential to treat the cause of the illness, not just the symptoms. Often, only a few days of antibiotic treatment are needed, and it is highly unlikely that there will be adverse fetal effects from the medication. NOTE: Quinolones are Category C pregnancy drugs: Adverse effects have been shown in some test animals but have not been demonstrated in humans. The benefits of treatment with a quinolone will most likely far outweigh any potential harm to the fetus. Remember, the nature and severity of your illness should determine the choice of treatment, not fetal risk. Effective treatment of your infection is the first priority, and keeping you healthy is also the best way to ensure a healthy baby.

CHAPTER 21
Traveling with Children

KEY POINTS:

▶ Children who travel should be up to date on their routine immunizations.

▶ Hepatitis A vaccine can be administered to children younger than the age of 2 years.

▶ The quinolone antibiotic ciprofloxacin is safe and effective for use in children.

▶ Azithromycin is an effective alternative to ciprofloxacin for treating travelers' diarrhea.

▶ The "BRAT" diet (bananas, rice, apple sauce, and toast) contains insufficient calories and nutrients.

▶ Children who are dehydrated recover more quickly, and feel better, when fed a normal diet as soon as possible.

▶ Children make great travelers. They are inquisitive, fun, and, when they choose, inexhaustible. Taking them on trips exposes them to new experiences, cultivates family togetherness, and builds memories that last a lifetime.

But traveling with children is never all fun and games. Parents must be aware of health and safety concerns, especially when traveling overseas, and even more so when visiting developing countries. Children may need immunizations even when adults do not. Children are susceptible to travelers' diarrhea, malaria, and other travel-related conditions. Children also acquire numerous "routine" illnesses whether or not they travel—for example, fevers, upper respiratory infections, and ear infections. If possible, parents should be familiar with the caliber of medical care in the area that they are visiting.

There are other issues to consider when traveling overseas. Infant car seats and seat belts are often not readily available. Toys bought overseas may not meet the same safety standards of those at home. Hiring local people to watch children may expose the children to infectious diseases (tuberculosis is a serious consideration). Children are vulnerable to severe sunburns during vacations in the tropics, and blistering sunburns are associated with an increased risk of skin cancer, such as melanoma, in later life. Swimming pools rarely have lifeguards. Teenagers often want to participate in potentially dangerous activities not available at home (e.g., parasailing and scuba diving).

Having alerted you to some of the health risks, the bottom line is that the benefits of traveling with children generally far outweigh the risks, provided that pre-travel preparation, and extra precautions are taken with respect to food, water, and insects, and common sense during travel.

VACCINATIONS FOR OVERSEAS TRAVEL

Vaccinating children for overseas travel involves two considerations: routine childhood vaccines and travel-related vaccines. For overseas travel, school-aged children are generally up-to-date with their routine vaccines and need no further injections. However, infants and preschool-aged children may need additional doses of such vaccines. "Childhood" diseases that no longer exist, or occur rarely, in this country are still prevalent in many developing countries and, sometimes, in developed countries. These diseases include diphtheria, pertussis (whooping cough), measles, mumps, and rubella (German measles), to mention the more common ones. Although children in the United States are routinely vaccinated against these diseases, the vaccines are administered at the age at which children respond with optimal, long-term protection. This is not necessarily the age at which children first become susceptible. Therefore, for travel, infants and children may need to be vaccinated at an earlier age than if they did not travel. However, when routine vaccinations are given at an earlier than usual age, or the intervals between doses of vaccines are shortened, the vaccines may give only partial immunity—which is better than no immunity at all—and the doses should be repeated at a later date. These additional doses cause no known untoward effects.

Up-to-date vaccination schedules are especially important for children who will have close contact with local children overseas. Parents should check their own immune status for childhood diseases. Traveling with children may increase parents' exposure to local children. Some childhood illnesses are more serious when contracted by an adult; for example, rubella and varicella (chickenpox) are especially serious for pregnant women.

Table 21.1   Changes in the Schedules for Routine Immunizations Due to Travel

Vaccine	Age Routinely Given	Accelerated Schedule for Travel
DTaP	2, 4, and 6 mos	6 wk, 10 wk, and 14 wk
Hepatitis B	birth, 1 mo, 6-12 mos	0, 1 mos, 2 mos (boosters at 12 mos)
Hib	2, 4, and 6 mos	6 wk, 10 wk, and 14 wk
MMR	12-15 mos	6 mos (measles)
Polio	2, 4, and 6 mos	6 wk, 9 wk, and 12 wk

NOTE: When vaccinations are given at younger than the recommended ages, and when the intervals between doses are shortened, vaccinations may need to be repeated at a later date.

Travel-Related Vaccines for Children

Cholera The cholera vaccine is no longer available in the United States. The risk of cholera to U.S. travelers of any age is extremely low. Breastfeeding is protective against cholera; careful preparation of formula and food from safe water and foodstuffs should protect non-breastfed infants.

Hepatitis A Hepatitis A is ubiquitous in countries with poor sanitation; children traveling to such countries should be protected. The disease in childhood rarely causes symptoms and, in fact, results in lifelong immunity. Infected children, especially those in diapers, can spread the disease to their caretakers. In the United States the hepatitis A vaccine (HAV) is approved for children 2 years of age and older (in Europe, 1 year and older).*

NOTE: Hepatitis A vaccine is safe in infants younger than 1 year of age, but is effective only after the disappearance of maternal antibodies. Infants vaccinated at ages 2, 4, and 6 months of age have shown 100% seroconversion, indicating that HAV (Havrix 360 ELISA units) is highly immunogenic in seronegative infants and could be included in the routine harmonized infant immunization schedule.

Japanese Encephalitis Japanese encephalitis (JE) is common throughout eastern Asia and is the leading cause of viral encephalitis worldwide. China, Japan, and other countries in the Far East vaccinate their children against this disease. However, this does not reduce the risk for travelers. Farm animals are the main reservoir for the virus, and mosquitoes spread the virus. Immunization is recommended for all children who will stay for several weeks or more in rural endemic areas, especially on or near farms, during transmission season. Reactions to the vaccination are common, possibly more so in children than in adults. JE vaccine is approved for children 1 year of age and older.

Meningococcal Meningitis This disease is rare among travelers. However, young children (and the elderly) may be more susceptible than other age groups. The effectiveness of the meningococcal vaccine in children is dependent on the child's age when the vaccine is administered. Protection may not be completely effective in children vaccinated between 3 months and 2 years, especially for vaccination before 3 months of age. The vaccine may be safely given to infants, but it may be less effective than in adults.

Rabies Pre-exposure rabies vaccine is indicated for prolonged stays in rural areas in developing countries where rabies is transmitted by domestic animals such as dogs and cats. The vaccine may be more important for children than for adults. In many areas, 40% of all cases of human rabies in local people occur in children younger than 14 years of age. Children tend to be fascinated by animals, use poor judgment around them, do not report minor bites, and, because of their height, may be more likely to suffer bites around the head and neck. Such wounds may be more likely to cause rabies. Pre-exposure rabies vaccination does not preclude proper wound care or post-exposure vaccination after an encounter with a possible rabid animal. But pre-exposure

---

*Children still officially too young for HAV are usually given immune globulin (IG)—the dose determined by the weight of the child and the length of exposure to hepatitis A. The disadvantage of IG is that it protects for no longer than 6 months. It also interferes with live attenuated virus vaccines such as measles, mumps, rubella, and varicella.

vaccination does eliminate the need for rabies immune globulin after an exposure, and it reduces the number of postexposure injections from five to two. NOTE: The newer preparations of rabies vaccine and rabies immune globulin may be difficult or impossible to find in developing countries.

Typhoid For typhoid fever, breastfeeding protects infants from contact with contaminated food and water. Careful preparation of formula and food from boiled, chlorinated, or filtered water can help protect non-breastfed infants and children up to 2 years of age. Because there is no vaccine currently available for use in children younger than 2 years of age, even more stringent preparation of formula, food, and water is necessary for those younger than 2 years of age to minimize their risk. The injectable TyphimVi typhoid vaccine is recommended for children more than 2 years of age traveling to areas where there is questionable sanitation.

Yellow Fever Yellow fever vaccine should not be administered to any infant less than 4 months of age, and children 4 to 6 months of age should be considered only under very unusual circumstances. Infants 6 to 9 months of age can receive the vaccine if they cannot avoid traveling to areas of risk and when a high level of protection against mosquito bites is not possible. Infants 9 months or older should be vaccinated as required or recommended for travel to South America or Africa. Unvaccinated children are at risk of acquiring the disease and should travel to infected areas only when travel is essential.

Tuberculosis Children should be tested for tuberculosis with the PPD skin test before and after travel to developing countries, especially when such travel is prolonged and closely exposes children to the local people. Tuberculosis vaccine (Bacille Calmette-Guérin, BCG) is almost never used in the United States. However, a recent review of the literature strongly suggests that BCG reduces, in children, both the incidence of serious TB infection and its spread to the central nervous system (brain and spinal cord coverings) and overwhelming infection. These latter complications are particularly common in young children who are newly infected. Most developing countries vaccinate all children at birth, and many European countries vaccinate children at risk, including those traveling to developing countries.

   Health-care professionals who advise parents about overseas travel with children must thoroughly familiarize themselves with the contraindications, side effects, and interactions of the various vaccines, other injectables, and medications that they administer or prescribe.

TRAVELERS' DIARRHEA

Studies of diarrhea among travelers to developing countries show that children, especially children younger than the age of 3, have a higher incidence of travelers' diarrhea than do adults, have more severe symptoms, and have symptoms that last longer. Children place their fingers and other objects in their mouths, swallow water while bathing and swimming, wash their hands much less frequently than adults, make improper food and beverage selections, and may be cared for by local caretakers. Better parental supervision can reduce the incidence of travelers' diarrhea, but lack of immunity to diarrhea-causing organisms may also be a factor. Treatment of diarrhea in children can be problematic: small children often refuse fluids when they need them the most; some effective medications given to adults may not be appropriate; and reliable medical facilities may not be at hand. Also, infants in diapers can spread the disease to the people who change those diapers—the parents.

Treating Dehydration

Fluid replacement and the prevention of dehydration historically have been considered the cornerstone of treatment of diarrhea in the pediatric traveler (although treatment with one of the newer antibiotics is now perhaps equally important). Correct treatment of diarrhea is imperative, starting after the first loose stool, but it is important to evaluate the seriousness of the situation. Is the diarrhea mild or copious? Is the child eating and drinking enough, despite having diarrhea? Children are not dehydrated if they take fluids well and are reasonably active and content, even if the diarrhea continues for a week. Not every episode of diarrhea calls for the administration of special formulas. Most of the time, just increasing the child's water intake, coupled with the regular intake of lightly salted food, takes care of the problem. Food increases the absorption of water, decreases the volume and frequency of stools, provides nutrients and calories, and speeds recovery. In other words, common sense treatment usually works.

However, what if the diarrhea is copious and severe, and the child isn't eating or drinking enough? Or the child has a fever and is generally quite sick? Symptoms of impending dehydration include continual vomiting and diarrhea, refusal to take or inability to retain fluids, and listlessness. Young children can dehydrate rapidly, sometimes in a matter of hours. In such cases, larger amounts of oral replacement fluids, or intravenous fluids, may become necessary, and hospitalization may be required. Parents traveling with small children should keep such eventualities in mind when choosing travel destinations. Fortunately, most cases of more severe diarrhea respond to the conscientious administration of an oral rehydration solution.

Some common treatments for diarrhea should be avoided, such as giving only clear fluids, and the BRAT* diet. These diets don't reduce stool volume, and are calorie deficient. Some other diets are also counterproductive. Soft drinks contain too much sugar and little or no sodium and potassium. Juice-like drinks are merely flavored sugar water. Gatorade and other sports drinks are intended to replace fluids lost by sweating and contain too low a concentration of sodium. Chicken broth contains much sodium but no glucose.

Treatment with Oral Rehydration Solutions Oral rehydration solutions (ORS solutions) contain the proper amounts of glucose (or starch), sodium, potassium, and base (citrate or bicarbonate) and are essential for keeping the body in metabolic balance when diarrhea is more severe. Premixed ORS solutions (PediaLyte, RiceLyte) are available at

---

*The BRAT diet (bananas, rice, apple sauce, and toast)—provides insufficient calories and nutrients, and most pediatricians now believe that this diet alone is too low in protein, fat, and energy content and impedes the recovery process. Children recover more quickly, and feel better, when fed a normal diet as soon as possible.

pharmacies in the United States and Canada, but these are bulky and are meant for home use, not for carrying abroad. For travel, there are small packets of ORS salts (WHO formula, CeraLyte) to which measured amounts of noncontaminated water are added. Travelers without these packets can easily prepare effective "homemade" ORS using table salt, sugar, and water. Instructions are found in Chapter 6.

Ideally, small children should take about 100 mL (about 3 ounces) of ORS with every loose stool or bout of vomiting. Solid food should be avoided as long as vomiting continues, which is rarely for more than 12 hours. If small children refuse to drink, they can be given smaller amounts every few minutes, by teaspoon or dropper. Amounts larger than 100 mL (3 ounces) should be avoided when children are vomiting; large amounts may induce vomiting. Unless vomiting occurs more frequently than every 45 minutes, water reaches the intestine and is absorbed. Infants should continue to breastfeed or drink formula and regular milk. Parents should watch for the return of urine output and improvement in the child's appearance and behavior, and restore a regular diet as soon as possible.

Cereal-based ORS (CB-ORS) is more effective than plain ORS. CB-ORS contains cooked starches (usually rice) in place of glucose. Starch causes more calories and water to be absorbed by the intestine. CB-ORS is available in the United States as a ready-to-drink solution (e.g., Ricelyte, available in most stores and pharmacies) and in packets (CeraLyte, available from Travel Medicine, Inc., at www.travmed.com). If RiceLyte is not available, children can be given plain water with one or more of the following: pretzels, salted crackers, mashed potatoes, rice cereal, or Cream of Wheat cereal. Drinks made with precooked infant rice cereal, unsweetened yogurt, or vegetable juices can also be used. Older children can be offered carbohydrates in the forms of rice, potatoes, cereal, pasta, and bread during the transition to their regular diet.

Anti-motility Drugs

Anti-motility drugs are not considered first-line treatment for diarrhea in infants and children. Loperamide (Imodium-AD) can cause drowsiness, abdominal distention, and ileus (stoppage of intestinal motility), so follow label instructions carefully.* Diphenoxylate (Lomotil) gives unpredictable results in children, especially in those who are dehydrated, and may result in serious, delayed opiate-related toxicity. This drug should be avoided. In moderate and severe diarrhea, anti-diarrheal drugs such as kaolin-pectate (Kaopectate) may reduce the number of stools but may do so by retaining fluids in the intestine, worsening electrolyte imbalance.

Pepto-Bismol (bismuth subsalicylate)

Studies reported in the New England Journal of Medicine have shown the efficacy of bismuth subsalicylate (BSS-Pepto-Bismol) along with oral rehydration for the treatment of infantile diarrhea. Infants given 100 to 150 mg/kg/day of BSS had significant reductions in their total stool output, total intake of oral rehydration solution, and duration of hospitalization. (Measurements of bismuth and salicylate concentrations in blood were well below levels considered toxic.)

*CAUTION: Not for children under 2 years of age.

278

Table 21.2   Child Dosages

>12 years	2 tbsp (1 dose cup, 30 mL)
9-12 years	1 tbsp (1/2 dose cup, 15 mL)
6-9 years	2 tsp (1/3 dose cup, 10 mL)
3-6 years	1 tsp (1/6 dose cup, 5 mL)
<3 years	1/2 tsp every 4 hours for a maximum of six doses/24 hours

Children older than age 3: Repeat dose hourly, as needed, to a maximum of 8 doses in any 24-hour period. Temporary, harmless darkening of the stools may occur. Do not give this medication to a child who has chickenpox or the flu because of the slight risk of Reye syndrome. NOTE: Reye syndrome has never been reported in association with the use of nonaspirin salicylates such as has been found in bismuth subsalicylate.

Antibiotics

Historically, oral rehydration therapy has been considered the cornerstone of treatment of diarrhea in children, with antibiotics relegated to a secondary role. This secondary status was because of questions of efficacy (because of antibiotic resistance) and/or safety (possibility of harmful side effects). Now, because of their remarkable effectiveness against almost all strains of bacteria that cause travelers' diarrhea and dysentery—and because of a re-evaluation of safety issues—the quinolone antibiotics have become accepted by many authorities as first-line therapy, especially in children with severe symptoms suggestive of enteroinvasive diarrhea.

The joint injuries observed in test animals have not been documented in infants and children given prolonged courses of quinolones for such disorders as cystic fibrosis, osteomyelitis, and chronic otitis media. It is now believed that the theoretical risk of joint damage does not justify arbitrarily withholding these antibiotics, especially for children with severe diarrhea or dysentery. A recent study in Israel of 210 cases of invasive diarrhea in children supports this conclusion. The children (35% were younger than 1 year of age) were treated with either oral liquid ciprofloxacin or intramuscular ceftriaxone. Clinical success was achieved in 99.5% of cases. Both drugs were equally effective. A clinical rheumatologist found no evidence of joint injury in patients given ciprofloxacin.

Although the issue is not entirely settled, most physicians now believe sick children deserve treatment with the most effective antibiotic. The antibiotics recommended for treating travelers' diarrhea, in order of effectiveness, are the following:

Quinolones   Furazolidone or cefixime
Azithromycin   Trimethoprim/sulfamethoxazole (Bactrim, co-trimoxazole)

Quinolones Ciprofloxacin is available in both liquid and tablet forms. In cases where there is vomiting, ciprofloxacin, ofloxacin, or levofloxacin can be given intravenously.

Ciprofloxacin (Cipro)—Ciprofloxacin is the quinolone most often prescribed for children. It has excellent activity against *Escherichia coli*, shigella, salmonella, and *Campylobacter*, bacteria that cause most cases of travelers' diarrhea and dysentery. Dosage: 250 to 500 mg twice daily for 1 to 3 days.

Ofloxacin (Floxin)—Ofloxacin is as effective as ciprofloxacin but has better activity against chlamydia and gram-positive bacteria, such as staphylococcus, streptococcus, and pneumococcus. Dosage: 200 to 400 mg twice daily for 1 to 3 days for diarrhea.

Levofloxacin (Levaquin)—This antibiotic is the active component of ofloxacin. It is also a useful antibiotic for the treatment of other infections such as sinusitis, some pneumonias, bacterial bronchitis, urinary tract infections, typhoid fever, uncomplicated skin infections, and chlamydia. Dosage: 250 to 500 mg once daily for 1 to 3 days for diarrhea. For pneumonia and cellulitis: 250 to 500 mg daily for 5 days

Ceftriaxone This cephalosporin antibiotic is effective against enteroinvasive organisms such as *E. coli*, shigella, and salmonella, but must be administered by injection. It is an appropriated drug for use in a hospital setting. It is not effective against *Campylobacter*.

Azithromycin (Zithromax) This drug is effective, especially for the treatment of mild-to-moderate diarrhea. Azithromycin has activity against salmonella and shigella—as well as enteroinvasive, enteropathogenic, enterohemorrhagic, and enterotoxigenic *E. coli*, the most common cause of travelers' diarrhea. In Thailand, azithromycin has been shown to be more effective than ciprofloxacin against *Campylobacter*. Child dosage: 10 mg/kg/day for 3 days.

Cefixime (Suprax) This is a broad-spectrum cephalosporin with activity against the usual organisms causing travelers' diarrhea (except *Campylobacter*). There are reports of shigella resistance. Cefixime is also a useful drug for treating ear infections. Child dosage: 8 mg/kg once daily for 3 to 5 days for diarrhea.

Furazolidone (Furoxone) Although not as rapidly effective as the quinolones, furazolidone has excellent activity against the majority of gastrointestinal pathogens, including *E. coli*, salmonella, shigella, *Campylobacter*, and the *Vibrio* species (which cause cholera). Furazolidone is also effective against *Giardia*. Child dosage: Children 5 years and older should receive 25 to 50 mg ($\frac{1}{4}$ to $\frac{1}{2}$ tablet) four times daily. Liquid furazolidone contains 50 mg per tbsp (15 mL). Side effects: Occasional nausea and vomiting. Not to be given to infants younger than 1 month of age.

5 years and older	$^1/_2$ to 1 tbsp four times daily
1 to 4 years	1 to $1^1/_2$ tsp four times daily
1 month to 1 year	$^1/_2$ to 1 tsp four times daily

Trimethoprim/Sulfamethoxazole (Co-trimoxazole, Bactrim) Most strains of *E. coli*, shigella, salmonella, and cholera bacteria are now resistant to TMP/SMX, and this antibiotic is now considered a last-choice drug. NOTE: TMP/SMX remains an effective treatment for cyclosporosis, a parasitic intestinal infection. Child dosage: Depending on the weight of the child, 1 to 4 tsp of pediatric suspension every 12 hours for 1 to 3 days. More than 88 lb, one double-strength (DS) tablet every 12 hours for 1 to 3 days. Side effects: GI upset, rash. TMP/SMX is safe for children older than age 2 months and can be taken by pregnant women.

CHILDREN, INSECTS, AND THE TROPICS

In the tropics, protecting children from insect bites is the first line of defense against malaria, dengue fever, and numerous other vector-borne diseases. Protection includes the following:

- Placing nets over baby carriages and cribs
- Eliminating standing water around living quarters
- Staying indoors at dusk and after dark
- Dressing children, between dusk and dawn, in long-sleeved clothing that fits over the neck, wrists, and ankles
- Not allowing children to go without shoes
- Covering exposed skin with an insect repellent containing DEET
- Spraying bed nets with a permethrin-containing insecticide
- Using a pyrethroid flying-insect spray in living and sleeping areas during evening and nighttime hours
- Sleeping in quarters that are air-conditioned, when possible

Use insect repellents containing 20% to 35% DEET. This is especially important in malarious areas. Products with higher concentrations are not much more effective and are more likely to produce skin rashes; neurologic symptoms are extremely rare and appear to be associated only with ingestion or extremely inappropriate overuse. DEET, when used correctly, is a safe product and carries no EPA or FDA warnings. Skin reactions to DEET can be minimized by applying it only to exposed skin, not using it on irritated skin, and washing it off when protection is no longer required. Permethrin insecticides, which are applied only to clothing or netting, have no known serious side effects.

MALARIA CHEMOPROPHYLAXIS

The effectiveness of preventive medication against malaria depends on the region of the world visited and the risk of acquiring malaria, especially chloroquine-resistant falci-parum malaria (CRFM).

Chloroquine Chloroquine is the drug of choice for chloroquine-sensitive malaria. In the United States, chloroquine is available only in bitter-tasting tablets. Dosage is calculated by body weight. Overseas, it is also available in syrup form. The concentration of chloroquine in syrup varies across countries. Chloroquine is generally well tolerated by children. Side effects are infrequent and tend to be mild. Reactions can be reduced by taking it with meals, or in divided, twice-weekly doses. Store chloroquine in a child-proof container out of the reach of children. The overdose of only one to two tablets can be fatal to a small child. NOTE: When calculating a child's dose of chloroquine, formulas state the dosage in either "salt" or "base."

Mefloquine Mefloquine is effective against most CRFM; however, mefloquine-resistant malaria is well documented in rural areas along the borders of Thailand. Doses of mefloquine for children are generally given as fractions of a tablet. No liquid preparation is available. Accurate dosing can be achieved by crushing tablets first and then dividing the powder. The powder can be given with apple sauce or a similar substance. Mefloquine was recently approved for children weighing as little as 5 kg, and most advisers would prescribe the drug even to a newborn who is traveling to a high-risk area of CRFM. Many small children vomit after taking mefloquine. The neuropsychological adverse effects of mefloquine that appear to be common among adults appear to be very rare among young children, or have not been reported.

Atovaquone/Proguanil (Malarone) This drug is the combination of atovaquone (250 mg) and proguanil (100 mg). Malarone is a welcome addition because it not only is 98% to 100% effective, but provides an alternative for persons intolerant of mefloquine or doxycycline, for children younger than 8 who cannot take doxycycline, and for those going on short trips (it is expensive), or are frequent travelers. Child dosage: In the United States a pediatric formulation is available and the prophylactic dosage is based on the weight of the child

10 to 20 kg	One pediatric-strength tablet
21 to 30 kg	Two pediatric-strength tablets
31 to 40 kg	Three pediatric-strength tablets
>10 kg	One adult strength tablet

Tablets should be taken with food or a milk-based drink at the same time each day. If vomiting occurs within 1 hour after dosing, a repeat dose should be taken. Side effects are minimal; they include stomach upset, cough, and skin rash.

Doxycycline Doxycycline is an alternative to mefloquine for the prophylaxis of CRFM. Doxycycline is contraindicated in children less than 8 years of age unless needed to treat a life-threatening illness, such as malaria. The drug can also exaggerate sunburn reactions; persons taking doxycycline should be instructed to avoid prolonged sun exposure and to use effective sunscreens that protect against UVA as well as UVB rays. Other side effects include yeast vaginitis (rare in children) and upset stomachs. The latter can be minimized by taking doxycycline with meals.

Lactating mothers taking anti-malarials secrete small amounts of the drug in their breast milk. The amount is insufficient to harm infants and insufficient to protect infants against malaria.

Treatment

Parents should be made aware that any unexplained fever should be considered a symptom of malaria in areas where malaria exists and must be evaluated immediately, ideally by experts in the disease. The problem is that children frequently have fevers because of viral diseases, medical experts are often not at hand, and antimalarial medication can mask other important infections. Emergency treatment with atovaquone/proguanil (Malarone), mefloquine (Lariam), or quinine, combined with doxycycline or clindamycin, should be administered when medical help is unavailable. Clear instructions for such eventualities must be provided for parents. See Chapter 7 for pediatric treatment doses of anti-malarial drugs.

ALTITUDE ILLNESS

The incidence of acute mountain sickness (AMS) in infants and young children is about the same as in adults, and, as in adults, the higher the altitude, the faster the ascent, the greater the incidence of AMS. Problems seem to develop more often in children who have had recent upper respiratory infections. Identifying AMS in young children can be problematic; children frequently become ill with vague viral illnesses that have symptoms similar to AMS—headaches (irritability), loss of appetite, inability to sleep, and fatigue, for example—and children cannot verbalize what is bothering them. Parents are advised that if children become ill, to assume that they are ill from altitude sickness and descend immediately. Acetazolamide (Diamox) may be helpful in reducing AMS when taken just before ascent.

AIR TRAVEL

Air travel appears to be safe for children with upper respiratory infections (URIs) and nasal allergies. Children do occasionally experience ear pain during flight, generally during descent, but less commonly than adults. Moreover, such pain does not cause permanent damage to the ear. The use of oral decongestants and nasal sprays for URIs and nasal allergies may help minimize pain, although some studies indicate that decongestants are not helpful in children. Nasal sprays may give some relief. Use sprays as directed and also at the onset of descent and then repeat 5 minutes later. Older children should blow their noses before using sprays.

Children with ear infections may have less risk of ear pain in flight than children without such infections. Ear infections often produce fluid in the middle ear. The fluid obliterates the middle ear space, and pressure differentials do not occur. Aerating tubes also prevent pressure differentials and pain.

Conventional wisdom recommends giving bottles or nursing infants who cry during flights. The conventional wisdom is that infants cry because they are experiencing barotrauma (pressure injury to the ear) or are dehydrated because of the low humidity aboard the aircraft, but barotrauma is rare and dehydration from low humidity alone does not occur. Low cabin humidity dries out the mucous membranes of the mouth and throat, creating a sensation of thirst. Giving frequent feedings may be counterproductive because at the cruising altitude of jet aircraft, the air in the intestine is already expanded 20% and feeding encourages air swallowing. Therefore, parents should not feed infants more often than they would at home.

CAR SAFETY

Heavy toys, sharp objects, or unused car seats should not be left loose on the back seat or on the ledge of the back window. These may become projectiles in the event of sudden stops or accidents. Some experts recommend seat restraints for large pets. Older children should also use seat belts in the back seat. Seat belts minimize roughhousing. However, in many developing countries, seat belts are difficult to find or are not available. Unruly children distract drivers. Worse, sometimes children accidentally poke drivers or end up in the driver's lap. Parents should keep extra car keys in their pockets. Small children lock doors better than they open them, and sometimes parents accidentally lock small children in cars. Parents should remind children not to dart out of the door and into the street when the car comes to a stop.

Car Sickness Motion sickness during automobile travel is more common in children than in adults. For susceptible children, parents should not give them large meals just prior to and during trips but should give frequent drinks of fruit juice or soda. When necessary, anti-motion sickness medication such as Dramamine (dimenhydrinate) may be effective.

Reading or coloring in moving vehicles may bring on motion sickness. For small children, car seats should be placed at a level where children can see out the window. Cars should be kept cool and well ventilated and no one should smoke. If a child complains of feeling ill, it's best to distract the child with an activity such as singing and not to talk about motion sickness.

LODGINGS

Parents should childproof rooms immediately by checking balconies and bathrooms, covering electrical outlets with furniture or tape, securing lamps and other objects that can be pulled off tables, and rearranging furniture with sharp edges. At night, a small light should be left on to help prevent injuries to children who get out of bed in unfamiliar surroundings. Keeping suitcases and clothes off the floor also helps prevent falls. Because poisonings often occur away from home, check that no medications or caustic substances are reachable. Avoid using syrup of ipecac—it is no longer recommended by poison control centers and may cause harm. Because hotel plumbing may be tricky, especially when the usual locations for hot and cold taps are reversed, children should be assisted with baths and showers. Even adults occasionally scald themselves by turning the wrong knob.

OUTDOORS AND WILDERNESS

Parents should stop at tourist offices and visitor centers for suggestions about safe and enjoyable activities and to obtain material about local health and safety issues— dangerous undercurrents at beaches, animals and plants to stay away from, for example. Frequently, the most common sources of mishaps in the national parks are knives, axes, and campfires.

Guidelines

- Teach children to sit down and stay put if they are separated from you. This facilitates your finding them. Have them carry a whistle for such emergencies; whistles are more effective for signaling than shouting.
- Have children wear loosely fitting long-sleeved shirts, long pants, and shoes and socks to minimize insect bites, sunburn (use a sunscreen with an SPF of 30 or greater), scratches from bushes, and exposure to poison ivy. When possible, bathe or shower children after outings. Look daily for insects embedded in the skin. Using soap helps prevent poison ivy, cleans cuts and bruises, and removes insect repellents and sunscreens.
- With the heat and humidity of the tropics, children need extra fluids and rest to avoid dehydration. The pace of travel should be slowed to accommodate the needs of children.
- Many children who drown or nearly drown do so not while swimming. They sometimes trip, slip, or otherwise fall off boats, docks, and piers, while adults are distracted or taking pictures. When possible, children should wear an age- and size-appropriate personal floatation device when playing near water.
- Shoes and socks protect feet against cuts, fungi, crawling insects, and the many insects that fly just above the ground. Clothing should be kept off the ground, but if it has been laid on the ground, it should be shaken vigorously to release insects. Insect bites can also occur when children strip leaves from trees and plants, shake bushes, kick logs, and turn over rocks. Use insect repellents when necessary, especially in wetlands in the spring.
- Children should be instructed not to drink natural water. Even crystal clear water in streams and lakes far from civilization may contain diarrhea-causing organisms. Ask knowledgeable local people before using well water. Illness may occur weeks later. In case of illness, physicians should always be informed where children have traveled.
- Animals often misinterpret the intentions of children who offer them food with outstretched hands, and especially when children make sudden moves as the animal nears. All animal bites and scratches should be reported to local game wardens and physicians.
- If small children eat unknown berries and plants, samples should be taken to show experts.

ILLNESS ABROAD

Medical Kits Bring a small medical kit (e.g., the Adventure Medical Family Traveler Kit, available at www.travelinghealthy.com) for basic first-aid treatment. You can stock the kit with additional items, such as those listed subsequently. Choosing a destination where there is no ready way of communicating with competent medical professionals adds an element of risk to the trip.

A typical medical kit should include the following:

- Medications that the child has used in the past year
- Antiseptic wipes, thermometer, and gauze bandages
- Insect repellent and sunscreen
- Packets of oral rehydration salts
- An antibiotic for general use or travelers' diarrhea (azithromycin or ciprofloxacin)
- An antihistamine (e.g., Benadryl syrup)
- Antibiotic and anti-fungal ointments
- Acetaminophen or ibuprofen for pain or fever
- Hydrocortisone ointment
- Malaria prophylaxis or standby treatment, as required by itinerary

NOTE: Syrup of ipecac is no longer recommended for children.

WORLD
MEDICAL GUIDE

Table of Contents

Disease Risk Summaries

Maps

Country Listings (A-Z)

Bulgaria, 381
Burkina Faso, 382
Burundi, 384
Cambodia, 386
Cameroon, 388
Canada, 392
Cape Verde, 393
Cayman Islands (British West Indies),
  396
Central African Republic, 397
Chad, 399
Chile, 400
China, People's Republic of, 402
Christmas Island (Australia), 408
Colombia, 409
Comoros Islands, 413
Congo, 414
Cook Islands (New Zealand), 416
Costa Rica, 417
Croatia, 420
Cuba, 421
Curaçao, 422
Czech Republic, 424
Denmark (including Greenland), 426
Djibouti, 427
Dominica, 428
Dominican Republic, 429
Ecuador, 431
Egypt, 436
El Salvador, 439
Estonia, 441
Ethiopia, 442
Fiji, 445
Finland, 446
France, 447
French Guiana, 449
French Polynesia, 452
Gabon, 453
Gambia, 455
Georgia, 458
Germany (Federal Republic of), 459
Ghana, 461
Great Britain, 464
Greece, 465

Grenada, 467
Guadeloupe (French West Indies), 469
Guatemala, 469
Guinea-Bissau, 472
Guyana, 474
Haiti, 476
Honduras, 478
Hong Kong (China), 481
Hungary, 482
India, 483
Indonesia, 487
Iran, 490
Iraq, 492
Ireland, 494
Israel, 495
Italy, 497
Ivory Coast (Côte d'Ivoire), 499
Jamaica, 503
Japan, 505
Jordan, 507
Kazakhstan, 509
Kenya, 512
Kiribati, 516
Kuwait, 518
Kyrgyzstan, 520
Laos, 523
Latvia, 526
Lebanon, 528
Lesotho, 529
Liberia, 531
Libya, 532
Lithuania, 535
Luxembourg, 537
Madagascar, 537
Malawi, 539
Malaysia, 542
Mali, 544
Martinique (French West Indies), 548
Mauritania, 549
Mauritius, 551
Mexico, 554
Micronesia, 558
Moldova, 560
Mongolia, 562

Disease Risk Summaries

The Caribbean

Immunizations: All travelers to the Caribbean should be up-to-date on their routine immunizations: tetanus-diphtheria (Td), measles-mumps-rubella (MMR), influenza, and varicella (chickenpox). Hepatitis A and hepatitis B vaccines are strongly recommended for all travelers. Typhoid fever, rabies, and yellow fever vaccines are recommended on an individual basis, according to the traveler's itinerary and possible exposure to disease.

AIDS/HIV: AIDS/HIV is spreading rapidly in the Bahamas and the Caribbean. The disease is spilling over to women from bisexuals and intravenous drug abusers, and through drug-related commercial sex. The highest incidence of AIDS/HIV, as well as the highest rates of heterosexually transmitted disease, are found in Haiti, the Dominican Republic, and the Bahamas.

Dengue fever: This mosquito-transmitted viral disease is widespread throughout the Caribbean, including Puerto Rico and the Virgin Islands. Transmission is year-round in coastal and lowland urban areas. Only Bermuda and the Cayman Islands are reported to be dengue-free.

Diarrheal disease: This disease is highly endemic throughout the region. Most cases of travelers' diarrhea are caused by bacteria such as enterotoxigenic *Escherichia coli* (ETEC), *Shigella*, *Campylobacter*, and *Salmonella* species. A quinolone antibiotic, combined with loperamide (Imodium), is recommended for the treatment of acute diarrhea. Persistent diarrhea may be due to a parasitic disease, such as giardiasis, amebiasis, or cryptosporidiosis. Outbreaks of vomiting and diarrhea, caused by the Norwalk virus (norovirus), have occurred on cruise ships from American ports. Treatment is supportive. Food safety measures, personal hygiene, and hand washing help limit the spread of these outbreaks.

Filariasis: This is a mosquito-transmitted disease. Highest risk occurs in Haiti and the Dominican Republic. Filariasis occurs (rarely) in the Lesser Antilles from Trinidad north to Guadeloupe. Travelers to these countries should take measures to prevent mosquito bites.

Hepatitis: Hepatitis A is endemic at moderate to high levels in most countries. Hepatitis A vaccine is recommended for all travelers. Hepatitis E may occur; levels are unclear. The hepatitis B carrier rate in the Caribbean varies from 0.8% to 4.1%. Hepatitis B is spread by infected blood, contaminated needles and unprotected sex. Vaccination is recommended for stays over 3 months; for anyone at occupational or social risk, and for anyone desiring maximal protection.

Leishmaniasis: Low to negligible risk. Currently, cutaneous and mucocutaneous leishmaniasis occurs only on the island of Hispaniola (Haiti and the Dominican Republic). Travelers should take measures to prevent insect (sand-fly) bites.

Leptospirosis: A public health concern in the Caribbean. Transmission of disease is through contact with water or moist soil that is contaminated with infected animal urine. The highest risk occurs in Barbados, Dominica, Jamaica, Saint Lucia, Saint Vincent, and Trinidad and Tobago.

Malaria: Malaria is present in Haiti and the Dominican Republic, where falciparum malaria accounts for approximately 99% of all cases. As of February 2005, the Centers for Disease Control and Prevention (CDC) has received reports of 21 new cases of falciparum malaria in travelers to resort areas of the Dominican Republic. All of these new cases had traveled to areas of the Dominican Republic where malaria had not previously been reported. The CDC recommends that all travelers to La Altagracia Province of the Dominican Republic, including the Punta Cana resort area, and all travelers to Haiti (all areas), take chloroquine prophylaxis. No cases of chloroquine-resistant falciparum malaria have been reported. In addition, travelers should take measures to prevent mosquito bites.

Rabies: There is a risk of rabies in Haiti, the Dominican Republic, and Grenada. Travelers to any country in the Caribbean, however, should avoid contact with stray animals, especially dogs, and seek immediate treatment of any animal bite. The following countries were declared rabies-free by the CDC in 1999: Antigua and Barbuda, Aruba, Bahamas, Barbados, Cayman Islands, Guadeloupe, Jamaica, Martinique, Montserrat, Netherlands Antilles (Bonaire, Curaçao, Saba, Saint Eustatius, and Saint Maarten), Saint Kitts and Nevis, Saint Lucia, Saint Martin, Saint Vincent and Grenadines, the United States, and British Virgin Islands.

Schistosomiasis: Limited or potential risk is present in Antigua, Guadeloupe, Martinique, Montserrat, Puerto Rico, and Saint Lucia. The disease may occur sporadically in the other islands. Travelers should avoid swimming, bathing, or wading in freshwater ponds or streams that may be snail infested.

Typhoid Fever: Typhoid vaccine is recommended for those traveling off the usual tourist routes, those visiting friends or relatives, and for long-stay visitors.

Yellow fever: Yellow fever activity is reported only in the remote forested areas of Trinidad and no human cases have been reported since 1980. The CDC recommends yellow fever vaccination for traveling within the rural endemic zone of this country.

Other diseases/health threats: Brucellosis, Chagas disease (low incidence; detected in Trinidad and Tobago), histoplasmosis, fascioliasis (confirmed in Guadeloupe), helminthic infections (ancylostomiasis, ascariasis, strongyloidiasis, and trichuriasis), syphilis (Bahamas, British Virgin Islands, Cayman Islands, and the Turks and Caicos have the highest rates), toxocariasis ("creeping eruption" from dog hookworm; reported from several islands), tuberculosis (endemic throughout the Caribbean).

Accidents and injuries: Accidents, especially motor vehicle crashes, are the leading cause of death among travelers younger than 55 years of age; cardiovascular diseases, such as heart attack, cause most fatalities in older travelers. Adequate medical care may not be readily available in some areas of the Caribbean. Travelers are advised to obtain supplemental travel health insurance with specific overseas coverage. The policy should pay for emergency medical transport when serious accident or illness requires treatment at a more advanced facility.

Marine Hazards: Swimming-related hazards include jellyfish, spiny sea urchins, and coral. Ciguatera poisoning is prevalent in the Caribbean and can result from eating coral reef fish such as grouper, snapper, sea bass, jack, and barracuda. Cooking does not destroy the ciguatoxin.

Scuba Diving: Divers' Alert Network (DAN) maintains a directory of all hyperbaric chambers in North America and the Caribbean. In association with Duke University Medical Center in North Carolina, DAN operates a 24-hour emergency phone number (919-684-8111) for members and nonmembers to call; their staff is available to answer questions and, if necessary, make referral to the closest functioning hyperbaric chamber.

Mexico and Central America

Immunizations: All travelers to Mexico and Central America should be up-to-date on their routine immunizations: tetanus-diphtheria (Td), measles-mumps-rubella (MMR), influenza, and varicella (chickenpox). Hepatitis A and hepatitis B vaccines are strongly recommended for all travelers. Typhoid fever, rabies, and yellow fever vaccines are recommended on an individual basis, according to the traveler's itinerary and possible risk of exposure.

AIDS/HIV: In Mexico and Central America, homosexual and bisexual activity is the prevailing mode of transmission, but the heterosexual transmission of HIV is increasing.

Chagas disease: Risk occurs primarily in those rural-agricultural areas of Central America where there are adobe-style huts and houses that can harbor the night-biting triatomid (assassin) bugs. Blood transfusions are also a potential source of infection.

Cholera: Persons who follow usual tourist itineraries and who observe food safety recommendations, even in countries reporting cholera, have virtually no risk. Risk increases for those who drink untreated water or eat poorly cooked or raw seafood in endemic areas. The risk of cholera to U.S. travelers is so low that vaccination is of questionable benefit. An oral cholera vaccine is available in Canada and Europe. NOTE: The oral cholera vaccine (Dukoral) provides up to 60% crossover protection against ETEC diarrhea, a common bacterial cause of travelers' diarrhea in this region.

Dengue fever: Dengue is widespread throughout Central America. In Mexico, dengue occurs primarily during July, August, and September. The *Aedes* mosquitoes, that transmit dengue, bite primarily at dusk and dawn and are present in populous urban areas as well as resort and rural areas. Prevention of dengue consists of taking protective measures against mosquito bites.

Helminthic diseases: Hookworm is common, especially in rural areas. Travelers should wear shoes to prevent transmission of this disease. Ascariasis and trichuriasis (roundworm and whipworm diseases), caused by the ingestion of food contaminated with the eggs of these worms, can be prevented by washing vegetables and adequately cooking all food. In Mexico and Central America, pork tapeworm disease (caused by the parasite *Taenia solium*) is common and can be prevented by thoroughly cooking food. Cysticercosis and neurocysticercosis, caused by the ingestion of pork tapeworm eggs, is prevalent. (Pork tapeworm eggs are transmitted by fecally contaminated food and/or water.)

Hepatitis: All travelers should receive hepatitis A vaccine before travel to these regions. The hepatitis B carrier rate in the general population of these regions is about 1% to 2%. Hepatitis B is spread by infected blood, contaminated needles, and unprotected sex. Vaccination is recommended for stays of more than 3 months; for anyone at occupational or social risk; for anyone desiring maximal protection. Outbreaks of hepatitis E, from contaminated drinking water, are reported from Mexico. There is no vaccine to prevent hepatitis E.

Leishmaniasis: Cutaneous leishmaniasis (chiclero ulcer), mucocutaneous leishmaniasis (espundia), and visceral leishmaniasis (kala-azar) occur in scattered areas of Mexico and Central America. These diseases are transmitted by sand flies (which bite in the evening and during the night). All travelers should take measures to prevent insect bites.

Malaria: There is low risk of malaria in Mexico. Most cases are confined to rural areas of the West Coast. There is risk of vivax malaria in other rural areas in Central America. Belize has the highest incidence, followed by Nicaragua and Guatemala. Malaria prophylaxis is not necessary when visiting resorts in Mexico, where personal protective measures against mosquito bites are recommended. There is no malaria in the major cities of Central America. Chloroquine prophylaxis is recommended for travelers visiting rural areas, including the northern areas of Panama. *Plasmodium vivax* accounts for >95% of malaria infections; the remainder are attributed to *Plasmodium falciparum*. Chloroquine-resistant malaria has not been reported except in southern Panama, where chloroquine-resistant *P. falciparum* can occur. All travelers should take measures to prevent mosquito bites. These precautions include applying a DEET-containing skin repellent, wearing permethrin-treated clothing, and, when appropriate, sleeping under a mosquito bed net.

Onchocerciasis: This is a form of filariasis prevalent in southern Mexico and Guatemala. There is low risk to tourists. Travelers should take measures to prevent insect (black fly) bites.

Rabies: This disease is present in all Central American countries, but the risk is highest in Mexico, El Salvador, Guatemala, and Honduras. Travelers should avoid contact with stray animals, especially dogs, and seek emergency treatment of any animal bite. Rabies vaccine is recommended for all persons planning a long stay (4 weeks or more) or extensive travel in rural areas of Mexico and Central America.

Travelers' diarrhea: There is a high risk of travelers' diarrhea throughout Mexico and Central America. The incidence in Belize and Costa Rica is lower, because of better sanitation. Travelers should observe all food and drink safety precautions. A quinolone antibiotic is recommended for self treatment of acute diarrhea. Diarrhea not responding to treatment with an antibiotic, or persistent diarrhea, may be due to a parasitic disease such as giardiasis, amebiasis, or cryptosporidiosis.

Typhoid fever: Typhoid vaccination is recommended for persons traveling for periods longer than 3 to 4 weeks in rural areas, and who will be staying in areas where there is substandard sanitation. The vaccine is especially important for those returning to their country of origin to visit family and friends.

Yellow fever: Yellow fever is potentially active in Panama, but is not reported. Vaccination is recommended for persons who plan to travel to the endemic areas in Panama (Chepo, Darien, or San Blas). The Canal Zone is free of yellow fever.

Other illnesses: Amebiasis (high incidence throughout Mexico and Central America), brucellosis (from consumption of contaminated dairy products or through occupational contact with infected animals), coccidiomycosis, histoplasmosis, gnathostomiasis (outbreaks in Mexico), toxocariasis, and toxoplasmosis.

Accidents and injuries: Accidents, especially motor vehicle crashes, are the leading cause of death among travelers younger than 55 years of age; cardiovascular diseases, such as heart attack, cause most fatalities in older travelers. Adequate medical care may not be readily available in many areas of Central America. Travelers are advised to obtain supplemental travel health insurance with specific overseas coverage. The policy should pay for emergency medical transport when serious accident or illness requires treatment at a more advanced facility.

Animal hazards: Scorpions, black widow spiders, brown recluse spiders, and several species of tarantulas are common in many areas of Mexico and Central America. The beaded lizard, Gila monster, and vampire bat are present in Mexico and elsewhere in the region.

Marine hazards: The Portuguese man-o'-war, stingrays, several species of poisonous fish, stinging anemones, coral and hydroids, and jellyfish are present in coastal waters and are a potential hazard to unprotected swimmers.

South America

Immunizations: All travelers to South America should be up-to-date on their routine immunizations: tetanus-diphtheria (Td), measles-mumps-rubella (MMR), influenza, and varicella (chickenpox). Hepatitis A and hepatitis B vaccines are strongly recommended for all travelers. Typhoid fever, rabies, and yellow fever vaccines are recommended on an individual basis, according to the traveler's itinerary and possible disease exposure.

AIDS/HIV: Homosexuality and bisexuality remain the prevailing modes of HIV transmission in South America, but there is a trend toward greater heterosexual transmission, especially in major cities in Brazil and Chile. HIV-1 prevalence is estimated at less than 1% of the general population of the countries of Latin America, but in some urban areas (e.g., Rio de Janeiro), 30% of female commercial sex workers and 80% of injecting drug users are HIV-positive. HIV-2, HTLV-1, and HTLV-2 viruses are reported in South America.

Bartonellosis (Oroya fever): This is a sand fly-transmitted illness found in arid river valleys on the northern slopes of the Andes (Peru, Ecuador, and Colombia) up to an elevation of 3,000 meters. There is no vaccine. Travelers should take measures to prevent insect bites.

Chagas disease: Occurs in all tropical areas of South America. Chagas disease is transmitted primarily in rural areas where there are adobe-style huts and houses that often harbor the night-biting triatomid (assassin) bugs. Travelers sleeping in such structures should take precautions against nighttime bites. These precautions include spraying sleeping quarters with an insecticide (such as Raid), sleeping away from walls, or sleeping under a bed net. Contaminated food and unscreened blood transfusions are also sources of infection.

Cholera: Disease activity is widespread but sporadic. The risk to travelers of acquiring cholera is considered extremely low (approximately 1:500,000 travelers). Prevention consists primarily in adhering to safe food and drink guidelines. NOTE: The oral cholera vaccine (Dukoral) provides up to 60% crossover protection against ETEC diarrhea, a common bacterial cause of travelers' diarrhea in this region.

Dengue fever: There have been dramatic increases in dengue fever and dengue hemorrhagic fever during the past decade in South America. Outbreaks and epidemics are reported from Brazil, Ecuador, Colombia, Peru, Venezuela, and other countries. *Aedes aegypti* mosquitoes, which transmit dengue, are present in populous urban areas as well as resort and rural areas. Prevention of dengue consists of taking protective measures against mosquito bites, especially at dusk and dawn when *Aedes* mosquitoes are most active.

Filariasis: Mosquito-borne; risk is present in parts of Brazil, French Guiana, Guyana, Suriname, and Venezuela. Travelers to risk areas should take measures to prevent insect (mosquito) bites.

Helminthic infections: Hookworm, roundworm, and whipworm are common, especially in rural areas.

Hepatitis A and E: All susceptible (nonimmune) travelers should receive the hepatitis A vaccine. Hepatitis E is endemic throughout South America, but data are scarce. Travelers should avoid contaminated drinking water.

Hepatitis B: The hepatitis B carrier rate in the Amazon Basin of Brazil is as high as 20%. High rates are also reported among aboriginal tribes in Venezuela and French Guiana. Other countries in South America have hepatitis B carrier rates of 1% to 3% in the general population. Hepatitis B is spread by infected blood, contaminated needles, and unprotected sex. Vaccination is recommended for stays longer than 3 months; for anyone at occupational or social risk; for anyone desiring maximal protection.

Leishmaniasis: Risk is present in most countries of tropical South America. Cutaneous, mucocutaneous, and visceral leishmaniasis (kala-azar) occur in many countries. Travelers to rural areas should take measures to prevent insect (sand fly) bites. Sand flies bite most actively between dusk and dawn and are found in greatest number on the periphery of rural forested areas.

Malaria: There is risk of malaria in most tropical regions of South America. Nearly one half of all cases are reported from Brazil; one third are reported from Bolivia, Colombia, Ecuador, Peru, and Venezuela. The highest rates occur in Guyana, French Guiana, the Amazon region of Brazil, and Peru. Chloroquine-resistant falciparum malaria is an increasing problem, especially in the Amazon Basin. Chemoprophylaxis with mefloquine, atovaquone/proguanil or doxycycline is currently recommended for travel to these areas. Travelers to regions of Argentina that border on Paraguay can take chloroquine prophylaxis. All travelers should also take anti-insect precautions. These precautions include applying a DEET-containing skin repellent, wearing permethrin-treated clothing, and sleeping under a mosquito bed net, preferably permethrin-treated.

Onchocerciasis: This form of filariasis is transmitted by black flies of the *Simulium* species. These flies are found near rivers, where they breed in surrounding vegetation. Disease is prevalent in Venezuela, Colombia, Ecuador, and northern Brazil. Travelers to these regions should take personal protective measures against insect (black fly) bites.

Rabies: Animal rabies has been reported from many countries, especially Argentina, Brazil, Colombia, and Ecuador. Human rabies in South America is usually transmitted by dogs, but an outbreak of vampire bat-transmitted rabies was reported in the Amazon jungle of Peru. Rabies vaccination is indicated following the unprovoked bite of a dog, cat, bat, or monkey. Bites by other animals should be evaluated on an individual basis. Immunization against rabies is recommended for extended travel to remote rural areas of South America.

Schistosomiasis: Risk is present in Brazil, Suriname, and north-central Venezuela. Travelers should avoid swimming, wading, or bathing in freshwater lakes, ponds, or streams that are possibly infested with schistosome-carrying snail larvae.

Travelers' diarrhea: This carries a high risk outside of deluxe hotels and resort areas. Lower risk occurs in Argentina and the Falkland Islands, where sanitation is generally better. Travelers should observe all food and drink safety precautions. A quinolone antibiotic (ciprofloxacin, ofloxacin, levofloxacin, etc) is recommended for the self treatment of acute diarrhea. Diarrhea not responding to treatment with an antibiotic, or persistent diarrhea, may be due to a parasitic disease such as giardiasis; treatment with metronidazole (Flagyl) or tinidazole (Fasigyn) may be considered. All cases of diarrhea should be treated with adequate fluid replacement.

Typhoid fever: The highest rates of typhoid fever in South America occur in Peru and Chile. Typhoid vaccination is recommended for persons traveling longer than 2 to 4 weeks in areas with substandard sanitation and for all those returning to their country of origin to visit friends and relatives. The typhoid vaccine is about 70% effective, so avoiding unsafe food and drink remains an important preventive measure.

Yellow fever: Risk is present in rural and jungle areas in all countries except Paraguay, Uruguay, Argentina, the Falkland Islands, and Chile. Vaccination is recommended for travel to rural areas of all yellow fever endemic zone countries. The estimated risk for unvaccinated travelers is approximately 1:25,000 per 2-week stay in an endemic area.

Other diseases/hazards: Brucellosis, echinococcosis (occurs in sheep-raising regions), coccidiomycosis, cysticercosis and neurocysticercosis (there is a very high incidence in Colombia), helminths (roundworm, hookworm, and whipworm infections are common in rural areas), histoplasmosis, human hantavirus infection (occurs throughout much of South America), leptospirosis, toxocariasis, trichinosis, and viral encephalitis. Portuguese man-o'-war, sea wasps, jellyfish, spiny sea urchins, stinging anemones, and sharp corals may be present in the coastal waters of these countries and pose a potential threat to swimmers. Carnivorous fish (including the piranha) may be found in freshwater bodies of some countries. Animal hazards include snakes (coral snakes, vipers), scorpions, black widow spiders, and large animals of the cat family, especially jaguars.

Accidents and injuries: There is a high risk of injury from motor vehicle, motorcycle, and moped accidents in the developing countries due to poor road conditions, chaotic traffic, lack of driver training, and poor vehicle maintenance. Rental vehicles and taxis may not be equipped with seat belts. All travelers should drive with extreme caution and avoid travel by road in rural areas after dark.

Europe, Eastern Europe, and Russia

Immunizations: All travelers to Europe and Russia should be up-to-date on their routine immunizations: tetanus-diphtheria (Td), measles-mumps-rubella (MMR), influenza, and varicella (chickenpox). Hepatitis A and hepatitis B vaccines are strongly recommended for all travelers. Typhoid fever, rabies, and tick-borne encephalitis vaccines are recommended on an individual basis, according to the traveler's itinerary and possible disease exposure.

AIDS/HIV: The countries with the highest incidences of AIDS and HIV are the Russian Federation, the Baltic States (Estonia, Latvia, and Lithuania), Bulgaria, Belarus, Moldova, Romania, and Ukraine. Injecting drug use and unsafe sex are driving the spread of HIV, but the virus is also moving from high-risk groups into the general population, where heterosexual contact is the main route of transmission. In Eastern Europe and Russia travelers should avoid unprotected sex with new partners, as well as unscreened blood transfusions and medical injections. (Many travelers now carry their own packets of sterile needles and syringes.) Blood supplies are reportedly screened in Czechoslovakia, Hungary, and Poland, but lack of public health funding may hamper complete screening for HIV and hepatitis B and C. Travelers should consider evacuation to a Western European medical facility when surgical care or blood transfusion is needed.

Diphtheria: Since the epidemic in Russia in the early nineties diphtheria has come under better control through improved childhood vaccination programs.

Ehrlichiosis: Cases of human granulocytic ehrlichiosis have been reported from Slovenia and the Netherlands.

European tick-borne encephalitis (TBE): The tick, *Ixodes ricinus*, the same tick that transmits Lyme disease, is the vector for this disease. Ticks are widely distributed in brushy and forested areas at elevations up to 1,500 meters. TBE occurs in all European countries (especially Austria, Germany, Switzerland, the Czech Republic, Hungary, the Balkans, and Eastern Europe) except the Benelux countries and the Iberian Peninsula. Transmission is maximal during spring and fall months. A vaccine is available in Europe and Canada.

Hemorrhagic fever with renal syndrome (HFRS): Cases of Hantavirus illness are reported in the Balkans and in eastern Europe. A milder form of HFRS (caused by Puumala virus) occurs in Scandinavia, other European countries, and European Russia. Travelers should avoid contact with rodent urine and rodent feces, which transmit the virus.

Hepatitis A: Hepatitis A vaccine is recommended for all travelers. There is increased risk of hepatitis A in Spain, Greece, the Balkans, Eastern Europe, and Russia.

Hepatitis B: The hepatitis B carrier rate in the general population of Europe varies, but is less than 1% in most western European countries. The carrier rate increases to 1% to 4% in Spain, Greece, Eastern Europe, and Russia. Hepatitis B is spread by infected blood, contaminated needles, and unprotected sex. Vaccination is recommended for stays longer than 3 months; for anyone at occupational or social risk; for anyone desiring maximal protection.

Leishmaniasis: Cutaneous and visceral leishmaniasis is present in the countries bordering the Mediterranean. Risk areas include Portugal, Spain, southern France, the Naples area, Majorca, the suburbs of Athens, and the Greek Isles. Travelers to these areas should take measures to prevent sand fly bites.

Lyme disease: Risk of transmission occurs throughout Europe in rural brushy, wooded, and forested areas up to elevations of 1,500 meters, especially in Scandinavia, Austria, Switzerland, southern Germany, and northern Italy. The ticks that transmit Lyme disease are most abundant and active April through September.

Malaria: There is no risk of malaria in Europe or Russia.

Mediterranean spotted fever (boutonneuse fever): Occurs in southern France and in the coastal regions of other Mediterranean countries, and also along the Black Sea coast, in brushy and/or forested areas below 1,000 meters elevation. Peak transmission period is July through September. Disease may be acquired in and around tick-infested houses and terrain, but more than 95% of cases are associated with contact with tick-carrying dogs.

Pertussis (whooping cough): Reported in the Netherlands. The *Bordetella pertussis* bacterium may be resistant to some vaccines and attacks adults as well as children.

Rabies: Occurs primarily in wild animals, especially foxes, in many rural areas of Europe. Countries free of human rabies include: Albania, Cyprus, Denmark, the Faeroe Islands, Finland, Gibraltar, Greece, Iceland, Ireland, Italy, the Isle of Man, Italy, Macedonia, Malta, Monaco, Norway, Portugal, Spain, Sweden, and the United Kingdom.

Sand fly fever and West Nile fever: Cases are reported from Albania and the Adriatic area.

Travelers' diarrhea: Low risk in most western European countries. Higher risk occurs in Spain, Greece, the Balkans, and Eastern Europe, especially Bulgaria, Hungary, and Romania. Giardiasis is a threat in Russia. Travelers to higher risk areas should drink only bottled, boiled, or treated water and avoid undercooked food. A quinolone antibiotic is recommended for the treatment of diarrhea.

Typhoid fever: Persons traveling extensively in Spain, Greece, Yugoslavia, and the Balkans, or the eastern European countries, especially Bulgaria, Hungary, and Romania, should consider typhoid vaccination.

Other illnesses/hazards: Brucellosis, echinococcosis (southern Europe), Legionnaire's disease (legionellosis outbreaks have been reported in tourists on package tours to Spain and Naples, Italy; contaminated water is the probable source), leptospirosis, listeriosis (from contaminated soft cheeses and meat; reported from France), tick-borne relapsing fever (risk in rocky, rural livestock areas), and soil-transmitted helminthic infections (roundworm, hookworm, and whipworm infections; reported in southern Europe). Raw cod ("lutefish") in Scandinavia may contain the fish tapeworm, *Diphyllobothrium latum*, a cause of anemia.

Road safety: Pedestrians should use extra caution when crossing the street in countries where there is left-sided traffic. There is a higher incidence of motor vehicle fatalities in Spain, Portugal, Yugoslavia, Greece, and eastern Europe. Seat belts should be worn at all times.

The Indian Subcontinent—Central Asia
(Afghanistan, Bangladesh, Bhutan, India, Kazakhstan, Kyrgystan, Nepal, Pakistan, Tadjikistan, Uzbekistan, and Turkmenistan)

Immunizations: All travelers to the Indian subcontinent should be up-to-date on their routine immunizations: tetanus-diphtheria (Td), measles-mumps-rubella (MMR), influenza, varicella (chickenpox), and polio. Hepatitis A and hepatitis B vaccines are strongly recommended for all travelers. Typhoid fever, rabies, meningococcal, Japanese B encephalitis, and oral cholera vaccines are recommended on an individual basis, according to the traveler's itinerary and possible disease exposure.

Recommended immunizations: Hepatitis A, hepatitis B, and typhoid. Depending on the length of stay and itinerary, rabies, Japanese encephalitis, meningitis, and/or cholera vaccines may be recommended for some people. A yellow fever vaccination certificate may be necessary if arriving from a country with active yellow fever, or from any country in a yellow fever endemic zone (e.g., Pakistan has this requirement).

AIDS/HIV: India is now considered the country that has the largest number of people infected with HIV in the world. Commercial sex workers continue to play a key part in the heterosexual spread of HIV, which is the dominant mode of transmission in India except in two regions (Nagaland and Manipur) where intravenous drug use is widespread. Between 30% and 60% of prostitutes and 15% of truck drivers are infected with HIV/AIDS in India. Another important mode of transmission is through contaminated blood and blood products and unsterile needles and syringes.

Cholera: This disease is active throughout the Indian subcontinent, but the threat to tourists is very low. Cholera is largely a disease of poverty and poor sanitation. The oral cholera vaccine is recommended primarily for travelers at significant risk, such as health-care or relief workers working in unsanitary environments. NOTE: The oral cholera vaccine (Dukoral) provides up to 60% crossover protection against ETEC diarrhea, a common bacterial cause of travelers' diarrhea in this region.

Dengue fever: Periodic epidemics of dengue and dengue hemorrhagic fever occur in India and other countries. To prevent dengue, travelers should take measures to prevent daytime mosquito bites.

Hepatitis: Hepatitis A vaccine is recommended for all travelers to this region. Hepatitis E may account for 70% of sporadic, acute viral hepatitis in these countries and is spread largely by sewage-contaminated water in rural areas. A vaccine against hepatitis E is not available. The hepatitis B carrier rate in the general population in this region is estimated at 5%. Vaccination is recommended for stays longer than 3 months; for anyone at occupational or social risk; for any traveler desiring maximal protection. Because the risk of illness or injury during travel cannot be predicted, *all* travelers should consider hepatitis B vaccine because of the risk of receiving a medical injection with an unsterile needle or syringe.

Influenza: Influenza is transmitted from November through March in areas north of the Tropic of Cancer and throughout the year in areas to the south. Vaccination is recommended for all travelers at risk

Japanese encephalitis (JE): This disease occurs throughout the year in India and Bangladesh, except in northern India where the risk is primarily April through November. The risk is low in the western states. Vaccination against Japanese encephalitis is recommended for travelers who will be staying more than 3 to 4 weeks in rural-agricultural endemic areas during the peak transmission period. Long-term urban expatriates should also be vaccinated on the assumption that rural travel will occur. In addition, personal protection measures against mosquito bites should be taken, especially in the evening.

Leishmaniasis: Risk for cutaneous leishmaniasis is present in Uzbekistan, Kazakhstan, and Turkmenistan. Cases of visceral leishmaniasis are reported in the northeastern states of India; sporadic cases of cutaneous leishmaniasis have been reported in the western states along the Pakistani-Indian border. Travelers to these regions should take measures to prevent sand fly bites.

Malaria: Limited foci of vivax malaria exist in Kazakhstan and Uzbekistan. In Tajikistan, cases are reported from the region of Khatlon Oblast. Turkmenistan reports vivax outbreaks in the Mary District; Kyrgyzstan reports malaria in southern and western areas bordering Tadjikistan and Uzbekistan; chloroquine prophylaxis is advised in the malarious risk areas. In Afghanistan, malaria occurs below 2,000 meters elevation, except there is no risk in Kabul; most cases of falciparum malaria have occurred in the eastern Afghanistan area along the border with Pakistan. Prophylaxis with atovaquone/proguanil, doxycycline, or mefloquine (A/P; DOX; MEF) is advised. Malaria is widespread in India, including Bombay and New Delhi; chloroquine-resistant falciparum malaria has been reported. Prophlyaxis with A/P; DOX; MEF is recommended for all travelers, especially those visiting friends and family.

Marine hazards: Stingrays, sea wasps, cones, jellyfish, sea urchins, and anemones are common in coastal waters and are potential hazards to unprotected swimmers.

Meningitis: Risk of meningococcal disease (Groups A and C) is present in the New Delhi region and adjacent southern areas, the site of the previous epidemics. The CDC does not currently recommend pre-travel vaccination with the meningococcal vaccine, but long-term travelers who expect close contact with the indigenous population should consider immunization with the quadrivalent meningococcal vaccine. NOTE: Meningitis was reported in Delhi in June 2005.

Polio: Polio remains active on the Indian sub-continent. All travelers should be fully immunized.

Rabies: India has the highest incidence of rabies in the world, with more than 30,000 human cases occurring annually. Travelers should seek immediate treatment of any animal bite, especially that of a dog. Rabies vaccination is indicated following the unprovoked bite of a dog, cat, bat, or monkey. Bites by other animals should be considered individually. Rabies vaccine is recommended for anyone planning long-term travel to this region, and for short-term travelers desiring extra protection, especially if they are visiting rural areas.

Tick-borne encephalitis (TBE): Peak transmission is April through June, especially in woods and forested areas. TBE is widespread in Europe. In Central Asia, it is termed "Russian spring-summer encephalitis."

Travelers' diarrhea: Year-round high risk in all countries. Water supplies are frequently obtained from wells that commonly are contaminated. Untreated sewage, industrial wastes, and agricultural runoffs contaminate many streams and rivers. Piped water supplies are quite limited and all water should be considered nonpotable, except in deluxe hotels. A quinolone antibiotic, combined with loperamide (Imodium), is recommended for the treatment of acute diarrhea. Persistent diarrhea may be due to a parasitic disease such as giardiasis, amebiasis, or cryptosporidiosis.

Tuberculosis: Tuberculosis is a major health problem throughout Asia. Travelers planning an extended stay should have a pre-departure TB skin test (PPD test) and be retested after returning from this country. Domestic employees hired by long-term visitors and expatriates should be screened for tuberculosis.

Typhoid fever: There is a high risk of typhoid fever in this region, especially in India. Typhoid vaccine is recommended for all travelers, but especially those traveling off the usual tourist routes, those visiting friends or relatives, and for long-stay visitors.

Yellow fever: There is no risk of yellow fever in the Indian subcontinent, but many countries may require a yellow fever vaccination certificate if arriving from an infected area.

Other illnesses/hazards: Arboviral diseases (Tahjna virus fever—mosquito-borne, the virus circulates through much of the former USSR; sand fly fever—limited to regions of southern central Asia (peak transmission April through October); West Nile virus fever—mosquito-borne, reported from Tajikistan; North Asian tick fever—occurs wherever tick vectors are found; boutonneuse fever—tick-borne, reported most commonly along the shores of the Caspian Sea; brucellosis (from unpasteurized dairy products); echinococcosis (dog feces are infective); legionellosis, leptospirosis, rickettsialpox, tick-borne relapsing fever (reported from Kirghizstan, Turkmenistan, and Uzbekistan); trichinosis, tularemia, and soil-transmitted and helminthic infections (roundworm, hookworm, and whipworm infections and strongyloidiasis).

Accidents and illness: Motor vehicle accidents, injuries and drowning are the leading causes of death among travelers younger than age of 55. Cardiovascular diseases cause most fatalities in older travelers. Medical care in these countries may not be adequate in cases of severe accident or illness. Travelers are advised to obtain supplemental travel health insurance with specific overseas coverage. The policy should provide for direct payment to the overseas hospital and/or physician at the time of service and include a medical evacuation benefit.

Animal Hazards: Animal hazards include snakes (kraits, cobras, coral snakes, vipers), scorpions, spiders, and leeches (abundant in the streams, marshes, and jungles).

North Africa

Immunizations: All travelers to North Africa should be up-to-date on their routine immunizations: tetanus-diphtheria (Td), measles-mumps-rubella (MMR), polio, influenza, and varicella (chickenpox). Hepatitis A and hepatitis B vaccines are strongly recommended for all travelers. Typhoid fever and rabies vaccines are recommended on an individual basis, according to the traveler's itinerary and possible disease exposure.

AIDS/HIV: There is a low prevalence of AIDS in North Africa.

Arboviral fevers: Few if any cases of dengue are reported from North Africa. Sand fly fever is widely distributed, especially in Egypt, Libya, and Tunisia. Rift Valley fever and West Nile fever are significant risks in Egypt. Crimean-Congo hemorrhagic fever and chikungunya fever: insufficient data are available to indicate whether or not these arboviral fevers have significant transmission in this region.

Filariasis: Occurs focally in the Nile Delta. Travelers to this region should take measures to prevent mosquito bites.

Hepatitis: All travelers to North Africa should receive hepatitis A vaccine. The hepatitis B carrier rate in the general population of these countries is estimated at 4% to 10%. Vaccination against hepatitis B is advised for all travelers to this region, especially those planning to stay for prolonged periods.

Leishmaniasis: Both cutaneous and visceral leishmaniasis (kala-azar) occurs in North Africa. Most cases are reported from the central and/or northern areas of Morocco, Algeria, Libya, and Tunisia. In Egypt, risk areas include the eastern Nile Delta, the Suez Canal zone, and northern Sinai. Travelers to these areas should take measures to prevent insect (sand fly) bites.

Malaria: This disease is not a major public health problem in North Africa. Malarious areas are found only in parts of Algeria and Egypt. *Plasmodium vivax* is the dominant species, but *Plasmodium falciparum* and *Plasmodium malariae* are also reported. There are no reports to date of chloroquine-resistant falciparum malaria. Chloroquine prophylaxis is recommended when traveling to malarious areas. All travelers to malarious areas should take personal protection measures against mosquito bites.

Mediterranean spotted fever (boutonneuse fever): Scattered cases are reported. Travelers are advised to avoid touching or petting dogs, which harbor dog ticks that transmit most cases of Mediterranean spotted fever.

Rabies: Animal rabies occurs in all countries. Human cases are also reported, usually from urban areas. Travelers should especially avoid contact with stray dogs and seek immediate treatment for any animal bite. Pre-exposure vaccination against rabies (three doses) should be considered by anyone planning long-term travel to this region.

Schistosomiasis: High risk occurs along the entire Nile River and in the Nile Delta region. Risk is present focally in Algeria (low risk), Libya, Tunisia, Morocco, and Western Sahara. Travelers to these countries should avoid swimming or wading in freshwater lakes, ponds, streams, or irrigation ditches.

Travelers' diarrhea: High risk outside of resort areas and first-class hotels. Piped water supplies in this region are frequently untreated and may be grossly contaminated. Travelers should observe all food and drink safety precautions. A quinolone antibiotic (ciprofloxacin, ofloxacin, levofloxacin, etc.) is recommended for the treatment of acute diarrhea. Diarrhea not responding to treatment with an antibiotic, or persistent diarrhea may be due to a parasitic disease such as giardiasis. Treatment with metronidazole (Flagyl) or tinidazole (Fasigyn) should be considered in cases of suspected parasitic disease.

Typhoid fever: Vaccination is recommended for extended travel outside the usual tourist routes of these countries and especially for those returning to their country of origin to visit friends and relatives.

Yellow fever: There is no risk of yellow fever in North Africa.

Other illnesses: Brucellosis (usually transmitted by raw goat or sheep milk), echinococcosis (a major health problem in central Tunisia, and occurs elsewhere), relapsing fever (louse-borne and tick-borne; reported in northern Sahara and coastal areas), tuberculosis (common), helminthic infections (roundworm, hookworm, and whipworm) are common in rural areas; incidence is estimated at 5%. Hepatitis C carriage rate is the highest in the world in Egypt due to a previous mass injection treatment campaign for schistosomiasis. In 1997, the carriage rate was estimated to be 18% of the population.

Sub-Saharan Africa

Immunizations: All travelers to sub-Saharan Africa should be up-to-date on their routine immunizations: tetanus-diphtheria (Td), measles-mumps-rubella (MMR), influenza, varicella (chickenpox), and polio. Hepatitis A and hepatitis B vaccines are strongly recommended for all travelers. Typhoid fever, rabies, meningococcal, and yellow fever vaccines are recommended on an individual basis, according to the traveler's itinerary and possible disease exposure.

African sleeping sickness (trypanosomiasis): This disease occurs in several countries of central and East Africa. Most risk to tourists occurs when visiting game parks. Travelers to rural areas should take measures to prevent insect (tsetse fly) bites. Unfortunately, insect repellents are not effective against this very aggressive fly.

AIDS/HIV: Widespread incidence of HIV infection in the countries of central and eastern Africa, where as many as 30% of the urban population is HIV-1 positive. In West Africa, HIV-2 is endemic and as many as 10% of the urban population is serologically positive. Travelers should avoid unsafe sexual contact, injections with unsterile needles and syringes, and unscreened blood transfusions. Travelers should consider carrying sterile needles and syringes in case an emergency medical injection is required.

Amebiasis: There is a high incidence of amebiasis in West and South Africa; to avoid amebiasis, travelers should drink only safe water and eat only well-cooked food. All fruit should be peeled before eating.

Cholera: This disease is reported to be active in many countries. Cholera occurs in areas with inadequate sanitation, such as urban slums and rural areas. The risk to tourists of acquiring cholera is considered to be very low, but may be increased in health-care and refugee camp aid workers These individuals should consider vaccination with the effective oral preparation available in Canada and Europe. NOTE: The oral cholera vaccine (Dukoral) provides up to 60% crossover protection against ETEC diarrhea, a common bacterial cause of travelers' diarrhea in this region.

Dengue fever: Very low risk. Although the *Aedes aegypti* mosquito that transmits dengue is found in most countries of Africa, cases of dengue appear to be rare.

Filariasis: Mosquito-borne Bancroftian filariasis is widespread in all countries, except southern Africa. To prevent filariasis, travelers should take measures to prevent mosquito bites.

Helminthic infections: There is widespread occurrence of hookworm, roundworm, and whipworm infections. *Strongyloides* infection is also prevalent. Travelers can prevent these infections by wearing shoes to prevent skin penetration by infectious worm larvae and cook food thoroughly to destroy infectious roundworm and whipworm eggs. Paragonimiasis (lung fluke disease) occurs in West Africa and is transmitted by the consumption of raw crustaceans.

Hepatitis: All nonimmune travelers should receive hepatitis A vaccine before visiting this region. The hepatitis B virus carrier rate in the countries of sub-Saharan Africa is estimated to exceed 10%. Vaccination is recommended for stays longer than 3 months; for anyone at occupational or social risk; for any traveler desiring maximal protection. Because the risk of illness or injury during travel cannot be predicted, all travelers should consider hepatitis B vaccine because of the risk of receiving a medical injection with an unsterile needle or syringe.

Lassa fever: Low risk to tourists. Lassa fever occurs primarily in West Africa (from Nigeria to Guinea). The virus of Lassa fever is believed to be spread by infective rat and rodent urine. Travelers can reduce exposure by eliminating rodents in the home.

Leishmaniasis: Epidemics of visceral leishmaniasis (kala-azar) have occurred in East Africa, Ethiopia, and Sudan, but sporadic cases also have been reported in Chad, Burkina Fasso, Central African Republic, Uganda, Zaire, and Zambia. Cutaneous leishmaniasis (Oriental sore) is widespread in Mali, Mauritania, Chad, and Central African Republic and is present, but less active, elsewhere, especially in the drier areas. To prevent leishmaniasis, travelers should take measures to prevent insect (sand fly) bites.

Loiasis: This form of filariasis is common in equatorial Africa, especially West and Central Africa. It is transmitted by the day-biting deer fly. Travelers should take protective measures against insect (fly) bites in rural areas.

Malaria: High risk in most countries, including urban areas. Transmission of disease is greater during and just after the rainy seasons when the mosquito population increases. Highest malaria attack rates for tourists are reported from East Africa, Ghana, Nigeria, and Malawi. Most malaria in sub-Saharan Africa is caused by *P. falciparum*, but *P. vivax* occurs in Ethiopia, Somalia, and Sudan. There is widespread occurrence of chloroquine-resistant *P. falciparum* throughout sub-Saharan Africa. Chemoprophylaxis with atovaquone/proguanil (Malarone), mefloquine (Lariam) or doxycycline is currently advised for people who travel to malarious areas. Travelers are reminded that no prophylactic drug provides 100% protection against all species of malaria. For this reason, travelers should also take careful measures to prevent mosquito bites. These measures include the frequent application of a DEET-containing insect repellent, the wearing of permethrin-treated clothing, and, if necessary, the use of permethrin-treated mosquito bed nets. Travelers should seek immediate medical consultation for a suspected attack of malaria, even if they have been taking prophylactic drugs. It is noteworthy that in sub-Saharan Africa, malaria blood films are often falsely positive. Travelers who are taking a recommended antimalarial drug for prophylaxis should not stop their medication in the face of a diagnosis of malaria regardless of the blood film results. NOTE: Risk of malaria is low or absent in Nairobi, the Ethiopian highlands, or on the islands of Cape Verde, Mauritius, Réunion, and the Seychelles.

Meningitis: Travelers (especially teachers, relief workers, missionaries, etc.) planning an extended visit to sub-Saharan Africa, especially during the dry season, November through June, should be vaccinated with the quadrivalent meningococcal vaccine.

Onchocerciasis: Widespread incidence in West and Central Africa, extending into Uganda, Sudan, and the Ethiopian highlands. Western Kenya is risk free. Travelers to risk areas should take measures to prevent blackfly bites. The blackfly is a daytime biter and is rarely found indoors.

Polio: There has been a resurgence of polio in west and central Africa, chiefly Nigeria, due to a breakdown in state-run immunization programs. Cases have now been reported from Benin, Botswana, Burkina Faso, Cameroon, Chad, Central African republic, Ghana, Guinea, Ivory Coast, Mali, Niger, Sudan, and Togo. Cases have recently been reported from Saudi Arabia and Yemen, brought there by Muslim pilgrims from Africa.

Rabies: Animal rabies has been reported from all countries. Most human cases are transmitted by dog bites, with risk occurring in both urban and rural areas. Jackals and mongooses should also be considered potentially rabid. Travelers should seek emergency treatment of any animal bite, especially if the bite was unprovoked. Pre-exposure rabies vaccination is recommended for all travelers (especially children) planning an extended visit or extensive travel in sub-Saharan Africa.

Schistosomiasis: Risk is present in all countries except for Cape Verde, Réunion, and the Seychelles. Travelers should avoid swimming, bathing, or wading in freshwater lakes, ponds, or streams.

Travelers' diarrhea: High risk outside first-class hotels and resorts. Most water sources should be considered potentially contaminated. Travelers should strictly observe safe food and drink precautions. A quinolone antibiotic (such as ciprofloxacin, ofloxacin, levofloxacin, etc.) is recommended for the self treatment of adults with diarrhea. Azithromycin or a quinolone is recommended for the treatment of children. Diarrhea not responding to treatment with an antibiotic, or persistent diarrhea, may be due to a parasitic disease such as giardiasis and treatment with metronidazole (Flagyl) or tinidazole (Fasigyn) should be considered.

Typhoid fever: Typhoid vaccine is recommended for all travelers, with the exception of short-term visitors who restrict their meals to major restaurants and hotels. Because the typhoid vaccines are only 60% to 70% effective, safe food and drink selection remains important.

West Nile fever, Chickungunya fever, and Rift Valley fever: These mosquito-transmitted diseases are avoided by taking personal protection measures against insect bites.

Yellow fever: This disease is currently reported active in nine countries—Angola, Cameroon, Gambia, Guinea, Kenya, Mali, Nigeria, Sudan, and Zaire. A vaccination certificate is absolutely required for entry to Benin, Burkina Fasso, Cameroon, Côte d'Ivoire (Ivory Coast), Gabon, Ghana, Liberia, Mali, Mauritania, Niger, Senegal, Sao Tome and Principe, and Togo, even if arriving directly from the United States or Canada. Travelers to the Cape Verde Islands, Equatorial Guinea, Gambia, Guinea-Bissau, Nigeria, and Sierra Leone will need a vaccination certificate if arriving from any "infected" or yellow fever endemic countries in Africa or Latin America.. The risk of yellow fever is estimated to be 1:2,500 during a 2-week stay between epidemics and 10-fold higher during epidemics.

Other diseases: African tick typhus (transmitted primarily by dog ticks), brucellosis, Crimean-Congo hemorrhagic fever (a tick-borne viral disease; occurs throughout Africa), cysticercosis and pork tapeworm disease, echinococcosis, leprosy, plague (human plague is reported from Madagascar, Malawi, Mozambique, Tanzania, Zaire, and Zimbabwe), syphilis, trachoma, typhus (louse borne), and acute hemorrhagic conjunctivitis are reported. Recently, Ebola virus and plague outbreaks have occurred in northern parts of the Democratic Republic of Congo.

Animal hazards: The puff adder, carpet viper, and spitting cobra are the most important species. The average tourist is at low risk; the overland traveler is at much higher potential risk of snake bite. Overland travelers should have prior knowledge of prevailing species and consider the need for access to cool-stored antivenom. Sterile needles, syringes, and intravenous administration sets are essential.

The Middle East

Immunizations: All travelers to the Middle East should be up-to-date on their routine immunizations: tetanus-diphtheria (Td), measles-mumps-rubella (MMR), influenza, varicella (chickenpox), and polio. Hepatitis A and hepatitis B vaccines are strongly recommended for all travelers. Typhoid fever, rabies, and meningococcal vaccines are recommended on an individual basis, according to the traveler's itinerary and possible disease exposure.

Cutaneous leishmaniasis: Risk is low, but this sand fly-transmitted disease is reported throughout the Middle East. Travelers should take protective measures to prevent insect (sand fly) bites from dusk to dawn. Hundreds of cases have been reported in U.S. troops stationed in Iraq.

Hepatitis: High risk. All nonimmune travelers should receive hepatitis A vaccine. The hepatitis B carrier rate in the general population of this region is estimated at 2% to 10%. Vaccination against hepatitis B is recommended for all visitors to this region, especially long-stay travelers. Hepatitis E is prevalent among guest workers in these countries and may possibly be a threat to travelers. Prevention of hepatitis E requires food and water precautions because there is no vaccine for this disease.

Malaria: The risk of malaria is low in this region. There is no malaria in Kuwait, Bahrain, Cyprus, Israel, Jordan, Lebanon, or Qatar. Vivax malaria is found in the northern third of Iraq below 1,500 meters elevation. In Saudi Arabia, malaria is confined to the extreme southwest, about 500 km south of Jeddah. The highest risk of malaria in the Middle East occurs during the rainy season, from December through March. Falciparum malaria accounts for 50% to 70% of cases, vivax the remainder. Chloroquine-resistant falciparum is reported in Yemen and Iran, and Saudi Arabia; mefloquine (Lariam), atovaquone/proguanil (Malarone) or doxycycline prophylaxis should be considered for travel to malarious areas of these countries. In other malarious regions, chloroquine prophylaxis is recommended. Personal protection measures against mosquito bites, including permethrin-impregnated bed nets, should be used by all travelers.

Polio: Outbreaks have been reported in Saudi Arabia and Yemen, associated with Muslim travels from sub-Saharan Africa.

Rabies: Animal rabies, mainly in dogs and foxes, is a problem in most countries, but human cases occur infrequently. Travelers should consider rabies vaccination if they will be in remote or rural areas for extended periods and unable to obtain prompt medical care after being bitten by a dog or wild animal.

Schistosomiasis: Risk is present in Yemen, Oman, Jordan, Iraq, Saudi Arabia, and Syria. Travelers should avoid swimming, bathing, or wading in freshwater lakes, ponds, streams, or irrigated areas in these regions.

Travelers' diarrhea: Medium to high risk throughout this region. Travelers should drink only commercially bottled, boiled, or chemically treated water, especially in rural areas. All food should be well cooked. Fruit should be peeled. A quinolone antibiotic (ciprofloxacin, ofloxacin, levofloxacin, etc.) is recommended for the self treatment of acute diarrhea. Diarrhea not responding to treatment with an antibiotic, or persistent diarrhea, may be due to a parasitic disease such as giardiasis, and treatment with metronidazole (Flagyl) or tinidazole (Fasigyn) should be considered. All cases of diarrhea should be treated with adequate fluid replacement.

Visceral leishmaniasis (kala-azar): Cases are reported throughout the region, especially from rural areas. All travelers to the Middle East are advised to take protective measures against insect (sand fly) bites.

Other diseases/hazards: Epidemic typhus, murine typhus, Q fever, sand fly fever (a viral illness transmitted by sand flies), Congo-Crimean hemorrhagic fever (a viral illness transmitted by ticks), brucellosis (transmitted by unpasteurized dairy products), echinococcosis, typhoid fever (most cases occur in the summer and early fall; multidrug-resistant strains of *Salmonella* bacteria are reported. Treatment drugs of choice are the quinolones and third generation cephalosporins). Tapeworm and hookworm disease and tuberculosis are reported from many areas. Meningitis (meningococcal serogroups A and W-135 serotypes) has occurred in sporadic epidemics in Saudi Arabia, among Muslim travelers to Mecca. The quadrivalent meningococcal vaccine is now required for entry to Saudia Arabia. Several cases of polio have recently been reported during the Hajj. All those attending the Hajj should have their polio immunization status up to date.

Southeast Asia

Immunizations: All travelers to Southeast Asia should be up-to-date on their routine immunizations: tetanus-diphtheria (Td), measles-mumps-rubella (MMR), influenza, varicella (chickenpox), and polio. Hepatitis A and hepatitis B vaccines are strongly recommended for all travelers. Typhoid fever, rabies, and Japanese B encephalitis vaccines are recommended on an individual basis, according to the traveler's itinerary and possible disease exposure.

AIDS/HIV: Although HIV was only recently introduced to Southeast Asia, it is spreading with alarming speed. Thailand has the highest incidence. The virus initially affected mostly homosexuals, but then spread quickly to IV drug users (IVDUs). The third wave of the epidemic now involves prostitutes and their heterosexual partners. As many as 70% of prostitutes in some rural areas of Thailand are now seropositive, and contact with infected prostitutes is spreading into the general population. In the Philippines, Malaysia, Singapore, Taiwan, Korea, and Indonesia, the HIV infection rate among prostitutes and the indigenous population is still relatively low. The potential for the eventual spread of AIDS in these areas, however, is considered high.

Avian (bird) flu (H5N1): Recent outbreaks of bird flu have been spreading throughout Thailand, Cambodia, and Vietnam. A small number of fatal cases have occurred among those exposed to live poultry. Travelers should avoid live bird markets and should consider carrying a course of Tamiflu (oseltamivir) for self treatment of presumed influenza. Also, they should carry a hand sanitizer (Purell) and use it liberally.

Cholera: Sporadic disease activity is reported in many Southeast Asian countries. Cholera occurs primarily in areas with inadequate sewage disposal and unsafe water supplies such as urban slums and rural areas. The risk to travelers of acquiring cholera is considered to be very low. Prevention consists of strict adherence to safe food and drink guidelines. NOTE: The oral cholera vaccine (Dukoral) provides up to 60% crossover protection against ETEC diarrhea, a common bacterial cause of travelers' diarrhea in this region.

Dengue fever: This disease is widespread throughout Southeast Asia in both sporadic and epidemic forms and in both urban and rural areas. There is a high incidence of dengue hemorrhagic fever in Bangkok. The *Aedes* mosquitoes, which transmit dengue, are most active at dusk and dawn. Travelers should also take measures to prevent mosquito bites.

Filariasis: The Bancroftian and Malayan forms are widespread in Southeast Asia. Filariasis is transmitted by four different species of mosquitoes. Insect precautions are recommended for rural travel. Travelers should apply a DEET-containing skin repellent and a permethrin clothing spray, and a mosquito bed net (permethrin treated) should be used to prevent bites while sleeping.

Helminthic infections (flukes): Oriental lung fluke disease (paragonimiasis) and liver fluke diseases (clonorchiasis, fascioliasis) are prevalent in the Indochina peninsula and the Philippines. Travelers should avoid eating raw, salted, or wine-soaked crustaceans such as freshwater crabs or crayfish (which can transmit clonorchiasis and paragonimiasis) and also avoid uncooked aquatic vegetables, such as watercress, which can transmit fascioliasis. Fasciolopsiasis (large intestinal fluke disease) can also be acquired through eating undercooked aquatic plants such as water chestnuts, bamboo shoots, and caltrops. These, too, should be avoided, if uncooked. Anisakiasis and capillariasis are other intestinal infections acquired by eating raw or undercooked fish (including fresh catch, crab, or squid). Cases have been reported from the Philippines, Thailand, Taiwan, and, recently, Indonesia.

Helminthic infections: Hookworm, roundworm, whipworm, and *Strongyloides* are highly prevalent in most rural areas of Southeast Asia. Travelers should wear shoes to prevent the hookworm and strongyloides larvae from penetrating the skin of the foot, and food should be thoroughly washed and/or cooked to destroy roundworm and whipworm eggs.

Hepatitis: All nonimmune travelers should receive hepatitis A vaccine before visiting Southeast Asia. The hepatitis B carrier rate in the general population of Southeast Asia is estimated at 10% to 20%. Vaccination against hepatitis B is recommended for all travelers, especially health-care workers, overseas corporate employees, expatriates, relief workers, teachers, and others who will have extended (more than 4 weeks) contact with the indigenous populations of the countries in this region. Hepatitis E is common and an important cause of severe illness and death in pregnancy. There is no vaccine to prevent hepatitis E.

Japanese encephalitis (JE): This disease is widespread throughout Asia. Japanese encephalitis may be transmitted seasonally, or year-round (in tropical regions). Vaccination against JE (three doses) is recommended for travelers who will be staying in, or visiting (longer than 30 days), rural-agricultural, rice-growing endemic areas during the peak transmission season. Depending on the epidemic circumstances, vaccine should be considered for persons spending less than 30 days whose activities, such as extensive outdoor activities in rural areas, place them at particularly high risk for exposure. All travelers to risk areas should also take measures to prevent mosquito bites between dusk and dawn.

Malaria: Both vivax and falciparum malaria occur in Southeast Asia. The falciparum-vivax ratio is usually about 2:1 in most areas, but may vary. Chloroquine- and multidrug-resistant *P. falciparum* is reported. In Borneo Kalamantan (Borneo), Papua New Guinea, Irian Jaya, Myanmar, Sumatra, and Sulewesa (Celebes), chloroquine-resistant *P. vivax* has been reported. Mefloquine (Lariam), atovaquone/proguanil (Malarone) or doxycycline prophylaxis is recommended when traveling to rural risk areas. All travelers to malarious areas should take measures to prevent insect bites. These measures include applying a DEET-containing skin repellent, wearing permethrin-treated clothing, and using, as needed, a mosquito bed net also treated with permethrin.

Polio: Reported active in Indonesia. All travelers should be fully immunized.

Rabies: Animal rabies has been reported from all countries in Southeast Asia. The highest risk occurs in Thailand. All travelers, especially children, should avoid touching or petting stray dogs. Travelers should seek immediate treatment of any animal bite. Rabies vaccination is indicated following the unprovoked bite of a dog, cat, bat, or monkey. Bites by other animals, including livestock, should be individually assessed. Pre-exposure vaccination against rabies should be considered before long-term travel to this region. This is especially true for travelers going to remote rural areas.

Schistosomiasis: There is low risk of schistosomiasis in most countries of Southeast Asia. Risk is present in the Philippines and in central Slaws (Indonesia) and also occurs in small foci in the Mekong Delta of Vietnam. There are several small foci among the aboriginal Malays in Peak and Pashing States in Malaysia. Travelers should avoid swimming or wading in freshwater lakes, ponds, or streams in these areas.

Scrub typhus: This chigger mite-transmitted disease is reported from many Asian countries. Chigger mites commonly inhabit second-growth forest, fruit, oil palm, or rubber plantations where there is tall grass. People who walk through tropical brush should inspect their skin for the presence of mites or ticks. Repellents and permethrin clothing spray should also be used in these areas.

Travelers' diarrhea: High risk in many areas, but some major cities (e.g., Singapore, Bangkok) in Southeast Asia are much safer than others. It is recommended that travelers to Southeast Asia drink only bottled, boiled, or treated water and consume only well-cooked food. Raw fish, crayfish, and crabs, as well as uncooked aquatic plants (e.g., watercress), should be strictly avoided. Travelers should carry a quinolone antibiotic (ciprofloxacin, ofloxacin, levofloxacin, etc.) with which to treat acute diarrhea. However, in Thailand, azithromycin (Zithromax) should be used because of the high prevalence of drug resistance. Diarrhea not responding to antibiotic treatment, or diarrhea that becomes persistent may be due to a parasitic disease such as giardiasis and treatment with metronidazole (Flagyl) or tinidazole (Fasigyn) should be considered. All cases of diarrhea should be treated with adequate fluid replacement.

Typhoid fever: Typhoid vaccine is recommended for all travelers, with the exception of short-term visitors who restrict their meals to major restaurants and hotels. Because the typhoid vaccines are only 60% to 70% effective, safe food and drink selection remains important.

Yellow fever: This disease does not occur in Asia, but many countries require a certificate of vaccination from travelers arriving from yellow fever-infected countries or from countries in the yellow fever endemic zones.

Other diseases/hazards: Other illnesses reported with varying frequency include anthrax, brucellosis, leprosy, leptospirosis, melioidosis, meningococcal meningitis, plague, toxoplasmosis, yaws, and tuberculosis. There is low risk to the average traveler of acquiring these illnesses. Sting rays, poisonous fish, sea anemones, the Indo-China man-of-war, and the very dangerous sea wasp are found along the coral reefs that fringe the countries of Southeast Asia. Swimmers should take sensible precautions to avoid these hazards.

Plant hazards: Bamboo, rattan, and large palm- or fern-like trees, which can cause serious puncture wounds and slow-healing lacerations, are widespread in the forested areas of these countries. Also common are the Regas family of trees, which are large forest trees whose black resinous sap can cause a potent poison ivy-type skin reaction. Stinging nettles, small thorny trees, and many species of euphorbs can also cause skin reactions.

Australia, New Zealand, Papua New Guinea, and Oceania (The Islands of Polynesia, Micronesia, and Melanesia)

Immunizations: All travelers to Australia, New Zealand, and the islands of the Pacific should be up-to-date on their routine immunizations: tetanus-diphtheria (Td), measles-mumps-rubella (MMR), influenza, and varicella (chickenpox). Hepatitis A and hepatitis B vaccines are strongly recommended for all travelers. Typhoid fever, rabies, and Japanese B encephalitis vaccines are recommended on an individual basis, according to the traveler's itinerary and possible disease exposure.

AIDS/HIV: A small number of AIDS cases and HIV infections have been reported from various areas. At present, AIDS is not considered a major public health problem in Australia, New Zealand, or Oceania.

Cholera: Sporadic cases regionwide. The risk to travelers of acquiring cholera is considered low. Prevention consists primarily in following safe food and drink guidelines. NOTE: The oral cholera vaccine (Dukoral) provides up to 60% crossover protection against ETEC diarrhea, a common bacterial cause of travelers' diarrhea in this region.

Dengue fever: Sporadic cases and epidemics occur in nearly all of the island groups of the South Pacific. Dengue is also reported in Northern Queensland (Australia). Peak infection rates occur during the rainy season months, December-January and May-June. Prevention of dengue consists of taking protective measures against mosquito bites.

Filariasis: Malayan filariasis is widespread in the rest of Oceania, including the Solomon Islands and Vanuatu. Up to 16% prevalence has been reported in French Polynesia. Hyperendemic foci has been reported in the Cook Islands. Travelers should take personal protection measures against mosquito bites.

Hepatitis: Hepatitis A is endemic at moderate to high levels, except for Australia and New Zealand, where the risk is low. The hepatitis B carrier rate in Oceania is estimated as high as 15%. Vaccination against hepatitis B is recommended for people planning an extended visit to Papua New Guinea or Oceania for stays longer than 3 months; for anyone at occupational or social risk; or for any traveler desiring maximal protection. There is a low risk of hepatitis B in Australia and New Zealand and vaccination is not routinely recommended.

Leptospirosis: Likely occurs region-wide. Most frequently reported from New Caledonia and French Polynesia. Also reported from Fiji, Micronesia, Solomon Islands, and Vanuatu.

Malaria: This disease occurs only in Papua New Guinea, the Solomon Islands, and Vanuatu. Falciparum malaria predominates over vivax approximately 2:1. Chloroquine- and multidrug-resistant *Plasmodium falciparum* malaria occurs. The recommended antimalarial prophylaxis for adult travelers is mefloquine, 250 mg weekly, except in Papua New Guinea where doxycycline, 100 mg daily, is recommended. Chloroquine-resistant

Plasmodium vivax has been reported from Papua New Guinea. There is no risk of malaria in Australia, New Zealand, or the other islands of Polynesia, Micronesia, or Melanesia.

Rabies: There is no indigenous rabies in Australia and Papua New Guinea. Most of Oceania is rabies free.

Travelers' diarrhea: Low risk in Australia and New Zealand. Moderate risk in French Polynesia. Higher risk in the Solomon Islands, Vanuatu, and Micronesia. Most risk occurs outside of first-class hotels and resorts. Travelers are best advised to drink only bottled, boiled, filtered, or treated water and consume only well-cooked food. A quinolone antibiotic is recommended for the treatment of acute diarrhea. Diarrhea not responding to antibiotic treatment may be due to a parasitic disease such as giardiasis, amebiasis, or cryptosporidiosis. Amebiasis and giardiasis are more common to the Solomon Islands, Kiribati, Vanuatu, and Micronesia, and less common in Fiji and the French Territories.

Typhoid fever: Typhoid outbreaks occurred in Vanuatu in 1987 and in Fiji in 1985. Travelers should consider typhoid vaccination before travel to Oceania. Typhoid is best prevented by strict adherence to safe food and drink guidelines.

Other illnesses/hazards: Angiostrongyliasis (human cases reported from Cook Islands, Fiji, French Polynesia, New Calendonia, Western Samoa, and Vanuatu), anisikiasis (endemic regionwide; associated with consumption of raw saltwater fish; cases have been reported from Kiribati), brucellosis, echinococcosis, paragonimiasis (enzootic on the Solomon Islands; likely more widespread), scrub typhus (reported in rural areas of the Solomon Islands and Vanuatu). Ross River fever (viral epidemic polyarthritis; mosquito-borne; endemic in northern and eastern Australia; now reported in the Central and South Pacific). Hookworm disease, roundworm disease, strongyloidiasis, and other helminthic infections are reported throughout Oceania. Tuberculosis (moderately endemic), trachoma, and yaws are reported (Oceania).

Marine hazards: Corals, jellyfish, sting rays, poisonous fish, sharks, and sea snakes are potential hazards to bathers. The box jellyfish, the most dangerous jellyfish in the world, and also the sea wasp are found in northern coastal waters of Australia. Four other varieties of jellyfish (jimble, Carukia, mauve stinger, and hairy stinger) should also be avoided. Swimmers should take sensible precautions to avoid these hazards.

NORTH AMERICA

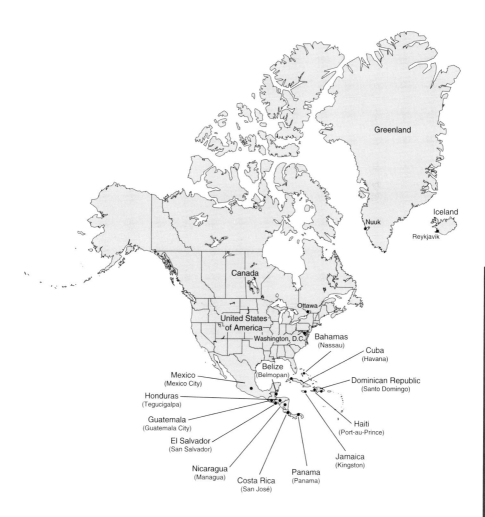

SOUTH AMERICA

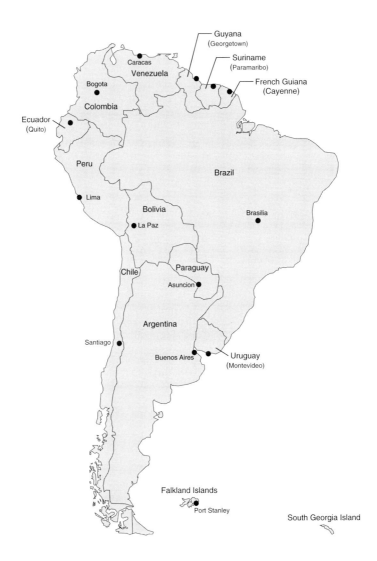

EUROPE

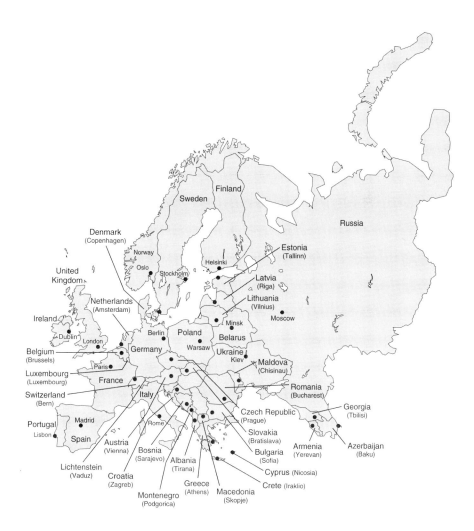

Finland

Sweden

Russia

Denmark
(Copenhagen)

Norway

Estonia
(Tallinn)

Helsinki

United
Kingdom

Oslo

Stockholm

Latvia
(Riga)

Netherlands
(Amsterdam)

Lithuania
(Vilnius)

Ireland

Minsk

Moscow

Dublin

Berlin

Poland

London

Belgium
(Brussels)

Germany

Warsaw

Belarus

Ukraine

Luxembourg
(Luxembourg)

Paris

Kiev

Moldova
(Chisinau)

France

Switzerland
(Bern)

Italy

Romania
(Bucharest)

Portugal

Madrid

Rome

Czech Republic
(Prague)

Georgia
(Tbilisi)

Lisbon

Spain

Slovakia
(Bratislava)

Armenia
(Yerevan)

Azerbaijan
(Baku)

Austria
(Vienna)

Bulgaria
(Sofia)

Lichtenstein
(Vaduz)

Bosnia
(Sarajevo)

Albania
(Tirana)

Cyprus (Nicosia)

Croatia
(Zagreb)

Greece
(Athens)

Crete (Iraklio)

Montenegro
(Podgorica)

Macedonia
(Skopje)

AFRICA

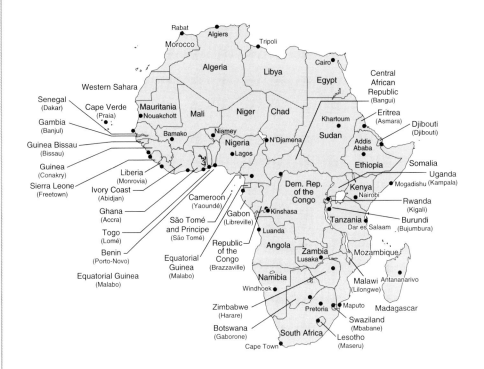

Rabat
Algiers
Tripoli
Morocco
Cairo
Algeria
Libya
Egypt
Central
African
Republic
Western Sahara
(Bangui)
Senegal
(Dakar)
Cape Verde
Mauritania
Niger
Chad
Eritrea
(Praia)
Nouakchott
Mali
(Asmara)
Khartoum
Djibouti
Gambia
Bamako
Niamey
(Djibouti)
(Banjul)
Nigeria
N'Djamena
Sudan
Guinea Bissau
Addis
(Bissau)
Lagos
Ababa
Guinea
Ethiopia
Somalia
(Conakry)
Liberia
Uganda
Sierra Leone
(Monrovia)
Dem. Rep.
Kenya
Mogadishu (Kampala)
(Freetown)
Ivory Coast
of the
Nairobi
Rwanda
(Abidjan)
Cameroon
Congo
(Kigali)
Ghana
(Yaoundé)
Gabon
Kinshasa
Tanzania
Burundi
(Accra)
São Tomé
(Libreville)
Dar es Salaam
(Bujumbura)
Togo
and Principe
Luanda
(Lomé)
(São Tomé)
Republic
Angola
Benin
of the
Zambia
Mozambique
(Porto-Novo)
Equatorial
Congo
Lusaka
Equatorial Guinea
Guinea
(Brazzaville)
(Malabo)
(Malabo)
Namibia
Malawi
Antananarivo
Windhoek
(Lilongwe)
Zimbabwe
Maputo
Madagascar
(Harare)
Pretoria
Swaziland
Botswana
(Mbabane)
(Gaborone)
South Africa
Lesotho
Cape Town
(Maseru)

ASIA

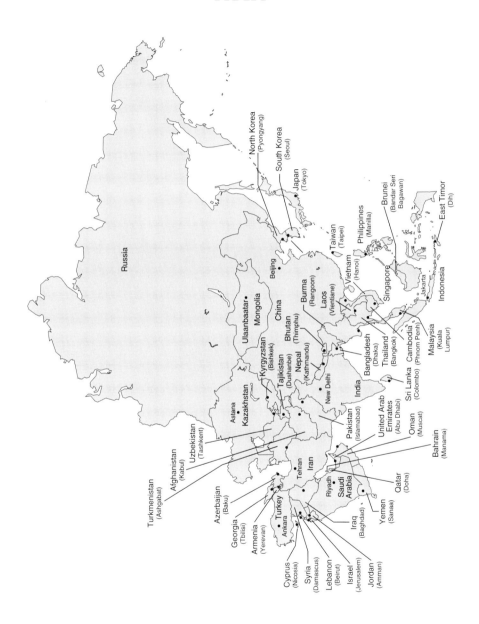

AUSTRALIA/OCEANIA

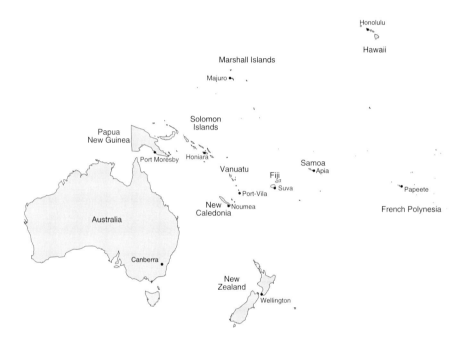

WORLD MEDICAL GUIDE—COUNTRY LISTINGS

Afghanistan

KABUL ★

CAPITAL:
Kabul

EMBASSY (IN U.S.):
2341 Wyoming Avenue, NW, Washington, DC 20008; Tel: 202-483-6410; Fax: 202-483-6488; Internet: http://www.embassyofafghanistan.org/main/consulate/visa.cfm

GMT:
+4 hours

TELEPHONE COUNTRY CODE:
93

USADIRECT:
None

ENTRY REQUIREMENTS
- **Passport/Visa**: A visa is required.
- **HIV Test**: Not required.
- **Vaccinations:** A yellow fever vaccination certificate is required when arriving from infected areas.

EMBASSIES/CONSULATES
- There is no American representation at this time. U.S. citizens who travel to Afghanistan should register with the U.S. Embassy in India, Pakistan, Tajikistan, Turkmenistan, or Uzbekistan. The nearest U.S. Embassies are in Islamabad, Pakistan and in Dushanbe, Tajikistan.
- **Canadian Embassy**: House 256, Street 15, Wazir-Akbar-Khan, Kabul, Afghanistan; Tel: 93-70-294-281; e-mail: homcanadakabul@yahoo.com.
- **British Embassy**: 15th Street, Roundabout Wazir Akbar Khan, PO Box 334, Kabul, Tel: 93-0-70-102-000, 00-873-762-854-939 (Satphone), Fax: 93-0-70-102-250 (Management), 93-0-70-102-274 (Political Section), e-mail: britishembassy.kabul@fco.gov.uk, Website: www.britishembassy.gov.uk/afghanistan

HOSPITALS/DOCTORS:
Local medical facilities are below Western standards and should be considered for use only for emergency care.

Current Advisories and Health Risks

CHOLERA: This disease is active in this country. People at high risk (e.g., relief, health-care workers) should consider immunization. Many countries, including Canada, license an oral cholera vaccine. The oral vaccine is not available in the United States.

HEPATITIS: All nonimmune travelers should receive hepatitis A vaccine before visiting this country. The hepatitis B carrier rate in the general population is estimated as high as 5%. Vaccination against hepatitis B should be considered by any traveler desiring maximal protection, or by a traveler who might be exposed to blood (for example, a health-care worker), have sexual contact with the local population, stay longer than 3 months, or be exposed through medical treatment.

HEPATITIS E: High risk. This disease is presumably widespread, especially in rural areas. Prevention consists of treating all drinking water to eliminate viruses. A vaccine is not available.

INFLUENZA: Influenza is transmitted from November through March. Vaccination is recommended for travel during this time.

JAPANESE ENCEPHALITIS (JE): Low risk; historically, this disease has occurred along the eastern borders. Travelers to rural areas should take measures to prevent mosquito bites.

LEISHMANIASIS: Cutaneous leishmaniasis occurs in rural and semirural areas, especially in the northern parts of the country at elevations between 400 and 800 meters. Major risk areas include the northern Afghan plains and the outskirts of Kabul. Other risk areas include Qandahar in the south and Herat in the west. There are sporadic cases of visceral leishmaniasis. All travelers should take measures to prevent insect (sand fly) bites.

MALARIA: Transmission generally occurs during the warmer months, May through October, with peak transmission during August and September. There is risk in all areas at altitudes lower than 2000 meters (6,500 feet) There is no malaria risk in Kabul. There may be malaria risk, however, in the urban areas in the south. *Plasmodium vivax* accounts for 95% to 98% of cases, but chloroquine-resistant falciparum malaria is reported, primarily along the border area with Pakistan.

All travelers should take one of the following drugs: atovaquone/proguanil (Malarone), mefloquine (Lariam), or doxycycline. Travelers should also take measures to prevent evening and nighttime mosquito bites.

POLIO: Reported active. All travelers should be fully immunized.

RABIES: Human cases occur sporadically. Rabies vaccine is recommended for those persons anticipating an extended stay, those whose work or activities may bring them into contact with animals, especially dogs, or when extra protection is desired. Prompt medical evaluation and treatment of any animal bite is essential.

TRAVELERS' DIARRHEA: High risk. Shigellosis is a major problem in this country. Only bottled, boiled, or treated water should be consumed. All food should be well cooked. A quinolone antibiotic is recommended for the treatment of diarrhea. Persistent diarrhea may be due to a parasitic infection such as giardiasis, amebiasis, or cryptosporidiosis.

TUBERCULOSIS: Tuberculosis is a major public health problem in this country. Travelers planning an extended stay should have a pre-departure TB skin test (PPD test) and be retested on return.

TYPHOID FEVER: Typhoid vaccine is recommended. Because the typhoid vaccines are only 60% to 70% effective, safe food and drink selection remain important.

OTHER DISEASES/HAZARDS: Brucellosis, diphtheria (recent cases are reported by the WHO), echinococcosis, leptospirosis (endemic in the northern and eastern plains), louse-borne typhus, pertussis, sand fly fever, Siberian tick typhus, scrub typhus, tick-borne relapsing fever, typhoid fever (highly endemic), tuberculosis, and intestinal helminthic (worm) infections.

Albania

CAPITAL:
Tirana
EMBASSY (IN U.S.):
202-223-4942
GMT:
+1 hour
TELEPHONE COUNTRY CODE:
355
USA DIRECT:
00-800-0010
ENTRY REQUIREMENTS
- **Passport/Visa:** Passport, visa, and birth certificate are required.
- **HIV Test:** Not required.
- **Vaccinations:** A yellow fever vaccination certificate is required from travelers older than 1 year of age arriving from infected areas.

EMBASSIES/CONSULATES
- **U.S. Embassy:** Rruga E Elbasanit 103, Tirana (Tel: 355-42-32875, Fax: 355-42-74957).
- **Canadian Embassy:** Rruga "Brigada VIII," Pallati 2, Apartamenti 1, PO Box 47, Tirana (Tel: 355-42-57274, 57275, 58344, and 58345, Fax: 355-42-57273.)
- **British Embassy:** Rruga Skenderbej 12, Tirana; Tel: 355-42-34973/4/5; Fax: 355-42-47697.

HOSPITALS/DOCTORS: Medical care in Albania is adequate for most problems. Travelers are advised to obtain supplemental travel health insurance with specific overseas coverage. The policy should provide for direct payment to the overseas hospital and/or physician at the time of service and include a medical evacuation benefit.
- Tirane Clinical Hospital #2 (900 beds); general medical/surgical facility; best treatment facility in Albania.
- ABC Health Center, Qemal Stafa #260, Tirana; Tel: 355-42-3-4105. This clinic serves the foreign and local communities of Tirana.

Current Advisories and Health Risks

For additional information, consult the Disease Risk Summary for Europe on page 300.

Algeria

CAPITAL:
Algiers

EMBASSY (IN U.S.):
2137 Wyoming Ave., NW, Washington, DC 20008
202-265-2800

GMT
+1 hour

TELEPHONE COUNTRY CODE:
213

INTERNET:
www.algeria-us.org

USADIRECT:
None

ENTRY REQUIREMENTS
- **Passport/Visa:** Valid passport and visa are required.
- **HIV Test:** Not required.
- **Vaccinations:** A yellow fever vaccination certificate is required for all travelers older than 1 year arriving from infected areas.

EMBASSIES/CONSULATES
- **U.S. Embassy**: 4 Chemin Cheikh Bachir El-Ibrahimi, Algiers. Tel: 213-21-691-425, 691-255, 691-186; Fax: 213-21-693-979.
- **Canadian Embassy**: 18, rue Mustapha-Khalef, Ben Aknoun, Alger-Gare, 16000 Alger. Tel: 213-21-914-951; 4960; Fax: 213-21-914-973; e-mail: alger@dfait-maeci.gc.ca
- **British Embassy**: 7th Floor, Hotel Hilton International, Palais des Expositions, Pins Maritimes, El Mohammadia, Algiers; Tel: 213-021-23-00-68, Fax: 213-021-23-00-67; e-mail: BritishEmbassy.Algiers@fco.gov.uk; Website: http://www.britishembassy. gov.uk/algeria.

HOSPITALS/DOCTORS
- University Hospital, Algiers (2,900 beds); all specialties.
- Institute Pasteur d'Algerie.
- University Hospital, Oran (2,200 beds); general medical/surgical facility; all specialties.

Current Advisories and Health Risks

CHOLERA: Sporadic cases of cholera may occur. Cholera vaccine is recommended primarily for people at high risk (e.g., relief workers) who work and live in highly endemic areas under less than adequate sanitary conditions.

HEPATITIS: All nonimmune travelers should receive hepatitis A vaccine. Hepatitis E presumably occurs, but levels are unclear. The hepatitis B carrier rate in the general population is estimated at 3%. Vaccination against hepatitis B virus (HBV) should be considered by anybody desiring maximal protection, or by a traveler who might be exposed to blood (e.g., a health-care worker), or have sexual contact with the local population, stay longer than 3 months, or be exposed to HBV through medical treatment.

INFLUENZA: Influenza is transmitted from November through March. Vaccination is recommended for travel during this time.

LEISHMANIASIS: Transmission occurs primarily from April to October. Cutaneous leishmaniasis is endemic in the semi-arid steppe region of the northern part of the Algerian Sahara. Major risk areas include Biskra (especially near Sidi Okba), Bechar (especially near Abadla), and M'sila Provinces. Visceral leishmaniasis (kala azar) occurs primarily in the less humid central and eastern parts of the northern coastal mountainous area; major foci are in the Grande Kabylie Region (Tizi Ouzou and Bejaia Provinces) and in the vicinities of Alger, Boumerdes, and Constantine.

MALARIA: Risk is primarily limited to the remote oases in the Sahara region of Adrar, Ouargla, and Tamanghasset Provinces from July through November. *Plasmodium vivax* accounts for more 90% of cases. Occasional cases are caused by *Plasmodium* malariae. Malaria chemoprophylaxis is not recommended for visits to any part of this country but mosquito-bite precautions should be observed.

MEDITERRANEAN SPOTTED (BOUTONNEUSE) FEVER (AFRICAN TICK TYPE): Presumed risk occurs primarily in suburban coastal areas. Precautions against tick bites should be taken.

RABIES: About 20 to 30 rabies cases are reported yearly. Human rabies is usually transmitted by dog bites, but bites by jackals and foxes should also be considered dangerous. Rabies vaccine should be considered for stays of over 3 months or for shorter stays if traveling to locations more than 24 hours travel from a reliable source of postexposure rabies vaccine. All animal bites or scratches should be medically evaluated.

SCHISTOSOMIASIS: Risk is present year-round. Urinary schistosomiasis occurs in two areas. One area occurs in the north, primarily in the Mitidja Plain near Alger, and also at Khemis El Khechna. The other area occurs in the southeast, in the Tassili N'Ajjer region. Travelers should avoid swimming or wading in freshwater lakes, ponds, or streams in these areas.

TRAVELERS' DIARRHEA: All water sources in Algeria should be considered potentially contaminated. Travelers should drink only bottled, boiled, or chemically treated water. A quinolone antibiotic, combined with loperamide (Imodium), is recommended for the treatment of acute diarrhea. Persistent diarrhea may be due to a parasitic infection such as giardiasis, amebiasis, or cryptosporidiosis.

TUBERCULOSIS: Tuberculosis is a major public health problem in this country. Travelers planning an extended stay should have a pre-departure TB skin test (PPD test) and be retested after leaving this country.

TYPHOID FEVER: Typhoid vaccine is recommended. Because the typhoid vaccines are only 60% to 70% effective, safe food and drink selection remain important.

- -

OTHER DISEASES/HAZARDS: AIDS/HIV (low reported incidence), brucellosis, echinococcosis (a major health problem countrywide, particularly in rural and highland areas), fascioliasis (sheep liver fluke disease; acquired by eating contaminated watercress), relapsing fever (tick- and louse-borne), sand fly fever (elevated risk in the coastal region and the steppe region of the northern part of the Algerian Sahara), trachoma, typhoid fever, tuberculosis, and intestinal helminthic infections (roundworm, hookworm, and whipworm diseases, as well as strongyloidiasis, are common in rural areas and among lower socioeconomic groups).

Angola ★ LUANDA

CAPITAL:
Luanda
EMBASSY (IN U.S.):
2100 16th St., NW
Washington, DC 20009
202-452-1042/3
Internet: www.angola.org
GMT:
+1 hour
TELEPHONE COUNTRY CODE:
244
USADIRECT:
0199
ENTRY REQUIREMENTS
- **Passport/Visa:** A valid passport and visa are required. Contact the Angolan embassy or consulate for additional information.
- **HIV Test:** Not required.
- **Vaccinations:** A yellow fever vaccination certificate is required for all travelers older than 1 year of age arriving from infected areas.
EMBASSIES/CONSULATES
- **U.S. Embassy**: Rua Houari Boumedienne, #32 Luanda. Tel: 244-2-447-028, 244-2-445-481; 24-hour duty officer 244-9-501-343; Fax: 244-2-446-924; e-mail: amembassyluanda@netangola.com.
- **Canadian Embassy**: Rua Rei Katyavala 113, Luanda; Tel: 244-2-448-366/71/77; Fax: 244-2-449-494; e-mail: consul.can@angonet.org.
- **British Embassy**: Rua Diogo Cao, 4, Caixa Postal 1244, Luanda; Tel: 244-2-334582, 334583, 392991, 387681; Fax: 244-2-333331; e-mail: postmaster@luanda.fco.gov.uk

- University Hospital, Luanda (500+ beds).
- Americo Boavioa (600 beds); general medical/surgical facility.
- NOTE: Medical care is substandard throughout the country, including medical care in the capital, Luanda.
- International SOS:
  - International SOS Angola, Limitada, Rua Luis Mota Feo, n 22, 1 Andar Luanda Angola; Admin Tel: 244-2-311742; Admin Fax: 244-2-310595
  - International Clinic—Ilha Clinica Sagrada Esperanca, Avenida Mortella—Mohamed, Ilha da Luanda, Angola; Clinic Mob: 244-923-330845; Clinic Fax: 244-2-309063, e-mail: internationalclinic@netangola.com
  - International Clinic—Gamek, Gamek Residential Camp, Lunda Sul, Luanda, Angola; Clinic Mob: 244-923-330843; Clinic Fax: 244-2-309063, Sales enquiries: 244-923-642601, e-mail: internationalclinic@netangola.com

Current Advisories and Health Risks

AIDS/HIV: The incidence of HIV is estimated at 5% of the general population, with a much higher incidence in young adults in the urban population. HIV is transmitted predominantly by heterosexual contact. All travelers are cautioned against unsafe sex, nonsterile medical or dental injections, and unscreened blood transfusions.

AFRICAN SLEEPING SICKNESS (TRYPANOSOMIASIS): African trypanosomiasis is epidemic in focal areas throughout the country. Cases of the Rhodesian form of trypanosomiasis have been reported in the southeast. The Gambian form of trypanosomiasis occurs primarily in the northwestern provinces of Zaire, Uige, Luanda, and Cuanza Norte, and as far south as Bengo Province. Travelers should take measures to prevent insect (tsetse fly) bites.

ANIMAL HAZARDS: Animal hazards include snakes (vipers, cobras, mambas), centipedes, scorpions, and black widow spiders.

CHIKUNGUNYA FEVER: This is a mosquito-borne viral illness, similar to dengue fever; human outbreaks in the region have occurred primarily in rural populations, but explosive urban outbreaks can also occur. Daytime mosquito bite protection measures are advised.

CHOLERA: This disease is active in this country and occurs year-round. Cholera is a rare disease in travelers from developed countries. Cholera vaccine is primarily recommended for people at high risk (e.g., health-care and relief workers) in highly endemic areas. Many countries, including Canada, license an oral cholera vaccine. The oral vaccine is not available in the United States.

DENGUE FEVER: Low apparent risk, but dengue does occur in urban and rural areas. Travelers are advised to take measures to prevent daytime mosquito bites.

HEPATITIS: All nonimmune travelers should receive hepatitis A vaccine. Hepatitis E presumably occurs, based on regional data, but its incidence is not known. The hepatitis B carrier rate in the general population is estimated to exceed 10%. Vaccination against hepatitis B virus (HBV) should be considered by anybody desiring maximal protection, or by a traveler who might be exposed to blood (e.g., a health-care worker), have sexual contact with the local population, stay longer than 3 months, or be exposed to HBV through medical treatment.

INFLUENZA: Transmitted year-round; vaccination is recommended.

MALARIA: Risk is present year-round throughout Angola, including urban areas and the enclave of Cabinda. Falciparum malaria accounts for 90% of cases, followed by *Plasmodium malariae*. Chloroquine-resistant falciparum malaria is prevalent. All travelers to Angola, including infants, children, and former residents of this country should take one of the following antimalarial drugs: atovaquone/proguanil, doxycycline, mefloquine, or (in special circumstances) primaquine. All travelers should take measures to prevent evening and nighttime mosquito bites. Insect-bite prevention measures include a DEET-containing repellent applied to exposed skin, insecticide (permethrin) spray applied to clothing, and use of a permethrin-treated bed net at night.

MENINGITIS: Angola lies south of the African "meningitis belt," but has reported outbreaks of type A meningococcal meningitis. Quadrivalent meningococcal vaccine is recommended for all travelers to Angola, November through June, who expect to have close contact with the local population.

ONCHOCERCIASIS: Transmitted by black flies near fast-flowing rivers. Risk areas lie particularly in the northern provinces of Cuanza Norte, Lunda, Malanje, Uige, and Zaire—and in the plateau region of the central province of Bie and the Cabinda exclave. Travelers should take precautions against insect bites.

POLIO: This disease is endemic. All travelers should be fully immunized.

RABIES: Considered a public health problem in many rural and urban areas; stray dogs are the primary cause of human infection. Pre-exposure rabies vaccine should be considered for stays longer than 3 months, or for shorter stays if traveling to locations more than 24 hours' travel from a reliable source of postexposure rabies vaccine. All animal bites or scratches should be medically evaluated and postexposure prophylaxis administered, as needed.

SCHISTOSOMIASIS: Infection rates for urinary schistosomiasis have been highest in the coastal provinces of Luanda, Bengo, and Benguela, decreasing in an eastward direction. Intestinal schistosomiasis, presumably distributed countrywide, is most prevalent in the southeastern province of Cuando Cubango. Travelers should avoid swimming, bathing, or wading in freshwater ponds, lakes, or streams.

TRAVELERS' DIARRHEA: High risk. Only major urban areas have access to public water systems, which serve primarily the former European sections. Water distribution systems may be damaged and contaminated. Travelers should all observe food and drink safety precautions. A quinolone antibiotic, plus loperamide (Imodium), is recommended for the treatment of acute diarrhea. Persistent diarrhea may be due to a parasitic disease, such as giardiasis or amebiasis.

TUBERCULOSIS: Tuberculosis a major health problem in this country. Travelers planning an extended stay should have a pre-departure TB skin test (PPD test) and be retested after returning to this country.

TYPHOID FEVER: Typhoid vaccine is recommended for travel to this country. The typhoid vaccine is 60% to 70% effective, so food and drink precautions should continue to be observed.

YELLOW FEVER: This disease is active in this country. The CDC recommends yellow fever vaccination for all travelers older than 9 months of age arriving from all countries.

OTHER DISEASES/HAZARDS: African tick typhus (contracted from dog ticks, often in urban areas, and bush ticks), brucellosis (from consumption of raw dairy products); Bancroftian filariasis (mosquito-borne—reported in the north; primarily Cabinda enclave and Zaire Province), leishmaniasis (low apparent risk; sporadic cases may have previously occurred); Marburg virus hemorrhagic fever (outbreak March 2005; reported in Uige Province, northern Angola; Ebola-family virus, spread by close contact with infected people), plague (flea borne; human cases last reported from Benguela Province), polio (this disease is currently active; all travelers should be fully immunized), relapsing fever (tick borne and louse-borne), toxoplasmosis; syphilis; tuberculosis (a major public health problem), typhoid fever, typhus (louse borne and flea borne), and intestinal worms (very common).

Argentina

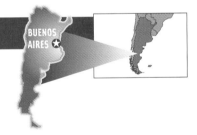

CAPITAL:
Buenos Aires
EMBASSY (IN U.S.):
1811 Q St., NW
Washington, DC 20009
202-238-6460
GMT:
−3 hours
TELEPHONE COUNTRY CODE:
54
USADIRECT:
0-800-555-4288
0-800-222-1288

ENTRY REQUIREMENTS

- **Passport/Visa**: U.S. citizens do not need a visa for a tourist/business stay of less than 90 days.
- **HIV Test**: Not required.
- **Vaccinations**: None required.

EMBASSIES/CONSULATES

- **U.S. Embassy**: 4300 Avenida Colombia, 1425 Buenos Aires. e-mail: BuenosAiresConsulate@state.gov; Website: embassy.state.gov/baires embassy.
- **Canadian Embassy**: 2828 Tagle, Buenos Aires. Tel: 11-4805-3032; Fax: 54-11-4806-1209; e-mail: bairs@dfait-maeci.gc.ca.
- **British Embassy**: Dr. Luis Agote 2412/52, 1425 Capital Federal, Buenos Aires, Tel: 54-11-4808-2200. Fax: 54-11-4808-2274, e-mail: askconsular.baires@fco.gov.uk; askcommercial.baires@fco.gov.uk; askinformation.baires@fco.gov.uk; www.britain.org.ar.

HOSPITALS/DOCTORS:

Medical insurance is recommended because there are no reciprocal health agreements with Canada or Europe. Medical facilities are generally of a high standard.

- **Clinica y Maternidad Suizo Argentina & The Swiss Medical Center**, Avenida Pueyrredón 1461-1118, Buenos Aires. 155-bed private hospital and medical center. Emergency services available 24 hours daily.
- **The British Hospital** (Hospital Britanico), Buenos Aires (400 beds), Perdriel 74, Buenos Aires; 243-bed private hospital, used by tourists and expatriates. 24-hour emergency services are available.
- **Mater Dei Hospital**, Buenos Aires (100 beds); most specialty services; used by the American community and other expatriates.

Current Advisories and Health Risks

CHAGAS DISEASE: Low risk to tourists, but about 60% of the country's area is endemic for Chagas disease. Risk occurs primarily in rural-agricultural areas and is associated with sleeping in adobe-style huts and houses that harbor the night-biting triatomid (assassin) bug. Prevention: Travelers should spray sleeping quarters with a contact insecticide, keep bed away from walls, and sleep under a permethrin-treated bed net. Unscreened blood transfusions are also a potential source of infection and should be avoided.

CHOLERA: This disease is reported in this country, but cholera is an extremely rare disease in travelers from developed countries. Cholera vaccine is recommended primarily for people at high risk (e.g., health-care, relief workers) who work and live in highly endemic areas under less than adequate sanitary conditions. Many countries, including Canada, license an oral cholera vaccine. The oral cholera vaccine is not available in the United States.

DENGUE FEVER: Low overall risk. Dengue may occur in the northeastern lowlands adjacent to Paraguay. Travelers to the northeast regions should take precautions against insect bites.

ECHINOCOCCOSIS: High incidence is reported in southern cattle/sheep rearing regions. Human prevalence is among the highest reported worldwide. Travelers to these regions should avoid contact with dogs to prevent accidental ingestion of infective eggs that are passed in dog feces. Strict personal hygiene, especially hand washing, is important and all travelers should pay close attention to food and drink guidelines to avoid ingestion of potentially contaminated food.

FOOD AND WATER SAFETY: Tap water is considered safe to drink. Drinking water outside main cities and towns may be contaminated and sterilization is advisable. Pasteurized milk and dairy products are safe for consumption, but travelers should avoid unpasteurized milk, a source of brucellosis. Local meat, poultry, seafood, fruit, and vegetables are generally considered safe to eat.

HEPATITIS: All nonimmune travelers should receive the hepatitis A vaccine. The hepatitis B carrier rate in the general population is estimated at about 1%. Vaccination against hepatitis B virus (HBV) should be considered by anybody desiring maximal protection, or by a traveler who might be exposed to blood (e.g., a health-care worker), or have sexual contact with the local population, stay longer than 3 months, or be exposed to HBV through medical treatment.

INFLUENZA: Influenza is transmitted from April through September in the Southern Hemisphere. Vaccination is recommended for travel to this country.

LEISHMANIASIS: Risk of cutaneous and mucocutaneous leishmaniasis is limited to the northern one third of the country, with the majority of cases reported from the Salta, Jujuy, Catamarca, and Santiago del Estero provinces. Occasional cases of visceral leishmaniasis have been reported from Salta and Chaco provinces. Travelers to these areas should take measures to prevent sand fly bites.

MALARIA: Risk is year-round in rural areas below 1,200 meters elevation in the rural areas of the Salta and Jujuy provinces (along Bolivian border) and the Misiones and Corrientes provinces (along border of Paraguay). Vivax malaria accounts for virtually 100% of cases. All travelers to malaria-risk areas in Argentina, including infants, children, and former residents of Argentina, should take chloroquine as their antimalarial drug. All travelers should also take measures to prevent evening and nighttime mosquito bites. Insect-bite prevention measures include a DEET-containing repellent applied to exposed skin, insecticide (permethrin) spray applied to clothing and gear, and use of a permethrin-treated bed net at night.

RABIES: Low risk; 18 to 20 human cases may occur annually from both urban and rural areas. Rabies vaccine is recommended only for those persons anticipating an extended stay, those whose work or activities may bring them into contact with animals (especially stray dogs), or when extra protection is desired. Prompt medical evaluation and treatment of any animal bite is essential, regardless of vaccination status.

TRAVELERS' DIARRHEA: Moderate risk outside of Buenos Aires and other urban areas. A quinolone antibiotic, combined with loperamide (Imodium), is recommended for the treatment of acute diarrhea. Persistent diarrhea may be due to a parasitic disease such as giardiasis, amebiasis, or cryptosporidiosis.

TYPHOID FEVER: Vaccination against typhoid fever is recommended for travelers venturing outside of tourist areas; long-term travelers; adventure travelers; and short-stay travelers wishing maximal protection. Because the typhoid vaccines are only 60% to 70% effective, safe food and drink selection remain important.

YELLOW FEVER: There is potential risk of yellow fever in northeastern forested areas, although no human cases have been reported recently. Yellow fever vaccine is recommended for travel to these rural areas, including the Iguassu Falls tourist resorts. NOTE: The Iguassu Falls area is shared by northeastern Argentina and the Matto Grosso do Sul state of Brazil. The CDC recommends yellow fever immunization for this area.

OTHER DISEASES/HAZARDS: Argentine hemorrhagic fever (viral disease transmitted by contact with infected rodent excreta; more common in agricultural areas of the moist pampas region of east-central Argentina), anthrax (mostly cutaneous; associated with farming and slaughterhouse exposure), arboviral fevers (mosquito-transmitted; eastern equine encephalitis, St. Louis encephalitis, Venezuelan encephalitis), brucellosis (high incidence; travelers should avoid unpasteurized cheese), fascioliasis (from consumption of contaminated wild watercress), hantaviral disease, leptospirosis, plague, schistosomiasis (endemic status unclear; officially not reported), trachoma (occurs in NE areas), trichinellosis, tuberculosis, strongyloidiasis, and other intestinal helminthic (worm) infections are reported.

Armenia

CAPITAL:
Yerevan
EMBASSY (IN U.S.):
202-319-2983
GMT:
+4 hours
ENTRY REQUIREMENTS
• **Passport/Visa**: required.
• **HIV Test**: Not required.
• **Required vaccinations**: None.
TELEPHONE COUNTRY CODE:
374
USA DIRECT:
0-800-111

- **U.S. Embassy**: 18 General Bagramian Street, Yerevan; Tel: 3741-151-551; Fax: 3741-151-550; Website: www.armeniaemb.org.
- **Canadian Embassy**: 25 Demirjian Street, Apt. 21, Yerevan; Tel: and Fax: 3741-567-903; Cellular: 3749-401-238.
- **British Embassy:** 34 Baghramyan Ave, Yerevan 375019; Tel: 3741-264301; Fax: 3741-264318; e-mail: britemb@arminco.com.

HOSPITALS/DOCTORS:

Travelers should contact the U.S. or Canadian embassy for medical referrals. In the event of serious medical conditions every effort should be made to go to a medical facility in Western Europe. Hospital accommodations are inadequate throughout this country and advanced technology is lacking.

Current Advisories and Health Risks

AIDS/HIV: AIDS cases are increasing and an epidemic may be in the making. The reasons include (1) an increase in IV drug abuse; (2) increases in prostitution and sexual promiscuity; (3) an increase in sexually transmitted diseases, (4) decreased availability of sterile needles and syringes, and (5) no education or prevention programs.

ACCIDENTS AND MEDICAL INSURANCE

- Accidents and injuries are the leading cause of death among travelers younger than age 55 and are most often caused by motor vehicle and motorcycle crashes; drownings, aircraft crashes, homicides, and burns are less common causes.
- Heart attacks cause most fatalities in older travelers.
- Infections cause only 1% of fatalities in overseas travelers, but, overall, infections are the most common cause of travel-related illness.
- Travelers are advised to obtain, before departure, supplemental travel health insurance with specific overseas coverage. The policy should provide for direct payment to the overseas hospital and/or physician at the time of service and include a medical evacuation benefit. The policy should also provide 24-hour hotline access to a multilingual assistance center that can help arrange and monitor delivery of medical care and determine if medical evacuation or air ambulance services are required.

ARBOVIRAL DISEASES

- Karelian fever (mosquito-borne; most cases occur July through September in the Karelian region).
- Tahjna virus fever (mosquito-borne; occurs sporadically from the Baltic region north to the Kolsky Peninsula).
- Sand fly fever (sand fly-borne; limited to Moldova and the Crimea).
- Dengue fever (mosquito-borne; cases previously reported from extreme southern regions).
- West Nile fever (mosquito-borne; virus reportedly circulates in the Volga Delta region from May through September).
- Sindbis virus fever (detected in the Volga Delta, July through August).

- All travelers should take measures to prevent evening and nighttime mosquito bites. Insect-bite prevention measures include a DEET-containing repellent applied to exposed skin, insecticide (permethrin) spray applied to clothing and gear, and use of a permethrin-treated bed net at night while sleeping.

CHOLERA:

- Sporadic cases of cholera may occur in this country. Cholera is an extremely rare disease in travelers from developed countries. Cholera vaccine is recommended primarily for people at high risk (e.g., relief workers) who work and live in highly endemic areas under less than adequate sanitary conditions.
- The oral cholera vaccine (Dukoral) provides up to 60% crossover protection against ETEC diarrhea.
- Many countries, including Canada, license an oral cholera vaccine. The oral vaccine is not available in the United States.
- Cholera vaccine is not "officially" required for entry into, or exit from, any country. Despite this, some countries, on occasion, require proof of cholera vaccination from travelers coming from cholera-infected countries. Anticipating such a situation, certain travelers may wish to carry a medical exemption letter from their health-care provider. Travel Medicine, Inc., recommends that travelers use the International Certificate of Vaccination (Yellow Card) for this purpose, having their health-care provider affirm that they are "exempt from cholera vaccine" and validate the exemption with both the provider's signature and the appropriate official stamp (the "Uniform Stamp" in the United States).

CRIMEAN-CONGO HEMORRHAGIC FEVER: Reported mostly from southern areas, but outbreaks have occurred in some areas of Rostov Oblast (near the sea of Azov), April through November. Risk areas are rural steppe, savannah, semi-desert, and foothill/low mountain habitats below 2,000 meters elevation.

DIPHTHERIA: An epidemic of diphtheria that began in 1990 in the Russian Federation has spread extensively, involving all countries of the former Soviet Union. Seventy percent of cases have occurred in persons older than 15 years. All travelers should be fully immunized against this disease. (The CDC estimates that 20% to 60% of Americans older than 20 years lack sufficient immunity to diphtheria.) Diphtheria vaccine in the United States is widely available and is administered in combination with the tetanus toxoid vaccine (Td vaccine).

FOOD AND WATER SAFETY: All water should be regarded as being a potential health risk. Water used for drinking, brushing teeth, or making ice should have first been boiled or otherwise sterilized. Eat only well-cooked meat and fish, preferably served hot. Pork, salad, and mayonnaise may carry increased risk. Vegetables should be cooked and fruit should be peeled. Milk is pasteurized and dairy products should be safe for consumption, however, the incidence of communicable diseases among livestock is increasing because of a breakdown in vaccination programs.

HEPATITIS: All nonimmune travelers should receive hepatitis A vaccine. Hepatitis E accounts for up to 18% of acute hepatitis in the south. The hepatitis B carrier rate in the general population of Russia is estimated at 3.8%. Vaccination against hepatitis B should be considered for stays longer than 3 months and by short-term travelers desiring maximal protection. Travelers should be aware that hepatitis B can be transmitted by unsafe sex and the use of contaminated needles and syringes. Blood supplies may be contaminated with hepatitis B and C viruses.

INFLUENZA: Influenza is transmitted from November through March. The flu vaccine is recommended for all travelers older than age 50; all travelers with chronic disease or a weakened immune system; travelers of any age wishing to decrease the risk of this illness; and pregnant women after the first trimester.

LEISHMANIASIS: Risk for cutaneous leishmaniasis primarily limited to southern regions, including portions of the Georgia Republic and the southern Ukraine, below 1,300 meters elevation. Visceral leishmaniasis is confined to areas along the southeastern coast of the Black Sea, the southeastern and southwestern coasts of the Caspian Sea and the border areas of Georgia and Azerbaijan. Travelers to these regions should take measures to prevent sand fly bites.

LYME DISEASE: Occurs focally in rural forested areas with the highest incidence in the Ural Mountain area. Risk presumably also occurs in the northwest and central areas.

MALARIA: Transmission currently is limited to the warmer months of June through September. Risk (exclusively *Plasmodium vivax*) exists in focal areas on the western border with Turkey. Risk is primarily in the Ararat Valley, with most cases in the Masis district and with minimal risk in the Artashat and Ararat districts. No risk exists in typical tourist destinations.
- Prophylaxis with chloroquine is recommended in risk areas.
- All travelers should take measures to prevent evening and nighttime mosquito bites. Insect-bite prevention measures include a DEET-containing repellent applied to exposed skin, insecticide (permethrin) spray applied to clothing and gear, and use of a permethrin-treated bed net at night while sleeping.

MEDITERRANEAN SPOTTED (BOUTONNEUSE) FEVER: Tick-borne; reported most commonly in the Black Sea coastal areas of the Caucasus, Transcaucasus, and the Crimea, and along the Caspian Sea coastline.

TICK-BORNE ENCEPHALITIS (TBE): Tick-borne encephalitis is transmitted from the Baltics to the Crimea. Peak transmission period is April through October. Risk is present primarily in rural brushy and forested areas below 1,500 meters elevation. Risk areas include the Urals and much of the northern, forested mountainous areas and the suburban "forests" bordering large cities. The highest number of cases are reported from the south-central areas, including Altay, Kemerovo, Novosibirsk Oblasts, and Krasnoyarsk Kray. Coinfection with Lyme disease is increasing. Travelers to endemic areas should take measures to prevent tick bites.

TRAVELERS' DIARRHEA: Moderate risk countrywide. A quinolone antibiotic, combined with loperamide (Imodium), is recommended for the treatment of acute diarrhea. Diarrhea not responding to antibiotic treatment may be due to a parasitic disease such as giardiasis, amebiasis, or cryptosporidiosis.

TUBERCULOSIS: Tuberculosis is a major public health problem in this country. Travelers planning an extended stay should have a pre-departure TB skin test (PPD test) and be retested after leaving this country.

TYPHOID FEVER: Typhoid fever is recommended for long-term travelers, adventure travelers, and those wishing maximum disease protection. Because the typhoid vaccines are only 60% to 70% effective, safe food and drink guidelines should continue to be observed.

OTHER DISEASES/HAZARDS: Anthrax (sporadic human cases occur, related to exposure to livestock in rural areas, especially southern areas), brucellosis (unpasteurized goat cheese should be avoided), echinococcosis (in southern and northeastern areas). *Echinococcus multilocularis* associated with reindeer culture in north), legionellosis; leptospirosis (a particular problem in fish-breeding areas of Rostov Province; extensive outbreaks have occurred in east central areas), North Asian tick typhus (also called Siberian tick typhus; occurs in the steppe areas bordering Kazakhstan, Georgia, and Azerbaijan; risk elevated May through June), opisthorchiasis (acquired from consumption of raw freshwater fish; reported from western European Russia), plague (flea-borne; usually occurs as isolated cases or small outbreaks in semi-arid areas of the southern republics of Azerbaijan, Armenia, and Georgia), rabies, rickettsialpox, tick-borne relapsing fever; (may occur south of 55 degrees north latitude), trichinosis (greatest risk in western Belarus and the Ukraine); tularemia ("rabbit fever"; risk may be elevated in the north), tuberculosis (40% rise in cases since 1995; incidence in Moscow has doubled since 1991), and helminthic infections (roundworm, hookworm, and whipworm infections and strongyloidiasis) reported, especially from the Transcaucasus, especially Azerbaijan.

Aruba

★ ORANJESTAD

CAPITAL:
Oranjestad
EMBASSY (IN U.S.):
202-244-5300
GMT:
−4 hours
TELEPHONE COUNTRY CODE:
297
USA DIRECT:
None

- **Passport/Visa**: Aruba is one of the Netherlands Antilles, an autonomous part of the Kingdom of the Netherlands. The Netherlands Antilles is a group of six Caribbean islands: Aruba, Bonaire, Curacao, Saba, Statia, and St. Maarten. Passport or proof of U.S. citizenship (i.e., certified birth certificate or voter registration card with photo ID) required. Visa not required for stay up to 14 days—may be extended to 90 days after arrival.
- **HIV Test**: Required by Aruba for immigrants.
- **Vaccinations**: Yellow fever vaccination required if traveling from an infected area.

EMBASSIES/CONSULATES

- **U.S. Embassy**: J.B. Gorsiraweg #1, Willemstad, Curacao; Tel: 599-9-461-3066; Fax: 599-9-461-6489; e-mail: cgcuracao@interneeds.net.
- **Canadian Embassy**: Maduro and Curiels Bank, N.V., Scharlooweg 55, Willemstad, Curacao; Tel: 599-9-466-1115/1121; Fax: 599-9-1122/1130.

HOSPITALS/DOCTORS:

- Oduber Hospital, Oranjestad: (279 beds). This hospital is regarded as one of the better medical facilities in the West Indies.
- Adequate care is available on Aruba, Curacao, and Saint Maarten but transfer to a more advanced medical facility should be considered for life-threatening medical or surgical conditions.

Current Advisories and Health Risks

ACCIDENTS AND MEDICAL INSURANCE

- Accidents and injuries are the leading cause of death among travelers younger than age 55 and are most often caused by motor vehicle and motorcycle crashes; drownings, aircraft crashes, homicides, and burns are less common causes.
- Heart attacks cause most fatalities in older travelers.
- Infections cause only 1% of fatalities in overseas travelers, but, overall, infections are the most common cause of travel-related illness.
- Travelers are advised to obtain, before departure, supplemental travel health insurance with specific overseas coverage. The policy should provide for direct payment to the overseas hospital and/or physician at the time of service and include a medical evacuation benefit. The policy should also provide 24-hour hotline access to a multilingual assistance center that can help arrange and monitor delivery of medical care and determine if medical evacuation or air ambulance services are required.

DENGUE FEVER: Dengue fever is widespread in the Caribbean. Travelers to the Netherlands Antilles should take measures to prevent daytime mosquito bites.

FOOD AND WATER SAFETY: Tap water is considered safe to drink. Milk is pasteurized and dairy products are safe for consumption. Local meat, poultry, seafood, fruit, and vegetables are generally considered safe to eat.

HEPATITIS: Nonimmune travelers should receive hepatitis A vaccine. Vaccination against hepatitis B should be considered for stays longer than 3 months or by those travelers desiring maximal protection. Travelers should be aware that hepatitis B can be transmitted by unsafe sex and the use of contaminated needles and syringes.

INFLUENZA: Influenza is transmitted year-round in the tropics. The flu vaccine is recommended for all travelers older than age 50; all travelers with any chronic disease or weakened immune system; travelers of any age wishing to decrease the risk of this illness; pregnant women after the first trimester.

MARINE HAZARDS

- Swimming-related hazards include jellyfish, spiny sea urchins, and corals.
- Ciguatera poisoning is prevalent and can result from eating reef fish such as grouper, snapper, sea bass, jack, and barracuda. The ciguatoxin is not destroyed by cooking.
- Scuba diving—Hyperbaric Chamber Referral: Divers' Alert Network (DAN) maintains an up-to-date list of all functioning hyperbaric chambers in North America and the Caribbean. DAN does not publish this list because at any one time a given chamber may be nonfunctioning, or its operator(s) may be away or otherwise unavailable. Through Duke University, DAN operates a 24-hour emergency phone line for anyone (members and nonmembers) to call and ask for diving accident assistance. Dive medicine physicians at Duke University Medical Center carry beepers, so someone is always on call to answer questions and, if necessary, make referral to the closest functioning hyperbaric chamber. In a diving emergency, or for the location of the nearest decompression chamber, call 919-684-8111.

TRAVELERS' DIARRHEA: Low to moderate risk. Food and water are generally safe on this island. A quinolone antibiotic, combined with loperamide (Imodium), are recommended for the treatment of acute diarrhea.

Australia

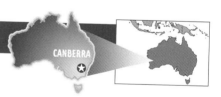

CAPITAL:
Canberra
EMBASSY (IN U.S.):
1601 Massachusetts Ave., NW
Washington, DC 20036
202-797-3000
GMT:
+10 hours
TELEPHONE COUNTRY CODE:
61
USADIRECT:
1-800-881-011 (Telstra)
1-800-551-155 (Optus)

- **Passport/Visa**: An ETA (Electronic Travel Authority) or nonelectronic label visa is required for tourist or business stays of up to 3 months.
- **HIV Test**: Required of all applicants for permanent residence age 15 or over. Tests taken in the U.S. are acceptable.
- **Vaccinations**: A yellow fever vaccination certificate is required of travelers older than 1 year if arriving within 6 days of having stayed overnight or longer in a country any part of which is infected.

EMBASSIES/CONSULATES

- **U.S. Embassy**: Moonah Place, Yarralumla; Tel: 61-2-6214-5600; Fax: 2-6273-3191; Website: www.usis-australia.gov.
- **Consulates**: Level 59, MLC Centre, 19-29 Martin Place, Sydney; Tel: 2-9373-9200; Fax: 2-9373-9184; Website: www.usconsydney.org. Consulate: 553 St. Kilda Road, Melbourne; Tel: 3-9526-5900; Fax: 3-9525-0769; Website: www.usis-australia.gov/melbourne. Consulate: Level 13, 16 St. Georges Terrace, Perth; Tel: 8-9231-9400; Fax: 8-9231-9444; Website: www.usis-australia.gov/perth.
- **Canadian Embassy**: Commonwealth Avenue, Canberra; Tel: 2-6270-4000; Fax: 6270-4081; e-mail: cnbra@dfait-maeci.gc.ca; Website: www.dfait-maeci.gc.ca/australia.
- **British High Commission**: Commonwealth Avenue, Yarralumla, Canberra, ACT 2600; Tel: 61-2-6270-6666, Fax: 61-2-6273-3236 (General), 61-2-6273-4360 (Economic), 61-2-6270-6653 (Chancery), e-mail: bhc.canberra@mail.uk.emb.gov.au, Website: www.britaus.net
- **Consular Section, Canberra**: Piccadilly House, 39 Brindabella Circuit, Brindabella Business Park, Canberra Airport, Canberra Act 2609, Tel: Passports/Entry Clearance 61-1902-941-555, e-mail: bhc.consular@mail.uk.emb.gov.au, Website: www.uk.emb.gov.au

HOSPITALS/DOCTORS

- Royal Melbourne Hospital (702 beds); most specialties and diagnostic capabilities; emergency services
- Traveler's Medical and Vaccination Centre, Melbourne
- Royal Prince Alfred Hospital, Sydney (1,532 beds); most specialties and diagnostic capabilities; emergency services; ICU
- Traveler's Medical and Vaccination Centre, Sydney
- Royal Darwin Hospital (648 beds); most specialties and diagnostic capabilities; emergency services
- Royal Perth Hospital (1,072 beds); ICU, CCU, burn unit; 24-hour emergency; ambulance service
- Traveler's Medical and Vaccination Centre, Perth; Tel: (9) 321-197
- Queen Elizabeth Hospital, Adelaide (Travel Clinic)
- Princess Alexandra Hospital, Brisbane (1,104 beds); many specialties; emergency and ambulance services

- International SOS:
  - International SOS (Australasia) Pty Ltd., Level 5, Challis House, 4 Martin Place, Sydney NSW 2000, Australia; Alarm Center Tel: 61-2-9372-2468; Alarm Center Fax: 61-2-9372-2455
  - International SOS (Australasia) Pty Ltd., Ground Floor 566 St Kilda Rd, Melbourne 3004, Australia; Admin Tel: 61-3-9526-7477; Admin Fax: 61-3-9526-7461

Current Health Risks and Advisories

ANIMAL HAZARDS: Animal hazards include snakes (death adder, Australian copperhead, Australian coral, and others), centipedes and scorpions, and spiders (red back, northern funnel-web, mouse, and brown recluse). Fresh- and saltwater crocodiles are present in Australia, but only the saltwater variety has been known to attack humans. Male platy-puses can inflict painful puncture wounds and should be avoided. Rogue scrub cattle (domestic animals gone wild) are particularly dangerous terrestrial animals and have been known to attack humans and vehicles without provocation.

CHOLERA: There is no risk of cholera in Australia.

DENGUE FEVER: Reported in parts of Northern Queensland and the Torres Strait Islands. Areas of greatest risk are along the coast from Cornavon to Port Darwin to Townsville. Peak infection rates occur during October to March through April. The *Aedes* mosqui-toes, which transmit dengue fever, bite during the daytime and are present in populous urban areas as well as resort and rural areas. Prevention of dengue consists of taking protective measures against daytime mosquito bites.

GIARDIASIS: Giardiasis is endemic in Tasmania and poses a risk to visitors, especially those who participate in wilderness activities such as bushwalking.

HEPATITIS: Hepatitis A is endemic at low levels. Nonimmune travelers should consider hepatitis A vaccine. Hepatitis E may occur but has not been reported. The carrier rate of the hepatitis B virus in the general population is 0.05% to 0.1%. Vaccination against he-patitis B virus (HBV) is recommended for long-stay travelers (>3 months); healthcare workers; travelers who may have sexual contact with the local population or be exposed to HBV through medical treatment or illicit drugs; anybody desiring maximal protection.

INFLUENZA: Influenza is transmitted from April through September in the Southern Hemisphere. Vaccination is recommended for travel during this time.

JAPANESE ENCEPHALITIS (JE): Limited risk exists on the outer islands of the Torres Strait and possibly in the adjacent Cape York Peninsula of the mainland. Transmission is pre-sumed to occur all year. Recommended for those spending more than 1 month in the Torres Strait Islands only. Evening and nighttime insect precautions are recommended.

MALARIA: There is no risk of malaria in Australia.

MARINE HAZARDS: The box jellyfish, the most dangerous jellyfish in the world, and also the sea wasp are found in northern coastal waters. Four other varieties of jellyfish (jimble, Carukia, mauve stinger, and hairy stinger) should also be avoided. The jellyfish population appears to be increasing, owing in part to over fishing of jellyfish predators, rising water temperatures, and pollution. Other hazards, including sharks, stingrays, and poisonous cone shells, are potential hazards in the coastal waters surrounding Australia. Swimmers should take sensible precautions to avoid these hazards.

RABIES: There are no reported cases of indigenous rabies in Australia.

TICK-BORNE DISEASES: Queensland tick typhus has been reported in travelers to the northern beaches of Sydney Harbour; cases of scrub typhus are reported from the tropical rain forests of Litchfield Park. A new tick-borne rickettsial disease, Flinders Island spotted fever, is reported to extend down the southeastern coastal areas of mainland Australia to Flinders Island and northern Tasmania.

TRAVELERS' DIARRHEA: Low risk. Water in major cities and urban areas is potable, but in rural areas and settlements the water may not meet strict standards of purification. A quinolone antibiotic is recommended for the treatment of acute diarrhea.

VIRAL ENCEPHALITIS: Outbreaks of Australian encephalitis (caused by the Murray Valley encephalitis virus) occur annually. Highest attack rates occur in the summer and fall (November through May), especially after periods of heavy rainfall. Most cases reported from Western Australia (tropical Kimberly region in the north of Western Australia), Victoria, and South Australia. A small number of cases occur in the Northern Territory. Mosquitoes transmit viral encephalitis. A small outbreak of Japanese encephalitis is reported from islands in the Torres Strait off the Australian mainland. All travelers should take precautions to prevent mosquito bites.

OTHER DISEASES/HAZARDS: Brucellosis (canned goat's milk in Australia need not be pasteurized and is a potential source of illness), Barmah forest disease (mosquito-borne viral disease), HIV (low risk of transmission), leptospirosis, Ross River fever (viral epidemic polyarthritis—mosquito borne; occurs throughout coastal Australia and in inland mosquito areas), melioidosis, and helminthic infections (endemic at low levels; hookworm disease, strongyloidiasis).

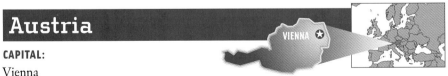

Austria

VIENNA ⭐

CAPITAL:
Vienna
EMBASSY (IN U.S.):
202-895-6767
GMT:
+1 hour

43
USADIRECT:
0-800-200-288
ENTRY REQUIREMENTS*
- **Passport/Visa**: A visa is not required for tourist/business stays up to 3 months.
- **HIV Test**: Testing is required of foreign workers applying for residence permits.
- **Vaccinations**: None required.

*Travelers should check with this country's embassy (or a consulate) in the United States, Canada, or the United Kingdom for any changes in these requirements.

EMBASSIES/CONSULATES
- **U.S. Embassy**: Boltzmanngasse 16 in the Ninth District; Tel: 43-1-31-339; Website: www.usembassy.at
- **Canadian Embassy**: Laurenzenberg 2, Vienna; Tel: 43-1-531-38-3000; Fax: 43-1-531-38-3905; e-mail: vienn@dfait-maeci.gc.ca, Website: www.kanada.at
- **British Embassy**: Jauresgasse 12, 1030 Vienna, Tel: 43-1-716-130, Fax: 43-1-716-13-2999 (Chancery), 43-1-716-13-6900 (Commercial), 43-1-716-13-2900 (Management), e-mail: press@britishembassy.at (Press & Public Affairs and Chancery), commerce@britishembassy.at, visa-consular@britishembassy.at (Consular and Visa enquiries), chancery@britishembassy.at (Political Section), Website: www.britishembassy.at

HOSPITALS/DOCTORS
- Vienna Municipal General Hospital (2,460 beds); major teaching facility; all specialties.
- Landeskrankenhaus Salzburg (1,300 beds); Müllner Hauptstraße 48, Salzburg; Major referral center with all specialties; 24-hour emergency services.
- For a physician referral in Vienna, contact the American Medical Society of Vienna, Tel: 43-(1)-424-568 or the Doctor's Board of Vienna—Service Department for Foreign Patients; Tel: 43-(1)-40-144. The Doctor's Board also provides 24-hour physician referral throughout Austria.

Current Advisories and Health Risks

FOOD AND WATER SAFETY: Milk is pasteurized and dairy products are safe for consumption. Local meat, poultry, seafood, fruit and vegetables are considered safe.

HEPATITIS: As a general precaution, the hepatitis A vaccine is recommended for all non-immune travelers. The hepatitis B carrier rate in the general population is less than 1%. Hepatitis B is spread by infected blood, contaminated needles, and unprotected sex. Vaccination is recommended for stays longer than 3 months; for anyone at occupational or social risk; for any traveler desiring maximal protection.

INFLUENZA: Influenza is transmitted from November through March. The flu vaccine is recommended for all travelers.

LYME DISEASE: Ticks transmitting Lyme disease are found primarily in forested areas at elevations below 1,000 meters, especially in the Danube River basin of eastern Austria.

Travelers are advised to take measures to prevent tick bites during the transmission season, March through September.

RABIES: No human cases have been reported recently, but foxes are a reservoir of the rabies virus.

SWIMMER'S ITCH: Cercarial dermatitis ("swimmer's itch") occurs in Austria in the summer months in warm-water lakes that harbor snails that contain bird or rodent schistosome larvae (called cercariae). The cercariae can penetrate the top layer of a swimmer's skin, causing a rash.

TICK-BORNE ENCEPHALITIS (TBE): This is a viral tick-transmitted disease present in the lowland forests of eastern and southeastern Austria, particularly in the areas around Klagenfurt, Graz, Wiener Neustadt, and Linz, as well in the Danube River valley west of Vienna. There is no apparent risk in the Tyrol and Voralberg provinces. Travelers to risk areas should take measures to prevent tick bites. The TBE vaccine (available in Canada and Europe) is recommended only for people at significant risk of exposure to tick-bites, for example, campers and hikers on extended trips, or forestry workers.

TRAVELERS' DIARRHEA: Low risk. Tap water supplied by municipal water systems is potable. Acute diarrhea is best treated with a quinolone antibiotic, combined with loperamide (Imodium).

OTHER DISEASES/HAZARDS: Leptospirosis (associated with exposure to livestock or swimming in lakes/streams), trichinosis (from eating wild boar), and tularemia (reported sporadically after contact with the meat of killed game).

Azerbaijan

BAKU ★

CAPITAL:
Baku
EMBASSY (IN U.S.):
9-9412-980-335
GMT:
+4 hours
TELEPHONE COUNTRY CODE:
994
USADIRECT:
None
ENTRY REQUIREMENTS
- **Passport/Visa:** Passport and visa required.
- **HIV Test:** Not required.
- **Vaccinations:** None required.

EMBASSIES/CONSULATES

- **U.S. Embassy**: Prospect Azadlig 83, Baku; Tel: 994-12-98-03-35, 36, or 37, 994-12-90-66-71, Website:www.usembassybaku.org.
- **Canadian Embassy:** Accredited to Canadian Embassy in Turkey. Cinnah Caddesi No. 58, Çankaya 06690, Ankara, Turkey; Tel: 90-312-409-2700; Fax: 90-312-409-2810; e-mail: ankra@international.gc.ca; Website: www.dfait-maeci.gc.ca/ankara.
- **British Embassy:** 45, Khagani Street, Baku AZ1000; Tel: 99-412-497-5188/89/90; Fax: 99-412-492-2739; e-mail: office@britemb.baku.az; Website: www.britishembassy.gov.uk/azerbaijan.

HOSPITALS/DOCTORS:

OMS Baku, 45 Islam Safarli Street, Baku. Tel: 12-973-150, 973-151. OMS Baku is a service provider for major oil companies and embassies in Azerbaijan.

The health service provides free medical treatment for all citizens. However, state-run services in Azerbaijan are limited and there is a lack of basic supplies and modern equipment. If a traveler becomes ill during an organized tour in Azerbaijan, emergency treatment is free, with small sums to be paid for medicines and hospital treatment. If a longer stay than originally planned becomes necessary because of illness, the visitor has to pay for all further treatment; therefore, travel insurance is recommended.

- International SOS: German Medical Center, 30 Rashid Behbutov Street, 370000 Baku, Azerbaijan; Clinic Tel: 994-12-4937-354; Clinic Fax: 994-12-4939-644

Current Advisories and Health Risks

AIDS/HIV: AIDS cases are increasing and an epidemic may be in the making. The reasons include (1) an increase in IV drug abuse; (2) increases in prostitution and sexual promiscuity; (3) an increase in sexually transmitted diseases; (4) decreased availability of sterile needles and syringes; and (5) no education or prevention programs.

ACCIDENTS AND MEDICAL INSURANCE

- Accidents and injuries are the leading cause of death among travelers younger than age of 55 and are most often caused by motor vehicle and motorcycle crashes; drownings, aircraft crashes, homicides, and burns are less common causes.
- Heart attacks cause most fatalities in older travelers.
- Infections cause only 1% of fatalities in overseas travelers, but, overall, infections are the most common cause of travel-related illness.
- Travelers are advised to obtain, before departure, supplemental travel health insurance with specific overseas coverage. The policy should provide for direct payment to the overseas hospital and/or physician at the time of service and should include a medical evacuation benefit. The policy should also provide 24-hour hotline access to a multilingual assistance center that can help arrange and monitor delivery of medical care and determine if medical evacuation or air ambulance services are required.

ARBOVIRAL FEVERS

- Karelian fever (mosquito-borne; most cases occur July through September in the Karelian region).

- Tahjna virus fever (mosquito-borne; occurs sporadically from the Baltic region north to the Kolsky Peninsula).
- Sand fly fever (sand fly-borne; limited to Moldova and the Crimea).
- Dengue fever (mosquito-borne; cases previously reported from extreme southern regions).
- West Nile virus (mosquito-borne; virus reportedly circulates in the Volga Delta region from May through September).
- Sindbis virus fever (detected in the Volga Delta; occurs July and August; incidence unclear).

NOTE: All travelers should take measures to prevent mosquito bites. Insect-bite prevention measures include a DEET-containing repellent applied to exposed skin, insecticide (permethrin) spray applied to clothing and gear, and use of a permethrin-treated bed net at night while sleeping.

CHOLERA: Sporadic cases of cholera may occur in this country. Cholera is an extremely rare disease in travelers from developed countries. Cholera vaccine is recommended primarily for people at high risk (e.g., relief workers) who work and live in highly endemic areas under less than adequate sanitary conditions.

- The oral cholera vaccine (Dukoral) provides up to 60% crossover protection against ETEC diarrhea, a common bacterial cause of travelers' diarrhea in this region.
- Many countries, including Canada, license an oral cholera vaccine. The oral vaccine is not available in the United States.
- Cholera vaccine is not "officially" required for entry into, or exit from, any country. Despite this, some countries, on occasion, require proof of cholera vaccination from travelers coming from cholera-infected countries. Anticipating such a situation, certain travelers may wish to carry a medical exemption letter from their health-care provider. Travel Medicine, Inc., recommends that travelers use the International Certificate of Vaccination (Yellow Card) for this purpose, having their health-care provider state that they are"exempt from cholera vaccine" and validate the exemption with both their signature and their official stamp (the "Uniform Stamp" in the United States).

CRIMEAN-CONGO HEMORRHAGIC FEVER: Reported mostly from southern areas, but outbreaks have occurred in some areas of Rostov Oblast (near the sea of Azov), April through November. Risk areas are rural steppe, savannah, semi-desert, and foothill/low mountain habitats below 2,000 meters elevation.

DIPHTHERIA: An epidemic of diphtheria that began in 1990 in the Russian Federation has spread extensively, involving all countries of the former Soviet Union. Seventy percent of cases have occurred in persons older than 15 years. All travelers to Russia and the New Independent States (NIS), especially adults, should be fully immunized against this disease. The CDC estimates that 20% to 60% of Americans older than 20 years lack sufficient immunity to diphtheria. Diphtheria vaccine in the United States is widely available and is administered in combination with the tetanus toxoid vaccine (Td vaccine).

348

HEPATITIS: All nonimmune travelers should receive hepatitis A vaccine. Hepatitis E accounts for up to 18% of acute hepatitis in the south. The hepatitis B carrier rate in the general population of Russia is estimated at 3.8%. Vaccination against hepatitis B should be considered for stays longer than 3 months and by short-term travelers desiring maximal protection. Travelers should be aware that hepatitis B can be transmitted by unsafe sex and the use of contaminated needles and syringes. Blood supplies may be contaminated with hepatitis B and C viruses.

INFLUENZA: Influenza is transmitted from November through March. The flu vaccine is recommended for all travelers older than age 50; all travelers with chronic disease or a weakened immune system; travelers of any age wishing to decrease the risk of this illness; and pregnant women after the first trimester.

LEISHMANIASIS: Risk for cutaneous leishmaniasis primarily limited to southern regions, including portions of the Georgia Republic and the southern Ukraine, below 1,300 meters elevation. Visceral leishmaniasis is confined to areas along the southeastern coast of the Black Sea, the southeastern and southwestern coasts of the Caspian Sea and the border areas of Georgia and Azerbaijan. Travelers to these regions should take measures to prevent sand fly bites.

LYME DISEASE: Lyme disease occurs focally in rural forested areas with the highest incidence in the Ural Mountains area. Risk presumably also occurs in the northwest and central areas. Travelers are advised to take measures to prevent tick bites during the peak transmission season, March through September.

MALARIA: Malaria risk, exclusively the vivax form, exists during the summer in southern lowland areas of Azerbaijan, as well as in the Khachmas region in the north. Sporadic cases have also been reported in the Baku suburbs.
- A weekly dose of 300 mg of chloroquine is the recommended prophylaxis for risk areas only.
- All travelers should take measures to prevent evening and nighttime mosquito bites. Insect-bite prevention measures include a DEET-containing repellent applied to exposed skin, insecticide (permethrin) spray applied to clothing and gear, and use of a permethrin-treated bed net at night while sleeping.

MEDITERRANEAN SPOTTED (BOUTONNEUSE) FEVER: Reported most commonly in the Black Sea coastal areas of the Caucasus, Transcaucasus, and the Crimea, and along the Caspian Sea coastline. Travelers should take measures to prevent tick bites.

TICK-BORNE ENCEPHALITIS (TBE): Tick-borne encephalitis is transmitted from the Baltics to the Crimea. Peak transmission period is April through October. Risk is present primarily in rural brushy and forested areas below 1,500 meters elevation. Highly enzootic foci occur throughout the Urals and much of the northern, forested mountainous areas, including suburban "forests" bordering large cities. Highest number of indigenous cases are reported from the south-central areas, including Altay, Kemerovo, Novosibirsk Oblasts, and Krasnoyarsk Kray. Coinfection with Lyme disease is increasing.

Travelers to risk areas are advised to take measures to prevent tick bites, especially during the peak transmission season, March through September. The TBE vaccine (available in Canada and Europe), is recommended only for people at significant risk of exposure to tick bites, e.g., campers and hikers on extended trips, or forestry workers.

TRAVELERS' DIARRHEA: High risk outside of first-class hotels. All water supplies are suspect, including municipal tap water, which may be untreated and grossly contaminated. Travelers should consume only bottled water or boiled or chemically treated water. Travelers should observe strict food and drink safety precautions. A quinolone antibiotic, combined with loperamide (Imodium), is recommended for the treatment of acute diarrhea. Diarrhea not responding to treatment with an antibiotic may be due to a parasitic disease, especially giardiasis.

TYPHOID FEVER: Typhoid fever is recommended for long-term travelers, adventure travelers, and those wishing maximal disease protection. Because the typhoid vaccines are only 60% to 70% effective, safe food and drink guidelines should continue to be observed.

OTHER DISEASES/HAZARDS: Anthrax (sporadic human cases occur, related to exposure to livestock in rural areas, especially southern areas), brucellosis (from unpasteurized dairy products), echinococcosis (in southern and northeastern areas). Echinococcus multilocularis is associated with the reindeer culture in north; legionellosis, leptospirosis (a particular problem in fish-breeding areas of the Rostov Province; extensive outbreaks have occurred in east central areas); North Asian tick typhus (also called Siberian tick typhus; occurs in the steppe areas bordering Kazakhstan, Georgia, and Azerbaijan; risk elevated in May and June), opisthorchiasis (acquired from consumption of raw freshwater fish; reported from western European Russia), plague (flea-borne; usually occurs as isolated cases or small outbreaks in semi-arid areas of the southern republics of Azerbaijan, Armenia, and Georgia), rabies, rickettsialpox, tick-borne relapsing fever (may occur south of 55 degrees north latitude), trichinosis (greatest risk in western Belarus and the Ukraine), tularemia ("rabbit fever"; risk may be elevated in the north), tuberculosis (40% rise in cases since 1995; incidence in Moscow has doubled since 1991), and helminthic infections (roundworm, hookworm, and whipworm infections and strongyloidiasis) reported especially from the Transcaucasus, especially Azerbaijan.

Bahamas

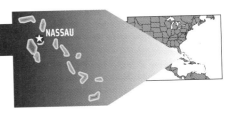

CAPITAL:
Nassau
EMBASSY (IN U.S.):
202-944-3390
GMT:
−5 hours

TELEPHONE COUNTRY CODE:
1-242
USADIRECT:
1-800-872-2881
ENTRY REQUIREMENTS
• **Passport/Visa**: Visa not required.
• **HIV Test**: Not required.
• **Vaccinations**: A yellow fever vaccination certificate is required from travelers older than 1 year of age coming from infected or endemic areas.
EMBASSIES/CONSULATES
• **U.S. Embassy**: Queen Street, downtown Nassau; Tel: 322-1181, after hours Tel: 328-2206.
• **Canadian Embassy**: Shirley Street, Shopping Plaza, Nassau; Tel: 393-2123 and 2124; Fax: 393-1305; e-mail: cdncon@bahamas.net.bs.
• **British High Commission**: Accredited to British High Commission in Jamaica. PO Box 575, 28 Trafalgar Road, Kingston 10, Jamaica; Tel: 1-876-510-0700; Fax: 1-876-511-5355; e-mail: bhckingston@cwjamaica.com.
HOSPITALS/DOCTORS:
• Princess Margaret Hospital, Nassau, New Providence: teaching hospital with most specialties, including ob/gyn; walk-in clinic; emergency medical services with four critical/trauma beds in ER.
• Rand Memorial Hospital, Freeport, Grand Bahama: basic care and most medical/surgical specialties; emergency medical services with a nine-bed ER.

Current Health Risks and Advisories

AIDS/HIV: The incidence of HIV/AIDS in the Bahamas is among the highest in the Caribbean. Transmission of HIV is most often heterosexual or from injecting drug use.

DENGUE FEVER: Low risk, but dengue fever is endemic throughout the Caribbean. All travelers should take measures to prevent daytime mosquito bites.

HEPATITIS: Nonimmune travelers should consider hepatitis A vaccination. Hepatitis B is spread by infected blood, contaminated needles, and unprotected sex. Vaccination is recommended for long-stay (more than 3 months) travelers; those who may be at occupational or social risk; anybody desiring maximal protection.

INFLUENZA: Influenza is transmitted throughout the year in the tropics. Vaccination is recommended.

MARINE HAZARDS
• Swimming related hazards include jellyfish, spiny sea urchins, and sharp coral.
• Ciguatera poisoning occurs and can result from eating coral reef fish such as grouper, snapper, sea bass, jack, and barracuda. The ciguatoxin is not destroyed by cooking.

- Scuba Diving—Hyperbaric Chamber Referral: Divers' Alert Network (DAN) maintains an up-to-date list of all functioning hyperbaric chambers in North America and the Caribbean. In a diving emergency, or for the location of the nearest decompression chamber, travelers should call 919-684-8111.

TRAVELERS' DIARRHEA: Low to moderate risk. A quinolone antibiotic, combined with loperamide (Imodium) is recommended for the treatment of acute diarrhea. Persistent diarrhea may be due to a parasitic infection such as giardiasis, amebiasis, or cryptosporidiosis.

OTHER DISEASES/HAZARDS: The hurricane season in the Caribbean occurs between June and November.

Bahrain

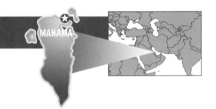

CAPITAL:
Manama

EMBASSY (IN U.S.):
202-342-0741

GMT:
+3 hours

TELEPHONE COUNTRY CODE:
973

USADIRECT:
800-001 or 800-000

ENTRY REQUIREMENTS

- **Passport/Visa:** Passport and visa required. Multi-entry tourist visa requires that the applicant submit a letter (for visa) or company letter (for business visa) on company letterhead guaranteeing full responsibility for all expenses, and stating a reason for visit and duration
- **HIV Test**: For all foreigners who are seeking work permits
- **Vaccinations**: A yellow fever vaccination certificate is required of travelers arriving from infected areas.

EMBASSIES/CONSULATES

- **U.S. Embassy:** Bldg. 979, Road # 3119, Zinj District (next to Al Ahli Sports Club), Manama; Tel: 273-300; Fax: 973-256-242; Website: www.usembassy.com.bh.
- **Canadian Embassy**: Accredited to Canadian Embassy in Saudi Arabia. Diplomatic Quarter, Riyadh, Saudi Arabia; Tel: 966-1-488-2288; Fax: 966-1-488-1997.
- **British Embassy:** 21 Government Avenue, Manama 306, PO Box 114, Kingdom of Bahrain, Tel: 973-17-574100, 973-17-574167 (Information), 973-17-9600274 (Emergency), Fax: 973-17-574161 (Chancery/Information), 973-17-574101 (Commercial), 973-17-574138 (Consular/Management), 973-17-574121 (Visa Section), e-mail: britemb@batelco.com.bh, Website: www.ukembassy.gov.bh.

HOSPITALS/DOCTORS:

Comprehensive medical services are available, with general and specialized hospitals in the main towns. An emergency health service is provided free of charge or at a nominal fee. Pharmacies are well equipped with supplies.

- American Mission Hospital, Manama, Bahrain; AMH has provided modern medical services to the residents of Bahrain and the Arabian Gulf for more than 100 years; Tel: 253447.
- International Hospital, Bahrain (300 beds); new civilian facility; most specialty services; emergency and surgical capabilities
- Salmaniya Medical Complex, Manama (620 beds); government teaching facility; all specialty services except neurosurgery
- International SOS: International SOS, Middle East Representative Office, 11th Floor, Building 722, Road 1708, Block 317, Diplomatic Area Manama, Bahrain; Tel: 973-17-532392; Fax: 973-17-530969

Current Advisories and Health Risks

HEPATITIS: Hepatitis A vaccine is recommended. Hepatitis E has not been reported. The hepatitis B carrier rate in the general population is 2%. Vaccination against hepatitis B should be considered for stays longer than 3 months and by short-term travelers desiring maximal protection.

INFLUENZA: Influenza is transmitted from November through March; flu vaccine is recommended for all travelers.

LEISHMANIASIS: Cutaneous leishmaniasis is reported, but levels are unclear. Travelers should take precautions against insect (sand fly) bites.

MALARIA: There is no risk of indigenous malaria in this country.

TRAVELERS' DIARRHEA: Tap water is potable. A quinolone antibiotic, combined with loperamide (Imodium), is recommended for the treatment of acute diarrhea.

Bangladesh

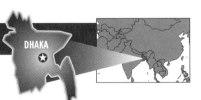

CAPITAL:
Dhaka
EMBASSY (IN U.S.):
202-342-8373
GMT:
+6 hours
TELEPHONE COUNTRY CODE:
880

ENTRY REQUIREMENTS

- **Passport/Visa**: A visa is not required for a tourist visit up to 15 days.
- **HIV Test**: Not required.
- **Vaccinations**: A yellow fever certificate is required of all persons (including infants) arriving by air or sea within 6 days of departure from an infected area, or a country with infection in any part, or a country where the WHO judges yellow fever to be endemic or present; required also for travelers arriving from or transiting to the following countries:

    Africa: Angola, Benin, Burkina Faso, Burundi, Cameroon, Central African Republic, Chad, Congo, Côte d'Ivoire, Democratic Republic of Congo, Equatorial Guinea, Ethiopia, Gabon, The Gambia, Ghana, Guinea, Guinea Bissau, Kenya, Liberia, Malawi, Mali, Mauritania, Niger, Nigeria, Rwanda, São Tomé and Principe, Senegal, Sierra Leone, Somalia, Sudan (south of 15 degrees N), Tanzania, Togo, Uganda, and Zambia.

    The Americas: Belize, Bolivia, Brazil, Colombia, Costa Rica, Ecuador, French Guiana, Guatemala, Guyana, Honduras, Nicaragua, Panama, Peru, Suriname, and Venezuela.

    Caribbean: Trinidad and Tobago.

    Any person (including infants) arriving by air or sea without a certificate within 6 days of departure from or transit through an infected area will be isolated up to 6 days.

EMBASSIES/CONSULATES

- **U.S. Embassy**: Diplomatic Enclave, Madani Avenue, Baridhara, Dhaka; Tel: 2-882-4700 through 4722; Website: www.usembassy-dhaka.org/state/embassy.htm.
- **Canadian Embassy**: House CWN 16/A, Road 48, Gulshan, Dhaka; Tel: 2-988-7091 through 988-7097; e-mail: dhaka@dfait-maeci.gc.ca; Website: www.dfait-maeci.gc.ca/dhaka.
- **British High Commission**: United Nations Road, Baridhara, Dhaka 1212; address: PO Box 6079, Dhaka 1212, Tel: 880-2-882-2705, Fax: 880-2-882-3437, 880-2-882-3666 (Immigration Section), 880-2-882-3437 (Consular), 880-2-881-6135, e-mail: ppabhc@citecho.net, Website: www.ukinbangladesh.org

HOSPITALS/DOCTORS:

Holy Family Hospital, Dhaka (286 beds); minimally equipped facility; should be used only for emergency stabilization.

Current Health Risks and Advisories

ANIMAL HAZARDS: Animal hazards include snakes (kraits, cobras, vipers), centipedes, scorpions, black widow spiders, brown recluse spiders, and large leeches (not poisonous, but can cause slow-healing ulcers). Other possible hazards include crocodiles, pythons, poisonous frogs and toads, lizards, tigers, leopards, and bears (sloth, Himalayan black, and Malayan sun).

CHOLERA: This disease is reported active in this country. Cholera, however, is an extremely rare disease in travelers from developed countries. Cholera vaccine is recommended primarily for people at high risk (e.g., relief workers) who work and live in highly endemic areas under less than adequate sanitary conditions.

Many countries, including Canada, license an oral cholera vaccine. The oral vaccine is not available in the United States.

DENGUE FEVER: Year-round risk, countrywide. Increased incidence of dengue occurs during the monsoon season, June through September. All travelers should take measures to prevent mosquito bites.

FILARIASIS: Bancroftian filariasis is reported, with 10% of the population infected. The prevalence is highest in the northern and central districts. Travelers should take measures to prevent mosquito bites.

FOOD AND WATER SAFETY: All water should be regarded as being potentially contaminated. Travelers should eat only well-cooked food, preferably served hot. Salad may carry increased risk. Vegetables should be cooked and fruit should be peeled before consumption.

HEPATITIS: All nonimmune travelers should receive hepatitis A vaccine. Hepatitis E, transmitted by contaminated drinking water, is endemic, with intermittent outbreaks. The hepatitis B carrier rate in the general population is estimated at 10%. Hepatitis B is spread by infected blood, contaminated needles, and unprotected sex. Vaccination is recommended for long-stay (more than 3 months) travelers; those who may be at occupational or social risk; anybody desiring maximal protection.

INFLUENZA: Influenza is transmitted year-round in the tropics. Vaccination is recommended for all travelers.

JAPANESE ENCEPHALITIS (JE): The risk of infection is greatest from June through October, countrywide, in rural agricultural areas. Sporadic cases of JE occur year-round. Vaccination against Japanese encephalitis is recommended for travelers who will be staying in rural-agricultural endemic areas more than several weeks. In addition, all travelers should take measures to prevent mosquito bites, especially in the evening. JE vaccine is not routinely recommended for travel exclusively to urban areas or if planning only short visits to the usual rural tourist sites.

LEISHMANIASIS: Visceral leishmaniasis (kala azar) is transmitted year-round, countrywide, including urban areas, with an increased incidence in the central delta districts of Mymensingh and Pabna. Travelers should take measures to prevent insect (sand fly) bites, especially in rural areas.

MALARIA: Risk is present year-round throughout this country. There is risk of malaria in all urban areas except Dhaka. Elevated risk occurs in the forested areas and foothills of the southeast and east bordering India and Burma. Falciparum malaria accounts for 50% to 75% of malaria cases in this country, vivax malaria, the remainder. Chloroquine-resistant falciparum malaria is confirmed in the eastern and northeastern regions. Prophylaxis with atovaquone/proguanil (Malarone), mefloquine (Lariam), or doxycycline is recommended. All travelers should take measures to prevent evening and nighttime mosquito bites.

RABIES: More than 2,000 human rabies deaths occur annually. All animal bites or scratches, especially from a dog, should be taken seriously, and immediate medical attention sought. Rabies vaccination may be required. Although rabies is rare among tourists, there is risk. No one should pet or pick up any stray animals. All children should be warned to avoid contact with unknown animals. Rabies vaccine is recommended for travel longer than 3 months, and for shorter stays for travelers who plan to venture off the usual tourist routes, where they may be more exposed to the stray dog population.

- -

TRAVELERS' DIARRHEA: High risk. Water supplies in Bangladesh are obtained from ditches, ponds, and streams in rural areas and from canals and ponds in urban areas of the country. Generally, water sources are contaminated with human and animal waste. In addition, the mineral content of the water (especially well water) is high. Travelers should observe strict food and drink guidelines. A quinolone antibiotic, combined with loperamide (Imodium), is recommended for the treatment of acute persistent diarrhea. Diarrhea may be due to a parasitic disease such as giardiasis, amebiasis, or cryptosporidiosis.

- -

TUBERCULOSIS: Tuberculosis (TB) a major health problem in this country. Travelers planning an extended stay should have a pre-departure TB skin test (PPD test) and be retested after leaving this country or returning home.

- -

TYPHOID FEVER: Typhoid vaccine is recommended for those traveling off the usual tourist routes, those visiting friends or relatives, and for long-stay visitors. Typhoid vaccines are 60% to 70% effective; safe food and drink precautions should continue to be observed.

- -

OTHER DISEASES/HAZARDS: Echinococcosis, influenza (transmitted year-round; vaccination recommended), sand fly fever (endemic countrywide at low levels), scrub typhus, tuberculosis (a major health problem), typhoid fever, and intestinal worms (whipworms, roundworms, hookworms) are reported.

Barbados

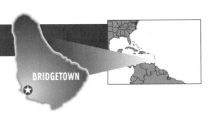

CAPITAL:
Bridgetown
EMBASSY (IN U.S.):
202-939-9200
GMT:
−4 hours
TELEPHONE COUNTRY CODE:
246
USADIRECT:
1-800-872-2881

ENTRY REQUIREMENTS

- **Passport/Visa**: U.S. citizens must enter Barbados using a valid U.S. passport. No visa is needed to enter Barbados for stays up to 28 days. For further information, travelers may contact the Embassy of Barbados, 2144 Wyoming Avenue, N.W., Washington, DC 20008, Tel: 202-939-9200, fax 202-332-7467, e-mail: barbados@oas.org or the consulates of Barbados in Los Angeles, Miami, or New York.
- **HIV Test**: Not required.
- **Vaccinations**: A yellow fever vaccination certificate is required from travelers older than 1 year of age coming from infected or endemic areas.

EMBASSIES/CONSULATES

- **U.S. Embassy**: Canadian Imperial Bank of Commerce Building, Broad Street. Tel: 246-436-4950.
- **U.S. Consulate**: American Life Insurance Company (ALICO) Building, Cheapside. Tel: 431-0225; Fax: 246-431-0179.
- **Canadian Embassy**: Bridgetown. Tel: 429-3550; Fax: 429-3780; e-mail: bdgtn@dfait-maeci.gc.ca; Website: www.dfait-maeci.gc.ca/bridgetown.
- **British High Commission:** Lower Collymore Rock (PO Box 676), Bridgetown; Tel: 1-246-430-7800; Fax: 1-246-430-7851.

HOSPITALS/DOCTORS:

Excellent medical facilities are available in Barbados, with both private and general wards. Barbados has a reciprocal health agreement with the United Kingdom. Medical insurance is recommended for all other nationals.

- Diagnostic Clinic & Hospital, St. Michael.
- Queen Elizabeth's Hospital, Bridgetown.
- Westgate Clinic, Bridgetown.

Current Advisories and Health Risks

See Disease Risk Summaries for the Caribbean and Mexico and Central America on pages 293 and 295.

Belarus

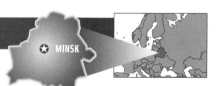

★ MINSK

CAPITAL:
Minsk
EMBASSY (IN U.S.):
202-986-1606
GMT:
+2/3 hours
TELEPHONE COUNTRY CODE:
375
USADIRECT:
8-800-101

ENTRY REQUIREMENTS

- **Passport/Visa**: Passport and visa required. Business visa requires 1 application form, 1 photo, and letter of invitation from a Belarusian organization, company or agency. Visitor visa (for stay of up to 30 days) requires one application form, one photo, and confirmation from receiving tourist organization in Belarus. Transit visa is required when traveling through Belarus. For information about student visas and other questions, contact the Embassy of the Republic of Belarus, 1619 New Hampshire Ave., NW, Washington, DC 20009; Tel: 202-986-1606.

 Visa applicants may need to meet specific requirements. Travelers should review the application and contact the Embassy of Belarus. According to the U.S. Department of State, HIV testing is required for all persons staying longer than 3 months. U.S. tests are acceptable.

EMBASSIES/CONSULATES

- **U.S. Embassy:** 46 Starovilenskaya Ulitsa. Tel: 375-172-10-12-83 or 234-77-61; Fax: 375-172-76-88-62.
- **Canadian Embassy**: Canada does not have an embassy in Belarus.
- **British Embassy:** 37 Karl Marx Street, 220030 Minsk; Tel: 375-172-105920; Fax: 375-172-292306; e-mail: britinfo@nsys.by; Website: www.britishembassy.gov.uk/belarus.

HOSPITALS/DOCTORS:

Medical care is substandard throughout the country including in Minsk. Adequate health insurance and medical evacuation coverage for all travelers are high priorities. In the event of serious medical conditions every effort should be made to go to Western Europe.

Current Advisories and Health Risks

See Disease Risk Summaries for Europe and Russia on page 300.

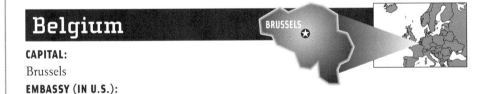

Belgium

CAPITAL:
Brussels
EMBASSY (IN U.S.):
202-333-6900
GMT:
+1 hour
TELEPHONE COUNTRY CODE:
32
USADIRECT:
0-800-100-10
ENTRY REQUIREMENTS
- **Passport/Visa**: A valid passport is required.
- **HIV Test**: Not required.
- **Vaccinations**: None required.

EMBASSIES/CONSULATES

- **U.S. Embassy:** 27 Boulevard du Regent, Brussels; Tel: 02-508-2111; Fax: 2-511-2725; Website: www.usinfo.be.
- **U.S. Consulate:** 25 Boulevard du Regent, Brussels. Fax: 02-513-0409.
- **Canadian Embassy:** 2, Avenue de Tervuren, Brussels; Tel: 2-741-0611; Fax: 2-741-0619; e-mail: bru@dfait-maeci.gc.ca; Website: www.dfait-maeci.gc.ca/brussels.
- **British Embassy:** Rue D'Arlon/Aarlenstraat 85, B-1040 Brussels; Tel: 32-2-287-6211; Website: www.britishembassy.gov.uk/belgium.

HOSPITALS/DOCTORS:

Medical care in Western Europe is of high quality and many physicians speak English. Travelers are advised to obtain supplemental travel health insurance with specific overseas coverage. The policy should provide for direct payment to the overseas hospital and/or physician at the time of service and include a medical evacuation benefit.

Hospital Universitaire St. Pierre, Brussels (567 beds); all specialties; emergency department; burn unit; considered one of Belgium's best hospitals.

Regionaal Ziekenhuis Lier (550-beds); Kolveniersevest, Belgium. Tel: 3-491-2345. All specialties, including neurosurgery; Emergency Department is open 7/24.

Alfons Van Gompel, MD, DTMH; Associate Professor of Tropical Medicine, Chief of the Polyclinic and Travel Clinic, Institute of Tropical Medicine, Kronenburgstraat 42/3, Antwerp, Belgium. Tel: 3-2476405; Fax: 3-2161431.

Current Advisories and Health Risks

All travelers should be up-to-date on their routine immunizations: tetanus-diphtheria (Td), measles-mumps-rubella (MMR), polio, influenza, and varicella (chickenpox). Immunization against hepatitis A and hepatitis B is recommended.

See Disease Risk Summary for Europe on page 300.

Belize

CAPITAL:
Belmopan

EMBASSY (IN U.S.):
202-332-9636

GMT:
−6 hours

TELEPHONE COUNTRY CODE:
501

USADIRECT:
811 (phones and pay phones); 555 (hotels)

ENTRY REQUIREMENTS

- **Passport/Visa:** No visa required for stays less than 30 days. Passports must be valid for at least 6 months.

- **HIV Test**: Testing required of travelers seeking permits for employment or immigration, or staying longer than 3 months.
- **Vaccinations**: A yellow fever vaccination certificate is required of all travelers arriving from infected areas.

EMBASSIES/CONSULATES
- **U.S. Embassy**: Gabourel Lane and Hutson Street, Belize City. Tel: 501-2-77161/62/63.
- **Canadian Embassy**: 85 North Front Street, Belize City. Tel: 501-231-060; Fax: 501-230-060; e-mail: cdncon.bze@btl.net.
- **British High Commission**: PO Box 91, Belmopan, Tel: 501-822-2146, Fax: 501-822-2761, e-mail: brithicom@btl.net, Website: www.britishhighbze.com

HOSPITALS/DOCTORS:
There are seven government hospitals—one in Belmopan, the capital, one in Belize City and one in each of the other five main district towns. Medical services in rural areas are provided by rural health-care centers, and mobile clinics operate in remote areas. International travelers are strongly advised to take out medical insurance before departing for Belize.
- Belize City Hospital; general medical/surgical faciity
- William J. Willitts, MD, DTM&H; Belize Diagnostic Center, 218 Leslie Street, Belize City; American, board-certified in internal medicine, gastroenterology, and travel medicine
- Scuba diving emergencies: A decompression chamber is located in San Pedro.

Current Health Risks and Advisories

CHOLERA: This disease is not reported active by the CDC, but occasional cases occur.

DENGUE FEVER: Year-round risk, countrywide, especially in urban areas. All travelers are advised to take measures to prevent mosquito bites.

HEPATITIS: Hepatitis A vaccine is recommended for all nonimmune travelers. Hepatitis E has been reported, but levels are unclear. Hepatitis B is spread by infected blood, contaminated needles, and unprotected sex. Vaccination is recommended for long-stay (more than 3 months) travelers; those who may be at occupational or social risk; anybody desiring maximal protection.

INFLUENZA: Influenza is transmitted year-round in the tropics. Vaccination is recommended.

LEISHMANIASIS: Year-round risk, especially in rural forested areas. Prevalence is highest in the central part of the country, lowest in the south. Increased transmission occurs May through December. Cases of cutaneous leishmaniasis have been reported among tourists and field-study participants. All travelers are advised to take measures to prevent insect (sand fly) bites.

MALARIA: Belize has the highest incidence of malaria in the Americas. Risk is present year-round in all rural areas of the country under 400 meters elevation, but especially during and after the rainy season. Overall, incidence is highest in the southern districts, but most falciparum cases are reported from the north. There is no risk of malaria in Belize City. *Plasmodium vivax* causes 96% of cases, *Plasmodium falciparum* 4%, but *P. falciparum* has been reported as high as 16% in some areas. Occasional cases are due to *Plasmodium malariae*. Chloroquine-resistant falciparum malaria has not been reported. Chloroquine prophylaxis is currently recommended for overnight visits to rural areas, rain forests, or the offshore islands. All travelers should take measures to prevent evening and nighttime mosquito bites.

MARINE HAZARDS: Swimming-related hazards include jellyfish, spiny sea urchins, and coral. Ciguatera poisoning is prevalent and can result from eating coral reef fish such as grouper, snapper, sea bass, jack, and barracuda. The ciguatoxin is not destroyed by cooking.

SCUBA DIVING-HYPERBARIC CHAMBER REFERRAL: A decompression chamber is located in San Pedro. Divers' Alert Network (DAN) maintains an up-to-date list of all hyperbaric chambers in North America and the Caribbean. In association with Duke University Medical Center in North Carolina, DAN operates a 24-hour emergency phone number (919-684-8111) for members and nonmembers to call and their staff is available to answer questions and, if necessary, make referral to the closest functioning hyperbaric chamber.

RABIES: Low risk. One or two cases of human rabies are reported each year. Dogs are main vectors, but vampire bats may also transmit disease. Travelers should avoid contact with dogs and seek immediate treatment of any unprovoked animal bite.

TRAVELERS' DIARRHEA: Moderate risk except for tourist resorts, where the risk is low. Raw sewage emptied into the ocean is a cause of beach contamination. Travelers should follow safe food and drink precautions. A quinolone antibiotic, combined with loperamide (Imodium), is recommended for the treatment of acute diarrhea.

TYPHOID FEVER: Typhoid vaccine is recommended for those traveling off the usual tourist routes, those visiting friends or relatives, and for long-stay visitors. Typhoid vaccines are 60% to 70% effective; safe food and drink precautions should continue to be observed.

OTHER DISEASES/HAZARDS: Amebiasis and giardiasis (low incidence), brucellosis, Chagas disease (endemic at low levels in Cayo district), cutaneous larva migrans (travelers should avoid walking barefoot on beaches or any place where cat and dog feces may contaminate the ground), cutaneous myiasis (caused by larvae of the human bot fly), cysticercosis, histoplasmosis (outbreaks associated with guano in bat caves), leptospirosis, tuberculosis (low incidence), typhoid fever (few officially reported cases), and intestinal helminthic infections (worms).

Benin

CAPITAL:
Porto-Novo

EMBASSY (IN U.S.):
202-232-6656

GMT:
+1 hour

TELEPHONE COUNTRY CODE:
229

USADIRECT:
102

ENTRY REQUIREMENTS
- **Passport/Visa**: Passport and visa required.
- **HIV Test:** Not required.
- **Vaccinations**: Yellow fever vaccine is required for all travelers older than 1 year of age arriving from all countries.

EMBASSIES/CONSULATES
- **U.S. Embassy:** Cotonou. Tel: 229-30-06-50, 30-05-13, or 30-17-92; Fax: 229-30-14-39, 30-19-74.
- **Canadian Embassy:** Accredited to Canadian Embassy in Côte d'Ivoire. Immeuble Trade Center, 23, avenue Noguès, Le Plateau, Abidjan, Côte d'Ivoire; Tel: 225-20-30-07-00; Fax: 225-20-30-07-20; e-mail: abdjn@international.gc.ca; Website: www.dfait-maeci.gc.ca/abidjan.
- **British High Commission:** Accredited to British Embassy in Nigeria. Shehu Shangari Way (North), Maitama, Abuja; Tel: 234-9-413-2010, 2011, 2796, 2880, 2883, 2887, 9817; Fax: 234-9-413-3552.

HOSPITALS/DOCTORS:
Medical facilities are limited, especially outside the major towns, and not all medicines are available. Doctors and hospitals often expect immediate cash payment for health services. Medical insurance is strongly recommended.
- General Hospital, Porto-Novo; general medical/surgical facility; ENT, pediatrics.
- General Hospital, Cotonou (350 beds); general medical/surgical facility; teaching hospital.

Current Advisories and Health Risks

IMMUNIZATIONS: All travelers should be up to date on their routine immunizations: tetanus-diphtheria (Td), measles-mumps-rubella (MMR), polio, influenza, and varicella (chickenpox). Immunizations against hepatitis A, hepatitis B, meningitis, rabies, and typhoid fever are recommended.

MALARIA: All travelers to Benin including infants, children, and former residents of this country should take one of the following antimalarial drugs: atovaquone/proguanil, doxycycline, mefloquine, or (in special circumstances) primaquine. Travelers should also take measures to prevent evening and nighttime mosquito bites. Insect-bite prevention measures include a DEET-containing repellent applied to exposed skin, insecticide (permethrin) spray applied to clothing, and use of a permethrin-treated bed net at night.

For additional information, consult the Disease Risk Summary for sub-Saharan Africa on page 307.

Bhutan

★ THIMPHU

CAPITAL:
Thimphu
EMBASSY (IN U.S.):
U.N. Mission: Tel: 212-826-1919
GMT:
+5 hours
TELEPHONE COUNTRY CODE
975
USADIRECT:
None
ENTRY REQUIREMENTS
- **Passport/Visa**: A visa is required. Contact the Bhutan Travel Service in New York City at 212-838-6382.
- **HIV Test**: Not required.
- **Vaccinations**: A yellow fever vaccination certificate is required from all travelers arriving from infected areas.

EMBASSIES/CONSULATES:
No formal diplomatic relations exist between the United States, Canada, United Kingdom, and Bhutan. The U.S. Embassy in New Delhi (Tel: 91-11-688-9033) handles informal diplomatic contact.

HOSPITALS/DOCTORS:
Medical care is substandard throughout the country including in Thimphu. Adequate medical evacuation coverage for all travelers is a high priority. In the event of serious medical conditions every effort should be made to go to Bangkok or Singapore.

Current Advisories and Health Risks

CHOLERA: This disease is active in this country. Cholera, however, is an extremely rare disease in travelers from developed countries. Cholera vaccine is recommended primarily for people at high risk (e.g., relief workers) who work and live in highly endemic areas under less than adequate sanitary conditions.

DENGUE FEVER: Likely endemic in southern plains region, year-round, with risk elevated during the rainy season, May through mid-October. Travelers should take precautions against daytime insect bites.

HEPATITIS: All nonimmune travelers should receive the hepatitis A vaccine. Hepatitis E is the predominant cause of acute adult hepatitis in Bhutan, and is transmitted by sewage-contaminated food and water. Sporadic outbreaks, as well as large epidemics, are reported. There is no hepatitis E vaccine. Travelers should follow safe food and drink guidelines. The hepatitis B carrier rate in the general population is estimated at 6%. Hepatitis B is transmitted by blood, unsafe sex, and contaminated needles and syringes. Vaccination against hepatitis B should be considered for stays exceeding 3 months; by anyone at occupational or social risk; by any traveler desiring maximal protection.

INFLUENZA: Flu is transmitted from November to March. Vaccination is recommended for travel at this time.

JAPANESE ENCEPHALITIS (JE): There is low-level risk of JE in the rural southern (terai) foothill districts, with transmission increased from May through mid-October. JE vaccine is recommended for stays of more than 3 to 4 weeks in rural agricultural (rice-growing, pig-farming) areas, or for repeated shorter visits to endemic areas of country, especially during the peak transmission season. Travelers should also take measures to prevent evening/nighttime mosquito bites.

LEISHMANIASIS: Visceral leishmaniasis is reported countrywide, with higher risk in the Bramaputra and Ganges River valleys. Travelers should take precautions against sand fly bites.

MALARIA: Endemic at moderate-to-high levels. Risk is present year-round in the south and southeastern districts bordering India, including urban areas. Risk generally limited to the Duars Plain and the mountain valleys of the Lesser Himalayas up to 1,700 meters elevation in the Chirang, Gaylegphug, Samchi, Samdrup Jongkhar, and Shemgang Districts. Risk may be elevated during the rainy season, May through mid-October. Thimbu is risk free. *P. falciparum* causes 45% of cases countrywide, *Plasmodium vivax* the remainder. Prophylaxis with atovaquone/proguanil (Malarone), mefloquine (Lariam), or doxycycline is recommended in risk areas. All travelers should take measures to prevent evening and nighttime mosquito bites.

RABIES: Highly prevalent. Dogs are the primary source of human infection. Medical attention should be sought for all animal bites or scratches. Although rabies is rare among tourists, there is risk. No one should pet or pick up any stray animals. Rabies pre-exposure vaccination is recommended for stays longer than 1 month and for short-term travelers who will be going to remote areas where medical care is not available within 24 hours.

SAND FLY FEVER: Endemic countrywide at low levels. Travelers should takes measures to prevent insect (sand fly) bites.

TRAVELERS' DIARRHEA: Water supplies in Bhutan are frequently contaminated as a result of substandard sanitary conditions. Prevention of diarrhea consists primarily in following strict adherence to safe food and drink guidelines. A quinolone antibiotic, combined with loperamide, is recommended for treating acute diarrhea. Persistent diarrhea may be due to a parasitic disease such as giardiasis or amebiasis.

TUBERCULOSIS: Tuberculosis a major health problem in this country. Travelers planning an extended stay should have a pre-departure TB skin test (PPD test) and be retested after leaving this country.Update changes

----

TYPHOID FEVER: Typhoid vaccine is recommended for travel outside of tourist areas. The typhoid vacccines are 60% to 70% effective. Food and drink precautions should continue to be observed.

OTHER DISEASES/HAZARDS: Brucellosis (reported in low numbers), leprosy (highly prevalent; an estimated five to ten cases/1,000 population), scabies, murine, and scrub typhus, typhoid fever, and intestinal worms (whipworms, roundworms, hookworms) are reported.

Bolivia

★ LA PAZ

CAPITAL:
La Paz
EMBASSY:
202-483-4410
GMT:
−4 hours
TELEPHONE COUNTRY CODE:
591
USADIRECT:
800-101-110
ENTRY REQUIREMENTS
- **Passport/Visa:** U.S. citizens do not need a visa for a 1-month stay. Tourist card issued on arrival. Passport required.
- **HIV Test:** Not required.
- **Vaccinations:** Yellow fever vaccine certificate required if traveling from an infected area. Bolivia recommends vaccination for travelers who are destined for risk areas, such as the departments of Beni, Cochabamba, Santa Cruz, and the subtropical part of La Paz Department.

EMBASSIES/CONSULATES
- **U.S. Embassy:** 2780 Avenida Arce, La Paz. Tel: 591-2-433-812 during business hours or 591-2-430-251 after-hours; Fax: 591-2-433-854, Website: www.megalink. com/usemblapaz.
- **Canadian Embassy:** Calle Victor Sangines 2678, Edificio Barcelona, Plaza España, La Paz. Tel: 591-2-415-021, 414-517, or 415-141; Fax: 591-2-414-453; e-mail: lapaz@ dfait-maeci.gc.ca.

- **British Embassy:** Avenida Arce No. 2732, Casilla (PO Box) 694, La Paz, Tel: 591-2-2433424; Fax: 591-2-2431073; e-mail: ppa@megalink.com (Embassy), dfid@zuper.net (DFID), Website: www.britishembassy.gov.uk/bolivia

HOSPITALS/DOCTORS

- Clinica Del Sur, 3539 Avenida Hernando Siles, La Paz. Highly rated 45-bed facility.
- Methodist Hospital, La Paz (113 beds); private hospital; limited emergency services.
- Trauma Klinik, San Miguel Calle Claudio Aliaga, La Paz. 17-bed facility provides above-average emergency care.
- In Cochabamba: Centro Medico Quirurgico Boliviano Belga; 60-bed hospital; emergency services are available 24 hours a day.
- In Santa Cruz: Clinica Angel Foianini, Avenida Irala; well-equipped 44-bed hospital often used by travelers and expatriates.

Current Advisories and Health Risks

ALTITUDE SICKNESS (AMS): Risk is present for those arriving in La Paz (altitude 3,500 meters) and/or traveling to the Altiplano zone in southwestern Bolivia where the altitude lies between 3,350 and 4,265 meters elevation. Travelers should consider taking acetazolamide (Diamox) prophylaxis before traveling to high altitudes. Descent to lower altitude is the best treatment for AMS.

CHAGAS DISEASE: Widely distributed in rural areas at elevations up to 3,600 meters, including portions of the Altiplano. In south central Cochabamba, up to 100% of villagers test positive for exposure. Risk occurs especially in those rural-agricultural areas where there are the adobe-style huts and houses that can harbor the night-biting triatomid (assassin) bugs. Travelers sleeping in such structures should take precautions against nighttime bites.

CHOLERA: Sporadic cases of cholera are reported. Cholera, however, is an extremely rare disease in travelers from developed countries. Cholera vaccine is recommended primarily for people at high risk (e.g., relief workers) who work and live in highly endemic areas under less than adequate sanitary conditions. Many countries, including Canada, license an oral cholera vaccine. The oral cholera vaccine is not available in the United States.

DENGUE FEVER: Risk occurs primarily in urban areas below 1,200 meters elevation. The most recent large outbreak of dengue occurred in southeastern Bolivia in the 1990s. To prevent dengue, travelers to all regions should take measures to prevent daytime mosquito bites.

HEPATITIS: Hepatitis A vaccine is recommended for all nonimmune travelers. Hepatitis B is spread by infected blood, contaminated needles, and unprotected sex. Vaccination is recommended for long-stay (more than 3 months) travelers; those who may be at occupational or social risk; anybody desiring maximal protection.

LEISHMANIASIS: Cutaneous and mucocutaneous leishmaniasis occurs year-round below 2,000 meters elevation. Risk is elevated in the Yungas region, the forested foothill valleys at 1,000 to 2,000 meters elevation east of the Andean Cordillera. A few cases of visceral leishmaniasis have been reported from the Yungas region, which is northeast of La Paz. All travelers to rural areas should take measures to prevent insect (sand fly) bites.

MALARIA: There is no risk of malaria in the highlands of La Paz, the provinces of Oruro and Potosi (southwestern portions of the country), and the cities of Cochabamba and Sucre. All other rural areas of the country below 1,000 meters elevation should be considered risk areas, especially the lowlands east of the Andean Cordillera and Pando Department. Limited risk may extend up to 2,500 meters elevation in some rural areas. Vivax malaria accounts for nearly 95% of all cases, whereas falciparum malaria accounts for the remainder. Falciparum malaria, however, may predominate in northern areas. Chloroquine-resistant falciparum malaria is becoming more prevalent in the north and along the Brazilian border. Prophylaxis with atovaquone/proguanil (Malarone), mefloquine (Lariam), or doxycycline is recommended in risk areas. All travelers should take measures to prevent evening and nighttime mosquito bites.

RABIES: Dogs are the primary source of human infection. Other sources include cats, vampire bats, and monkeys. All animal bites or scratches should be taken seriously, and medically evaluated. Although rabies is rare among tourists, there is risk. No one should pet or pick up any stray animals. All children should be warned to avoid contact with unknown animals. Rabies pre-exposure vaccination is recommended for stays longer than 3 months and for short-term travelers who will be going to remote areas where quality medical attention is not available within 24 hours.

TRAVELERS' DIARRHEA: High risk outside of deluxe hotels and tourist resorts. Travelers should follow all food and drink precautions. A quinolone antibiotic, combined with loperamide (Imodium), is recommended for the treatment of acute diarrhea. Persistent diarrhea may be due to a parasitic disease such as giardiasis, amebiasis, or cryptosporidiosis.

TUBERCULOSIS: Tuberculosis (TB) a major health problem in this country. Travelers planning an extended stay should have a pre-departure TB skin test (PPD test) and be retested after leaving this country or returning home.

TYPHOID FEVER: Typhoid vaccine is recommended for those traveling off the usual tourist routes, those visiting friends or relatives, and for long-stay visitors. Typhoid vaccines are 60% to 70% effective; safe food and drink precautions should continue to be observed.

YELLOW FEVER: This disease is active in jungle areas east of the Andean highlands. A yellow fever vaccination is recommended for all travelers who are destined for high-risk areas (the Departments of Beni, Cochabamba, La Paz, and Santa Cruz).

OTHER DISEASES/HAZARDS: AIDS (low incidence), Bolivian hemorrhagic fever (low risk, but potentially fatal; outbreak occurred in 1990s in El Beni Department. The virus is transmitted by aerosolized rodent urine. Risk may be increased by sleeping in primitive shelters near rodent habitats. Person-to-person transmission can also occur. Brucellosis, coccidiomycosis (endemic near border with Paraguay), echinococcosis (occurs primarily in sheep-raising regions of the Altiplano), fascioliasis (liver fluke disease; high incidence in northwestern Altiplano), Lyme disease (may occur), tuberculosis (a serious public health problem; highest incidence in South America), strongyloidiasis and other helminthic (worm) infections, toxoplasmosis, typhoid fever, and typhus (louse borne).

Bonaire

KRALENDIJK

CAPITAL:
Kralendijk
EMBASSY (IN U.S.):
202-244-5300
GMT:
−4 hours
TELEPHONE COUNTRY CODE:
599
USADIRECT:
001-800-872-2881
To place calls from Bonaire, Curacao, Saba, St. Eustatius, and St. Maarten.
ENTRY REQUIREMENTS
- **Passport/Visa:** Bonaire is one of the Netherlands Antilles, an autonomous part of the Kingdom of the Netherlands. The Netherlands Antilles is a group of six Caribbean islands: Aruba, Bonaire, Curacao, Saba, Statia, and St. Maarten. Passport or proof of U.S. citizenship (i.e., certified birth certificate or voter registration card with photo ID) required. Visa not required for stay up to 14 days, extendible to 90 days after arrival.
- **HIV Test:** Required by Aruba for immigrants intending to stay.
- **Vaccinations:** Yellow fever vaccination required if traveling from an infected area.
EMBASSIES/CONSULATES
- **U.S. Embassy:** J.B. Gorsiraweg #1, Willemstad, Curacao; Tel: 599-9-461-3066; Fax: 599-9-461-6489; e-mail: cgcuracao@interneeds.net.
- **Canadian Embassy:** Maduro and Curiels Bank, N.V., Scharlooweg 55, Willemstad, Curacao; Tel: 599-9-466-1115/1121; Fax: 599-9-1122/1130.
HOSPITALS/DOCTORS
Adequate medical care is available on Aruba, Curacao, and Saint Maarten but is not up to the standards of industrialized countries. Medical care is substandard on other islands, namely Bonaire, Saba, and Statia.
- The San Francisco Hospital is equipped to deal with emergencies and has a decompression chamber for scuba diving emergencies.

Current Advisories and Health Risks

For additional information, consult Disease Risk Summaries for the Caribbean on page 293.

Bosnia and Herzegovina

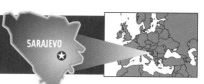

SARAJEVO ✪

CAPITAL:
Sarajevo
EMBASSY (IN U.S.):
U.S. Embassy, Sarajevo: 387-71-659-992
GMT:
+1 hour
TELEPHONE COUNTRY CODE:
387
USADIRECT:
00-800-0010
ENTRY REQUIREMENTS
• **Passport:** Required. A visa is not required for tourist stays up to 3 months.
• **HIV Test:** Not required.
• **Vaccinations:** None required.
EMBASSIES/CONSULATES
• **U.S. Embassy:** Lipasina 43, Sarajevo; Tel: 387-33-445-700; Fax: 387-33-659-722; Website: www.usis.com.ba.
• **Canadian Embassy:** Logavina 7, Sarajevo; Tel: 387-33-447-900; Fax: 387-447-901; e-mail: sjevo@dfait-maeci.gc.ca.
• **British Embassy:** Tina Ujevica 8, Sarajevo; Tel: 00-387-33-28-2200; Fax: 00-387-33-20-4780; e-mail: britemb@bih.net.ba; Website: www.britishembassy.ba.
HOSPITALS/DOCTORS
• Medical care is substandard throughout the country, including major cities. Hospital accommodations are inadequate and advanced technology is lacking. Shortages of routine medications and supplies may be encountered.
• All international travelers are advised to take out full medical insurance. Adequate evacuation coverage is a high priority. In the event of serious medical conditions every effort should be made to go to Western Europe.
• There is a reciprocal health agreement with the United Kingdom. Hospital treatment, some dental treatment, and other medical treatment are normally free. Prescribed medicines must be paid for.

Current Advisories and Health Risks

AIDS/HIV: Increased cases reported especially from eastern Europe (mainly Romania and Bulgaria). Infected blood and contaminated needles and syringes are important sources of infection. Travelers should consider carrying sterile needles and syringes and should avoid, if possible, blood transfusions and medical injections. Travelers should consider evacuation to a European medical facility when surgical care, or blood transfusions, are needed.

ACCIDENTS, ILLNESS, AND MEDICAL INSURANCE

- Accidents and injuries are the leading cause of death among travelers younger than the age of 55 and are most often caused by motor vehicle and motorcycle crashes, drownings, aircraft crashes, homicides, and burns are less common causes.
- Heart attacks cause most fatalities in older travelers.
- Infections cause only 1% of fatalities in overseas travelers, but, overall, infections are the most common cause of travel-related illness.
- Travelers are advised to obtain, before departure, supplemental travel health insurance with specific overseas coverage. The policy should provide for direct payment to the overseas hospital and/or physician at the time of service and include a medical evacuation benefit. The policy should also provide 24-hour hotline access to a multilingual assistance center that can help arrange and monitor delivery of medical care and determine if medical evacuation or air ambulance services are required.

CRIMEAN-CONGO HEMORRHAGIC FEVER: This is a viral encephalitis transmitted by ticks. Transmission season is primarily April through August, with peak activity April through May. Travelers are advised to take measures to prevent tick bites.

EHRLICHIOSIS: Cases of human granulocytic ehrlichiosis have been reported from Slovenia and the Netherlands.

EUROPEAN TICK-BORNE ENCEPHALITIS (TBE): The tick vector for this disease (the same tick that transmits Lyme disease), is widely distributed in brushy and forested areas at elevations up to 1,500 meters in rural wooded areas, exclusively in the regions around the Sava River in the far north of the country. Risk exists only between April and October. The TBE vaccine is available in Europe and by special release in Canada and is recommended only for those with intense outdoor exposure in risk areas for a period of longer than 3 weeks, especially if hiking or camping, or undertaking similar outdoor activities. Tick-bite precautions are also recommended.

HEMORRHAGIC FEVER WITH RENAL SYNDROME (HFRS): Cases of Hantaan virus illness are reported in the Balkans. Travelers should avoid contact with rodent urine or rodent feces, which transmit the virus.

HEPATITIS: All nonimmune travelers should receive hepatitis A vaccine. The hepatitis B carrier rate is 1% to 4%. Hepatitis B vaccine should be considered for stays longer than 3 months and for travelers wanting increased protection. Travelers should be aware that the risk of hepatitis B is increased by unsafe sex and the use of unsterile needles and syringes.

LYME DISEASE: Risk of transmission occurs throughout Europe in rural brushy, wooded, and forested areas up to 1,500 meters elevation. Presumably there is risk in the Balkans. The ticks that transmit Lyme disease are most abundant and active April through September. Travelers should be advised to take measures to prevent tick bites. Prevention measures include applying a DEET-containing repellent on exposed skin and wearing permethrin-treated clothing.

MALARIA: There is no risk of malaria in Europe.

MEDITERRANEAN SPOTTED (BOUTONNEUSE) FEVER: Risk is unclear, but this disease occurs in southern France and in the coastal regions of other Mediterranean countries, and also along the Black Sea coast, in brushy and/or forested areas below 1,000 meters elevation. Peak transmission period is July through September. Disease may be acquired in and around tick-infested houses and terrain, but more than 95% of cases are associated with contact with tick-carrying dogs.

ROAD SAFETY

• Seat belts should be worn at all times.

• Bosnia-Herzegovina is among the rare countries in Europe that have fewer than 10 kilometers of four-lane highway. The existing, two-lane roads between major cities are quite narrow at places, lack guard rails, and are full of curves. Travel by road should be considered risky because roads are not well maintained, particularly in winter. Driving in winter is hazardous due to fog, heavy snow, and ice. Overland travel should be undertaken with a four-wheel drive vehicle equipped with spare parts, tires, and fuel, as well as food, water, blankets, torches, and a medical kit.

SAND FLY FEVER AND WEST NILE FEVER: Cases have been reported from the Adriatic area, but the risk is unclear. Travelers should be advised to prevent nighttime insect bites.

TRAVELERS' DIARRHEA: Higher risk occurs in Spain, Greece, the Balkans, and eastern Europe. Travelers should drink only bottled, boiled, or treated water and avoid undercooked food. A quinolone antibiotic, combined with loperamide (Imodium), is recommended for the treatment of diarrhea.

TYPHOID FEVER: Persons traveling extensively in the Balkan States should consider typhoid vaccination. Typhoid vaccine is 60% to 70% effective, so careful selection of food and drink remains important.

Botswana

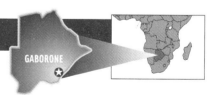

CAPITAL:
Gaborone
EMBASSY (IN U.S.):
202-244-4990/4991
GMT:
+2 hours
TELEPHONE COUNTRY CODE:
267
USADIRECT:
None

- **Passport/Visa:** No visa for stays up to 90 days.
- **HIV Test:** Not required.
- **Vaccinations:** Yellow fever vaccination required if traveling from an infected area and older than 1 year of age. Required also for travelers arriving from countries in the yellow fever endemic zones.

*Travelers should check with this country's embassy (or a consulate) in the United States, Canada, or the United Kingdom for any changes in these requirements.

EMBASSIES/CONSULATES

- **U.S. Embassy:** Embassy Drive, Government Enclave, Gaborone; Tel: 353-982, Fax: 356-947.
- **Canadian Embassy:** Vision Hire Building, Queens Road, Plot 182, Gaborone; Tel: & Fax: 30-44-11, e-mail: canada.consul@info.bw.
- **British High Commission:** Private Bag 0023, Gaborone; Tel: 267-395-2841; Fax: 267-395-6105; e-mail: bhc@botsnet.bw; Website: www.britishhighcommission.gov.uk/botswana.

HOSPITALS/DOCTORS

- Princess Marina Hospital, Gaborone (237 beds); general medical and surgical services.
- Medical care is substandard throughout the country even in the best private medical facilities in Gaborone and Francistown. In the event of serious medical conditions, every effort should be made to go to Johannesburg, South Africa. There are hospitals in all main towns. All main towns have chemists, and pharmaceutical supplies are readily available. Health insurance is essential. There is a government medical scheme and medicines supplied by government hospitals are free.
- The dust and heat may cause problems for asthmatics and people with allergies to dust. Those with sensitive skin should take precautions. Botswana's altitude, 1000 meters (3300 ft) above sea level, reduces the filtering effect of the atmosphere. Hats and sunscreen are advised.
- International SOS: MRI Centre, Physical Location, Plot 10 216, Unit 1, Mandela Road, Gaborone, Botswana; Alarm Center Tel: 267-3901-601; Admin Fax: 267-316-4728

Current Health Risks and Advisories

AIDS/HIV: The HIV prevalence rate is 36% in the 15 to 49 age group. Heterosexual contact is the predominant mode of transmission.

AFRICAN SLEEPING SICKNESS (TRYPANOSOMIASIS): Incidence data not available. Sporadic cases have been reported in the northern areas, including cases among foreign visitors to the Okavango swamps in the northwest district of Ngamiland. All travelers should take measures to prevent insect (tsetse fly) bites.

ANIMAL HAZARDS: Animal hazards include snakes (vipers, cobras), centipedes, scorpions, and black widow spiders.

CHOLERA: Sporadic cases occur, with occasional outbreaks. Cholera, however, is an extremely rare disease in travelers from developed countries. Cholera vaccine is recommended primarily for people at high risk (e.g., relief workers) who work and live in highly endemic areas under less than adequate sanitary conditions.

HEPATITIS: All nonimmune travelers should receive hepatitis A vaccine. Hepatitis E is endemic, with outbreaks reported in north-central areas. Incidence of hepatitis B in the general population is between 5% and 19%. Hepatitis B is spread by infected blood, contaminated needles, and unprotected sex. Vaccination is recommended for stays longer than 3 months; for anyone at occupational or social risk; for any traveler desiring maximal protection. Because the risk of illness or injury during travel cannot be predicted, some experts believe that *all* travelers should be immunized against hepatitis B owing to the risk of receiving a medical injection with an unsterile needle or syringe.

INFLUENZA: Influenza is transmitted year-round in the tropics. The flu vaccine is recommended for all travelers.

LEISHMANIASIS: Very low risk. Sporadic cases have been reported in the medical literature.

MALARIA: Moderate seasonal risk in northern areas and sporadic risk in southeastern border areas. Increased transmission occurs during and just after the rainy season, October to mid-April. Malaria is moderately endemic in northern areas, including the Boteti, Chobe, Ngamiland, Okavango, and Tutume districts/subdivisions. Limited transmission occurs in the southeastern border with South Africa, extending along the Molopo River bordering South Africa. Gaborone is essentially risk free, except in years with very heavy rain fall. *Plasmodium falciparum* accounts for 95% of malaria cases. Prophylaxis with atovaquone/proguanil (Malarone), mefloquine (Lariam), or doxycycline is recommended in risk areas. All travelers should take measures to prevent evening and nighttime mosquito bites.

POLIO: Recent cases of poliomyelitis in Benin, Botswana, Chad, Côte d'Ivoire, Burkina Faso, Cameroon, Central African Republic, Guinea, and Sudan have been linked to recent outbreaks of polio in the northern Nigeria. All travelers to Botswana should be fully immunized against this disease.

RABIES: Dogs are the primary source of human infection. Rabid jackals are also a potential threat, especially in the rural eastern areas. All animal bites or scratches should be taken seriously and immediate medical attention should be sought.

SCHISTOSOMIASIS: Risk areas of urinary schistosomiasis are widely distributed along the eastern border from Francistown to Lobatse, with scattered foci in the north. Risk areas for intestinal schistosomiasis are confined to the Okavango Delta marshlands in the northwest district of Ngamiland and the northeastern Chobe drainage system, including the Kasane vicinity. Travelers to these areas should avoid swimming, bathing, or wading in freshwater ponds, lakes, or streams.

TRAVELERS' DIARRHEA: High risk. Water from deep boreholes may be unpalatable due to high salinity. Indiscriminate disposal of human waste causes serious contamination of ground water in many villages, and in some towns. Piped water is available in many communities but many water treatment and distribution systems are poorly maintained and may be contaminated. Travelers should observe safe food and drink precautions. A quinolone antibiotic, combined with loperamide (Imodium), is recommended for the treatment of acute diarrhea. Persistent diarrhea may be due to a parasitic infection such as giardiasis, amebiasis, or cryptosporidiosis.

- -

TUBERCULOSIS: Tuberculosis (TB) a major health problem in this country. Travelers planning an extended stay should have a pre-departure TB skin test (PPD test) and be retested after returning from this country.

- -

TYPHOID FEVER: Typhoid vaccine is recommended for those traveling off the usual tourist routes, those visiting friends or relatives, and for long-stay visitors. Because the typhoid vaccines are only 60% to 70% effective, safe food and drink selection remains important.

- -

OTHER DISEASES/HAZARDS: African tick typhus (contracted from dog ticks, often in urban areas; disease also transmitted by bush ticks), arboviral fevers (mosquito transmitted; West Nile and Rift Valley fever may occur; explosive urban outbreaks of chikungunya fever have occurred, but human cases are primarily reported from rural areas), brucellosis, leptospirosis, tick-borne relapsing fever, flea- and louse-borne typhus, tuberculosis (a major health problem), trachoma, typhoid fever, and intestinal helminthic (worm) infections (common).

Brazil

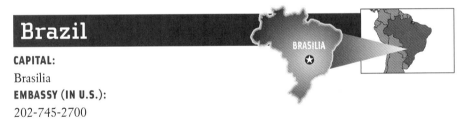

BRASÍLIA

CAPITAL:
Brasilia

EMBASSY (IN U.S.):
202-745-2700

GMT:
−3 hours

TELEPHONE COUNTRY CODE:
55

USADIRECT:
0800-890-0288 or 0800-888-8288

ENTRY REQUIREMENTS

- **Passport/Visa:** A valid passport and visa are required.
- **HIV Test:** Not required.
- **Vaccinations:** A yellow fever vaccination certificate is required from travelers older than 9 months of age arriving from an infected area, unless the traveler has a medical waiver. A certificate is also required if arriving from Africa from Angola, Cameroon, Democratic Republic of Congo, Gabon, The Gambia, Ghana, Guinea, Liberia,

Nigeria, Sierra Leone, and Sudan. Vaccination is also required if arriving from Bolivia, Colombia, Ecuador, or Peru.

EMBASSIES/CONSULATES

- **U.S. Embassy:** Avenida das Nacoes, Lote 3, Brasilia. Tel: 55-61-321-7272; Website: www.embaixada-americana.org.br.
- **Canadian Embassy:** Setor de Embaixadas Sul, Avenida das Naçoes, Lote 16, 70359-900, Brasilia DF. Tel: 55-61-321-2171; e-mail: brsla@dfait-maeci.gc.ca; Website: www.dfait-maeci.gc.ca/brazil/brasilia/bsa-menu-e.html.
- **British Embassy:** Setor de Embaixadas Sul, Quadra 801, Conjunto K, CEP 70200-010, Brasilia—DF, Tel: 55-61-329-2300, Fax: 55-61-329-2369, e-mail: contact@uk.org.br, Website: www.uk.org.br

HOSPITALS/DOCTORS

- Brasilia: Hospital de Base (600 beds); most specialty services including trauma; 24-hour emergency department.
- Casa de Saude Santa Lucia; some specialty and emergency services.
- Sao Paulo: Hospital Samaritano; 24-hour emergency services.
- Clinica Hamermesz; highly recommended by expatriates.
- Albert Einstein Hospital. Excellent facility, but nurses may be undertrained.
- Rio de Janeiro: Hospital Miguel Couto (117 beds); some specialty services including trauma and emergency.
- Hospital Souza Aguiar (480 beds); most specialty services including orthopedics, trauma, and emergency.
- The Evangelical Hospital; efficient, capable facility.
- Hospital Israelita Albert Sabin, 56, rua Lucio de Mendonca, Tijuca, Rio de Janeiro.
- Anapolis (Goias): Hospital Evengelico; mission hospital staffed by British expatriates.
- Cuiaba (Mato Grosso State): Sao Rafael Hospital; advanced facility with CT, MRI ultrasound.
- Manaus: Adventist Hospital, Mineiros (Goias).

Current Advisories and Health Risks

AIDS/HIV: Brazil has the highest HIV/AIDS rate in South America. Most cases are reported from Rio de Janeiro and Sao Paulo. Behaviors responsible for HIV transmission include heterosexual and same-sex contact, commercial sex, and injecting drug use.

CHAGAS DISEASE: Risk is present in most rural areas of eastern and southern Brazil. This disease is transmitted primarily in well-populated rural-agricultural areas where there are adobe-style huts and houses that often harbor the night-biting triatomid (assassin) bugs. Travelers sleeping in such structures should take measures to prevent nighttime bites.

CHOLERA: This disease is active in this country. Cholera, however, is an extremely rare disease in travelers from developed countries. Cholera vaccine is recommended primarily for people at high risk (e.g., relief workers) who work and live in highly endemic areas under less than adequate sanitary conditions. Many countries, including Canada, license an oral cholera vaccine. The oral vaccine is not available in the United States.

DENGUE FEVER: Mosquito transmitted. Most recent outbreaks have occurred from December through June in southern areas. Risk may be elevated from April through August in more northern areas. Risk is present year-round in Rio de Janeiro State and Sao Paulo and Ceara States. Travelers should take precautions against daytime mosquito bites.

FILARIASIS: Focally endemic in northeastern urban coastal areas, including Belem, Maceio, and Recife. Travelers to these regions should take measures to prevent insect (mosquito) bites.

HEPATITIS: Hepatitis A vaccine is recommended for all nonimmune travelers. The overall hepatitis B carrier rate is between 1% to 2%, but may approach 20% in some areas of the Amazon Basin. Hepatitis B is spread by infected blood, contaminated needles, and unprotected sex. Vaccination is recommended for long-stay (longer than 3 months) travelers; those who may be at occupational or social risk; anybody desiring maximal protection.

INFLUENZA: Influenza is transmitted year-round in the tropics. Vaccination is recommended.

INSECT-TRANSMITTED VIRAL DISEASES: Oropouche fever (vectored by biting midges; explosive outbreaks occur), Mayaro virus disease (dengue-like illness, mosquito-vectored; attack rates up to 20% in the Amazon Basin, including Paro State), eastern equine encephalitis, St. Louis encephalitis, Western equine encephalitis, and Venezuelan equine encephalitis are reported. At least 30 other insect-borne viral illnesses are associated with illness in humans.

LEISHMANIASIS: Cutaneous, mucocutaneous, and visceral leishmaniasis occur in rural and peri-urban areas. Cutaneous leishmaniasis and mucocutaneous leishmaniasis occur nearly countrywide in rural and peri-urban areas with risk elevated in the more humid areas of northern, north-central, and central states; most visceral leishmaniasis occurs in the semi-arid northeastern states (with sharp increases in Maranhao, Piaui, and Rio Grande do Norte States), but has also been reported as far west and south as extreme western Mato Grosso do Sul State and Rio de Janiero State, respectively. All travelers to these regions should take protective measures to prevent insect (sand fly) bites.

MALARIA: Risk occurs in the States of Acre, Rondônia, Amapá, Amazonas, Roraima, and Tocantins. Parts of states of Maranhaõ (western part), Mato Grosso (northern part), and Pará (except Belem City). There is also transmission in urban areas, including large cities such as Porto Velho, Boa Vista, Macapa, Manaus, Santarem, and Maraba. Countrywide, *Plasmodium falciparum* accounts for 40% of officially reported malaria cases. Nearly all other cases are caused by *Plasmodium vivax*. Chloroquine-resistant falciparum malaria is a major problem in the Amazon region. Prophylaxis with atovaquone/proguanil

(Malarone), mefloquine (Lariam), or doxycycline is recommended in risk areas. All travelers should take measures to prevent evening and nighttime mosquito bites.

ONCHOCERCIASIS: Risk is present near swift-flowing streams in densely forested highlands in northern Amazonas and Poraima States. Travelers to these areas should take measures to prevent insect (black fly) bites.

PLAGUE: From 35 to 150 cases are reported annually, mostly from the drier northern and eastern states from Bahia and Ceara south to Minas Gerais. Travelers to these regions should avoid close contact with rodents (which may be carrying infective fleas). Prophylaxis with tetracycline is protective.

RABIES: High risk, relative to other South American countries. From 40 to 120 human cases are reported annually, usually transmitted by stray dogs. Vampire bats have also been implicated. Most risk occurs in the northeastern states, but cases are also reported countrywide from both urban and rural areas. Rabies vaccine should be considered for stays longer than 3 months or for shorter stays if traveling to locations more than 24 hours from a reliable source of postexposure rabies vaccine. All animal bites or scratches should be medically evaluated.

SCHISTOSOMIASIS: Intestinal schistosomiasis is a major public health problem. Most cases are reported from the Minas Gerais and Bahia states. Risk is present in northern and eastern states from Maranhao south to Parana, including both urban and rural areas. There is no apparent risk in the Amazon Basin. Travelers to risk areas should avoid swimming, wading, or bathing in freshwater ponds, lakes, or streams.

TRAVELERS' DIARRHEA: High risk outside of resorts and first-class hotels. Travelers should follow all food and drink precautions. A quinolone antibiotic, combined with loperamide (Imodium), is recommended for the treatment of diarrhea. Persistent diarrhea may be due to a parasitic disease such as giardiasis, amebiasis, or cryptosporidiosis.

TUBERCULOSIS: Tuberculosis (TB) a major health problem in this country. Travelers planning an extended stay should have a pre-departure TB skin test (PPD test) and be retested after leaving this country or returning home.

TYPHOID FEVER: Typhoid vaccine is recommended for those traveling off the usual tourist routes, those visiting friends or relatives, and for long-stay visitors. Typhoid vaccines are 60% to 70% effective; safe food and drink precautions should continue to be observed.

YELLOW FEVER: Brazil recommends vaccination for travelers destined for endemic zones including rural areas in the states of Acre, Amapá, Amazonas, Goiás, Maranhão, Mato Grosso, Mato Grosso do Sul, Pará, Rondônia, Roraima and Tocantins, and certain areas of Bahia, Minas Gerais, Parana, Piauí, Rio Grande do Sul, Santa Catarina, and São Paulo.

OTHER DISEASES/HAZARDS: Angiostrongyliasis, brucellosis, cutaneous larva migrans, cryptococcosis, cysticercosis (an important health problem in northeastern Brazil, and probably elsewhere), echinococcosis, human monocytic ehrlichiosis, hepatic capillariasis (from ingestion of embryonated eggs in food or dirt), leprosy (highly endemic in Recife area), leptospirosis (mostly in rat-infested urban slums), mansonellosis, measles, meningitis (epidemics reported from Sao Paulo; most cases due to serogroup B meningococci), respiratory syncytial virus (the most common cause of bronchiolitis in children), relapsing fever trachoma, toxocariasis, tuberculosis (a serious public health problem; 25% of children in some areas may be infected), strongyloidiasis, and other helminthic (worm) infections.

British Virgin Islands

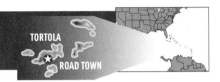

TORTOLA
ROAD TOWN

CAPITAL:
Road Town
EMBASSY (IN U.S.):
202-462-1340
GMT:
−4 hours
TELEPHONE COUNTRY CODE:
809
USADIRECT:
1-800-872-2881
ENTRY REQUIREMENTS
• **Passport/Visa:** A Visa is not required for stays less than 90 days.
• **HIV Test:** All immigrants and work permit applicants are required to have HIV testing.
• **Vaccinations:** None required.
EMBASSIES/CONSULATES:
Accredited to U.S. and Canadian Embassies in Bridgetown, Barbados (see page 357).
HOSPITALS/DOCTORS:
Limited, but adequate, care is available for most problems. All serious accidents or injuries should be evacuated by air ambulance to San Juan or Miami. Travelers are advised to obtain supplemental travel health insurance with specific overseas coverage. The policy should provide for direct payment to the overseas hospital and/or physician at the time of service and include a medical evacuation benefit.
• Peebles Hospital, Tortola (50 beds); limited medical/surgical services.
CURRENT ADVISORIES AND HEALTH RISKS
For additional information, consult Disease Risk Summaries for Mexico and Central America on page 295.

Brunei Darussalam

CAPITAL:
Bandar Seri Begawan

EMBASSY (IN U.S.):
202-342-0159

GMT:
+8 hours

TELEPHONE COUNTRY CODE
673

USADIRECT:
800-1111

ENTRY REQUIREMENTS
- **Passport/Visa:** A valid passport, visa, and tourist card are required.
- **HIV Test:** Required for all persons applying for work permits.
- **Vaccinations:** A yellow fever vaccination certificate is required for travelers older than 1 year of age coming from infected areas or who have passed through partly or wholly endemic areas within the preceding 6 days.

EMBASSIES/CONSULATES
- **U.S. Embassy:** 3rd floor, Teck Guan Plaza, Jalan Sultan, Bandar Seri Begawan. Tel: 673-2-229-670; Fax: 673-2-225-293; e-mail: amembbsb@brunet.bn.
- **Canadian Embassy:** 5th Floor, Jalan McArthur Building, No. 1, Jalan McArthur, Bandar Seri Begawan. Tel: 673-2-22-00-43; Fax: 673-2-22-00-40; e-mail: bsbgn@dfait-maeci.gc.ca; Website: www.dfait-maeci.gc.ca/Brunei.
- **British High Commission:** PO Box 2197, Bandar Seri Begawan 8674; Tel: 673-2-222231/223121; Fax: 673-2-234315; e-mail: brithc@brunet.bn; Website: www.britishhighcommission.gov.uk/brunei.

HOSPITALS/DOCTORS:
Adequate medical care is available in Brunei for most problems, but in the event of a serious medical condition, transport to a medical facility in Singapore may be indicated. Travelers are advised to obtain supplemental travel health insurance with specific overseas coverage. The policy should provide for direct payment to the overseas hospital and/or physician at the time of service and include a medical evacuation benefit.

Current Advisories and Health Risks

CHOLERA: Vaccination not recommended. Sporadic cases occur, but the risk to travelers is low.

DENGUE FEVER: There is risk of both dengue fever and dengue hemorrhagic fever in both urban and rural areas. The mosquitoes that transmit dengue bite primarily during the daytime.

HEPATITIS: All travelers should receive hepatitis A vaccine. The hepatitis B carrier rate in the general population is estimated at 10% to 12%. Hepatitis B is spread by infected blood, contaminated needles, and unsafe sex. Vaccination is recommended for stays longer than 3 months; for anyone at occupational or social risk; for any traveler desiring maximal protection.

INFLUENZA: Influenza is transmitted from November through March. The flu vaccine is recommended for all travelers who may be at risk.

JAPANESE ENCEPHALITIS (JE): Transmission occurs year-round, but the risk is low. Vaccination is recommended for travelers who will be staying in rural-agricultural areas for extended periods (more than 4 weeks) during the peak transmission season.

RABIES: WHO reported Brunei rabies free in 1997 through 1998, but this does not eliminate risk. All animal bites, especially those from a dog, must be medically evaluated.

MALARIA: There is no risk of malaria within this country.

TRAVELERS' DIARRHEA: The food and drink in first-class restaurants and hotels are considered generally safe. A quinolone antibiotic, combined with loperamide (Imodium), is recommended for the treatment of acute diarrhea. Persistent diarrhea may be due to a parasitic disease, such as giardiasis or amebiasis.

TUBERCULOSIS: Tuberculosis (TB) is a health problem in this country. Travelers planning an extended stay should have a pre-departure TB skin test (PPD test) and be retested after returning from this country.

TYPHOID FEVER: Typhoid vaccine is recommended for all travelers, with the exception of short-term visitors who restrict their meals to major restaurants and hotels. Because the typhoid vaccines are only 60% to 70% effective, safe food and drink selection remains important.

OTHER DISEASES/HAZARDS: AIDS/HIV (low incidence; some risk associated with unprotected sexual contact, injecting drug use, or unscreened blood transfusions), fasciolopsiasis (giant intestinal fluke; risk associated with ingesting aquatic plants), other helminthic infections (hookworm, roundworm), filariasis (transmitted by mosquitoes), mite-borne typhus (scrub typhus), melioidosis, and typhoid fever are reported. Animal hazards include various snakes and leeches. Marine hazards include stonefish, lionfish, and the box jellyfish, whose stings are potentially life threatening. Antivenom exists but may not be readily available.

Bulgaria

★ SOFIA

CAPITAL:
Sofia
EMBASSY (IN U.S.):
202-387-7969
GMT:
+1 hour
TELEPHONE COUNTRY CODE:
359
USADIRECT:
00-800-0010

ENTRY REQUIREMENTS

- **Passport/Visa:** Passport required. Visa not required for a stay of up to 30 days. Border tax $20 (U.S.) must be paid when entering Bulgaria. For persons staying longer than 30 days, obtain a visa in advance. Under Bulgarian law, an AIDS test is required for all intending immigrants and may be required for foreigners staying longer than a month for purposes of study or work; U.S. test is accepted. All travelers, except those staying in a private boarding house or hotel, etc., are required to register with the regional passport office or the police within 48 hours after their arrival in Bulgaria. For more information, contact the Consular Section of the Embassy of the Republic of Bulgaria, 1621 22nd St., NW, Washington, DC 20008 (202/387-7969)
- **HIV Test:** Testing required for all foreigners staying longer than one month for purpose of study or work.
- **Vaccinations:** None required.

EMBASSIES/CONSULATES

- **U.S. Embassy:** 1 Saborna St., Sofia. Tel: 359-2-937-5100; Fax: 359-2-981-8977; Website: www.usembassy.bg. Consulate: 1 Kapitan Andreev St, Sofia. Tel: 359-2-963-2022; Fax: 359-2-963-2859.
- **Canadian Embassy:** Sofia.Tel: 359-2-943-3700; Fax: 359-943-3707; e-mail: canada@mail.techno-link.com.
- **British Embassy:** 9 Moskovska Street, Sofia; Tel: 359-2-933-9222; Fax: 933-9219; Website: www.british-embassy.bg

HOSPITALS/DOCTORS:

Medical care in Bulgaria is below Western standards. Travelers are advised to obtain supplemental travel health insurance with specific overseas coverage. The policy should provide for direct payment to the overseas hospital and/or physician at the time of service and include a medical evacuation benefit.

- Institute of Traumatology and Orthopedics, Sofia (400 beds); specialized treatment center for the entire country.

Current Advisories and Health Risks

For additional information, consult the Disease Risk Summary for Europe on page 300.

Burkina Faso

CAPITAL:
Ouagadougou
EMBASSY (IN U.S.):
202-332-5577
GMT:
+0 hour
TELEPHONE COUNTRY CODE:
226
USADIRECT:
None
ENTRY REQUIREMENTS*
• **Passport/Visa:** Valid passport and visa are required.
• **HIV Test:** Not required.
• **Vaccinations:** A yellow fever vaccination certificate is required for all travelers arriving from all countries, including the United States and Canada.
*Travelers should check with this country's embassy (or a consulate) in the United States, Canada, or the United Kingdom for any changes in these requirements.
EMBASSIES/CONSULATES
• **U.S. Embassy:** Avenue John F. Kennedy, Ouagadougou. Tel: 226-30-67-23/24/25; Fax: 226-31-23-68.
• **Canadian Embassy:** rue Agostino Néto, Ouagadougou, Province du Kadiogo. Tel: 226-31-18-94; Fax: 226-31-19-00; e-mail: ouaga@dfait-maeci.gc.ca.
• **British Honorary Consul:** Mr. Yves Pichot, British Consulate, Hotel Yibi, 10 BP 13593, Ouagadougou. Tel: 226-50-30-73-23; Fax: 226-50-30-59-00; e-mail: ypi@cenatrin.bf
HOSPITALS/DOCTORS:
Travelers should contact the U.S. or Canadian embassies for medical referrals. Medical evacuation insurance is strongly recommended.

Current Advisories and Health Risks

AIDS/HIV: Heterosexual contact is the predominant mode of transmission. HIV prevalence estimated at 17% of the high-risk urban population. All travelers are cautioned against unsafe sex, unsterile medical or dental injections, and unnecessary blood transfusions.

AFRICAN SLEEPING SICKNESS (TRYPANOSOMIASIS): Disease activity has been reported in the vicinities of Banfora and Bobo Diolasso in the southwest, and the Koudougou vicinity west of Ouagadougou. Travelers should take protective measures against insect (tsetse fly) bites.

CHOLERA: This disease is active in this country. Cholera vaccine is recommended primarily for people at high risk (e.g., relief workers) who work and live in highly endemic areas under less than adequate sanitary conditions.

FILARIASIS: Bancroftian filariasis is endemic. Travelers should take measures to prevent mosquito bites.

HEPATITIS: All susceptible travelers should receive hepatitis A vaccine. The hepatitis B carrier rate in the general population exceeds 10%. Hepatitis B is spread by infected blood, contaminated needles, and unsafe sex. Vaccination is recommended for stays longer than 3 months; for anyone at occupational or social risk; for any traveler desiring maximal protection. Because the risk of illness or injury during travel cannot be predicted, some experts believe that *all* travelers should be immunized against hepatitis B because of the risk of receiving a medical injection with an unsterile needle or syringe.

INFLUENZA: Influenza is transmitted year-round in the tropics. The flu vaccine is recommended for all travelers.

LEISHMANIASIS: Low risk. Cutaneous leishmaniasis has been reported in the western and eastern areas, and a focus has been previously identified near Arabinda (northeastern province of Soum). Travelers should take precautions against insect (sand fly) bites.

MALARIA: Risk is present throughout this country year-round, including urban areas. Risk is elevated during and immediately following the rainy season, June through October. Falciparum malaria accounts for 85% to 95% of cases, followed by *Plasmodium ovale.* Multidrug resistant falciparum malaria is reported. Prophylaxis with atovaquone/proguanil (Malarone), mefloquine (Lariam), or doxycycline is recommended. All travelers should take measures to prevent evening and nighttime mosquito bites.

MENINGITIS: Serogroup W-135 meningococcal disease has been confirmed in some districts. Quadrivalent meningitis vaccine, which protects against serogroups A, C, Y, and W-135, is recommended for travelers staying longer than 1 month during the dry season, December to June, and should be considered for shorter stays, any time of the year if extensive, close contact with the local population is anticipated.

ONCHOCERCIASIS: Highest transmission rates occur near fast-flowing rivers. Incidence is declining, due to black fly control programs. Travelers should take measures to prevent insect (black fly) bites.

POLIO: This disease is endemic. All travelers should be fully immunized.

RABIES: Sporadic cases of human rabies are reported countrywide. All animal bites or scratches, especially from a dog, should be treated immediately; rabies vaccination may be required. Rabies vaccine is recommended for travel longer than 3 months, for shorter stays for travelers who plan to venture off the usual tourist routes, or when travelers desire extra protection.

SCHISTOSOMIASIS: Urinary schistosomiasis is widely distributed, especially in the eastern one third of this country, with focal areas of risk in all major river basins. Intestinal schistosomiasis is widely distributed in the southwest, with scattered foci in other areas. Travelers should avoid swimming, wading, or bathing in freshwater lakes, ponds, or streams.

TRAVELERS' DIARRHEA: All surface water sources should be considered potentially contaminated. Water from deep wells is usually free of bacterial contamination, but may contain high levels of minerals and sediment. Travelers should observe all food and drink precautions. A quinolone antibiotic, combined with loperamide (Imodium), is recommended for the treatment of acute diarrhea. Persistent diarrhea may be due to a parasitic infection such as giardiasis, amebiasis, or cryptosporidiosis.

TUBERCULOSIS: Tuberculosis (TB) a major health problem in this country. Travelers planning an extended stay should have a pre-departure TB skin test (PPD test) and be retested after returning from this country.

TYPHOID FEVER: Typhoid vaccine is recommended for those traveling off the usual tourist routes, those visiting friends or relatives, and for long-stay visitors. Because the typhoid vaccines are only 60% to 70% effective, safe food and drink selection remains important.

YELLOW FEVER: Outbreaks of yellow fever were reported in 2003 in Burkina Faso. There are no reports of recent outbreaks. Yellow fever vaccination is required for all travelers older than 1 year of age entering this country.

OTHER DISEASES/HAZARDS: African tick typhus (transmitted by dog ticks and bush ticks), anthrax (mostly cutaneous), brucellosis (usually from consumption of unpasteurized dairy products), dracunculiasis (risk is countrywide), Lassa fever (rare, sporadic cases; transmitted from infected rodents via dried urine/feces, usually in dust in rural dwellings), leprosy (overall prevalence 2 cases/1,000 population), leptospirosis, loiasis, louse-borne (epidemic) typhus and relapsing fever, tuberculosis (a major health problem), intestinal worms (common), and typhoid fever are reported.

Burundi

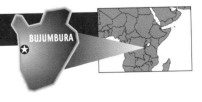

CAPITAL:
Bujumbura
EMBASSY (IN U.S.):
202-342-2574
GMT:
+2 hours

TELEPHONE COUNTRY CODE:
257

USADIRECT:
None

ENTRY REQUIREMENTS

- **Passport/Visa:** Passport and visa required. For specific requirements, consult the Embassy of the Republic of Burundi, Suite 212, 2233 Wisconsin Ave., NW, Washington, DC 20007 (202-342-2574) or Permanent Mission of Burundi to the U.N. (212-499-0001 thru 0006).
- **HIV Test:** Not required.
- **Vaccinations:** A yellow fever vaccination certificate is required for all travelers older than 1 year of age arriving from infected areas.

EMBASSIES/CONSULATES

- **U.S. Embassy:** Avenue des Etats-Unis, B.P. 34, Bujumbura. Tel: 257-223-454; Fax: 257-222-926.
- **Consulate of Canada:** 4708, Boulevard de l'uprona, Bujumbura, Burundi; Tel.: 257 24-58-98; Fax: 257 24-58-99; e-mail: consulat.canada@usan-bu.net.
- **British Embassy:** Accredited to British Embassy in Ghana. Parcelle No 1131, Boulevard de l'Umuganda, Kacyiru Sud, BP 576 Kigali; Tel: 250-585771, 585773, 584098, 586072; Fax: 250-582044, 511586.

HOSPITALS/DOCTORS:

Medical care in Burundi is well below Western standards. Travelers are advised to obtain supplemental travel health insurance with specific overseas coverage. The policy should provide for direct payment to the overseas hospital and/or physician at the time of service and include a medical evacuation benefit.

- Hospital Prince Regent Charles; general medical/surgical facility; ICU.
- Clinique Prince Louis Rwagasore (13 beds).
- Travelers should contact the U.S. Embassy for physician referrals.

Current Advisories and Health Risks

IMMUNIZATIONS: All travelers should be up-to-date on their routine immunizations: tetanus-diphtheria (Td), measles-mumps-rubella (MMR), polio, influenza, and varicella (chickenpox). Immunization against hepatitis A, hepatitis B, meningitis, rabies, and typhoid fever are recommended.

MALARIA: Risk is present year-round throughout this country, including urban areas. Transmission is highest during and immediately after the rainy seasons, September through December and March through May. Peak transmission in the Rusizi Valley occurs during the drier months of May through September. Risk may be lower in locations above 1,800 meters elevation. Falciparum malaria accounts for approximately 80% of cases, followed by *Plasmodium malariae* in as many as 20% of cases. Chloroquine-resistant falciparum malaria is reported. Prophylaxis with atovaquone/proguanil (Malarone), mefloquine (Lariam), or doxycycline is recommended.

INSECT-BITE PREVENTION: All travelers should take measures to prevent evening and nighttime mosquito bites. Insect-bite prevention measures include a DEET-containing repellent applied to exposed skin, insecticide (permethrin) spray applied to clothing and gear, and use of a permethrin-treated bed net at night while sleeping.

For additional information, consult the Disease Risk Summary for sub-Saharan Africa on page 307.

Cambodia

CAPITAL:
Phnom Penh
EMBASSY (IN U.S.):
202-726-7742
GMT:
+7 hours
TELEPHONE COUNTRY CODE:
855
USADIRECT:
1-800-881-001
ENTRY REQUIREMENTS
- **Passport/Visa:** A visa is required.
- **HIV Test:** Not required.
- **Vaccinations:** A yellow fever vaccination certificate is required if travelers are arriving from an infected area.

EMBASSIES/CONSULATES
- **U.S. Embassy**: no. 16, Street 228 (between streets 51 and 63), Phnom Penh; Tel: 855-23-216-436 or 218-931.
- **Canadian Embassy:** Villa 11, R.V. Senei Vinnavaut Oum (Street 254), Chaktamouk Ward, Daun Penh District, Phnom Penh 23; Tel: 855-23-213-470; e-mail: pnmpn@dfait-maeci.gc.ca.
- **British Embassy:** 27-29 Street 75, Phnom Penh; Tel: 855-23-427124, 428295; Fax: 855-23-427125; e-mail: BRITEMB@bigpond.com.kh; Website: www.britishembassy. gov.uk/cambodia.

HOSPITALS/DOCTORS
- 7 Jan 1979 Hospital, Phnom Penh (500 beds); some specialties; emergency services; preferred hospital in this country.
- Battambang Provincial Hospital (325 beds).
- Raffles Medical Center, Hotel Sofitel Cambodiana, Phnom Penh. Private hotel-based clinic; convenient; used by expatriates.
- International SOS: International SOS (Cambodia) Pte Ltd., House 161, Street 51, Sang-Kat Boeung Peng, Khon Doun Penh, Phnom Penh, Cambodia; Clinic/Admin Tel: 755-23-216-911; Clinic/Admin Fax: 755-23-215-711

Current Advisories and Health Risks

ACCIDENTS AND ILLNESS: Accidents are the leading cause of death among travelers younger than age 55; cardiovascular disease accounts for most fatalities in older travelers. Infections cause less than 1% of fatalities in travelers, but are the most common cause of travel-related illness.

AIDS/HIV: Cambodia has the highest HIV infection rate in Asia. Initially driven by an extensive commercial sex industry, prevalence is now fueled by transmission between casual, noncommercial partners and between spouses as new infections develop when men who engage in commercial sex bring the infection home. There is a very low rate of injecting drug use as a cause of HIV transmission.

ANIMAL HAZARDS: Animal hazards include snakes (cobras, vipers), spiders (black and brown widow), crocodiles, and leeches.

CHOLERA: This disease is reported active in this country, but the threat to tourists is very low. Vaccination is not routinely recommended.

DENGUE FEVER: Endemic at high levels year-round. Increased risk may occur in urban areas. The *Aedes* mosquitoes, which transmit dengue, bite primarily during the daytime and are present in populous urban areas as well as resort and rural areas. All travelers are advised to take precautions against mosquito bites.

HEPATITIS: There is a high risk of hepatitis A in this country. All nonimmune travelers should receive hepatitis A vaccine. Water-borne outbreaks of hepatitis E are reported, but data are scarce. The hepatitis B carrier rate in the general population is estimated to exceed 10%. Hepatitis B is transmitted by blood, unsafe sex, and contaminated needles and syringes. Vaccination against hepatitis B should be considered for stays longer than 3 months; by anyone at occupational or social risk; by any traveler desiring maximal protection.

INFLUENZA: Influenza is transmitted year-round in the tropics. The flu vaccine is recommended for all travelers to this country.

JAPANESE ENCEPHALITIS (JE): Sporadic cases occur throughout the year, primarily in rural areas, but occasionally near or within urban areas. Vaccination should be considered by travelers planning an extended stay (more than 3 to 4 weeks) in rural-agricultural areas during the peak transmission season, June through October.

MALARIA: Risk is present year-round throughout this country, especially in the forested areas along the borders, mountainous areas, and rural areas. Moderate risk is present in the central region and with lower risk from Tonle Sap Lake, down the Mekong River to the Vietnamese border. There is no risk in Phnom Penh. Falciparum malaria accounts for 90% of cases; vivax malaria the remainder. Mefloquine-resistant falciparum malaria is common in western Cambodia, especially along the Thai-Cambodian border. Prophylaxis with atovaquone/proguanil (Malarone) or doxycycline is recommended. All travelers should take measures to prevent evening and nighttime mosquito bites.

MARINE HAZARDS: Stingrays, jellyfish, and several species of poisonous fish are common in the country's coastal waters and are potential hazards to unprotected swimmers.

RABIES: Sporadic cases of human rabies are reported countrywide, and the risk of human rabies is increased in rural areas. All animal bites or scratches, especially from a dog, should be medically evaluated. Rabies vaccine is recommended for travel longer than 3 months, for shorter stays for travelers who plan to venture off the usual tourist routes where they may be more exposed to the stray dog population, or when travelers desire extra protection. The State Department recommends vaccination for all expatriate corporate employees and their families, especially the children.

SCHISTOSOMIASIS: Risk is present year-round, especially along the Mekong and Mun Rivers and in Battambang Province. Travelers should avoid swimming, bathing, or wading in freshwater lakes, ponds, or streams.

TRAVELERS' DIARRHEA: Travelers should observe strict food and drink safety precautions. A quinolone antibiotic, combined with loperamide (Imodium), is recommended for the treatment of acute diarrhea. Persistent diarrhea may be due to a parasitic disease such as giardiasis or amebiasis.

TUBERCULOSIS: Tuberculosis a major health problem in this country. Travelers planning an extended stay should have a pre-departure TB skin test (PPD test) and be retested after leaving this country. Domestic help hired by long-stay visitors should be screened for TB.

TYPHOID FEVER: Typhoid vaccine is recommended, especially for long-term travelers, adventure travelers, those visiting friends or family, and those wishing maximal disease protection. Because the typhoid vaccines are only 60% to 70% effective, safe food and drink guidelines should continue to be observed.

OTHER DISEASES/HAZARDS: Anthrax (may be associated with eating infected buffalo meat), chikungunya fever (regionally endemic, with outbreaks), echinococcosis, filariasis (endemic; current levels unclear), leprosy (highly endemic), leptospirosis, plague, rabies, scrub typhus, tuberculosis (highly endemic), and soil-transmitted helminthic (worm) diseases (ascariasis, hookworm disease, strongyloidiasis). Other helminthic infections (fasciolopsiasis, gnathostomiasis, opisthorchiasis, and clonorchiasis) are reported.

Cameroon

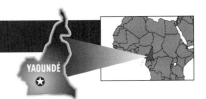

CAPITAL:
Yaoundé
EMBASSY (IN U.S.):
202-265-8790
GMT:
+1 hour

TELEPHONE COUNTRY CODE:
237
USADIRECT:
None
ENTRY REQUIREMENTS
- **Passport/Visa:** Valid passport and visa are required.
- **HIV Test:** Not required.
- **Vaccinations:** A yellow fever vaccination certificate is required from all travelers older than 1 year of age arriving from all countries.
- Travelers should check with this country's embassy (or a consulate) in the United States, Canada, or the United Kingdom for any changes in these requirements.

EMBASSIES/CONSULATES
- **U.S. Embassy:** Rue Nachtigal, Yaoundé. Tel: 23-40-14, Fax: 237-23-07-53.
- **Canadian Embassy:** Immeuble Stamatiades, Place de l'Hôtel de Ville, Yaoundé. Tel: 23-23-11; Fax: 237-22-10-90; e-mail: yunde@dfait-maeci.gc.ca.
- **British High Commission:** Avenue Winston Churchill, BP 547, Yaoundé; Tel: 237-2-22-05-45/2-22-07-96; Fax: 237-2-22-01-48; e-mail: BHCyaounde@fco.gov.uk.

HOSPITALS/DOCTORS
- Polyclinic Bonanjo, Douala; ambulatory care clinic; can also stabilize patients before medical evacuation.
- LaQuintinie Hospital, Douala (930 beds); general medical services; ICU; X-ray.
- University of Yaoundé Medical Center; general medical services.
- Central Hospital, Yaoundé (554 beds); general medical services; blood bank.
- Polyclinique Sende, Yaoundé; general medical services.

CURRENT ADVISORIES AND HEALTH RISKS

AIDS/HIV: By the year 2010, AIDS mortality is estimated to more than double. Heterosexual contact is the predominant means of HIV transmission. HIV prevalence is estimated at 9% of the urban population and 45%, or higher, among commercial sex workers. All travelers are cautioned against unsafe sex, unsterile medical or dental injections, and unnecessary blood transfusions.

AFRICAN SLEEPING SICKNESS (TRYPANOSOMIASIS): Most risk is found in the vicinities of Bafia (Mbam Division, Centre Province) and Fontem/Mamfe (Manyu/Fontem Division, Sud-Ouest Province). Mbam Division reports the most cases of sleeping sickness. Potential areas for recurrence include Extreme-Nord Province bordering Chad, and Est Province, bordering the Nola vicinity of the Central African Republic. Travelers to risk areas should take measures to prevent insect (tsetse fly) bites.

ANIMAL HAZARDS: Common animal hazards include snakes (vipers, mambas, cobras), centipedes, scorpions, and black widow spiders.

CHOLERA: This disease is active in this country. The risk of cholera, however, is extremely low in travelers from developed countries. Cholera vaccine is recommended primarily for travelers at high risk who work and live in highly endemic areas under less than adequate sanitary conditions.

HEPATITIS: Hepatitis A vaccine is recommended for all travelers. The hepatitis E virus is endemic, but levels are unclear. The hepatitis B carrier rate in the general population is estimated at 10% to 12%. Hepatitis B is spread by infected blood, contaminated needles, and unprotected sex. Vaccination is recommended for stays longer than 3 months; for anyone at occupational or social risk; for any traveler desiring maximal protection. The risk of illness or injury during travel cannot be predicted, some experts believe that *all* travelers should be immunized against hepatitis B owing to the risk of receiving a medical injection with an unsterile needle or syringe.

INFLUENZA: Influenza is transmitted year-round in the tropics. The flu vaccine is recommended for all travelers.

LEISHMANIASIS: Cutaneous leishmaniasis is endemic in northern Cameroon, but risk may exist focally countrywide. Foci of cutaneous leishmaniasis occur in the north in the vicinity of Mokolo (50 kilometers west of Maroua) and also may occur in areas bordering Chad (including the N'Djamena vicinity); other foci historically have been reported from the eastern areas. A recently identified focus of visceral leishmaniasis has been reported from Kousseri in Extreme-Nord Province.

LOIASIS: Highly endemic foci presumably persist in southern rain forest and swamp forest areas. All travelers should take measures to prevent insect (deer fly) bites.

MALARIA: Risk is present year-round throughout this country, including urban areas. Risk is elevated during and immediately following the rainy seasons (March through June and September through November in the south; June through September in the more arid north). Falciparum malaria accounts for approximately 90% of malaria in this country. Chloroquine-resistant falciparum malaria is prevalent. Prophylaxis with atovaquone/proguanil (Malarone), mefloquine (Lariam), or doxycycline is recommended. All travelers should take measures to prevent mosquito bites, especially during the evening and at night.

MENINGITIS: Northern Cameroon lies within the sub-Saharan meningitis belt. Meningococcal vaccine is recommended for travelers staying longer than 1 month during the dry season, December to June, and should be considered for shorter stays, any time of the year if extensive, close contact with the local population is anticipated.

ONCHOCERCIASIS: Highly endemic foci presumably persist along fast-flowing rivers in the south and the southwest and in the savanna area of northern Cameroon. All travelers should take measures to prevent insect (black fly) bites, especially in the vicinity of rivers.

PARAGONIMIASIS (LUNG FLUKE DISEASE): This disease is endemic; travelers should avoid eating uncooked freshwater crustaceans, such as crabs.

POLIOMYELITIS (POLIO): Recent cases of poliomyelitis in Cameroon and also Benin, Botswana, Chad, Côte d'Ivoire, Burkina Faso, Central African Republic, Guinea, and Sudan have been linked to recent outbreaks of polio in northern Nigeria. All travelers to Cameroon should be fully immunized against this disease.

RABIES: Rabies is a public health problem in many rural and urban areas, including Yaoundé. Immediate medical attention should be sought for all animal bites or scratches, especially from a dog. Rabies vaccine is recommended for travel longer than 3 months, and for shorter stays if travelers plan to venture off the usual tourist routes.

SCHISTOSOMIASIS: Urinary and intestinal schistosomiasis are highly endemic in the north and in the southwest. Intestinal schistosomiasis is endemic in Nord Province and in Center-Sud Province. Areas also infested include Yaoundé, Edea, and Douala. Travelers should avoid swimming, bathing, or wading in freshwater ponds, lakes, or streams.

TRAVELERS' DIARRHEA: High risk. Several urban areas in the south, including Douala, Yaoundé, and Mbalmayo, have treatment plants and piped water systems, but improper operation and poor maintenance of the plants allow bacterial recontamination. All water sources should be considered potentially contaminated. A quinolone antibiotic, combined with loperamide (Imodium), is recommended for the treatment of acute diarrhea. Persistent diarrhea may be due to a parasitic infection such as giardiasis, amebiasis, or cryptosporidiosis.

TUBERCULOSIS: Tuberculosis (TB) is a major health problem in this country. Travelers planning an extended stay should have a pre-departure TB skin test (PPD test) and be retested after returning from this country.

TYPHOID FEVER: Typhoid vaccine is recommended for those traveling off the usual tourist routes, those visiting friends or relatives, and for long-stay visitors. Because the typhoid vaccines are only 60% to 70% effective, safe food and drink selection remains important.

YELLOW FEVER: Yellow fever vaccination is required to enter this country. This country is in the Yellow Fever Endemic Zone. A valid yellow fever vaccination certificate may be required for ongoing travel to other countries in Africa, Asia, and South America.

OTHER DISEASES/HAZARDS: Brucellosis (from consumption of raw dairy products or occupational exposure), Bancroftian filariasis (mosquito-borne), cutaneous larva migrans, Lassa fever (current endemic status unclear), leprosy (up to 1.9 cases/1,000 population), mansonellosis, toxoplasmosis, tuberculosis (a major health problem), typhus (murine- and louse-borne), relapsing fever (louse-borne), Rift Valley fever, typhoid fever, and intestinal worms.

Canada

CAPITAL:
Ottawa

EMBASSY (IN U.S.):
202-682-1740

GMT:
−5 hours

TELEPHONE COUNTRY CODE:
1

USADIRECT:
1-800-CALL ATT

ENTRY REQUIREMENTS

- **Passport/Visa:** Americans visiting Canada are required to carry proof of citizenship. Acceptable documents are (1) a passport; (2) an original birth certificate, or a notarized copy; (3) a voter's registration card; (4) a Selective Service card; (5) a naturalization certificate; or (6) a baptismal certificate for infants. A driver's license is not accepted as proof of citizenship, but may be used to verify the other documents. Children younger than age 16 must have written travel permission if not accompanied by a parent or guardian. For further information, contact the Canadian Embassy in Washington, DC at 202-682-1770.
- **HIV Test:** Not required.
- **Vaccinations:** None required.

EMBASSIES/CONSULATES

- **U.S. Embassy:** Ottawa, 100 Wellington Street; Tel: 613-238-5335.
- **Canadian Embassy:** 501 Pennsylvania Ave., N.W., Washington, DC 20001; Tel: 202-682-1740.
- **British High Commission:** 80 Elgin Street, Ottawa, Ontario K1P 5K7; Tel: 1-613-237-1530; Fax: 1-613-237-7980.

HOSPITALS/DOCTORS:
Medical care in Canada is of high quality. Travelers to this country are advised to obtain supplemental travel health insurance that provides for direct payment to the hospital and/or physician at the time of service and also includes a medical evacuation benefit.

- International SOS: International SOS Canada Inc., 80 Tiverton Court, Suite 401, Markham, Ontario, L3R 0G4 Canada; Admin Tel: 1-905-940-2444; Admin Fax: 1-905-940-3551.

Current Advisories and Health Risks

ACCIDENTS AND ILLNESS: Motor vehicle accidents, injuries, and drowning are the leading causes of death among travelers younger than age 55. Cardiovascular diseases cause most fatalities in older travelers. Infectious diseases are responsible for less than 1% of fatalities in travelers.

HEPATITIS: All travelers should be vaccinated against hepatitis A. There is a high carrier rate of the hepatitis B virus in the Inuit population in northern Canada. Hepatitis B is spread by infected blood, contaminated needles, and unsafe sex. Vaccination is recommended for stays longer than 3 months; for anyone at occupational or social risk; for any traveler desiring maximal protection.

INFLUENZA: All travelers should be immunized for protection during the flu season, which lasts from October to April.

INSECT-BITE PREVENTION: Black flies, mosquitoes, and other biting insects can be a significant problem during the spring and summer months. Campers, hikers, and other outdoor enthusiasts can protect themselves by applying a DEET repellent to exposed skin and wearing permethrin-treated clothing. Also useful are head nets and mesh jackets, as well as bed nets at night.

INTESTINAL PARASITES: Giardiasis and cryptosporidiosis occur in wilderness areas, but the risk to campers and hikers is not clearly defined. Rural streams, lakes, and ponds may be contaminated from human or animal sewage and filtration of drinking water is advised; chlorination alone is not adequate for removing *Giardia* and *Cryptosporidium* oocysts from drinking water.

Hand washing reduces person-to-person transmission of these diseases. Community outbreaks of cryptosporidiosis sporadically have occurred after breakdowns in municipal water treatment systems.

RABIES: Very low risk to humans. Less than 5% of human cases are transmitted by dogs. Most rabies in Canada is confined to animals, particularly arctic foxes and red foxes. Travelers should seek immediate treatment for any unprovoked animal bite, particularly if from a fox, raccoon, skunk, or bat. Other wild animals in Canada that can potentially transmit rabies include groundhogs, wolves, bobcats, and black bears.

Cape Verde

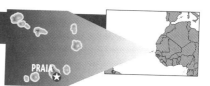

CAPITAL:
Praia

EMBASSY (IN U.S.):
202-965-6820

GMT:
+1 hour

TELEPHONE COUNTRY CODE:
238

USADIRECT:
0-800-2288

- **Passport/Visa:** Passport and visa required.
- **HIV Test:** Not required.
- **Vaccinations:** Required for travelers coming from infected countries or from Senegal.

EMBASSIES/CONSULATES
- **U.S. Embassy:** Rua Abilio M. Macedo 81, Praia, Island of Santiago; Tel: 61-56-16 or 17; Fax: 61-13-55.
- **Canadian Embassy:** Accredited to Canadian Embassy in Dakar, Senegal (see page 643).
- **British Embassy:** Accredited to British Embassy in Senegal. 20 Rue du Docteur Guillet, (Boite Postale 6025), Dakar; Tel: 221-823-7392, 823-9971; Fax: 221-823-2766, 823-8415; e-mail: britemb@sentoo.sn.

HOSPITALS/DOCTORS:
Local medical treatment varies in quality and can be inadequate, including medical care in the capital of Paria.

Current Advisories and Health Risks

ACCIDENTS, ILLNESS, AND MEDICAL INSURANCE:
- Accidents and injuries are the leading cause of death among travelers younger than age 55 and are most often caused by motor vehicle and motorcycle crashes, drownings, aircraft crashes, homicides, and burns are less common causes.
- Heart attacks cause most fatalities in older travelers.
- Infections cause only 1% of fatalities in overseas travelers, but, overall, infections are the most common cause of travel-related illness.
- Travelers are advised to obtain, before departure, supplemental travel health insurance with specific overseas coverage. The policy should provide for direct payment to the overseas hospital and/or physician at the time of service and include a medical evacuation benefit. The policy should also provide 24-hour hotline access to a multilingual assistance center that can help arrange and monitor delivery of medical care and determine if medical evacuation or air ambulance services are required.

CHOLERA: This disease is reported active at this time, but the risk is low. Cholera is an extremely rare disease in travelers from developed countries. Cholera vaccine is recommended primarily for people at high risk (e.g., relief workers) who work and live in highly endemic areas under less than adequate sanitary conditions.
- The oral cholera vaccine (Dukoral) provides up to 60% crossover protection against ETEC diarrhea.
- Many countries, including Canada, license an oral cholera vaccine. The oral vaccine is not available in the United States.
- Cholera vaccine is not "officially" required for entry into, or exit from, any country. Despite this, some countries, on occasion, require proof of cholera vaccination from travelers coming from cholera-infected countries. Anticipating such a situation, certain travelers may wish to carry a medical exemption letter from their health-care provider. Travel

Medicine, Inc., recommends that travelers use the International Certificate of Vaccination (Yellow Card) for this purpose, having their health-care provider affirm that they are "exempt from cholera vaccine" and validate the exemption with both the provider's signature and the appropriate official stamp (the "Uniform Stamp" in the United States).

HEPATITIS: Hepatitis A vaccine is recommended for all travelers. The hepatitis E virus is endemic, but levels are unclear. Hepatitis B vaccine is recommended for stays longer than 3 months and for short-term travelers wanting increased protection. Travelers should be aware that the risk of hepatitis B is increased by unsafe sex and the use of unsterile needles and syringes.

INFLUENZA: Influenza is transmitted year-round in the tropics. The flu vaccine is recommended for all travelers older than age 50; all travelers with any chronic disease or weakened immune system; travelers of any age wishing to decrease the risk of this illness; pregnant women after the first trimester.

MALARIA: Since September 2001, local health officials have reported 66 cases of *Plasmodium falciparum* malaria, including one death due to complications of cerebral malaria, in the Praia area of Sao Tiago, in the Cape Verde Islands. Most case-patients resided in Fontao, a suburb northwest of Praia proper, and the rest resided in nearby Terra Branca. Imported malaria cases from other countries in West Africa might have initiated the outbreak.

- Malaria prophylaxis is not routinely recommended at this time.
- All travelers should take measures to prevent evening and nighttime mosquito bites. Insect-bite prevention measures include a DEET-containing repellent applied to exposed skin, insecticide (permethrin) spray applied to clothing and gear, and use of a permethrin-treated bed net at night while sleeping.

TRAVELERS' DIARRHEA: High risk. All water sources should be considered potentially contaminated. A quinolone antibiotic, combined with loperamide (Imodium), is recommended for the treatment of acute diarrhea. Diarrhea not responding to treatment with an antibiotic, or chronic diarrhea, may be due to a parasitic disease such as giardiasis, amebiasis, or cryptosporidiosis.

TUBERCULOSIS: Tuberculosis is a significant health problem in this country. Travelers planning an extended stay should have a pre-departure TB skin test (PPD test) and be retested after leaving this country.

TYPHOID FEVER: Typhoid vaccine is recommended for travel to this country. The typhoid vaccine is 60% to 70% effective, so food and drink precautions should continue to be observed.

YELLOW FEVER: This disease is not active in this country. A yellow fever vaccination certificate is required for travelers coming from infected countries or from Kenya, Mali, or Senegal. Certificate not required or recommended for other travelers.

Cayman Islands (British West Indies)

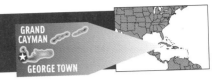

GRAND CAYMAN
GEORGE TOWN

CAPITAL:

Grand Cayman

EMBASSY

202-462-1340 (British Embassy)

GMT:

−5 hours

TELEPHONE COUNTRY CODE:

345

USADIRECT:

1-800-872-2881

ENTRY REQUIREMENTS

- **Passport/Visa:** The Cayman Islands are overseas territory of the United Kingdom. These islands include Anguilla, Cayman Islands, Montserrat, and Turks and Caicos. Proof of U.S. citizenship, photo ID, onward/return ticket and sufficient funds required for tourist stay up to 6 months. Consult the British Embassy (202-588-7800) for further information.
- **HIV Test:** Not required.
- **Vaccinations:** None required.

EMBASSIES/CONSULATES:

The Cayman Islands is an overseas territory of Britain. The United States does not maintain an embassy in the Cayman Islands. The Cayman Islands are accredited to the Canadian High Commission in Kingston, Jamaica. Tel: 876-926-1500.

HOSPITALS/DOCTORS:

Medical care is adequate for most health problems. Travelers are advised to obtain supplemental travel health insurance with specific overseas coverage. The policy should provide for direct payment to the overseas hospital and/or physician at the time of service and include a medical evacuation benefit.

- Georgetown Hospital (128 beds), Grand Cayman; Tel: 949-8600; newly expanded and renovated; includes maternity, surgical, medical, and pediatric units. The emergency room is open 24 hours with a physician on duty at all times. The hospital maintains a two-man, double-lock decompression chamber for diving emergencies. Georgetown Hospital is affiliated with Baptist Hospital of Miami for patient referrals involving advanced care or treatment and can arrange Learjet emergency medical air transport.
- There are two private medical centers on Grand Cayman, the Professional Medical Centre (345-949-6066) and the the Cayman Medical and Surgical Centre (345-949-8150).

Current Advisories and Health Risks

For additional information, consult Disease Risk Summaries for Mexico and Central America on page 295.

Central African Republic

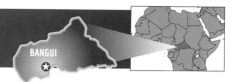

BANGUI

CAPITAL:
Bangui
EMBASSY (IN U.S.):
202-483-7800
GMT:
+1 hour
TELEPHONE COUNTRY CODE:
236
USADIRECT:
None
ENTRY REQUIREMENTS*
- **Passport/Visa:** A visa is required.
- **HIV Test:** Not required.
- **Vaccinations:** A yellow fever vaccination certificate is required from all travelers older than 1 year of age arriving from all countries.

*Travelers should check with this country's embassy (or a consulate) in the United States, Canada, or the United Kingdom for any changes in these requirements.

EMBASSIES/CONSULATES
- **U.S. Embassy:** Bangui at Avenue David Dacko; Tel: 236-61-02-00; Fax: 236-61-44-94.
- **Canadian Embassy:** Quartier Assana, Bangui; Tel: 236-61-09-73; Fax: 236-61-40-74.
- **British High Commission:** Accredited to British Embassy in Cameroon. Avenue Winston Churchill, BP 547, Yaoundé; Tel: 237-2-22-05-45/2-22-07-96; Fax: 237-2-22-01-48; e-mail: BHCyaounde@fco.gov.uk.

HOSPITALS/DOCTORS
- National University Hospital Center, Bangui; general medical/surgical facility; some French military medical officers on staff.
- American Lutheran Church Missionary Hospital. Bouar; general medical services.
- Clinicas las Condes, Bangui.

Current Advisories and Health Risks

AIDS/HIV: HIV/AIDS is present in more than 10% of the adult population countrywide and over 20% of the high-risk urban population. Heterosexual transmission is the predominate means of transmission. All travelers are cautioned against unsafe sex, medical or dental injections, and blood transfusions.

AFRICAN SLEEPING SICKNESS (TRYPANOSOMIASIS): Risk areas include the Ouham Valley in the northwest, the Nola vicinity (extreme southwest near the Cameroon border), and the southeast. Travelers should take measures to prevent insect (tsetse fly) bites.

ANIMAL HAZARDS: Animal hazards include snakes (boomslang, viper, cobra), centipedes, scorpions, and spiders (black widow, brown recluse).

CHOLERA: This disease is reported active in this country, but the threat to tourists is very low. Cholera vaccine is recommended primarily for people at high risk (e.g., relief workers) who work and live in highly endemic areas under less than adequate sanitary conditions. Many countries, including Canada, license an oral cholera vaccine. The oral vaccine is not available in the United States.

HEPATITIS: High risk. All nonimmune travelers should receive hepatitis A vaccine. Hepatitis E: As many as 20% of cases of acute infectious hepatitis are antibody-positive for hepatitis E. The hepatitis B carrier rate in the general population is estimated at 15%. Hepatitis B is spread by infected blood, contaminated needles, and unprotected sex. Vaccination is recommended for stays longer than 3 months; for anyone at occupational or social risk; for any traveler desiring maximal protection. The risk of illness or injury during travel cannot be predicted. Some experts believe that *all* travelers should be immunized against hepatitis B because of the risk of receiving a medical injection with an unsterile needle or syringe.

INFLUENZA: Influenza is transmitted year-round in the tropics. The flu vaccine is recommended for all travelers.

LEISHMANIASIS: Sporadic cases of cutaneous leishmaniasis have been reported in the northwest and southwest. Visceral leishmaniasis may occur in the southwest. Travelers should take measures to prevent sand fly bites.

LOIASIS: Highly endemic focus in southwestern rain forest and swamp forest areas. Travelers should take measures to prevent insect (deer fly) bites.

MALARIA: Risk is present year-round throughout this country, including urban areas. Chloroquine-resistant falciparum malaria accounts for most cases. Prophylaxis with atovaquone/proguanil (Malarone), mefloquine (Lariam), or doxycycline is recommended. All travelers should take measures to prevent evening and nighttime mosquito bites.

MENINGITIS: Central African Republic lies within the sub-Saharan meningitis belt. Outbreaks of Group A meningococcal disease occur sporadically. Quadrivalent meningitis vaccine, which protects against meningococcal serogroups A, C, Y, W-135, is recommended for all travelers staying longer than 1 month during the dry season, December to June, and should be considered for shorter stays during the dry season if close contact with the local population is anticipated.

RABIES: Sporadic cases of human rabies are reported countrywide. All animal bites or scratches, especially from a dog, should be treated immediately. Although rabies is rare among tourists, there is risk. No one should pet or pick up any stray animals. All children should be warned to avoid contact with unknown animals. Rabies vaccine is recommended for travel longer than 3 months, for shorter stays for travelers who plan to venture off the usual tourist routes where they may be more exposed to the stray dog population, or when travelers desire extra protection.

SCHISTOSOMIASIS: Widespread throughout most of the country. The highest infection rates are reported in the northwest. Travelers should avoid freshwater exposure.

TRAVELERS' DIARRHEA: All water, including piped water from municipal treatment facilities, is considered contaminated. Travelers should observe all food and drink safety precautions. A quinolone antibiotic, combined with loperamide (Imodium) is recommended for the treatment of acute diarrhea. Persistent diarrhea may be due to a parasitic infection such as giardiasis, amebiasis, or cryptosporidiosis.

TUBERCULOSIS: Tuberculosis (TB) a major health problem in this country. Travelers planning an extended stay should have a pre-departure TB skin test (PPD test) and be retested after returning from this country.

TYPHOID FEVER: Typhoid vaccine is recommended for those traveling off the usual tourist routes, those visiting friends or relatives, and for long-stay visitors. Because the typhoid vaccines are only 60% to 70% effective, safe food and drink selection remains important.

YELLOW FEVER: A yellow fever vaccination certificate is required for all travelers entering this country.

OTHER DISEASES/HAZARDS: African tick typhus (contracted from dog ticks, often in urban areas, and bush ticks), brucellosis (usually from the consumption of unpasteurized dairy products), filariasis (mosquito-borne), Lassa fever (low risk; current endemic status unclear), leprosy (high incidence; up to 2.7 cases/1,000 population), rabies (transmitted primarily by dogs in urban and rural areas), toxoplasmosis, tuberculosis (a major health problem), typhoid fever, and intestinal worms (very common).

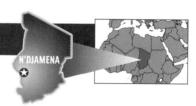

Chad

CAPITAL:
N'Djamena
EMBASSY (IN U.S.):
202-462-4009
GMT:
+1 hour
TELEPHONE COUNTRY CODE:
235
USADIRECT:
None

- **Passport/Visa:** Valid passport and visa are required.
- **HIV Test:** Not required.
- **Vaccinations:** None required. The CDC recommends yellow fever immunization for all travelers older than 9 months of age, arriving from any country.

EMBASSIES/CONSULATES

- **U.S. Embassy:** N'Djamena. Avenue Felix Eboue; Tel: 51-62-18/32-69. Canadian Embassy (Cameroon); Tel: 237-221-090.
- **Canadian Embassy:** Accredited to the Canadian Embassy in Cameroon; Tel: 011-237-223-2311.
- **British High Commission:** Accredited to British Embassy in Cameroon. Avenue Winston Churchill, BP 547, Yaoundé; Tel: 237-2-22-05-45/2-22-07-96; Fax: 237-2-22-01-48; e-mail: BHCyaounde@fco.gov.uk.

HOSPITALS/DOCTORS:

Medical care in Chad is below Western standards. Travelers are advised to obtain, before departure, supplemental travel health insurance with specific overseas coverage. The policy should provide for direct payment to the overseas hospital and/or physician at the time of service and include a medical evacuation benefit.

- N'Djamena Central Hospital (620 beds); general medical services; some specialties.
- Sahr Hospital (325 beds); general medical facility. Travelers should contact the U.S. Embassy for physician referrals.
- International SOS: Le Centre Médical International, Route de l'Aéroport, BP 1215, N'Djamena, Chad; Clinic/Admin Tel: 235-52-25-01; Clinic/Admin Fax: 235-52-25-03, Medical Emergencies: 235-27-19-13.

Current Advisories and Health Risks

Malaria risk is present year-round throughout this country, including urban areas. Prophylaxis with atovaquone/proguanil (Malarone), mefloquine (Lariam), or doxycycline is recommended. Chad lies within the "meningitis belt" of sub-Saharan Africa. Quadrivalent meningitis vaccine is advised for those travelers anticipating close, extended contact with the indigenous population.

See Disease Risk Summary for sub-Saharan Africa for additional advisories on page 307.

Chile

SANTIAGO

CAPITAL:
Santiago
EMBASSY (IN U.S.):
202-785-1746
GMT:
−4 hours

TELEPHONE COUNTRY CODE:

56

USADIRECT:

800-225-288

800-360-311

ENTRY REQUIREMENTS

- **Passport/Visa:** U.S. citizens do not need a visa for a 3-month stay. Travel to frontier areas for scientific, technical, or mountaineering activities requires 90-day prior authorization.
- **HIV Test:** Not required.
- **Vaccinations:** Yellow fever vaccine may be required for entry to Easter Island.

EMBASSIES/CONSULATES

- **U.S. Embassy:** Avenida Andres Bello 2800, Santiago. Tel: 56-2-335-6550, 232-2600; Tel: after hours 56-2-330-3321; Fax: 56-2-330-3005; e-mail: SantiagoAmcit@state.gov; Website: www.usembassy.cl.
- **Canadian Embassy:** Nueva Tajamar 481, Torre Norte, 12th Floor, Las Condes, Santiago. Tel: 56-2-362-9660; Fax: 56-362-9393; e-mail: stago@dfait-maeci.gc.ca; Website: www.dfait-maeci.gc.ca/santiago.
- **British Embassy:** Av. El Bosque Norte 0125, Casilla 72-D, Santiago; Tel: 56-2-370-4100; e-mail: chancery.santiago@fco.gov.uk; Website: www.britemb.cl.

HOSPITALS/DOCTORS:

Jose Joaquin Aguirre Hospital (1,700 beds); general medical/surgical facility; Clinica las Condes, Santiago. La Clinica Francesca, Concepcion. La Clinica Sanitorio Aleman, Concepcion.

Current Advisories and Health Risks

AIDS/HIV: Relatively low rates of HIV infection are reported, but the incidence is increasing, especially in urban areas. Seventy-two percent of cases of AIDS are currently due to homo- and bisexual transmission. Cases due to heterosexual transmission are increasing.

ACCIDENTS, ILLNESS, AND MEDICAL INSURANCE: Accidents and injuries are the leading cause of death among travelers younger than age 55 and are most often caused by motor vehicle and motorcycle crashes; drownings, aircraft crashes, homicides, and burns are less common causes. Important safety rules to follow are (1) Do not drive at night; (2) Do not rent a motorcycle, moped, bicycle, or motorbike, even if you are experienced; and (3) Don't swim alone, at night, or if intoxicated.

- Heart attacks cause most fatalities in older travelers.
- Infections cause only 1% of fatalities in overseas travelers, but, overall, infections are the most common cause of travel-related illness.

MEDICAL INSURANCE: Travelers are advised to obtain, before departure, supplemental travel health insurance with specific overseas coverage. The policy should provide for direct payment to the overseas hospital and/or physician at the time of service and include a medical evacuation benefit. The policy should also provide 24-hour hotline access to a multilingual assistance center that can help arrange and monitor delivery of medical care and determine if medical evacuation or air ambulance services are required.

ANIMAL HAZARDS: Animal hazards include black widow and brown widow spiders. There are no venomous land snakes on the mainland of Chile. Portuguese man-o'-war, sea wasps, and several species of stingrays are found in the country's coastal waters and are potential hazards to swimmers.

CHAGAS DISEASE: No cases reported since 1999. Nonetheless, travelers to rural areas should sleep under a mosquito net (well tucked in), sleep away from walls if in an adobe-style house, and spray sleeping quarters with an insecticide (such as RAID Flying Insect Spray) before retiring. Unscreened blood transfusions are also a potential source of infection. The rate of contaminated blood reported by Chilean blood banks is in the 1.9% to 6.5% range.

CHOLERA: This disease is active in this country, but the threat to tourists is very low. Cholera is an extremely rare disease in travelers from developed countries. Cholera vaccine is recommended primarily for people at high risk (e.g., relief workers) who work and live in highly endemic areas under less than adequate sanitary conditions.

- The oral cholera vaccine (Dukoral) provides up to 60% crossover protection against ETEC diarrhea.
- Many countries, including Canada, license an oral cholera vaccine. The oral vaccine is not available in the United States.
- Cholera vaccine is not "officially" required for entry into, or exit from, any country. Despite this, some countries, on occasion, require proof of cholera vaccination from travelers coming from cholera-infected countries. Anticipating such a situation, certain travelers may wish to carry a medical exemption letter from their health-care provider. Travel Medicine, Inc., recommends that travelers use the International Certificate of Vaccination (Yellow Card) for this purpose.

See Disease Risk Summary for South America for additional advisories on page 297.

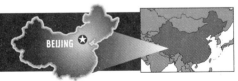

China, People's Republic of

BEIJING ✪

CAPITAL:
Beijing
EMBASSY (IN U.S.):
2201 Wisconsin Ave., NW, Washington, DC 20007
202-338-6688
www.china-embassy.org
GMT:
+8 hours
TELEPHONE COUNTRY CODE:
86

USADIRECT:

108-888 (northern China, Beijing)

108-11 (southern and central China, Shanghai, and Guangzhou regions)

ENTRY REQUIREMENTS

- **Passport/Visa:** Tourist visas are issued only after receipt of a confirmation letter from a Chinese tour agency or letter of invitation from a relative in China.
- **HIV Test:** Required for persons staying more than 6 months. Persons discovered to be carrying drugs for HIV treatment (antiretrovirals) may not be allowed entry into China. Narcotic-containing drugs, legally prescribed for personal use, may be prohibited.
- **Vaccinations:** A valid yellow fever vaccination certificate is required from all travelers arriving from infected areas.

EMBASSIES/CONSULATES*

- **U.S. Embassy:** 2 Xiu Shui Dong Jie, Beijing; Tel: 86-10-6532-3431, 6532-3831; Fax: 86-10-6532-4153, 6532-3178; Website: www.usembassy-china.org.cn.
- **Canadian Embassy:** 19 Dong Zhi Men Wai, Chao Yang District, Beijing; Tel: 86-10-6532-353; Fax: 86-10-6532-5544, e-mail: bejing-cs@dfait-maeci.gc.ca; Website: www.canada.org.cn.
- **British Embassy:** 11 Guang Hua Lu, Jian Guo Men Wai, Beijing 100600, Tel: 86-10-5192-4000, Fax: 86-10-6532-1937, e-mail: info@britishcentre.org.cn; Website: www.britishembassy.org.cn.

*Travelers should check with this country's embassy (or nearest consulate) in the U.S., Canada, or the UK for any changes in requirements.

HOSPITALS/DOCTORS:

- The quality of medical facilities is uneven. Competent, trained doctors and nurses are available in the major metropolitan centers, and more Western-style medical clinics for foreigners are opening. Chinese hospitals are often spartan and medical technology may not be up-to-date. Most hotels have their own clinics or access to doctors. Hotels will also help guests buy medicine or refer them to a hospital. Doctors and hospitals expect cash payment and may not accept checks or credit cards.
- The Sino-German Clinic, Beijing (located in the Landmark Building); staffed by Chinese, German, and U.S. physicians; open 24 hours.
- Medex Assistance Corp., Regus Office 19, Beijing Lufthansa Center, #50 Liangmaqiou Rd., Beijing. 86-10-6465-1264.
- Shanghai Center Clinic (World Link Medical Center facility), Shanghai Center, 1376, Nanjing Xi Lu, Suite 203, Shanghai. Tel: 86-21-6279-7688.
- The Shanghai Center Clinic is the preferred outpatient medical facility for travelers covered by International SOS.
- Hong Qiao Clinic (World Link Medical Center facility) in Mandarine City, 10 minutes from Shanghai Int'l. Airport; Tel: 86-21-6405-5788.
- Guangzhou International SOS Clinic, Guangdong Provincial Hospital of TCM, Guangzhou; Tel: 86-20-8735-1051.
- Hong Kong International SOS Clinic, 27/F Soundwill Plaza, 38 Russell Street, Causeway Bay, Hong Kong; Tel: 85-2-2528-9998.

- GlobalDoctor, Ltd., an Australian company, has opened clinics staffed by English-speaking doctors within the VIP wards of government-run hospitals in Chengdu, Nanjing, Beijing, Xian, and Shenzhen. GlobalDoctor contact number in Australia: Tel: 61-8-922-630-88.
- International SOS:
  - Beijing International (SOS) Clinic, Building "C" BITIC Leasing Center, No 1 North Road, Xing Fu San Cun, Chaoyang District, Beijing, P.R. China 100027; Alarm Center Tel: 76-10-6462-9100; Alarm Center Fax: 76-10-6462-9111; Clinic Tel: 76-10-6462-9112; Clinic Fax: 76-10-6462-9111.
  - International SOS China Ltd. - Guangzhou Room 1502, Dongshan Plaza, 69 Xian Lie Zhong Road, Guangzhou, 510095, P. R. China; Admin Tel: 7620-7732-6253; Admin Fax: 7620-7732-6417.
  - International SOS (HK) Ltd., 16/F World Trade Centre, 280 Gloucester Road, Causeway Bay, Hong Kong (SAR); Alarm Center Tel: 752-2528-9900; Alarm Center Fax: 752-2528-9933.
  - International SOS Nanjing Clinic, Nanjing Hilton Hotel, Ground floor, 319 Zhongshan Donglu, Nanjing, 210016 , P.R. China; Clinic Tel: 76-25-7480-2842; Clinic Fax: 76-25-7480-2843.
  - International SOS (China) Ltd. Shanghai Branch Unit E-G, 22/F Sun Tong Infoport Plaza, 55 Huaihai Road (W), Shanghai 200030, People's Republic of China; Alarm Center Tel: 76-21-6295-0099; Alarm Center Fax: 76-21-5298-9096.
  - Shekou International SOS Clinic, G/F CMIT Building, 9 Industrial Road South, Shekou, Shenzhen 51/8067, P.R. China; Clinic Tel: 76-755-2669-3667; Clinic Fax: 76-755-2667-4780.
  - Tianjin International SOS Clinic, Sheraton Tianjin Hotel, Zi Jin Shan Road, He Xi District, Tianjin 300074, People's Republic of China; Clinic Tel: 7622-2352-0143; Clinic Fax: 7622-2352-0145.

Current Advisories and Health Risks

AIDS/HIV: The spread of HIV is an increasingly serious public health problem. Yunnan Province has the highest incidence. Injecting drug users account for 60% to 70% of those infected countrywide.

ACCIDENTS: Road accidents and drowning are the most common causes of fatalities in travelers. Important safety rules to follow are (1) Do not drive at night; (2) Do not rent a motorcycle, moped, bicycle, or motorbike, even if you are experienced; and (3) Do not swim alone, at night, or if intoxicated.

ACUTE MOUNTAIN SICKNESS (AMS): Risk occurs at elevations above 8,000 feet. Acetozolamide (Diamox) prophylaxis should be considered when traveling to Tibet and to high-altitude destinations in the Qinghai, Xinjiang, Sichuan, Yannan, and Gansu Provinces. Immediate descent is the best treatment for more severe AMS.

AIR POLLUTION: Severe air pollution exists in Beijing and other large industrial cities. Pollutants include windblown dust and dirt, soot from coal-burning stoves and furnaces, and exhaust from motor vehicles. Because of the widespread burning of soft coal, especially in cities with heavy industry, there is the potential for exacerbation of respiratory illnesses such as bronchitis, asthma, and emphysema.

CHOLERA: This disease is reported active in this country, but the threat to tourists is very low. Cholera vaccine is recommended primarily for people at high risk (e.g., relief workers) who work and live in highly endemic areas under less than adequate sanitary conditions. Many countries, including Canada, license an oral cholera vaccine. The oral vaccine is not available in the United States.

DENGUE FEVER: Dengue occurs as frequent, often widespread, outbreaks. The incidence is highest in southeastern China, south of 42 degrees north latitude. Elevated risk occurs in coastal urban areas below 1,500 meters elevation. Most disease transmission occurs during the summer months; in the tropical provinces; however, the transmission period extends from March through November. The *Aedes* mosquitoes, which transmit dengue, are daytime biters. Prevention of dengue fever consists of taking protective measures against mosquito bites.

ECHINOCOCCOSIS: Human alveolar hydatid disease, a potentially fatal disease caused by larvae of the canine tapeworm *Echinococcus multilocularis*, is common throughout western and northwestern China. This disease is caused by the larval stage of the fox tapeworm and is spread to humans by close contact with infected domesticated dogs and cats or by contact with fox/canine feces.

FILARIASIS: Both the Bancroftian and Malayan forms are reported in the southwestern provinces. Travelers to these areas should take measures to prevent mosquito bites.

HELMINTHIC (WORM) DISEASES: Moderately to highly endemic in rural and urban areas. Diseases caused by soil-transmitted helminths (hookworm disease, strongyloidiasis) can be prevented by wearing shoes and not walking barefoot outdoors. Food-transmitted roundworm infections (ascariasis, trichuriasis) can be prevented by washing salads and/or vegetables or thoroughly cooking food to destroy infective eggs. Lung fluke and liver fluke disease (paragonimiasis, clonorchiasis) can be prevented by not eating raw freshwater crabs, crayfish, or fish. Fasciolopsiasis (large intestinal fluke disease) and fascioliasis (sheep liver fluke disease) can be prevented by not eating undercooked or raw water plants, such as watercress and other aquatic vegetables. Anisakiasis can be avoided by not eating raw saltwater fish, including raw octopus and squid; capillariasis can be prevented by avoiding raw or undercooked freshwater fish.

HEPATITIS: There is a high risk of hepatitis A in China and all nonimmune travelers should receive hepatitis A vaccine. Hepatitis E is a leading cause of sporadic acute viral hepatitis in China. A high incidence is reported in rural areas. Transmission is primarily by contaminated drinking water. All travelers, especially in rural areas, should drink only boiled, bottled, or chemically treated water. The hepatitis B carrier rate in the general population is estimated at 10%, but the incidence may be higher. In Guangdong Province, the hepatitis B virus (HBV) may infect as many as 75% of the populace. Hepatitis B is spread by infected blood, contaminated needles, and unprotected sex. Vaccination is recommended for long-stay travelers (longer than 3 months); those who may be at occupational or social risk, and anybody desiring maximal protection.

INFLUENZA: Influenza is transmitted November through March in temperate areas. Vaccination is recommended for travelers to China.

JAPANESE ENCEPHALITIS (JE): This mosquito-transmitted disease is present in all regions, except in Qinghai Province, Xinjiang Province, and Tibet (Xizang). The risk of JE is greatest in rural pig-breeding agricultural areas of the central and eastern provinces, especially during the warm, rainy months from May to September. Risk of JE is year-round in the tropical southern provinces. There is low risk of transmission in urban areas due to the relative absence of mosquitoes. Vaccination against Japanese encephalitis is recommended for travelers who will be staying in rural-agricultural endemic areas for extended periods (more than 3 to 4 weeks).

LEISHMANIASIS: Visceral leishmaniasis (kala-azar) occurs in the temperate central and northeastern provinces, mainly Gansu, Shaanxi, Shanxi, Shandong and Sichuan Provinces, and Xinjiang and Nei Mongol Autonomous Regions. Most cases reported are from Gansu Province. Risk of disease transmission is elevated from May through October, when sand flies are more active. Cutaneous leishmaniasis has been reported from the Xinjiang Autonomous Region. All travelers to these areas should avoid sand fly bites when visiting these areas.

LYME DISEASE: Lyme disease occurs mostly in northern and northeastern provinces through the warmer months. Sporadic cases are reported from other forested regions. Measures to prevent tick bites are recommended.

MALARIA: The highest prevalence of malaria in China is reported in the rural east and south. Seven provinces (Guangdong, Guizhou, Yunnan, Guangxi, Hainin, Sichuan, and Fujian) account for 76% of all cases. Less than 1% of cases are reported from the north and northeast.

- Urban and densely populated areas are normally malaria free. Travelers to cities and popular tourist areas, including Yangtze River cruises, are not at risk and do not need chemoprophylaxis.
- Chloroquine-resistant falciparum malaria is present only on Hainan Island, in Yunnan Province and sporadically in Guangxi Province. These areas are in the southwest of China and the risk is minimal in large cities.
- Vivax malaria alone occurs in a few isolated areas in the "flood" plains of the Yangtze (Chang Jiang) and Yellow (Huang He) rivers—specifically within the provinces of Fujian, Guangxi, Guizhou, Sichuan, and Xizang (along the valley of the Zangbo river). Isolated cases occasionally occur in other parts of the country.

• Prevention—Prophylaxis with atovaquone/proguanil (Malarone), mefloquine (Lariam), or doxycycline is recommended in Hainin, Yunnan, and Guangxi Provinces. Chloroquine is recommended in all other risk areas. All travelers should take measures to prevent evening and nighttime mosquito bites.

MENINGITIS: An outbreak of Group C meningococcal meningitis was reported in 11 cities in Anhui Province in 2005. Students 13 to 18 years of age were predominantly affected. In the past, most cases of meningococcal disease in China were caused by serogroup A. Travelers to this region should consider vaccination if they expect prolonged close contact with the local population.

RABIES: A higher than average incidence of rabies is reported in urban and rural areas, with stray dogs the main threat. All animal bites or scratches, especially from a dog, should be taken seriously, and immediate medical attention sought. Rabies vaccination may be required. Although rabies is rare among tourists, there is risk. No one should pet or pick up any stray animals. All children should be warned to avoid contact with unknown animals. Rabies vaccine is recommended for travel longer than 3 months, and for shorter stays for travelers who plan to venture off the usual tourist routes, where they may be more exposed to the stray dog population.

SCHISTOSOMIASIS: Year-round risk occurs in southern tropical areas and June through August in temperate areas. Schistosomiasis is widespread south of 35 degrees north latitude, including the provinces of Anhui, Hubei, Jiangsu, Hunan, Jiangxi, Sichuan, Yunnan, and Zhejiang. Major endemic areas include the Yangtze River Valley, including tributaries and adjacent lakes. All travelers should avoid swimming, wading, or bathing in freshwater lakes, ponds, or streams.

SCRUB TYPHUS: Year-round incidence in warmer southern areas. Scrub typhus is transmitted by mites; insect-bite protection is recommended.

TRAVELERS' DIARRHEA: Moderate to high risk. In urban and resort areas, most hotels have generally safe restaurants and potable water. Travelers should observe food and drink safety precautions and drink only boiled, bottled, or chemically treated water and consume only well-cooked food. Raw fish and shellfish, and undercooked aquatic plants (e.g., watercress salad), should be avoided. A quinolone antibiotic, combined with loperamide (Imodium), is recommended for the treatment of acute diarrhea. Persistent diarrhea may be due to a parasitic disease such as giardiasis, amebiasis, or cryptosporidiosis.

TUBERCULOSIS: Tuberculosis is a major public health problem in this country. Travelers planning an extended stay should have a pre-departure TB skin test (PPD test) and be retested after leaving this country.

TYPHOID FEVER: Typhoid vaccine is recommended for those traveling off the usual tourist routes, visiting friends or relatives, and long-stay visitors. Because the typhoid vaccines are only 60% to 70% effective, food and drink precautions should also be observed.

OTHER DISEASES/HAZARDS: Anthrax (mostly cutaneous; associated with animal contact); brucellosis, Crimean-Congo; hemorrhagic fever (low endemicity; in Xinjiang Province only); Chikungunya fever, leptospirosis (periodic outbreaks countrywide; highest incidence in Yunnan Province); Lyme disease (human cases reported from Henan, Jiangsu, Fujian, Anhui, and Heilomgiang Provinces, and Xinjiang Autonomous Region); melioidosis (endemic in Guangdong and Hainin Provinces, and Guangxi Autonomous Region; risk elevated June through August); plague (reported in Gansu, Qinghai, and Yunnan Provinces and Nei Mongol and Xinjiang, and Xizang Autonomous Regions); Russian spring-summer encephalitis (presumably occurs in northern China, especially Inner Mongolia); Siberian tick typhus; tuberculosis (highly endemic); trachoma (widespread); and murine and epidemic (louse-borne) typhus (low risk).

Christmas Island
(Australia)

CAPITAL:
The Settlement
EMBASSY (IN U.S.):
202-638-3800
1-800-874-5100
GMT:
+7 hours
TELEPHONE COUNTRY CODE:
6724
USADIRECT:
None
ENTRY REQUIREMENTS
• **Passport/Visa:** A passport is required.
• **Vaccinations:** Same requirements as for Australia.
• **HIV Test:** Same requirements as for Australia.
EMBASSIES/CONSULATES:
Neither the United States, Canada, nor the United Kingdom has an embassy on the Christmas Island. A territory of Australia, Christmas Island is located in the Indian Ocean, about 870 miles (1,400 km) northwest of Australia. The climate is tropical, and temperatures average 81°F (27°C) throughout the year.
HOSPITALS/DOCTORS:
Adequate medical care is available in The Settlement in several small hospitals. Given the remote location, adequate evacuation coverage for all travelers is a high priority. In the event of serious medical conditions, every effort should be made to go to Australia.

Current Advisories and Health Risks

ACCIDENTS, ILLNESS, AND MEDICAL INSURANCE

- Accidents and injuries are the leading cause of death among travelers younger than age 55 and are most often caused by motor vehicle and motorcycle crashes; drownings, aircraft crashes, homicides, and burns are less common causes.
- Heart attacks cause most fatalities in older travelers.
- Infections cause only 1% of fatalities in overseas travelers, but, overall, infections are the most common cause of travel-related illness.
- Travelers are advised to obtain, before departure, supplemental travel health insurance with specific overseas coverage. The policy should provide for direct payment to the overseas hospital and/or physician at the time of service and include a medical evacuation benefit. The policy should also provide 24-hour hotline access to a multilingual assistance center that can help arrange and monitor delivery of medical care and determine if medical evacuation or air ambulance services are required.

DENGUE FEVER: This disease is present. Travelers should take protective measures against mosquito bites.

HEPATITIS: Nonimmune travelers should receive hepatitis A vaccine. Vaccination against hepatitis B should be considered for stays longer than 3 months and by short-term travelers desiring maximal protection. Travelers should be aware that hepatitis B can be transmitted by unsafe sex and the use of contaminated needles and syringes.

INFLUENZA: Influenza is transmitted year-round in the tropics. The flu vaccine is recommended for all travelers older than age 50; all travelers with chronic disease or a weakened immune system; travelers of any age wishing to decrease the risk of this illness; pregnant women after the first trimester.

MALARIA: No risk.

MARINE HAZARDS

- Swimming-related hazards include jellyfish, spiny sea urchins, and coral.
- Ciguatera poisoning is prevalent and can result from eating coral reef fish such as grouper, snapper, sea bass, jack, and barracuda. The ciguatoxin is not destroyed by cooking.

TRAVELERS' DIARRHEA: Low risk. A quinolone antibiotic, combined with loperamide (Imodium), is recommended for the treatment of diarrhea.

Colombia

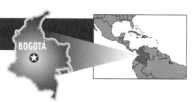

CAPITAL:
Bogotá
EMBASSY (IN U.S.):
202-387-8338

ENTRY REQUIREMENTS

- **Passport/Visa:** A visa is required for stays exceeding 30 days. All travelers should read the most recent State Department Travel Warning for this country. Passport required.
- **HIV Test:** Not required.
- **Vaccinations:** No vaccinations are required for entry.

EMBASSIES/CONSULATES

- **U.S. Embassy:** Avenida El Dorado and Carrera 50, Bogotá. Tel: 57-1-315-0811 during business hours or 315-2109/2110 for emergencies during nonbusiness hours; Fax: 57-1-315-2196/2197; Website: usembassy.state.gov/bogota.

  U.S. Consulate: Calle 77B, No. 57-141, Centro Empresarial Las Americas, Barranquilla, Atlantico. Tel: 57-5-353-2001; Fax: 5-353-5216; e-mail: conagent@metrotel.net.co.
- **Canadian Embassy:** Cra. 7, No. 115-3, Bogotá; Tel: 57-1-657-9800; Fax: 57-1-657-9912; e-mail: bgota@dfait-maeci.gc.ca. Website: www.dfait-maeci.gc.ca/bogota.
- **British Embassy:** Edificio ING Barings, Carrera 9 No 76-49 Piso 9, Bogotá; Tel: 57-1-326-8300; e-mail: britain@cable.net.co.

HOSPITALS/DOCTORS:

- San Ignacio University Hospital, Santafé de Bogotá, Colombia. Tel: 57-1-288-8188. Private hospital (264 beds) affiliated with Javeriana University School of Medicine. All specialties, including major trauma.
- Fundacion Santa Fe de; Calle 116 #9-02, Santafé de Bogotá; general hospital (170 beds) with good reputation; Tel: 57-1-629-0766. 24-hour emergency services; renal dialysis; limited trauma capability.

Current Advisories and Health Risks

AIDS/HIV: HIV prevalence estimated at up to 41% of homosexual males and 30% of prostitutes. Heterosexual contacts now responsible for spreading more cases than homosexual contacts.

ACUTE MOUNTAIN SICKNESS (AMS): Risk is present for those arriving in Bogotá (altitude 2,600 meters) or traveling to the Central Highlands where the elevation exceeds 3,000 meters in many areas. Travelers should consider acetazolamide prophylaxis and gradual acclimatization. The best treatment of moderate-to-severe AMS is immediate descent to a lower altitude.

BARTONELLOSIS (OROYA FEVER): This severe bacterial disease is transmitted by sand flies between 800 and 3,000 meters elevation in the southwestern areas. Treatment of the first phase of the disease (fever and anemia phase) is effective with chloramphenicol, penicillin, or tetracycline. The second phase (skin lesion phase) is best treated with rifampin or streptomycin. Travelers are advised to take insect-bite prevention measures to prevent sand fly bites.

CHAGAS DISEASE: Widely distributed below 2,700 meters elevation in northern and western areas (primarily west of the eastern Andean foothills). Elevated risk in Norte de Santander Department. Risk of transmission occurs primarily in those rural-agricultural areas where there are adobe-style huts and houses that often harbor the night-biting triatomid (assassin) bugs. Travelers sleeping in such structures should take precautions against nighttime bites.

CHOLERA: Sporadic cases of this disease occur. Cholera, however, is an extremely rare disease in international travelers from developed countries, such as the United States and Canada. Cholera vaccine (no longer available in the United States) is recommended primarily for travelers at high risk who work and live in highly endemic areas under less than adequate sanitary conditions.

• The oral cholera vaccine (Dukoral) provides up to 60% crossover protection against ETEC diarrhea.

Cholera vaccine is not "officially" required for entry into, or exit from, any country. Despite this, some countries, on occasion, require proof of cholera immunization from travelers coming from cholera-infected countries. Anticipating such a situation, travelers may wish to carry a medical exemption letter from their health-care provider. If possible, it is advisable to contact the embassy or consulate at the destination country to confirm the requirement for cholera vaccination (if any) and the acceptability of a medical exemption letter.

DENGUE FEVER: Year-round risk (elevated during local rainy seasons) in widely scattered urban and periurban areas below 1,800 meters elevation. Risk may be elevated in the northern, north-central (Magdalena River Valley), and western areas. All travelers are advised to take measures to prevent mosquito bites.

HEPATITIS: All nonimmune travelers should receive hepatitis A vaccine before visiting this country. The hepatitis B carrier rate in the general population is estimated to be 1.3% and as high as 20% in high-risk groups (e.g., prostitutes, drug addicts) and in the Amazon Basin. Hepatitis B vaccine is recommended for stays longer than 3 months and for short-term travelers wanting increased protection. Travelers should be aware that the risk of hepatitis B is increased by unsafe sex and the use of unsterile needles and syringes.

INFLUENZA: Influenza is transmitted year-round in the tropics. The flu vaccine is recommended for all travelers older than age 50; all travelers with any chronic or immuno-compromising conditions; travelers of any age wishing to decrease the risk of this illness; pregnant women after the first trimester.

LEISHMANIASIS: Risk of cutaneous leishmaniasis (the cause of 95% of cases) is widely distributed in many jungle and forested highland areas up to 1,500 meters elevation. Many cases are reported in the Pacific coastal region. Visceral leishmaniasis risk occurs below 900 meters elevation in the valleys of the Magdalena River and its tributaries in southern Cundinamarca County. All travelers should take measures to prevent insect (sand fly) bites.

MALARIA: There is no risk of malaria in Bogotá Department, the major urban areas, and the islands of San Andres and Providencia. Elsewhere, this disease is highly endemic countrywide year-round in rural areas below 800 meters elevation. Malaria activity varies markedly among regions and from year to year within specific areas. Risk may be elevated during and immediately following local rainy seasons. Vivax malaria accounts for 60% of cases overall; the remainder are falciparum malaria. (In some Pacific coastal areas, however, falciparum accounts for 98% of cases.) Chloroquine-resistant falciparum malaria is reported in all malarious areas. In addition, there are now reports of chloroquine-resistant vivax malaria. Unconfirmed mefloquine resistance has been reported in the Amazonian region. Atovaquone/proguanil (Malarone), mefloquine (Lariam), or doxycycline prophylaxis is recommended when traveling to malaria risk areas.

RABIES: Rabies is a relatively minor health threat in this country, but there is risk. Human rabies is usually transmitted by dog bites, but bats also transmit the disease. Rabies vaccine should be considered for stays of longer than 3 months or for shorter stays if traveling to locations more than 24 hours from a reliable source of postexposure rabies vaccine. All animal bites or scratches while in this country should be medically evaluated.

ROCKY MOUNTAIN SPOTTED FEVER: This rickettsial disease also occurs outside the United States.

OTHER DISEASES/HAZARDS: Brucellosis (increased incidence in Uraba region of Antioquia Department), coccidiomycosis, cysticercosis, echinococcosis, filariasis (mosquito-borne; a small focus is reported near Cartegena), leptospirosis, mansonellosis (black fly-borne; endemic areas limited to riverine valleys in extreme eastern and southern Colombia), onchocerciasis (black fly-borne; endemic in the south-central Pacific coastal area), paragonimiasis (lung fluke disease; transmitted by infected raw freshwater crabs or crayfish), tuberculosis (a serious public health problem), viral encephalitis (mosquito-transmitted), and strongyloidiasis and other helminthic infections are reported. Animal hazards include snakes (vipers, coral snakes), centipedes, scorpions, and spiders (black widow, brown recluse, banana, wolf). Caimans and crocodiles are abundant and electric eels and poisonous frogs are found in the country's freshwaters. Pumas, jaguars, wild boar, and large tropical rodents also occur in Colombia. Sea wasps, Portuguese man-of-war, sea wasps, and stingrays are found in the coastal waters of Colombia and could be a hazard to swimmers.

Comoros Islands

★ MORONI

CAPITAL:
Moroni
EMBASSY (IN U.S.):
212-972-8010
GMT:
+3 hours
TELEPHONE COUNTRY CODE:
269
USADIRECT:
None
ENTRY REQUIREMENTS
- **Passport/Visa:** Passport and onward/return ticket required. For specific requirements, consult the Federal and Islamic Republic of Comoros, 336 East 45th St., 2nd Floor, New York, NY 10017; Tel: 212-972-8010.
- **HIV Test:** Not required.
- **Vaccinations:** None required.

EMBASSIES/CONSULATES
- **U.S. Embassy:** None.
- **Canadian Embassy:** Accredited to the Canadian High Commission in Tanzania; Tel: 225-22-211-2831/2/3/4.
- **British Embassy:** Accredited to British Embassy in Madagascar. Lot II 164 Ter, Alarobia – Amboniloha, BP 167, Antananarivo 101; Tel: 261-20-22-49378/79/80; Fax: 261-20-22-49381; e-mail: ukembant@simicro.mg

HOSPITALS/DOCTORS:
Medical care in the Comoros Islands is substandard. Travelers are advised to obtain, before departure, supplemental travel health insurance with specific overseas coverage. The policy should provide for direct payment to the overseas hospital and/or physician at the time of service and include a medical evacuation benefit.

Current Advisories and Health Risks

MALARIA: Risk of falciparum malaria is present countrywide, including urban areas. Prophylaxis with atovaquone/proguanil (Malarone), mefloquine (Lariam), or doxycycline is recommended. All travelers should take measures to prevent mosquito bites.

See Disease Risk Summary for sub-Saharan Africa for additional health advisories.

Congo

CAPITAL:
Brazzaville

EMBASSY (IN U.S.):
202-726-0825

GMT:
+1 hour

TELEPHONE COUNTRY CODE:
242

USADIRECT:
None

ENTRY REQUIREMENTS

- **Passport/Visa:** Valid passport and visa are required. Return or onward ticket required.
- **HIV Test:** Not required.
- **Vaccinations:** A yellow fever vaccination certificate is required from all travelers older than 1 year of age arriving from all countries.

EMBASSIES/CONSULATES

- **U.S. Embassy:** Brazzaville. Avenue Amilcar Cabral; Tel: 832-070/832-624.
- **Canadian Embassy:** Zaire. Tel: [243] (12) 27551.
- **British Embassy:** 83 Avenue du Roi Baudouin, Kinshasa; Tel: 243-98169100, 98169111, 98169200; Fax: 243-8846102; e-mail: ambrit@ic.cd.

HOSPITALS/DOCTORS

- Centre Medical Guenin, Pointe-Noire. Small (9 bed) facility that offers limited care. Emergency services are available 24 hours daily.
- Brazzaville General Hospital (900 beds); general medical services.
- Travelers should contact the U.S. Embassy for physician referral.

Current Advisories and Health Risks

AIDS/HIV: Massive population mobility has increased the vulnerability to HIV/AIDS throughout the subregion; the vulnerability of adolescent girls and women has also increased, in large part due to sexual and gender-based violence. In general, adults older than 30 years have the highest infection rate: nearly 10% of men 35 to 49 years old, and 7% of women 25 to 39 years old, are living with the disease.

AFRICAN SLEEPING SICKNESS (TRYPANOSOMIASIS): This disease is currently active. Major risk areas include the southern savanna of Niari and Bouenza Regions, along the Congo River north of Brazzaville to north of Betou, and in the northwest (Etoumbi vicinity) and the extreme southwest of Cuvette Region (Okoyo vicinity); risk also occurs along the Lefini River. All travelers to these regions should take measures to prevent insect (tsetse fly) bites.

ANIMAL HAZARDS: Animal hazards include snakes (mambas, adders, vipers, cobras), centipedes, scorpions, and black widow spiders.

CHOLERA: Although this disease is active in this country, the threat to tourists is very low. Cholera is an extremely rare disease in travelers from developed countries. Cholera vaccine is recommended primarily for people at high risk (e.g., relief workers) who work and live in highly endemic areas under less than adequate sanitary conditions. Many countries, including Canada, license an oral cholera vaccine. The oral vaccine is not available in the United States.

EBOLA VIRUS HEMORRHAGIC FEVER: Sporadic outbreaks occur. The Ebola virus is acquired by direct contact with the body fluids or secretions of infected patients. It is not transmitted by insect bites.

MARBURG VIRUS HEMORRHAGIC FEVER: Outbreaks of Marburg hemorrhagic fever were reported in 1998. Although the geographic area to which the virus is native is unknown, this area appears to include at least parts of Uganda and Western Kenya, and perhaps Zimbabwe. As with the Ebola virus, the actual animal host for Marburg virus remains a mystery. Humans who become ill can spread the disease, especially in a setting of close contact, such as in a hospital.

HEPATITIS: All susceptible travelers should receive hepatitis A vaccine. The hepatitis B carrier rate in the general population is estimated as high as 17.5%. Hepatitis B is spread by infected blood, contaminated needles, and unsafe sex. Vaccination is recommended for stays longer than 3 months; for anyone at occupational or social risk; for any traveler desiring maximal protection. The risk of illness or injury during travel cannot be predicted and some experts believe that *all* travelers should be immunized against hepatitis B because of the risk of receiving a medical injection with an unsterile needle or syringe.

INFLUENZA: Influenza is transmitted year-round in the tropics. The flu vaccine is recommended for all travelers.

LOIASIS: Areas in the rain forest and villages in the Chaillu mountains are highly endemic. Travelers should take personal protection measures against biting deer flies.

MALARIA: Risk is present year-round countrywide, including urban areas. Risk is elevated during and just after the rainy season—April through October north of the equator and October through May south of the equator. Prophylaxis with atovaquone/proguanil (Malarone), mefloquine (Lariam), or doxycycline is recommended. All travelers should take measures to prevent evening and nighttime mosquito bites.

ONCHOCERCIASIS: High prevalence in two southwestern areas: the Djoue River basin and the bank region of the Congo River. Travelers should take personal protection measures against insect (black fly) bites.

SCHISTOSOMIASIS: Risk of urinary schistosomiasis is present in the southwestern regions of Bouenza, Niari, and Kouilou, as well as the Brazzaville vicinity. Less risk occurs in the northern areas of the country. Travelers should avoid swimming, bathing, or wading in freshwater lakes, ponds, or streams.

TRAVELERS' DIARRHEA: High risk. Rural villages and towns obtain water from untreated sources. Travelers should observe all food and drink safety precautions. A quinolone antibiotic, combined with loperamide (Imodium), is recommended for the treatment of acute diarrhea. Persistent diarrhea may be due to a parasitic disease such as giardiasis, amebiasis, or cryptosporidiosis.

TUBERCULOSIS: Tuberculosis (TB) is a major health problem in this country. Travelers planning an extended stay should have a pre-departure TB skin test (PPD test) and be retested after returning from this country.

TYPHOID FEVER: Typhoid vaccine is recommended for those traveling off the usual tourist routes, those visiting friends or relatives, and for long-stay visitors. Because the typhoid vaccines are only 60% to 70% effective, safe food and drink selection remains important.

YELLOW FEVER: Sporadic outbreaks occur. A *yellow fever vaccination certificate is required* to enter this country.

OTHER DISEASES/HAZARDS: Brucellosis (from consumption of raw dairy products or occupational exposure), Chikungunya fever (mosquito-transmitted; cyclic outbreaks occur regionally), mansonellosis (mosquito-borne form of filariasis), leprosy, leptospirosis, paragonimiasis (from eating raw crabs), human monkeypox, rabies, toxoplasmosis, tuberculosis (a major health problem), and intestinal helminths (very common).

Cook Islands (New Zealand)

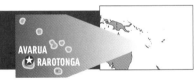

CAPITAL:
Avarua, Rarotonga
EMBASSY (IN U.S.):
202-328-6628
GMT:
−10 hours
TELEPHONE COUNTRY CODE:
682
USADIRECT:
09-111

ENTRY REQUIREMENTS

- **Passport/Visa:** Passport, proof of sufficient funds, and onward/return ticket required. Visa not needed for visit up to 31 days. For longer stays and further information, contact the Consulate for the Cook Islands, Kamehameha Schools, #16, Kapalama Heights, Honolulu, HI 96817 (808-847-6377). The Cook Islands are self-governing in free association with New Zealand; the Cook Islands are fully responsible for internal affairs; New Zealand retains responsibility for external affairs and defense.
- **HIV Test:** Not required.
- **Vaccinations:** None required.

EMBASSIES/CONSULATES:

There are no local embassies. The U.S. Embassy in Wellington, New Zealand, has jurisdiction for this region. Cook Island is accredited to the Canadian Embassy in Sydney, Australia.

HOSPITALS/DOCTORS:

Medical care in the Cook Islands is adequate for most conditions, but transport among islands is a problem. In the event of serious accident or injury, travelers should consider evacuation to a country with more advanced medical facilities. Travelers are advised to obtain supplemental travel health insurance with specific overseas coverage. The policy should provide for direct payment to the overseas hospital and/or physician at the time of service and include a medical evacuation benefit.

- Avarua Hospital/Rarotonga General Hospital, Avarua; Tel: 22-664
- Mauke Hospital, Mauke, Southern Cook Islands; Tel: 35-664

Hospitals on other islands (minimal standard of care):

- Aitutaki Hospital, Aitutaki Tel: 31-041
- Mangaia Hospital, Mangaia Tel: 34-027
- Atiu Hospital, Atiu Tel: 33-664

Current Advisories and Health Risks

MALARIA: There is no risk of malaria in the Cook Islands.

See Disease Risk Summary for Oceania on page 315.

Costa Rica

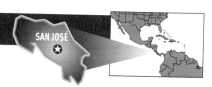

CAPITAL:
San José

EMBASSY (IN U.S.): (CONSULAR SEC.):
202-328-6628

GMT:
−6 hours

TELEPHONE COUNTRY CODE:
506

0-800-011-4114

ENTRY REQUIREMENTS*

- **Passport/Visa:** A visa is not required for travelers holding U.S. or Canadian passports.
- **HIV Test:** Testing required of travelers staying more than 90 days.
- **Vaccinations:** No vaccinations are required to enter this country.

*Travelers should check with this country's embassy (or a consulate) in the United States, Canada, or the United Kingdom for any changes in these requirements.

EMBASSIES/CONSULATES

- **U.S. Embassy:** Pavas, San José. Tel: 506-220-3050; usembassy.or.cr.
- **Canadian Embassy:** Oficentro La Sabana, Building No. 5, Centro Colon, San José, Tel: 506-296-4149; Fax: 506-296-4270; e-mail: sjose@dfait-maeci.gc.ca; Website: www.dfait-maeci.gc.ca/sanjose
- **British Embassy:** Apartado 815, Edificio Centro Colon (11th Floor), San José 1007; Tel: 506-258-2025; Fax: 506-233-9938; e-mail: britemb@racsa.co.cr; Website: www.britishembassycr.com.

HOSPITALS/DOCTORS:

- Hospital Clinica Biblica; private hospital with extensive medical/surgical capabilities, including cardiac surgery, 24-hour emergency department, and ambulance service. CT and MRI are now available. Hospital-based physician group is 90% English-speaking; many staff physicians have received advanced training in the United States. Hospital Clinica Biblica is used by embassy personnel, tourists, and expatriates. Address: Calle Central and Ave. 14.
- Dr. Max Gutreiman Goldberg, Hospital San José CIMA
- Autopista Prospero Fernandez (500 meters west of the toll station), Torre Medica, 4th Floor, Suite 4, San José
- Dr. Roberto Herrera Guido (pediatrics), Hospital San José CIMA, Autopista Prospero Fernandez, Torre Medica, San José.

Current Advisories and Health Risks

CHOLERA: Sporadic cases of this disease occur. Cholera, however, is an extremely rare disease in travelers from developed countries. Cholera vaccine is recommended only for those at high risk who work and live in highly endemic areas under less than adequate sanitary conditions.

DENGUE FEVER: Year-round risk, countrywide, below 1,300 meters elevation in urbanized areas. Risk is elevated in coastal provinces. To prevent dengue travelers should take measures to prevent mosquito bites.

HEPATITIS: Hepatitis A vaccine is recommended for all nonimmune travelers. The hepatitis B carrier rate in the population is less than 1%. Hepatitis B is spread by infected blood, contaminated needles, and unprotected sex. Vaccination is recommended for stays longer than 3 months; for those at occupational or social risk; for anybody desiring maximal protection.

INFLUENZA: Influenza is transmitted year-round in the tropics. The flu vaccine is recommended for all travelers.

LEISHMANIASIS: The potential for transmission of cutaneous leishmaniasis is present in most rural forested areas below 800 meters elevation. There is increased transmission from May through July. Incidence is highest in areas bordering Panama. Travelers must take precautions against insect (sand fly) bites.

LEPTOSPIROSIS: Risk has been associated with sports activities, such as white-water rafting, where there is exposure to contaminated water in flooded rivers.

MALARIA: Low risk occurs year-round in rural areas below 500 meters elevation. There is no risk in the central highlands (Cartago and San José Provinces). Risk is increased during, and just after, the rainy season, May through November, peaking during September and October. Risk may be elevated in the Atlantic coastal lowlands and along the northern border with Nicaragua. Seventy percent of malaria cases are reported from Limon Province on the Atlantic coast. Vivax malaria accounts for more than 97% of cases. No cases of drug-resistant falciparum malaria have been reported. Chloroquine prophylaxis is not routinely recommended for tourists going to Costa Rica but should be considered by anyone staying overnight near the border with Nicaragua. Measures to prevent mosquito bites should be taken, especially from dusk to dawn.

TRAVELERS' DIARRHEA: Low risk in most areas. The tap water in San José and major resorts is potable. A quinolone antibiotic is recommended for the treatment of acute diarrhea. Persistent diarrhea may be due to a parasitic infection such as giardiasis, amebiasis, or cryptosporidiosis.

TYPHOID FEVER: Typhoid vaccine is recommended for those traveling off the usual tourist routes, those visiting friends or relatives, and for long-stay visitors. Because the typhoid vaccines are only 60% to 70% effective, safe food and drink selection remains important.

YELLOW FEVER: Costa Rica is in the Yellow Fever Endemic Zone, but this disease is not active. Vaccination not required or recommended.

OTHER DISEASES/HAZARDS: Abdominal angiostrongyliasis, brucellosis, Chagas disease (occurs sporadically in rural areas of Alajuela, Guanacaste, Heredia, and San José Provinces at elevations below 1,300 meters, but is not considered a major public health problem), cysticercosis, filariasis (transmitted by black flies; endemic near Puerto Limon), fascioliasis (liver fluke disease; from contaminated water plants), filariasis (mosquito-transmitted; reported in Puerto Limon), paragonimiasis (lung fluke disease; from ingestion of raw freshwater crabs or crayfish), rabies (very low risk), tick-borne rickettsioses (Rocky Mountain spotted fever reported from Limon Province; tick-borne relapsing fever), Venezuelan equine encephalitis, and strongyloidiasis and other helminthic infections are reported.

Croatia

CAPITAL:
Zagreb
EMBASSY (IN U.S.):
202-588-5899
GMT:
+1 hour
TELEPHONE COUNTRY CODE:
385
USADIRECT:
0-800-220-111
ENTRY REQUIREMENTS
- **Passport/Visa:** Passport required. Visa not required for tourist/business stay of up to 90 days. For stays over 3 months, a visa is required and should be obtained in advance. For additional information, consult the Embassy of Croatia, 2343 Massachusetts Ave., NW, Washington, DC 20008 (202-588-8933)
- **HIV Test:** Not required.
- **Vaccinations:** None required.

EMBASSIES/CONSULATES
- **U.S. Embassy:** Andrije Hebranga 2, Zagreb; Tel: 1-455-5500; Website: www.usembassy.hr.
- **Canadian Embassy:** Prilaz Gjure Dezelica 4, Zagreb; Tel: 1-488-1200, 488-1211; Fax: 1-488-1230; e-mail: zagrb@dfait-maeci.gc.ca.
- **British Embassy:** UI Ivana Lucica 4, 10000 Zagreb; Tel: 385-1-600-9100; Fax: 385-1-600-9111; e-mail: british.embassyzagreb@fco.gov.uk.

HOSPITALS/DOCTORS:
Health facilities in Croatia, although generally of Western caliber, are under severe strain. Some medicines are in short supply. Doctors and hospitals may expect immediate cash payment for health services. Travelers to Croatia are advised to obtain supplemental travel health insurance with specific overseas coverage. The policy should provide for direct payment to the overseas hospital and/or physician at the time of service and include a medical evacuation benefit. The U.S. Embassy in Zagreb mauntains a referral list of doctors and hospitals. Go to www.mdtravelhealth.com/destinations/europe/croatia.html.

Current Advisories and Health Risks

All travelers should be up to date on tetanus-diphtheria, measles-mumps-rubella, polio, and varicella immunizations.

For additional information, consult the Disease Risk Summary for Europe on page 300.

Cuba

CAPITAL:
Havana
EMBASSY (IN U.S.):
202-797-8518
GMT:
−5 hours
TELEPHONE COUNTRY CODE:
53
USADIRECT:
None
ENTRY REQUIREMENTS

- **Passport/Visa:** Passport and visa required. For specific requirements, travelers should consult the Cuban Interests Section, 2630 16th St., NW, Washington, DC 20009 (202-797-8518). **Attention:** U.S. citizens need a U.S. Treasury Dept. license in order to engage in any transactions related to travel to and within Cuba (this includes the use of U.S. currency). Before planning any travel to Cuba, U.S. citizens should contact the Licensing Division, Office of Foreign Assets Control, U.S. Department of Treasury (202-622-2480) or www.treas.gov/ofac.
- **HIV Test:** AIDS test required for those staying longer than 90 days.
- **Vaccinations:** None required.

EMBASSIES/CONSULATES:
U.S. Interest Section, Havana. Calzado, between Calles L and M, Vedado. Tel: 32-0551-59. The United States does not maintain formal diplomatic relations with Cuba.

- **Canadian Embassy:** Calle 30 No. 518, Miramar (Playa), Ciudad de la Habana, Cuba; Tel: (53-7) 204-2516; Fax: (53-7) 204-1069 (immigration section); Website: www.havana.gc.ca.
- **British Embassy:** Calle 34 No. 702/4 entre 7ma Avenida y 17, Miramar, Havana; Tel: 53-7-204-1771; Fax: 53-7-204-8104; e-mail: embrit@ceniai.inf.cu.

HOSPITALS/DOCTORS:
There is a well-organized and accessible health-care system in Cuba and neighborhood-based family medicine is widely available. Travelers are advised to obtain, before departure, supplemental travel health insurance with specific overseas coverage. The policy should provide for direct payment to the overseas hospital and/or physician at the time of service and include a medical evacuation benefit.

Current Advisories and Health Risks

CHOLERA: This disease is reported active in this country, but the threat to tourists is very low. Cholera is an extremely rare disease in travelers from developed countries. Cholera vaccine is recommended primarily for people at high risk who work and live in highly endemic areas under less than adequate sanitary conditions.

DENGUE FEVER: The incidence of dengue fever is widespread. Dengue hemorrhagic fever is reported. Travelers should take measures to prevent daytime mosquito bites.

FASCIOLIASIS (LIVER FLUKE DISEASE): Human fascioliasis is endemic, with Cuba having the highest infectivity rates in the Caribbean. Visitors should avoid aquatic vegetables, such as watercress, and thoroughly cook goat and sheep livers before consumption.

FOOD AND WATER SAFETY: Main water sources are chlorinated and, although relatively safe, may cause mild abdominal upsets. Bottled water is available and is advised. Milk is pasteurized and dairy products are safe for consumption. Local meat, poultry, seafoods, and fruit are generally considered safe to eat.

HEPATITIS: Hepatitis A vaccine is recommended. The hepatitis B carrier rate in the general population is estimated at 0.8%. Hepatitis B is spread by infected blood, contaminated needles, and unsafe sex. Vaccination is recommended for stays longer than 3 months; for anyone at occupational or social risk; for any traveler desiring maximal protection. The risk of illness or injury during travel cannot be predicted and some experts believe that *all* travelers should be immunized against hepatitis B because of the risk of receiving a medical injection with an unsterile needle or syringe.

TRAVELERS' DIARRHEA: Medium risk. A quinolone antibiotic is recommended for acute diarrhea. Persistent diarrhea may be due to a parasitic infection such as giardiasis, amebiasis, or cryptosporidiosis.

TYPHOID FEVER: Typhoid vaccine is recommended for those traveling off the usual tourist routes, those visiting friends or relatives, and for long-stay visitors. Because the typhoid vaccines are only 60% to 70% effective, safe food and drink selection remains important.

Curaçao

CAPITAL:
Willemstad
EMBASSY (IN U.S.):
202-244-5300
GMT:
+1 hour
TELEPHONE COUNTRY CODE:
599
USADIRECT:
001-800-872-2881

ENTRY REQUIREMENTS

- **Passport/Visa:** Curaçao is one of the Netherlands Antilles, an autonomous part of the Kingdom of the Netherlands. The Netherlands Antilles is a group of six Caribbean islands: Aruba, Bonaire, Curaçao, Saba, Statia, and St. Maarten. Passport or proof of U.S. citizenship (e.g., certified birth certificate or voter registration card with photo ID) required. Visa not required for stay up to 14 days, extendible to 90 days after arrival.
- **HIV Test:** Required by Aruba for intending immigrants.
- **Vaccinations:** Yellow fever vaccination required if traveling from an infected area.

EMBASSIES/CONSULATES

- **U.S. Embassy:** J.B. Gorsiraweg #1, Willemstad, Curaçao; Tel: 599-9-461-3066; Fax: 599-9-461-6489; e-mail: cgcuracao@interneeds.net.
- **Canadian Embassy:** Maduro and Curiels Bank, N.V., Scharlooweg 55, Willemstad, Curaçao; Tel: 599-9-466-1115/1121; Fax: 599-9-1122/1130.
- **British Consulate:** Jan Sofat 38, Willemstad, Curaçao; Tel: 599-9-747-3322; Fax: 599-9-747-3330.

HOSPITALS/DOCTORS:

There are three hospitals on Curaçao. The largest, St Elizabeth, is well equipped. Travel health insurance is recommended.

Current Advisories and Health Risks

ACCIDENTS, ILLNESS, AND MEDICAL INSURANCE

- Accidents and injuries are the leading cause of death among travelers younger than age 55 and are most often caused by motor vehicle and motorcycle crashes; drownings, aircraft crashes, homicides, and burns are less common causes.
- Heart attacks cause most fatalities in older travelers.
- Infections cause only 1% of fatalities in overseas travelers, but, overall, infections are the most common cause of travel-related illness.
- Travelers are advised to obtain, before departure, supplemental travel health insurance with specific overseas coverage. The policy should provide for direct payment to the overseas hospital and/or physician at the time of service and include a medical evacuation benefit. The policy should also provide 24-hour hotline access to a multilingual assistance center that can help arrange and monitor delivery of medical care and determine if medical evacuation or air ambulance services are required.

DENGUE FEVER: Dengue fever is widespread in the Caribbean. Travelers to the Netherland Antilles should take measures to prevent daytime mosquito bites.

FOOD AND WATER SAFETY: All main water on the island is distilled from sea water and is safe to drink. Bottled mineral water is widely available. Milk is pasteurized and dairy products are safe for consumption. Local meat, poultry, seafood, fruits, and vegetables are generally considered safe to eat.

HEPATITIS: Nonimmune travelers should receive hepatitis A vaccine. Vaccination against hepatitis B should be considered for stays longer than 3 months or by those travelers desiring maximal protection. Travelers should be aware that hepatitis B can be transmitted by unsafe sex and the use of contaminated needles and syringes.

INFLUENZA: Influenza is transmitted year-round in the tropics. The flu vaccine is recommended for all travelers older than age 50; all travelers with any chronic disease or weakened immune system; travelers of any age wishing to decrease the risk of this illness; pregnant women after the first trimester.

MALARIA: No risk.

MARINE HAZARDS
- Swimming related hazards include jellyfish, spiny sea urchins, and corals.
- Ciguatera poisoning is prevalent and can result from eating reef fish such as grouper, snapper, sea bass, jack, and barracuda. The ciguatoxin is not destroyed by cooking.
- Scuba diving—Hyperbaric Chamber Referral: Divers' Alert Network (DAN) maintains an up-to-date list of all functioning hyperbaric chambers in North America and the Caribbean. DAN does not publish this list because at any one time a given chamber may be nonfunctioning, or its operator(s) may be away or otherwise unavailable. Through Duke University, DAN operates a 24-hour emergency phone line for anyone (members and nonmembers) to call and ask for diving accident assistance. Dive medicine physicians at Duke University Medical Center carry beepers, so someone is always on call to answer questions and, if necessary, make referral to the closest functioning hyperbaric chamber. In a diving emergency, or for the location of the nearest decompression chamber, call 919-684-8111.

TRAVELERS' DIARRHEA: Low to moderate risk. Food and water are generally safe on this island. A quinolone antibiotic, combined with loperamide (Imodium), are recommended for the treatment of acute diarrhea.

YELLOW FEVER: No risk. A yellow fever vaccination certificate is required if traveling from an infected area.

Czech Republic

★ PRAGUE

CAPITAL:
Prague
EMBASSY (IN U.S.):
202-363-6315
GMT:
+1 hour
TELEPHONE COUNTRY CODE:
42
USADIRECT:
00-420-001-01

ENTRY REQUIREMENTS

- **Passport/Visa:** A visa is not required for stays up to 30 days.
- **HIV Test:** Not required.
- **Vaccinations:** None required.

EMBASSIES/CONSULATES

- **U.S. Embassy:** Trziste 15, Prague; Tel: 0-2-5753-0663; Website: www.usembassy.cz.
- **Canadian Embassy:** Mickiewiczova 6, 125-33, Prague; Tel: 0-2-7210-1800; Fax: 420-2-7210-1890; e-mail: canada@canada.cz
- **British Embassy:** Thunovska 14, 118 00 Prague 1; Tel: 420-2-5740-2111; Fax: 420-2-5740-2296; e-mail: info@britain.cz.

HOSPITALS/DOCTORS:

There are numerous private clinics and doctors on call to serve the medical needs of travelers.

- UNICARE Medical Center: Na Dlouhem lanu 11, Prague; Tel: 42-23535-6553; Branch office (pediatrics and general medicine): Kosatcova, Pruhonice; Tel: & Fax: 42-26775-0427; Unicare Medical Center is a private medical center providing basic outpatient care and services including referrals and an escort system to the best facilities in Prague. Emergency care (for noncritical emergencies) is available 24 hours/day, with staff members on call for foreign and local patients.
- Canadian Medical Centres, 1/30 Veleslavinska; Outpatient care in a modern, private medical clinic. English-speaking Czech physicians provide primary care on a drop-in basis, or as part of a membership package.
- American Medical Centers, Janovskeho 48, Prague; Tel: 02-807-756; 24-hour emergency services and walk-in clinic with English-speaking physicians. The American Medical Center Prague offers routine outpatient care as well as limited emergency and first-aid care 24-hours daily; it also has 7 overnight beds. The clinic does not handle major trauma but can stabilize and evacuate critically injured patients. It has cardiac monitoring, defibrillators, and oxygen. Staff members speak English. The clinic is located in downtown Prague.
- International SOS:
  - International SOS Assistance (CZ) s.r.o., Vaclavske namesti 62, 110 00 Prague 1, Czech Republic; Alarm Center Med Tel: 420-222-111-155; Alarm Center Med Fax: 420-222-111-156
  - BaltAssist Ltd., Physical Location, Vaike-Ameerika 8, Room 313, 10129 Tallinn, Estonia; Admin Tel: 372-524-4426; Admin Fax: 372-656-7894

Current Advisories and Health Risks

AIDS/HIV: Unlike the Russian Federation and some other countries in Eastern Europe, sex between men is the predominant mode of HIV transmission in the Czech Republic, Hungary, Slovenia, and the Slovak Republic.

HEPATITIS: There is a higher incidence of hepatitis A in Eastern Europe than elsewhere in Europe. Hepatitis A vaccine is recommended for nonimmune travelers. Hepatitis B is spread by infected blood, contaminated needles, and unsafe sex. Vaccination is recommended for stays longer than 3 months; for anyone at occupational or social risk; for any traveler desiring maximal protection. The risk of illness or injury during travel cannot be predicted and some experts believe that *all* travelers should be immunized against hepatitis B because of the risk of receiving a medical injection with an unsterile needle or syringe.

INFLUENZA: Influenza season is from November to April. The flu vaccine is recommended for all travelers.

LYME DISEASE: Lyme disease is transmitted in all regions of the country, including the parks in Prague and other cities, primarily during the warmer months, April through September. Travelers should take measures to prevent tick bites.

TICK-BORNE ENCEPHALITIS (TBE): European tick-borne encephalitis (TBE) occurs April through October in lowland forested areas, with a higher incidence south of Prague in the Vlatva (Moldau) River basin, north of Brno, in the vicinity of Plzen, and in the Danube River basin near Bratislava. The TBE vaccine (available in Europe and Canada) is recommended only for people who expect to have extensive exposure to ticks in rural areas (e.g., hikers, campers). All travelers to rural areas should take precautions to prevent tick bites.

TRAVELERS' DIARRHEA: Low to moderate risk. Water supplies in urban areas are potable. A quinolone antibiotic, plus loperamide (Imodium), is recommended for the treatment of acute diarrhea. Persistent diarrhea may be due to a parasitic infection such as giardiasis, amebiasis, or cryptosporidiosis.

TYPHOID FEVER: Typhoid vaccine is recommended for those traveling off the usual tourist routes, those visiting friends or relatives, and for long-stay visitors. Because the typhoid vaccines are only 60% to 70% effective, safe food and drink selection remains important.

OTHER DISEASES/HAZARDS: Brucellosis, echinococcosis, rabies (moderately enzootic, with foxes serving as primary zoonotic reservoirs; approximately 60% of domestic animal rabies occurs in stray cats), tularemia, and intestinal helminthic infections. Listeriosis, transmitted through the consumption of contaminated meat and milk products, has been reported in South Bohemia and North Moravia.

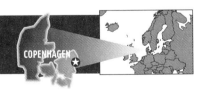

Denmark (including Greenland)

CAPITAL:
Copenhagen
EMBASSY (IN U.S.):
202-234-4300

GMT:

+1 hour

TELEPHONE COUNTRY CODE:

45

USADIRECT:

8001-0010

ENTRY REQUIREMENTS

- **Passport/Visa:** Passport required. Visa not required for a stay of up to 90 days. Contact the Danish Embassy, 3200 Whitehaven Street NW, Washington, DC. 20008; 202-234-4300.
- **HIV Test:** Not required.
- **Vaccinations:** None required.

EMBASSIES/CONSULATES

- **U.S. Embassy:** Dag Hammarskjolds Alle 24, Copenhagen. Tel: 35-55-31-44; Fax: 45-35-43-02-23; Website: www.usembassy.dk.
- **Canadian Embassy:** Kr. Bernikowsgade 1, Copenhagen K. Tel: 33-48-32-00; Fax: 45-33-48-32-20/21; e-mail: copen@dfait-maeci.gc.ca, Website: www.canada.dk.
- **British Embassy:** Kastelsvej 36/38/40, DK-2100 Copenhagen Ø; Tel: 45-35-44-52-00; Fax: 45-35-44-52-93; e-mail: info@britishembassy.dk; Website: www.britishembassy.dk.

HOSPITALS/DOCTORS:

- Medical facilities widely available. In Greenland and the Faroe Islands, facilities are limited and evacuation is required for serious illness/injury. Supplemental health insurance, including air evacuation and special insurance for arctic areas when visiting Greenland and the Faroe Islands, is advisable.
- Bispebjerb Hospital, Copenhagen (1,150 beds); emergency department and trauma unit

Current Advisories and Health Risks

- All travelers should be up to date on tetanus-diphtheria, measles-mumps-rubella, polio, and varicella immunizations.
- Tick-borne encephalitis is not endemic in Denmark.

For additional information, consult the Disease Risk Summary for Europe on page 300.

Djibouti

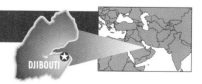

CAPITAL:

Djibouti

EMBASSY (IN U.S.):

202-331-0270

GMT:

+3 hours

253

USADIRECT:

None

ENTRY REQUIREMENTS

- **Passport/Visa:** Valid passport and visa are required.
- **HIV Test**: Not required.
- **Vaccinations:** A yellow fever vaccination certificate is required for all travelers older than 1 year of age arriving from infected areas.

EMBASSIES/CONSULATES

- **U.S. Embassy:** Djibouti; Villa Plateau du Serpent Boulevard; Tel: 353-849, 353-995, 352-916.
- **Canadian Embassy:** Accredited to the Canadian Embassy in Ethiopia; Tel: 251-1-151-100.
- **British Embassy:** Accredited to the British Embassy in Ethiopia. Consular Section, Comoros Street, PO Box 858, Addis Ababa, Ethiopia; Tel: 251-1-612354; Fax: 251-1-614154.

HOSPITALS/DOCTORS:

Medical care in Djibouti is below Western standards. Travelers are advised to obtain supplemental travel health insurance with specific overseas coverage. The policy should provide for direct payment to the overseas hospital and/or physician at the time of service and include a medical evacuation benefit.

- Peltier Hospital, Djibouti City (700 beds); limited emergency and surgical facilities; old and poorly maintained buildings.

Current Advisories and Health Risks

MALARIA: Present year-round, countrywide, including urban areas. Higher malaria risk occurs from November through March. There is only minimal risk of malaria in Djibouti City. Prophylaxis with atovaquone/proguanil (Malarone), mefloquine (Lariam) or doxycycline is recommended.

POLIO: This disease is active in parts of Africa and Saudi Arabia. All travelers should be fully immunized. A polio booster is recommended for adult travelers.

For additional information, consult the Disease Risk Summary for sub-Saharan Africa on page 307.

Dominica

CAPITAL:

Roseau

EMBASSY (IN U.S.):

202-364-6781

GMT:

−4 hours

TELEPHONE COUNTRY CODE:

809

USADIRECT:

1-800-872-2881

ENTRY REQUIREMENTS

- **Passport/Visa:** Passport or proof of U.S. citizenship and photo ID, and return/onward ticket required for tourist stay of up to 21 days. For longer stays and other information, consult the Consulate of the Commonwealth of Dominica, 3216 New Mexico Ave., NW, Washington, DC 20016 (202-364-6791).
- **HIV Test:** Not required.
- **Vaccinations:** A yellow fever vaccination certificate is required for travelers over 1 year of age coming from infected or endemic areas.

EMBASSIES/CONSULATES:

Neither the United States nor Canada has an embassy in the Commonwealth of Dominica.

- **British High Commission:** Lower Collymore Rock (PO Box 676), Bridgetown, Barbados; Tel: 1-246-430-7800; e-mail: britishhc@sunbeach.net.

HOSPITALS/DOCTORS:

Basic medical care in Dominica is adequate for most needs. All emergencies should be flown by air ambulance to a location where a higher level of care is available. Travelers are advised to obtain supplemental travel health insurance with specific overseas coverage. The policy should provide for direct payment to the overseas hospital and/or physician at the time of service and include a medical evacuation benefit.

- General Hospital, Portsmouth (50 beds); limited medical services.
- Princess Margaret Hospital, Roseau (247 beds); general medical/surgical facility.

Current Advisories and Health Risks

For additional information, consult Disease Risk Summaries for the Caribbean and Mexico and Central America on pages 293 and 295.

Dominican Republic

CAPITAL:

Santo Domingo

EMBASSY

202-332-6280

GMT:

−4 hours

TELEPHONE COUNTRY CODE:

809

1-800-872-2881

ENTRY REQUIREMENTS
- **Passport/Visa:** Tourist card or visa required.
- **HIV Test:** Not required.
- **Vaccinations:** None required.

EMBASSIES/CONSULATES
- **U.S. Embassy:** Calle Cesar Nicolas Penson and Calle Leopoldo Navarro, Santo Domingo. Tel: 809-221-2171, after hours: 809-221-8100; Website: usemb.gov.do/acs.htm.
- **Canadian Embassy:** Capitán Eugenio de Marchena No. 39, La Esperilla, Santo Domingo Tel: 809-685-1136; Fax: 682-2691; e-mail: sdmgo@dfait-maeci.gc.ca.
- **British Embassy:** Ave 27 de Febrero No 233, Edificio Cerominas Pepín, Santo Domingo; Tel: 1-809-472-7111; Fax: 1-809-472-7190; e-mail: brit.emb.sadom@codetel.net.do.

HOSPITALS/DOCTORS
- Clinica Abreu (76 beds); general medical/surgical facility; emergency department; frequently used by embassy personnel.
- Centro Medico Universidad Hospital (200 beds); general medical/surgical facility.
- Private medical care is excellent, but expensive. Travelers are advised to obtain, before departure, supplemental travel health insurance with specific overseas coverage. The policy should provide for direct payment to the overseas hospital and/or physician at the time of service and include a medical evacuation benefit.

Health Risks and Advisories

HEPATITIS: Nonimmune travelers should receive hepatitis A vaccine. Vaccination against hepatitis B should be considered for stays longer than 3 months or by those travelers desiring maximal protection. Travelers should be aware that hepatitis B can be transmitted by unsafe sex and the use of contaminated needles and syringes.

INFLUENZA: Influenza is transmitted year-round in the tropics. The flu vaccine is recommended for all travelers to this country.

MALARIA: The CDC recommends that all travelers to La Altagracia Province and Duarte Province, including travelers to the Punta Cana resort area, should take an antimalarial drug. In addition, an antimalarial drug is recommended for travelers to rural areas in all parts of the country. Chloroquine is the recommended drug for the Dominican Republic. All travelers should take measures to prevent evening and nighttime mosquito bites. Insect-bite prevention measures include a DEET-containing repellent applied to exposed skin, insecticide (permethrin) spray applied to clothing and gear, and use of a permethrin-treated bed net.

MARINE HAZARDS: Swimming-related hazards include jellyfish, spiny sea urchins, and coral.

CIGUATERA POISONING: Most reported cases of ciguatera poisoning have involved travelers who ate fish in the Caribbean while on holiday. These cases included consuming grouper in the Dominican Republic, kingfish in Jamaica, barracuda in Haiti, and a fish casserole in Cuba. Any reef fish can cause ciguatera poisoning, but species such as barracuda, moray eel, grouper, red snapper, jack, sturgeon, and sea bass are the most commonly involved. The occurrence of toxic fish is sporadic, and not all fish of a given species or from a given locality will be toxic. The ciguatoxin is not destroyed by cooking.

SCUBA DIVING: Divers' Alert Network (DAN) maintains an up-to-date list of all hyperbaric chambers in North America and the Caribbean. In association with Duke University Medical Center in North Carolina, DAN operates a 24-hour emergency phone number (919-684-8111) for members and nonmembers to call and their staff is available to answer questions and, if necessary, make referral to the closest functioning hyperbaric chamber.

TRAVELERS' DIARRHEA: High risk outside of deluxe resorts, but cases of shigellosis (dysentery) have been reported in tourists staying in such facilities. Acute diarrhea should be treated with a quinolone antibiotic combined with loperamide. Persistent diarrhea may be due to a parasitic infection such as giardiasis, amebiasis, cryptosporidiosis or cyclosporiasis.

FILARIASIS: Mosquito-transmitted; lymphatic filariasis continues to be prevalent in the Caribbean region, particularly Guyana, Haiti, and the Dominican Republic.

LEISHMANIASIS: The Dominican Republic is the only country in the West Indies where an autochthonous focus of cutaneous leishmaniasis has been discovered within the last 20 years. Most of the cases are of the diffuse clinical type, but subclinical or mild cases are apparently common. The responsible agent is a new species of *Leishmania* and the suspected vector is *Leishmania cristophei*, the only human-biting sand fly on the island. Travelers are advised to take measures to prevent insect bites.

SCHISTOSOMIASIS: This is a parasitic infection that may be found in fresh water in parts of the Dominican Republic. Travelers should not swim in fresh water, except in chlorinated swimming pools or bodies of water known to be safe.

Ecuador

CAPITAL:
Quito
EMBASSY (IN U.S.):
202-234-7200

GMT:
−5 hours
TELEPHONE COUNTRY CODE:
593
USADIRECT:
1-999-119
1-800-225-528
ENTRY REQUIREMENTS
- **Passport/Visa:** A passport and return/onward ticket are required to obtain an entry permit valid for 90 days.
- **HIV Test:** Testing may be required for students or long-term visitors. Travelers should contact the Ecuadorian Embassy in Washington, DC, for information; Tel: 202-234-7200.
- **Vaccinations:** A yellow fever vaccination certificate is required for travelers older than 1 year of age arriving from a yellow fever-infected area.

EMBASSIES/CONSULATES
- **U.S. Embassy:** corner of Avenida 12 de Octubre and Avenida Patria (across from the Casa de la Cultura); Tel: 593-2-562-890, ext. 480, or 561-749 for after-hours emergencies; Fax: 593-2-561-524; Website: www.usembassy.org.ec.
- **U.S. Consulate:** corner of 9 de Octubre and Garcia Moreno (near the Hotel Oro Verde); Tel: 593-4-323-570, or 321-152 for after-hours emergencies; Fax: 593-4-320-904.
- **Canadian Embassy:** Edificio Josueth Gonzalez, 4th Floor, Av. 6 de diciembre 2816, PO Box 17-11-6512 (CCI), Quito; Tel: 593-2-506-162 or 232-114; Fax: 503-108; e-mail: quito@dfait-maeci.gc.ca.
- **British Embassy:** Citiplaza Building, Naciones Unidas Ave & República de El Salvador 14th Floor; Tel: 593-2-2-970-800-/-970-801; Fax: 593-2-2-970-807; e-mail: britembq@interactive.net.ec.

HOSPITALS/DOCTORS
- Hospital Vozandes Quito (75 beds); 254 Villa Lengua, Quito. Tel: 593-2-26-2142. This is a preferred facility for travelers who have infectious or tropical diseases. Emergency care is available 24 hours a day.
- Metropolitano Hospital (120-beds), Avenida Mariana de Jesús y Nicolas Arteta y Calisto, Quito; Tel: 593-2-26-1520, 2-26-9030. This facility can handle trauma and cardiac emergencies 24 hours a day. MRI and CT are available.
- Hospital Clinica Pichincha, Avendas Veintimilla y Paez, Quito; Tel: 593-2-56-2408, 2-56-2410. Hospital Clinica Pichincha is a small hospital (100 beds) known mainly for cardiology and intensive care; general medical services are not on the same level as other major hospitals in Quito. Emergency services are available 24 hours a day.

Current Advisories and Health Risks

AIDS/HIV: Incidence of HIV infection appears relatively low at the present time. Highest incidence reported in the port city of Guayaquil.

ACCIDENTS, ILLNESS, AND MEDICAL INSURANCE

- Accidents and injuries are the leading cause of death among travelers under the age of 55 and are most often caused by motor vehicle and motorcycle crashes; drownings, aircraft crashes, homicides, and burns are less common causes.
- Heart attacks cause most fatalities in older travelers.
- Infections cause only 1% of fatalities in overseas travelers, but, overall, infections are the most common cause of travel-related illness.
- Travelers are advised to obtain, before departure, supplemental travel health insurance with specific overseas coverage. The policy should provide for direct payment to the overseas hospital and/or physician at the time of service and include a medical evacuation benefit. The policy should also provide 24-hour hotline access to a multilingual assistance center that can help arrange and monitor delivery of medical care and determine if medical evacuation or air ambulance services are required.

ALTITUDE SICKNESS (AMS): Extreme variations in altitude occur in this country. Risk of altitude sickness (acute mountain sickness—AMS) is present for tourists arriving in Quito (altitude 3,000 meters) and other high-altitude destinations. Travelers to high altitudes should consider prophylaxis with acetazolamide (Diamox), as well as gradual ascent if going to higher altitudes. The best treatment for AMS is immediate descent to a lower altitude.

BARTONELLOSIS (OROYA FEVER): The severe febrile form of this disease with hemolysis (Oroyo fever) has been reported for decades in the highland provinces and cities bordering Peru, including the villages of Zumba, Ibarra, and Zaruma. Transmission of this disease by sand flies occurs primarily between 500 and 3,000 meters elevation. In the coastal lowland province of Manabi, however, there are a growing number of cases of cutaneous bartonellosis, characterized only by chronic verrucous skin lesions.

CHAGAS DISEASE: Widely distributed in rural areas, but more common in the Pacific coastal provinces of Manabi and Guayas. Risk of transmission occurs in rural-agricultural areas where there are adobe-style huts and houses that potentially harbor the night-biting triatomid (assassin) bugs. Travelers sleeping in such structures should take measures to prevent nighttime bites. Contaminated food and unscreened blood transfusions are also potential sources of infection.

CHOLERA: This disease is reported active in this country, but the threat to tourists is very low. Cholera is an extremely rare disease in travelers from developed countries. Cholera vaccine is recommended primarily for people at high risk who work and live in highly endemic areas under less than adequate sanitary conditions.

- The oral cholera vaccine (Dukoral) provides up to 60% crossover protection against ETEC diarrhea.
- Many countries, including Canada, license an oral cholera vaccine. The oral vaccine is not available in the United States.
- Cholera vaccine is not "officially" required for entry into, or exit from, any country. Despite this, some countries, on occasion, require proof of cholera immunization from

travelers coming from cholera-infected countries. Anticipating such a situation, travelers may wish to carry a medical exemption letter from their health-care provider. If possible, it is advisable to contact the embassy or consulate at the destination country to confirm the requirement for cholera vaccination (if any) and the acceptability of a medical exemption letter.

DENGUE FEVER: The greatest risk of infection occurs in the coastal urban areas, especially in Guayas, Loja, and Esmeraldas Provinces, but dengue is also endemic in urban and rural areas throughout this country. The *Aedes aegypti* mosquitoes, which transmit dengue, bite primarily during the daytime.

FASCIOLIASIS (LIVER FLUKE DISEASE): This disease is not uncommon in the highlands of western Ecuador, especially in Chimborazo, Cotopaxi, and Azuay. Domestic livestock are the primary host. Travelers should avoid uncooked foods.

HEPATITIS: All nonimmune travelers should receive hepatitis A vaccine before visiting this country. Hepatitis E is regionally endemic. The overall hepatitis B carrier rate in the general population is estimated at 2%, with much higher rates among the indigenous groups of the Amazon Basin. Hepatitis B vaccine is recommended for stays longer than 3 months and for short-term travelers wanting increased protection. Travelers should be aware that the risk of hepatitis B is increased by unsafe sex and the use of unsterile needles and syringes. An outbreak of fulminant hepatitis D has been reported in the Waorani tribe of the Amazon Basin.

LEISHMANIASIS: This disease is considered a public health problem in rural areas under 2,000 meters elevation on the Pacific coast, the Andean plains, and the eastern Amazonian lowland (particularly in Imbabura and Pichincha Provinces, as well as Zamora, Esmeraldas, and Manabi Provinces). Over 90% of cases are cutaneous, the rest mucocutaneous. "Uta," a form of cutaneous leishmaniasis, may occur at elevations up to 3,000 meters. Visceral leishmaniasis has not been confirmed.

MALARIA: This disease occurs countrywide in coastal and rural areas below 2,000 meters elevation; overall risk may be elevated in the northern lowlands on both sides of the Andes. Travelers visiting only Quito, the central highland tourist areas (including Cotopaxi volcano), Cuenca, Guayaquil city, or the Galapagos Islands are not at risk and do not require prophylaxis. In malarious areas, risk may be increased February through August. The coastal provinces of Esmeraldas, Guayas (including Guayaquil), and Manabi account for two thirds of all officially reported malaria, followed by Los Rios, Pinchincha, and Napo Provinces. Other provinces with malaria include El Oro, Morona-Santiago, Pastaza, Sucumbios, and Zamora-Chinchipe. Countrywide, 65% to 70% of malaria is vivax, 30% to 35% is falciparum, but falciparum causes up to 70% of malaria in Manabi Province. Chloroquine-resistant *Plasmodium falciparum* likely occurs in all malarious areas.

- Prophylaxis with atovaquone/proguanil (Malarone), mefloquine (Lariam), or doxycycline is recommended.
- All travelers should take measures to prevent evening and nighttime mosquito bites.

ONCHOCERCIASIS: This disease occurs along river systems in Esmeraldas Province (northwestern Ecuador). Infection rates up to 95% are reported among some Amerindian communities in the Santiago River basin. Outbreaks are reported spreading from Esmeraldas Province to other parts of the country. All travelers to rural areas with fast-flowing rivers should take measures to prevent insect (black fly) bites.

PARAGONIMIASIS (LUNG FLUKE DISEASE): This may be one of the most prevalent and least recognizable public health problems in Ecuador. Nearly one half of Ecuador's rural population is estimated to be infected. Risk may be elevated in the northern and western coastal areas including Esmeraldas and Manabi Provinces. All travelers should avoid eating uncooked crustacea, especially raw freshwater crabs and crayfish, which harbor the infective cercariae.

RABIES: Human rabies occurs countrywide in both urban and rural areas. Most cases are reported from the western provinces of Guayas, especially in and around Guayaquil. Rabid dogs are the primary threat. Rabid bats are reported in the province of Napo. Although rabies is rare among tourists, there is risk. No one should pet or pick up any stray animals. All children should be warned to avoid contact with unknown animals.

- All animal bites or scratches, especially from a dog, should be taken seriously and immediate medical attention sought, even if the traveler has previously been vaccinated against rabies. Additional rabies vaccine may be required. Medical evacuation to a medical facility stocking rabies vaccine may be necessary if adequate vaccines are not available.

- Rabies vaccine is recommended for travel longer than 3 months, for shorter stays for travelers who plan to venture off the usual tourist routes where they may be more exposed to the stray dog population, or when travelers desire extra protection.

TRAVELERS' DIARRHEA: High risk. Contaminated water is a major problem throughout Ecuador. Even the two largest cities, Quito and Guayaquil, do not have reliable sources of safe, potable water. Travelers should follow food and drink precautions. A quinolone antibiotic is recommended for the treatment of diarrhea. Diarrhea not responding to antibiotic treatment may be due to a parasitic disease such as giardiasis, amebiasis, or cryptosporidiosis.

TUBERCULOSIS: Tuberculosis (TB) is a major public health problem in this country. Travelers planning an extended stay should have a pre-departure TB skin test (PPD test) and be retested after leaving this country.

TYPHOID FEVER: Typhoid vaccine is recommended. Focal outbreaks occur throughout the country. Large outbreaks have occurred in Quito. Because the typhoid vaccines are only 60% to 70% effective, safe food and drink selection remain important.

YELLOW FEVER: This disease is currently active in this country. Provinces reporting yellow fever activity include Morona-Santiago, Napo, Pastaza, Sucumbios, and Zamora-Chinchipe. Vaccination is recommended for travel outside urban areas. This country is in the Yellow Fever Endemic Zone. Although yellow fever vaccination is not required for entry into this country if arriving from the United States or Canada, it may be required for ongoing travel to other countries in Latin America, Africa, the Middle East, or Asia.

Egypt

CAPITAL:
Cairo
EMBASSY (IN U.S.):
202-895-5400
GMT:
+2 hours
TELEPHONE COUNTRY CODE:
20
USADIRECT:
510-0200 (Cairo)
02-510-0200
ENTRY REQUIREMENTS
• **Passport/Visa:** Passport and visa required.
• **HIV Test:** Foreigners applying for study, training, or work permits must have been tested; spouses of applicants are exempt.
• **Vaccinations:** A yellow fever vaccination certificate is required from all travelers arriving from a country any part of which is infected and be older than 1 year of age. Required also for travelers arriving from or transiting:

Africa: Angola, Benin, Burkina Faso, Burundi, Cameroon, the Central African Republic, Chad, Congo, Côte d'Ivoire, Democratic Republic of Congo, Equatorial Guinea, Ethiopia, Gabon, The Gambia, Ghana, Guinea, Guinea Bissau, Kenya, Liberia, Mali, Niger, Nigeria, Rwanda, São Tomé and Principe, Senegal, Sierra Leone, Somalia, Sudan (south of 15 degrees N), Tanzania, Togo, Uganda, and Zambia.

Americas: Belize, Bolivia, Brazil, Colombia, Costa Rica, Ecuador, French Guiana, Guyana, Panama, Peru, Suriname, and Venezuela.

Caribbean: Trinidad and Tobago.

Air passengers in transit but coming from these countries or areas without a certificate will be detained in the precincts of the airport until they resume their journey. All travelers arriving from Sudan are required to possess a vaccination certificate or location certificate issued by a Sudanese official center stating that they have not been in Sudan south of latitude 15 degrees N within the preceding 6 days.
EMBASSIES/CONSULATES
• **U.S. Embassy:** 5 Latin America Street, Garden City, Cairo. Tel: 20-2-795-7371 or 20-2-797-2301; Fax: 20-2-797-2472; e-mail: consularcairo@state.gov; Website: www.usembassy.egnet.net.
• **Canadian Embassy:** 5 El Saraya El Kobra Square, Arab African International Bank Building, Cairo. Tel: 20-2-794-3110; Fax: 20-2-796-3548; e-mail: cairo@dfait-maeci.gc.ca.

- **British Embassy:** 7, Ahmed Ragheb Street, Garden City, Cairo; Tel: 20-2-794-0850, 794-0852/8; e-mail: info@britishembassy.org.eg; Website: www.britishembassy.org.eg.

HOSPITALS/DOCTORS

- Facilities have many Western trained medical professionals. The U.S. Embassy in Cairo provides a list of local hospitals and English-speaking physicians. Most medical facilities are adequate for non-emergencies in tourist areas. Emergency and intensive care facilities are limited, but some in Cairo are of high quality.
- Al-Salam Hospital, Cairo (300 beds); Private civilian hospital; quality of care probably Egypt's best; most major specialties; ambulance service.
- El Nasr City Medical Center, Cairo (600 beds); government hospital; sophisticated diagnostics and most medical specialties; ambulance service.
- Cleopatra Hospital, Heliopolis, Cairo (80 beds); 24-hour trauma and emergency services; high-quality care.

Current Advisories and Health Risks

ANIMAL HAZARDS: Animal hazards include snakes (cobras, vipers), scorpions, and black widow spiders.

ARBOVIRAL FEVERS: West Nile fever, Rift Valley fever, and sand fly fever are regularly reported. The highest transmission rates are June through October with more risk in the Nile River Delta and Nile Valley, with risk increasing from north to south. There is negligible risk of dengue fever in Egypt. All travelers to this country, particularly to the Nile Valley and Nile Delta, should take measures to prevent mosquito and sand fly bites.

CHOLERA: Low risk to travelers. Vaccination is not routinely recommended.

FILARIASIS: Reported primarily from the eastern Nile Delta, including Ad Daqahliyah, Al Qalyubiyah, and Ash Sharqiyah Governorates, and possibly Asyu't Governorate. Travelers are advised to take measures to prevent mosquito bites.

HEPATITIS: All nonimmune travelers should receive the hepatitis A vaccine. Hepatitis E is endemic, with 30% of cases of acute viral hepatitis caused by this virus. The hepatitis B carrier rate is estimated to be 4% of the population. Hepatitis B is spread by infected blood, contaminated needles, and unprotected sex. Vaccination is recommended for long-stay (over 3 months) travelers; those who may be at occupational or social risk, and anybody desiring maximal protection. The hepatitis C virus is widespread, with prevalence rates up to 67% in some areas. There is a high risk of hepatitis C from blood transfusions.

INFLUENZA: Influenza is transmitted November through March. Vaccination is recommended.

INTESTINAL HELMINTHS (WORMS): Fascioliasis (liver fluke disease) is common in Cairo and the Nile Delta. Aquatic plants (e.g., wild watercress) are a source of infection, but the disease can also be transmitted by undercooked sheep and goat livers. Eating Fessikh (salted raw fish) puts the traveler at risk for acquiring heterophyiasis, an exotic infection of tiny flukes. Ascariasis (roundworm infection), ancylostomiasis (hookworm disease), trichuriasis (whipworm infection), and taeniasis (pork tapeworm disease) are common in rural areas of the Nile River Delta and Nile River Valley.

LEISHMANIASIS: Cutaneous leishmaniasis is focally distributed countrywide in rural and peri-urban areas, including Cairo. Primary risk areas include the Nile River Delta, the Suez Canal Zone, and the Sinai Peninsula (primarily northeastern Sinai). Visceral leishmaniasis possibly occurs near Alexandria. Travelers should take measures to prevent insect (sand fly) bites, including the use of permethrin-treated bed nets.

MALARIA: Risk exists in scattered rural areas of Al Faiyum Governorate, particularly Sennoris District. Transmission occurs primarily during the summer and fall (June to October). Possible risk exists in the Nile River Delta, along the Suez Canal, the northern Red Sea coast, part of southern Egypt (the rural areas near Aswan), and scattered oases (including Siwa Oasis and El Gara, a small oasis near Siwa). Urban centers, including Cairo and Alexandria, are risk free. Falciparum malaria is endemic only in the El Faiyum Governorate, where it predominates. Chloroquine prophylaxis is recommended only for those traveling to oases in the El Faiyum area. All travelers should take measures to prevent evening and nighttime mosquito bites.

MENINGITIS: Significant outbreaks of meningococcal disease have occurred in Egypt, involving primarily group A disease, but groups B and C are also reported. The risk for travelers is low; vaccination is not currently recommended.

POLIO: This disease is endemic. All travelers should be fully immunized.

RABIES: Primarily a risk in urban areas, including Cairo. Stray dogs are the primary source of human exposure, but jackals are also a reservoir of infection. Rabies vaccine should be considered for stays of longer than 3 months or for shorter stays if traveling to locations more than 24 hours from a reliable source of postexposure rabies vaccine. All animal bites or scratches while in this country should be medically evaluated.

SCHISTOSOMIASIS: This disease is widespread in Egypt and is a major public health problem. Urinary and intestinal schistosomiasis are found in the Nile River Delta, throughout the Nile Valley (particularly in the canals and irrigation ditches in rural farming areas), and along the Suez Canal. Areas above the Aswan Dam are heavily infected. Travelers should avoid swimming or wading in freshwater lakes, streams, or irrigated areas. Well-maintained, chlorinated swimming pools, however, are safe.

TRAVELERS' DIARRHEA: High risk outside of deluxe hotels and resorts. A quinolone antibiotic, combined with loperamide (Imodium), is recommended for the treatment of acute diarrhea. Persistent diarrhea may be due to a parasitic disease such as amebiasis, giardiasis, or cryptosporidiosis.

TUBERCULOSIS: Tuberculosis (TB) is a major health problem in this country. Travelers planning an extended stay should have a pre-departure TB skin test (PPD test) and be retested after leaving this country or returning home.

TYPHOID FEVER: Typhoid vaccine is recommended for those traveling off the usual tourist routes, those visiting friends or relatives, and for long-stay visitors. Typhoid vaccines are 60% to 70% effective; safe food and drink precautions should continue to be observed.

OTHER DISEASES/HAZARDS: Anthrax (cutaneous form; usually from exposure to infected, freshly slaughtered animals), AIDS (low risk; HIV prevalence is reported as less than 1% of the population), Mediterranean spotted fever (low risk; also known as boutonneuse fever and African tick typhus; reported from Ghiza and the Sharqiya and Aswan Governorates), brucellosis (usually from ingestion of unpasteurized goat/sheep milk and cheese), cholera (sporadic outbreaks occur), echinococcosis, filariasis (endemic in eastern Nile Delta and possibly in Asyut Governorate), flea-borne typhus, leprosy, leptospirosis, toxoplasmosis, trachoma, tuberculosis, typhoid fever (reported countrywide; elevated risk in populated areas with poor sanitation), murine typhus (flea-borne).

El Salvador

CAPITAL:
San Salvador
EMBASSY (IN U.S.):
202-331-4032
GMT:
−6 hours
TELEPHONE COUNTRY CODE:
503
USADIRECT:
800-1288
800-1785
ENTRY REQUIREMENTS

- **Passport/Visa:** A multiple-entry visa can be obtained by travelers staying longer than 30 days.
- **HIV Test:** Not required.
- **Vaccinations:** A yellow fever vaccination certificate is required from travelers older than 6 months of age coming from infected or endemic areas.

EMBASSIES/CONSULATES

- **U.S. Embassy**: San Salvador. Final Boulevard Santa Elena, Urbanizacion Santa Elena, Antiguo Cuscatlan; Tel: 278-4444.
- **Canadian Embassy**: Centro Financiero Gigante, 63 Av. Sur y Alameda Roosevelt, Local 6, Nivel Lobby II, San Salvador; Tel: 503-279-4655; Fax: 503-279-0765; e-mail: ssal@dfait-maeci.gc.ca.
- **British Embassy:** Accredited to the British Embassy in Guatemala. 16 Calle 00-55, Zona 10, Edificio Torre Internacional, Nivel 11, Guatemala City; Tel: 502-2367-5425-29; Fax: 502-2367-5430; e-mail: embassy@intelnett.com.

Policlinica Salvadorena Hospital (103 beds); some specialties; emergency services; ICU; CCU.

Current Advisories and Health Risks

CHAGAS DISEASE: Occurs in all rural areas under 1,500 meters elevation where there are adobe-style dwellings that potentially harbor the night-biting triatomid (assassin) bugs. Travelers sleeping in such structures should take precautions against nighttime bites.

CHOLERA: This disease is reported active in this country, but the threat to tourists is very low. Cholera is an extremely rare disease in travelers from developed countries. Cholera vaccine is recommended only for travelers at high risk who work and live in highly endemic areas under less than adequate sanitary conditions.
- The manufacture and availability of the injectable cholera vaccine in the United States ceased in June 2000.
- Many countries, including Canada, license an oral cholera vaccine. The oral cholera vaccine is not available in the United States.
- Cholera vaccine is not "officially" required for entry into, or exit from, any country.

DENGUE FEVER: Year-round risk, elevated June through December. Most cases occur in urban areas at lower elevations in the vicinity of San Salvador and in the eastern regions bordering Honduras. Travelers should take measures to prevent daytime mosquito bites.

HEPATITIS: Hepatitis A vaccine is advised for all nonimmune travelers. Hepatitis E may occur, but data are lacking. The carrier rate of the hepatitis B virus is estimated at 1.2% in the general population. Hepatitis B vaccine should be considered for stays longer than 3 months and by short-term travelers desiring maximal protection. Travelers should be aware that hepatitis B can be transmitted by unsafe sex and the use of contaminated needles and syringes.

LEISHMANIASIS: Cutaneous leishmaniasis is reported from the Rio Lempa valley. Most risk occurs in forested rural areas. There is risk of visceral leishmaniasis in the warm, dry valleys near the Honduran border. Travelers should avoid insect (sand fly) bites.

MALARIA: Risk is present year-round in rural areas below 1,000 meters elevation. Greatest risk is in coastal areas below 600 meters elevation and is minimal in northern and central zones. There is no risk of malaria in urban areas. This disease is highly active. Vivax malaria accounts for 98% of cases. Chloroquine prophylaxis is recommended for travel in rural areas.

RABIES: About 10 to 12 human deaths annually are reported. Rabid vampire bats are common, but dogs are the primary source of human infection. Rabies vaccination is indicated following the unprovoked bite of a dog, cat, bat, monkey, or other animal. Vaccination against rabies is recommended for long-term travel to this country.

TRAVELERS' DIARRHEA: Piped water supplies may be contaminated. Travelers should observe all food and drink safety precautions. A quinolone antibiotic is recommended for the treatment of acute diarrhea. Diarrhea not responding to treatment with an antibiotic, or chronic diarrhea, may be due to a parasitic disease such as giardiasis, amebiasis, or cryptosporidiosis.

OTHER DISEASES/HAZARDS: Anthrax, brucellosis, coccidiomycosis, cysticercosis, leptospirosis, measles, relapsing fever (tick-borne), syphilis, AIDS (low number of cases reported), tuberculosis (highly endemic), typhoid fever, strongyloidiasis and other helminthic infections, and typhus are reported. Hazardous animals include venomous snakes, scorpions, spiders, and biting bats.

Estonia

CAPITAL:
Tallinn
EMBASSY (IN U.S.):
202-588-0101
GMT:
+2 hours
TELEPHONE COUNTRY CODE:
372
USADIRECT:
800-12-001
ENTRY REQUIREMENTS
• **Passport/Visa:** Passport required. Visas are not required for stays of up to 90 days, but for longer stays, a residency permit is required. For further information, contact the Estonian Embassy, temporarily located at 1730 M St., NW, Suite 503, Washington, DC 20036; Tel: 202-588-0101) or the Consulate General of Estonia, 600 Third Ave., 26th Floor, New York, NY 10016; Tel: 212-883-0636. Website: www.estemb.org.
• **HIV Test:** Test required for persons seeking residency permits; U.S. tests results accepted.
• **Vaccinations:** None required.
EMBASSIES/CONSULATES
• **U.S. Embassy**: Kentmanni 20, Tallinn; Tel: 372-668-8100; Fax: 372-668-8267; Website: www.usemb.ee.
• **Canadian Embassy**: Toom Kooli 13, 2nd Floor, 10130 Tallinn; Tel: 372-627-3310-11; Fax: 627-3312; e-mail: canembt@zzz.ee.
• **British Embassy:** Wismari 6, 10136 Tallinn; Tel: 372-667-4700; e-mail: information@britishembassy.ee; Website: www.britishembassy.ee.
HOSPITALS/DOCTORS:
Medical facilities are improving but still are not up to Western standards. There are many highly trained medical professionals, but hospitals and clinics suffer from lack of

equipment. Travelers are advised to obtain supplemental travel health insurance with specific overseas coverage. The policy should provide for direct payment to the overseas hospital and/or physician at the time of service and include a medical evacuation benefit.
• Tallinn Central Hospital, Ravi Strut 18, Tallinn (500 beds); Tel: 372-2-620-7000; public hospital with 24-hour emergency services and other specialties.

Current Advisories & Health Risks

For additional information, consult the Disease Risk Summary for Europe on page 300.

Ethiopia

CAPITAL:
Addis Ababa
EMBASSY (IN U.S.):
202-234-2281
GMT:
+3 hours
TELEPHONE COUNTRY CODE:
251
USADIRECT:
None
ENTRY REQUIREMENTS
• **Passport/Visa:** Passport and visa required. Exit visas are required of all visitors remaining in Ethiopia for more than 30 days. For longer stays and other information, contact the Embassy of Ethiopia, 3506 International Dr., NW, Washington, DC 20008; Tel: 202-364-1200. Website: www.ethiopianembassy.org
• **HIV Test:** Not required.
• **Vaccinations:** A yellow fever vaccination certificate is required for all travelers older than 1 year of age arriving from yellow fever-infected areas.
EMBASSIES/CONSULATES
• **U.S. Embassy:** Entoto Avenue, Addis Ababa; Tel: 251-1-550-666, ext. 316/336; Fax: 251-1-551-094; Website: www.telecom.net.et/~usemb-et.
• **Canadian Embassy:** Old Airport Area, Higher 23, Kebele 12, House Number 122, Addis Ababa; Tel: 251-1-71-30-22; Fax: 71-30-33; e-mail: addis@dfait-maeci.gc.ca.
• **British Embassy:** Fikre Mariam Abatechan Street, PO Box 858, Addis Ababa; Tel: 251-1-61-23-54; Fax: 251-1-61-05-88; e-mail: BritishEmbassy.AddisAbaba@fco.gov.uk.
HOSPITALS/DOCTORS:
Medical facilities are of very poor quality and poorly maintained. Even the best hospitals in Addis Ababa have antiquated equipment and shortages of supplies and medicine. Travelers to Ethiopia are advised to obtain supplemental travel health insurance with specific overseas coverage. The policy should provide for direct payment to the overseas hospital and/or physician at the time of service and include a medical evacuation benefit. Any traveler with a serious medical problem, or injury, should be evacuated to Nairobi, Kenya.

- Empress Zauditu Memorial Hospital, Addis Ababa (207 beds); basic diagnostic and treatment services.
- Mekan Hiwet Hospital, Addis Ababa (750 beds); basic treatment and emergency services; surgical capabilities.

Current Advisories and Health Risks

AFRICAN SLEEPING SICKNESS (TRYPANOSOMIASIS): Areas of transmission of the Rhodesian form of sleeping sickness occur in southwestern Ethiopia in Gamo, Gofa, Ilubabor, Kefa, and Welega Administrative Divisions. Gambien sleeping sickness may occur in areas adjacent to southern Sudan. Travelers to these areas should take measures to prevent insect (tsetse fly) bites.

ANIMAL HAZARDS: Animal hazards include snakes (vipers, cobras, mambas), centipedes, scorpions, and black widow spiders.

ARBOVIRAL FEVERS: Dengue fever most likely occurs in the coastal regions. Sand fly fever, West Nile fever, Chikungunya fever, Sindbis fever, and Rift Valley fever may occur. Travelers should take precautions against mosquito bites.

CHOLERA: This disease is active in this country but is a rare disease in travelers from developed countries. Cholera vaccine is recommended primarily for people at high risk (e.g., health-care, relief workers) who work and live in highly endemic areas under less than adequate sanitary conditions. Many countries, including Canada, license an oral cholera vaccine. The oral vaccine is not available in the United States.

ARBOVIRAL FEVER: Dengue most likely occurs in the coastal regions. Sand fly fever, West Nile fever, Chikungunya fever, Sindbis fever, and Rift Valley fever may also occur, but levels are unclear. Travelers should take measures to prevent insect bites.

HEPATITIS: The hepatitis A vaccine is recommended for all travelers. Hepatitis E is endemic, but the levels are unclear. The hepatitis B carrier rate in the general population is estimated at 11%. Hepatitis B is spread by infected blood, contaminated needles, and unprotected sex. Vaccination is recommended for stays longer than 3 months; for anyone at occupational or social risk; for anyone desiring maximal protection.

INFLUENZA: Influenza is transmitted from November through March in areas north of the Tropic of Cancer and throughout the year in areas south of that. The flu vaccine is recommended for all travelers at risk.

LEISHMANIASIS: Widespread incidence, with focal distribution countrywide. Cutaneous leishmaniasis occurs in most areas of the Ethiopian highland plateau (elevation 1,500 to 2,700 meters), including Addis Ababa. Areas of risk for visceral leishmaniasis (kala-azar) include the northwestern, southwestern, and southern lowlands, and the northeastern low-lying arid areas along the Red Sea coast. Travelers to these areas should take measures to prevent insect (sand fly) bites.

MALARIA: Transmission occurs year-round in most lowlands and urban areas below 1,500 to 2,000 meters elevation, especially in areas near or around lakes, swamps, streams, and irrigation ditches. Risk is elevated during and immediately following the rainy season (from June through September). There is no malaria in Addis Ababa (elevation 2,450 meters) or the Ethiopian highlands. Prophylaxis with atovaquone/proguanil (Malarone), mefloquine (Lariam), or doxycycline is recommended.

MENINGITIS: Ethiopia lies within the African "meningitis belt." Vaccination with the quadrivalent meningococcal vaccine is advised for all travelers, especially those anticipating close, extended contact with the indigenous population.

ONCHOCERCIASIS: Black fly-borne; occurs primarily along rivers in the Angered Valley and Humera area in Gonder, western Gojam, and most of Kefa, Ilubabor, and Welega Administrative Divisions; additional foci may occur in lowland areas of Gonder, Gama, Gofa, and Western Shewa and Sidamo Administrative Divisions.

POLIO: This disease is active in this country. The WHO also reports recent cases of poliomyelitis in Benin, Botswana, Burkina Faso, the Central African Republic, Chad, Côte d'Ivoire, Guinea, and Sudan that have been linked to outbreaks of polio in northern Nigeria. All travelers to Ethiopia should be fully immunized against polio.

RABIES: Higher than average risk. There is a large stray dog population, especially in Addis Ababa and other urban areas, that is primarily responsible for disease transmission. Travelers should seek immediate treatment of any animal bite, especially if from a dog. Rabies vaccine is recommended for anyone planning long-term travel to this country, and for short-term travelers desiring extra protection, especially if going to rural areas where the risk of animal bites is higher and where medical care is less readily available.

SCHISTOSOMIASIS: Intestinal schistosomiasis is widely distributed in highland areas, primarily occurring in agricultural communities along streams between 1,300 and 2,000 meters elevation. Limited areas of urinary schistosomiasis are confined to the warmer lowland areas (below 800 meters elevation). Travelers should avoid swimming or wading in freshwater lakes, ponds, or streams.

TRAVELERS' DIARRHEA Most rural water supplies consist of unprotected wells, streams, or natural springs. In urban areas, piped water is commonly available at public distribution points, but may be contaminated. Travelers should observe all food and drink safety precautions. A quinolone antibiotic, combined with loperamide (Imodium) is recommended for the treatment of acute diarrhea. Persistent diarrhea may be due to a parasitic disease such as giardiasis, amebiasis, or cryptosporidiosis.

TUBERCULOSIS: Tuberculosis (TB) is a major health problem in this country. Travelers planning an extended stay should have a pre-departure TB skin test (PPD test) and be retested after returning home.

TYPHOID FEVER: Typhoid vaccine is recommended for all travelers, with the exception of short-term visitors who restrict their meals to major restaurants and hotels. Because the typhoid vaccines are only 60% to 70% effective, safe food and drink selection remains important.

YELLOW FEVER: Yellow fever vaccine is recommended for all travelers older than 9 months of age.

OTHER DISEASES/HAZARDS: African tick typhus, anthrax (in Gonder region), brucellosis, echinococcosis (high prevalence among nomadic pastoralists in the southwest), filariasis (endemic focus of Bancroftian filariasis at Gambela), leptospirosis, relapsing fever (tick-borne and louse-borne); toxoplasmosis, trachoma (up to one half of the population infected), typhus (louse-borne and flea-borne; endemic in highlands), and intestinal helminthic infections (very common).

Fiji

CAPITAL:
Suva
EMBASSY (IN U.S.):
202-337-8320
GMT:
+12 hours
TELEPHONE COUNTRY CODE:
679
USADIRECT:
004-890-1001

ENTRY REQUIREMENTS

- **Passport/Visa:** Passport, proof of sufficient funds and onward/return ticket required. Visa not required for stay of up to 4 months. Contact the Embassy of Fiji, 2233 Wisconsin Ave, NW., #240, Washington, DC, 20007; Tel: 202-337-8320, or Fiji Mission to UN in NYC.
- **HIV Test:** Not required.
- **Vaccinations:** A yellow fever vaccination certificate is required for travelers older than 1 year of age entering Fiji within 10 days of having stayed overnight or longer in infected areas.

EMBASSIES/CONSULATES

- **U.S. Embassy:** Suva. 31 Loftus St; Tel: 314-466.
- **Canadian Embassy:** Nadi Airport, Nadi; Tel: 721-936 or 722-400, 724-489; e-mail: HonConFiji@is.com.fj.
- **British High Commission:** Victoria House, Gladstone Road, Suva (PO Box 1355); Tel: 679-3229100; Fax: 679-3229132; Website: http://www.britishhighcommission. gov.uk/fiji.

HOSPITALS/DOCTORS:
Medical facilities are adequate for routine medical problems. Travelers with serious medical emergencies should be evacuated to Australia.
Travelers to Fiji are advised to obtain supplemental travel health insurance with specific overseas coverage. The policy should provide for direct payment to the overseas hospital and/or physician at the time of service and include a medical evacuation benefit.
- The main hospitals are located in Suva, Lautoka, Sigatoka, Ba, Savusavu, Taveuni, Labasa and Levuka, with clinics and medical representations elsewhere throughout the islands.
- Colonial War Memorial Hospital, Suva (500 beds); Tel: 679-31-3444. This is a teaching hospital and the main medical facility in Fiji. There is a hyperbaric chamber onsite for the treatment of diving-related injuries.

Current Advisories and Health Risks

All travelers should be up to date on their routine immunizations: tetanus-diphtheria (Td), measles-mumps-rubella (MMR), polio, and varicella (chickenpox). Immunization against hepatitis A, hepatitis B, influenza, and typhoid fever is recommended.

For additional information, consult the Disease Risk Summary for Oceania on page 315.

Finland

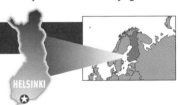

CAPITAL:
Helsinki
EMBASSY (IN U.S.):
202-298-5800
GMT:
+2 hours
TELEPHONE COUNTRY CODE:
358
USADIRECT:
0-8001-10015
ENTRY REQUIREMENTS
- **Passport/Visa:** Passport required. Tourist/business visa not required for stay of up to 90 days.
- **HIV Test:** Not required.
- **Vaccinations:** None required.

EMBASSIES/CONSULATES
- **U.S. Embassy:** Itainen Puistotie 14B, Helsinki. Tel: 9-171931; Fax: 358-9-652057; e-mail: consular@usembassy.fi; Website: www.usembassy.fi.
- **Canadian Embassy:** Pohjoisesplanadi 25 B, Helsinki. Tel: 09-17-11-41; Fax: 60-10-60; e-mail: hsnki@dfait-maeci.gc.ca; Website: www.canada.fi.
- **British Embassy:** Itainen Puistotie 17, 00140, Helsinki; Tel: 358-9-2286-5100; e-mail: info@britishembassy.fi; Website: www.britishembassy.fi.

HOSPITALS/DOCTORS:
Medical care is of high quality and many physicians speak English. There are five universities with medical schools; these tend to deal with the more specialized treatments. Travelers to Finland are advised to obtain supplemental travel health insurance with specific overseas coverage. The policy should provide for direct payment to the overseas hospital and/or physician at the time of service and include a medical evacuation benefit.
• Helsinki University Central Hospital; Tel: 9-1912-2177.

Current Advisories and Health Risks

IMMUNIZATIONS: All travelers should be up to date on their routine immunizations: tetanus-diphtheria (Td), measles-mumps-rubella (MMR), polio, influenza, and varicella (chickenpox). Hepatitis A and B vaccines are recommended.

LYME DISEASE: This disease is reported in brushy and forested areas, April through October, in the southern coastal regions and Aland Islands at elevations below 1,500 meters. Travelers should take tick bite precautions.

TICK-BORNE ENCEPHALITIS (TBE): Rare cases are transmitted April through October by ticks found in brushy and wooded areas, mostly in forested areas along the coast of the Gulf of Finland from Kotka to the border with Russia, and all the islands south of Turku, including the Aland islands. There is no risk in the Helsinki area. A TBE vaccine is available in Canada and Europe, but is recommended only for those who will have prolonged or intense exposure (e.g., hiking or camping for 2 to 3 weeks or more) in rural endemic areas.

TRAVELERS' DIARRHEA: Low risk. Tap water throughout Finland is potable. A quinolone antibitotic, combined with loperamide (Imodium), is recommended for the treatment of acute diarrhea.

OTHER ILLNESSES/HAZARDS: Although smoking and drug abuse are significantly less frequent in Finland than in Europe on average, alcoholism is a public health problem and a burden on health facilities. Driving a motor vehicle accident while intoxicated may result in heavy penalties and possible incarceration. Finland has one of the lowest infant mortality rates in the world, but the life expectancy of Finnish men is deteriorated by cardiovascular disease, excessive consumption of alcohol, and accidents.

For additional information, consult the Disease Risk Summary for Europe on page 300.

France

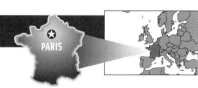

CAPITAL:
Paris
EMBASSY (IN U.S.):
202-944-6000

GMT:
+1 hour
TELEPHONE COUNTRY CODE:
33
USADIRECT:
0-800-99-0011

ENTRY REQUIREMENTS
- **Passport/Visa:** Visas not required for tourists; business stays up to 3 months.
- **HIV Test:** Not required for tourists.
- **Vaccinations:** None required.

EMBASSIES/CONSULATES
- **U.S. Embassy:** 2, Rue St. Florentin, Place de la Concorde, Paris. Tel: 01-43-12-22; Fax: 01-42-61-61-40; Website: www.amb-usa.fr;
- **Canadian Embassy:** 4 Rue Jean Rey, Paris; Tel: 33-01-4059-3300/2; Fax: 01 4059-3310.
- **British Embassy:** 35 rue du Faubourg St. Honoré, 75383 Paris Cedex 08; Tel: 33-1-44-51-31-00; Fax: 33-1-44-51-34-83; Website: http://www.amb-grandebretagne.fr.

HOSPITALS/DOCTORS
- The American Hospital, Paris; 63 Blvd. Victor Hugo, Neuilly-sur-Seine; Tel: 01-47-47-70-15 for emergency advice as well as physician or outpatient clinic referrals. All specialties; bilingual staff; 85% have had additional training in the United States; large corporate and international clientele; the hospital has angioplasty and coronary artery bypass grafting surgery (CABG) capabilities; emergency department with English-speaking doctors; open 24 hours.
- International SOS: International SOS (France) S.A., Immeuble "Le Ravel", 12-14 rue d'Alsace – B.P. 322, 92306 LEVALLOIS-PERRET Cedex, France; Alarm Center Tel: 33-1-5563-3155; Alarm Center Fax: 33-1-5563-3156.

Medical care in Western Europe is of high quality and many physicians speak English. Travelers are advised to obtain, before departure, supplemental travel health insurance with specific overseas coverage. The policy should provide for direct payment to the overseas hospital and/or physician at the time of service and include a medical evacuation benefit.

Current Advisories and Health Risks

HEPATITIS: Low risk. Hepatitis A vaccination is not considered necessary for routine travel to France but nonimmune travelers may wish to be immunized. The carrier rate of the hepatitis B virus in the general population is less than 1%. Hepatitis B is spread by infected blood, contaminated needles and syringes, and unprotected sex. Vaccination is recommended for stays longer than 3 months; for anyone at occupational or social risk; for any traveler desiring maximal protection.

INFLUENZA: Influenza is transmitted from November through March. The flu vaccine is recommended for all travelers to this country.

LEISHMANIASIS: Low risk, but visceral and cutaneous leishmaniasis do occur in rural areas of southern France, primarily in the departments of Bouche-de-Rhone, Provence, and Alpes-Maritimes, and on Corsica. Transmission occurs between May and November, peaking in July and August. Travelers should take measures to prevent insect (sand fly) bites.

LISTERIOSIS: Outbreaks of listeriosis, caused by consumption of unpasteurized dairy products, especially soft cheeses, such as Brie, have been reported. Young children, pregnant women, and travelers with compromised immunity should avoid soft cheese products.

LYME DISEASE: Low risk, but transmission occurs in wooded, brushy areas or in broadleaf (oak) forests. Risk is elevated in eastern France. Travelers to rural areas countrywide should take measures to avoid tick bites.

MEDITERRANEAN SPOTTED (BOUTONNEUSE) FEVER: This rickettsial disease, transmitted by dog ticks, occurs in southern France in regions below 1,000 meters elevation. Peak transmission occurs July through September. The primary endemic areas are the Mediterranean coast (especially the vicinity of Marseille and the island of Corsica. Disease may be acquired in and around tick-infested houses and terrain, but more than 95% of cases are associated with contact with dogs.

RABIES: No human cases are reported, but rabies is reported enzootic in the fox population. All unprovoked animal bites should be medically evaluated for possible rabies.

TRAVELERS' DIARRHEA: Low risk. Tap water throughout France is potable.

OTHER DISEASES/HAZARDS: Brucellosis, echinococcosis, fascioliasis (cases reported from Orne and Manche Departments in Normandy), leptospirosis, legionellosis, giardiasis, human alveolar echinococcosis (cases reported from the Franche-Comte region; the red fox is the definitive host), tick-borne meningoencephalitis (due to Rickettsia slovaca; reported in central France/Pyrenees mountains), toxoplasmosis (from ingesting undercooked beef), trichinosis (outbreaks associated with consumption of poorly cooked horse meat have occurred), tick-borne encephalitis occurs; risk is elevated in the Alsace region.

French Guiana

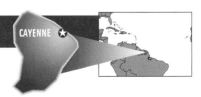

CAYENNE ★

CAPITAL:
Cayenne
EMBASSY (IN U.S.):
202-944-6000
GMT:
−3 hours

594
0-800-99-0011

ENTRY REQUIREMENTS

- **Passport/Visa:** Passport required. Visa not required for tourist/business stays of up to 3 months. For further information, contact the Consulate General of France, 4101 Reservoir Rd., NW, Washington, DC 20007; Tel: 202-944-6200.
- **HIV Test:** Not required.
- **Vaccinations:** A yellow fever vaccination certificate is required for all travelers older than 1 year of age arriving from all countries.

EMBASSIES/CONSULATES:

The United States maintains no diplomatic representation in French Guiana, which is an overseas department of France. For assistance in French Guiana, U.S. citizens may contact the U.S. Embassy in Paramaribo, Suriname (Tel: 597-477-881) which has consular jurisdiction in this area.

- **Canadian High Commission:** Accredited to the Canadian High Commission in Guyana. High and Young Streets, Georgetown, Guyana; Postal Address: PO Box 10880, Georgetown, Guyana; Tel: 592-227-2081/2/3/4/5; Fax: 592-225-8380; e-mail: grgtn@international.gc.ca; Website: www.georgetown.gc.ca.
- **British Consulate:** Tel: 594-31-10-34; Fax: 594-30-40-94.

HOSPITALS/DOCTORS:

Medical care in French Guiana is limited. Hospital facilities are available only in larger urban areas. Windows in patients' rooms frequently are not glass-paned but are fitted with wooden slats, letting in insects.

- Clinique Saint Paul, Cayenne (81 beds); general medical/surgical facility; ob/gyn; cardiology; pediatrics.

Current Advisories and Health Risks

All travelers should be up to date on their routine immunizations: tetanus-diphtheria (Td), measles-mumps-rubella (MMR), polio, influenza, and varicella (chickenpox). Immunization against hepatitis A, hepatitis B, and typhoid fever is recommended.

AIDS/HIV: Endemic at moderate levels. The primary risk factor for HIV infection is multiple heterosexual contacts, with HIV seropositivity highest among Haitian immigrants.

ANIMAL HAZARDS: Animal hazards include snakes (vipers), centipedes, scorpions, black widow spiders, brown recluse spiders, banana spiders, pruning spiders, and wolf spiders.

CHOLERA: Sporadic cases occur. Vaccination is not routinely recommended for tourist travel.

DENGUE FEVER: Risk is present, with intermittent epidemics. All travelers should take measures to prevent daytime mosquito bites.

HEPATITIS: Hepatitis A vaccination is recommended for all travelers. The hepatitis B carrier rate in the population is 2% to 13% with the higher rates in some rural areas. Hepatitis B is spread by infected blood, contaminated needles, and unprotected sex. Vaccination is recommended for stays longer than 3 months; for anyone at occupational or social risk; for anyone desiring maximal protection.

LEISHMANIASIS: Cutaneous leishmaniasis has become a public health problem, primarily among people living in forested areas. Transmission occurs primarily from November through May with the highest risk of transmission during periods of lowest rainfall, October through December. Most cases of leishmaniasis occur in the eastern half of the country. U.S. military units undergoing jungle training have experienced attack rates exceeding 50% during a 3- to 4-week exposure. Travelers to forested areas should take protective measures against sand flies, which bite from dusk to dawn.

MALARIA: Risk is present in all areas of this country year-round. The highest incidence of malaria occurs in territories bordering Brazil (Oiapoque River valley) and Suriname (Maroni River valley). The risk of vivax malaria is greatest in the east and along the coast. Prophylaxis with atovaquone/proguanil (Malarone), mefloquine (Lariam), or doxycycline is recommended.

MARINE HAZARDS: Electric eels and various carnivorous fish (including piranha) may be found in the country's fresh waters. Vampire bats are also present in this country. Portuguese man-of-war, sea wasps, and stingrays are found in the coastal waters and could be a hazard to swimmers.

RABIES: Sporadic cases occur. Dogs are the primary source of infection although vampire bats have also transmitted the disease. Rabies vaccination is recommended for long-term travelers to this country.

TRAVELERS' DIARRHEA: Water in Cayenne is considered generally safe for consumption. A quinolone antibiotic, combined with loperamide (Imodium) is recommended for the treatment of diarrhea. Persistent diarrhea may be due to a parasitic disease such as giardiasis or amebiasis.

TUBERCULOSIS: Tuberculosis (TB) is a major health problem in this country. Travelers planning an extended stay should have a pre-departure TB skin test (PPD test) and be retested after returning from this country.

TYPHOID FEVER: Typhoid vaccine is recommended for all travelers, with the exception of short-term visitors who restrict their meals to major restaurants and hotels. Because the typhoid vaccines are only 60% to 70% effective, safe food and drink selection remains important.

YELLOW FEVER: A yellow fever vaccination certificate is required for entry to this country. This country is in the Yellow Fever Endemic Zone.

OTHER DISEASES/HAZARDS: Brucellosis (common; from ingestion of unpasteurized dairy products), filariasis (endemic in coastal urban areas), leptospirosis, leprosy (countrywide prevalence), polio (no longer a threat in Latin America), syphilis, tungiasis, strongyloidiasis, and other helminthic infections.

French Polynesia

PAPEETE

CAPITAL:
Papeete

EMBASSY (IN U.S.):
202-944-6200

GMT:
−10 hours

TELEPHONE COUNTRY CODE:
689

USADIRECT:
None

ENTRY REQUIREMENTS

- **Passport/Visa:** No visa required for stays of less than 30 days. French Polynesia is a French overseas territory.
- **HIV Test:** Not required.
- **Vaccinations:** A yellow fever vaccination certificate is required of travelers arriving from infected areas.

EMBASSIES/CONSULATES:

There is no U.S. Embassy or diplomatic post on the island of Tahiti, nor any of the other islands. For assistance, travelers should contact the U.S. Embassy in Suva, Fiji; Tel: 679-314-466.

- **Canadian Embassy:** Accredited to the Australian Consulate General in New Caledonia. Immeuble Foch, 7th Floor, 19 Avenue du Maréchal Foch, Nouméa, New Caledonia; PO Box 22, Nouméa, 98845, New Caledonia; Tel: 687-27-2414; Fax: 687-27-8001.
- **British Consulate:** Tel: 689-70-63-82; Fax: 689-42-00-50.

HOSPITALS/DOCTORS:

French Polynesia enjoys a high standard of health, with medical and dental services adequate for most medical problems, pharmacies, private clinics, and a large government hospital in Tahiti. The outer islands have hospitals or dispensaries and a few private practitioners. Travelers are advised to obtain, before departure, supplemental travel health insurance with specific overseas coverage. The policy should provide for direct payment to the overseas hospital and/or physician at the time of service and include a medical evacuation benefit.

Current Advisories and Health Risks

AIDS/HIV: A small number of AIDS cases and HIV infections have been reported. The hospital blood supply is screened for HIV and is considered safe.

452

DENGUE FEVER: This disease occurs sporadically. Highest risk is during the rainy season months. Travelers should take measures to prevent daytime mosquito bites.

FILARIASIS: Moderately high rates (up to 19%) of Malayan filariasis reported in the general population. Travelers should take protective measures against mosquito bites.

HEPATITIS: Hepatitis A vaccine is recommended for all travelers. The hepatitis B carrier rate in the general population of Oceania is estimated at 5.5% to 15%. Hepatitis B is spread by infected blood, contaminated needles, and unprotected sex. Vaccination is recommended for stays longer than 3 months; for anyone at occupational or social risk; for anyone desiring maximal protection.

INFLUENZA: Influenza is transmitted year-round in the tropics; flu vaccine is recommended for all travelers.

MALARIA: There is no risk of malaria in French Polynesia.

MARINE HAZARDS: Swimming-related hazards include jellyfish, spiny sea urchins, and coral. Ciguatera poisoning is prevalent and can result from eating coral reef fish such as grouper, snapper, sea bass, jack, and barracuda. The ciguatoxin is not destroyed by cooking.

TRAVELERS' DIARRHEA: Low to medium risk. The tap water on most of the main islands is generally safe, but travelers are advised to drink bottled, boiled, or treated water. A quinolone antibiotic, combined with loperamide (Imodium), is recommended for the treatment of acute diarrhea. Persistent diarrhea may be due to a parasitic infection such as giardiasis, amebiasis, or cryptosporidiosis.

TYPHOID FEVER: Outbreaks of typhoid fever have been reported, but the incidence is low. Typhoid vaccine is recommended for travelers venturing outside of tourist areas; adventure travelers; long-term travelers; those wishing maximal disease protection. Because the typhoid vaccines are only 60% to 70% effective, safe food and drink selection remains important.

Gabon

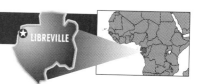

LIBREVILLE

CAPITAL:
Libreville
EMBASSY (IN U.S.):
202-797-1000
GMT:
+1 hour
TELEPHONE COUNTRY CODE:
241

00-001
ENTRY REQUIREMENTS
- **Passport/Visa:** Passport and visa required. Visa for a stay of up to 4 months, requires two application forms, two photos, vaccination certificate for yellow fever, letter from a sponsor or hotel in Gabon, and a $60 fee. Business visas also require company letter. For longer stays and other information contact the Embassy of the Gabonese Republic, 2034 20th St., Suite 200, NW, Washington, DC 20009; Tel: 202/797-1000 or 1021.
- **HIV Test:** Not required.
- **Vaccinations:** A yellow fever vaccination certificate is required from all travelers older than 1 year of age arriving from all countries.

EMBASSIES/CONSULATES
- **U.S. Embassy:** Boulevard de la Mer, Centre Ville, Libreville; Tel: 76-20-03/4 or 74-34-92.
- **Canadian Embassy:** Quartier Batterie IV, Libreville; Tel: 73-73-54; Fax: 73-73-88; e-mail: lbrve@dfait-maeci.gc.ca.
- **British High Commission:** Accredited to the British Embassy in Cameroon. Avenue Winston Churchill, BP 547, Yaoundé; Tel: 237-2-22-05-45/2-22-07-96; Fax: 237-2-22-01-48; e-mail: BHCyaounde@fco.gov.uk.

HOSPITALS/DOCTORS:
Medical care in this country is substandard. Travelers to Gabon are advised to obtain supplemental travel health insurance with specific overseas coverage. The policy should provide for direct payment to the overseas hospital and/or physician at the time of service and include a medical evacuation benefit.
- The Albert Schweitzer Hospital, Lambarene; world famous missionary hospital provides basic medical/surgical treatments.
- Libreville General Hospital (630 beds); general medical/surgical facility; maternity wing.
- Bongolo Evangelical Hospital, La Bomba (80 beds); missionary hospital; emergency care available.

Current Advisories and Health Risks

IMMUNIZATIONS: All travelers should be up to date on their routine immunizations: tetanus-diphtheria (Td), measles-mumps-rubella (MMR), polio, influenza, and varicella (chickenpox). Immunization against hepatitis A, hepatitis B, and typhoid fever is recommended. Rabies vaccine is recommended for long-term (over 1 month) travelers. A yellow fever vaccination certificate is required to enter this country.

MALARIA: Risk is present year-round, countrywide, including urban areas. Risk is elevated during and immediately after the rainy seasons (October through December and February through April). Prophylaxis with atovaquone/proguanil (Malarone), mefloquine (Lariam), or doxycycline is recommended.

SLEEPING SICKNESS: Risk areas for sleeping sickness (trypanosomiasis) persist along the coast, primarily the Komo estuary around Libreville, and the mouth of the Ogooue River near Port Gentil. Travelers should take measures to prevent insect (tsetse fly) bites.

SCHISTOSOMIASIS: Foci of disease are scattered throughout all provinces, with a major focus in the Libreville area. Travelers should avoid swimming, bathing, or wading in freshwater lakes, ponds, or streams.

For additional information, consult the Disease Risk Summary for sub-Saharan Africa on page 307.

Gambia

CAPITAL:
Banjul
EMBASSY (IN U.S.):
202-785-1399
GMT:
+0 hours
TELEPHONE COUNTRY CODE:
220
USADIRECT:
00111
ENTRY REQUIREMENTS
• **Passport/Visa:** Passport and visa required.
• **HIV Test:** Not required.
• **Vaccinations:** A yellow fever vaccination certificate is required of all travelers arriving from infected or endemic countries.
EMBASSIES/CONSULATES
• **U.S. Embassy:** Kairaba Avenue in Fajara, Banjul; Tel: 392856, 392858 or 391971; Fax: 392475.
• **Canadian Embassy:** Accredited to Canadian Embassy in Senegal. Corner of Galliéni and Brière-de-l'Isle Streets, Dakar, Senegal; Tel: 221 889-47-00; Fax: 221 889-47-20; e-mail: dakar@international.gc.ca;Website: www.dakar.gc.ca.
• **British High Commission:** 48 Atlantic Road, Fajara (PO Box 507), Banjul; Tel: 220-4495133, 4495134; Fax: 220-4496134; e-mail: bhcbanjul@gamtel.gm.
HOSPITALS/DOCTORS:
Travelers should contact the U.S. Embassy in Banjul for hospital/physician referrals.

Current Advisories and Health Risks

AIDS/HIV: Incidence of HIV-1 and HIV-2 is increasing. Transmission is predominantly heterosexual; prevalences estimated to be 0.1% and 2%, respectively, among low-risk urban populations, and 14% and 27%, respectively, among high-risk urban populations. Travelers should avoid unsafe sex, unsterile needles and syringes, and unscreened blood transfusions.

ACCIDENTS, ILLNESS, AND MEDICAL INSURANCE:

- Accidents and injuries are the leading cause of death among travelers younger than age 55 and are most often caused by motor vehicle and motorcycle crashes; drownings, aircraft crashes, homicides, and burns are less common causes.
- Heart attacks cause most fatalities in older travelers.
- Infections cause only 1% of fatalities in overseas travelers, but, overall, infections are the most common cause of travel-related illness.
- Travelers are advised to obtain, before departure, supplemental travel health insurance with specific overseas coverage. The policy should provide for direct payment to the overseas hospital and/or physician at the time of service and include a medical evacuation benefit. The policy should also provide 24-hour hotline access to a multilingual assistance center that can help arrange and monitor delivery of medical care and determine if medical evacuation or air ambulance services are required.

AFRICAN SLEEPING SICKNESS (TRYPANOSOMIASIS): Low-level transmission occurs countrywide, but levels are unclear. Travelers should take precautions against insect (tsetse fly) bites.

ARBOVIRAL DISEASES: There is evidence of chikungunya fever, West Nile fever, dengue fever, Rift Vally fever and Crimean-Congo hemorrhagic fever in this country, but levels are unclear. Travelers should take measures to prevent insect bites.

CHOLERA: This disease is reported active in this country, but the threat to tourists is very low. Cholera is an extremely rare disease in travelers from developed countries. Cholera vaccine is recommended primarily for people at high risk who work and live in highly endemic areas under less than adequate sanitary conditions.

- The oral cholera vaccine (Dukoral) provides up to 60% crossover protection against ETEC diarrhea.
- Many countries, including Canada, license an oral cholera vaccine. The oral vaccine is not available in the United States.
- Cholera vaccine is not "officially" required for entry into, or exit from, any country.

HEPATITIS: Hepatitis A vaccine is recommended for all nonimmune travelers. Hepatitis E levels are unclear. The hepatitis B carrier rate in the general population is estimated as high as 16%. Vaccination against hepatitis B should be considered for stays longer than 3 months and by short-term travelers desiring maximal protection. Travelers should be aware that hepatitis B can be transmitted by unsafe sex and the use of contaminated needles and syringes. Hepatitis C is likely endemic.

INFLUENZA: Influenza is transmitted year-round in the tropics. The flu vaccine is recommended for all travelers older than age 50; all travelers with chronic disease or a weakened immune system; travelers of any age wishing to decrease the risk of this illness; pregnant women after the first trimester.

456

LEISHMANIASIS: Transmission occurs primarily from April through October. Risk may occur countrywide. Sporadic cases of cutaneous and visceral leishmaniasis have been reported from clinics in the Farafenni and Banjul vicinities. Travelers should take precautions to prevent insect (sand fly) bites.

MALARIA: The risk of malaria is countrywide, including urban areas, with the peak transmission immediately following the rainy season, June through October. Chloroquine-resistant *Plasmodium falciparum* is prevalent countrywide.
- Prophylaxis with atovaquone/proguanil (Malarone), mefloquine (Lariam), or doxycycline is recommended for all travelers.
- All travelers should take measures to prevent insect bites, especially in the evening and at night.

MENINGITIS: This country is in the "meningitis belt." Meningitis vaccine is recommended for all travelers staying longer than 1 month during the dry season, December to June, and should be considered for short-term travel if contact with the indigenous population is expected.

POLIO: This disease is likely endemic. All travelers should be immunized.

RABIES: Sporadic cases of human rabies are reported countrywide. All animal bites or scratches, especially from a dog, should be taken seriously and immediate medical attention sought. Although rabies is rare among tourists, there is risk. No one should pet or pick up any stray animals. All children should be warned to avoid contact with unknown animals. Rabies vaccine is recommended for travel longer than 3 months; for shorter stays for travelers who plan to venture off the usual tourist routes where they may be more exposed to the stray dog population; or when travelers desire extra protection.

SCHISTOSOMIASIS: Transmitted year-round; risk may be elevated during and immediately following the rainy season (usually June through October). Foci of *Schistosoma haematobium* likely are distributed primarily along the Gambia River. Limited foci of *Schistosoma mansoni* have been reported in the extreme southwestern corner of the Gambia, including the Banjul vicinity. Travelers should avoid bathing or swimming in freshwater lakes, ponds, or streams.

TRAVELERS' DIARRHEA: High risk, except in tourist hotels in Banjul. Travelers should treat acute diarrhea with a quinolone antibiotic, plus loperamide (Imodium).

TUBERCULOSIS: Tuberculosis is a major public health problem in this country. Travelers planning an extended stay should have a pre-departure TB skin test (PPD test) and be retested after leaving this country.

TYPHOID FEVER: Vaccination against typhoid fever is recommended for travelers venturing outside of tourist areas; long-term travelers; adventure travelers; those wishing maximal disease protection. Because the typhoid vaccines are only 60% to 70% effective, safe food and drink selection remains important.

YELLOW FEVER: This disease is active in the Upper River Division. Risk is considered to exist countrywide except in Banjul. In 2001, a tourist from Belgium died from yellow fever after visiting Gambia. Yellow fever vaccine is recommended for travelers to this country.

OTHER DISEASES/HAZARDS: African tick typhus (focally distributed; contracted from dog ticks—often in urban areas—and bush ticks); anthrax (cutaneous and gastrointestinal forms reported); Bancroftian filariasis (mosquito-borne; likely endemic at low levels); onchocerciasis (black fly-borne; highly endemic foci have been reported along fast-flowing rivers in the east).

Georgia

TBILISI

CAPITAL:
Tbilisi
EMBASSY (IN U.S.):
202-393-6060
TELEPHONE COUNTRY CODE:
995
GMT:
+3 hours
USADIRECT:
8^0288. ^ indicates second dial tone.

ENTRY REQUIREMENTS

- **Passport/Visa:** Passport, visa and letter of invitation required. Visa requires passport (not a photocopy), one application, one photo, and processing fee ($40 to $70). Please provide SASE or prepaid airbill for return of documents. For additional information, contact the Embassy of the Republic of Georgia, 1615 New Hampshire Ave., NW, Suite 300, Washington, DC 20009; Tel: 202-393-6060.
- **HIV Test:** Required for all foreigners staying longer than 1 month.
- **Vaccinations:** None required.

EMBASSIES/CONSULATES

- **U.S. Embassy:** 25 Atoneli Street, Tbilisi, 0105, Georgia; Tel: 995-32-98-99-67; Fax: 995-32-93-37-59; e-mail: consulate-tbilisi@state.gov; Website: http://georgia. usembassy.gov.
- **Canadian Embassy:** Accredited to the Canadian Embassy in Turkey. Cinnah Caddesi No. 58, Çankaya 06690, Ankara, Turkey; Tel: 90-312-409-2700; Fax: 90-312-409-2810; e-mail: ankra@international.gc.ca; Website: www.dfait-maeci.gc.ca/ankara.
- **British Embassy:** GMT Plaza, 4 Freedom Square, 0105 Tbilisi; Tel: 995-32-274747; Fax: 995-32-274792; e-mail: British.Embassy.Tbilisi@fco.gov.uk.

HOSPITALS/DOCTORS:
Medical care in Georgia is below Western standards. Travelers are advised to obtain supplemental travel health insurance with specific overseas coverage. The policy should

provide for direct payment to the overseas hospital and/or physician at the time of service and include a medical evacuation benefit.

Current Advisories and Health Risks

MALARIA: Risk is present in southeastern parts of the country in the districts of Lagodekhi, Sighnaghi, Dedophilistskaro, Saraejo, Gardabani, and Marneuli in the Kakheti and Kveno Kartli regions. There is no risk in Tbilisi. Chloroquine prophylaxis is recommended.

For additional information, consult the Disease Risk Summary for Europe on page 300.

Germany (Federal Republic of)

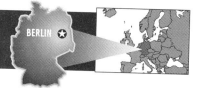

CAPITAL:
Berlin

EMBASSY (IN U.S.):
4645 Reservoir Rd., NW
Washington, DC 20007
202-298-4393
Website: www.germany-info.org

GMT:
+1 hour

TELEPHONE COUNTRY CODE:
49

USADIRECT:
0800-225-5288

ENTRY REQUIREMENTS
• **Passport/Visa:** A valid passport is required.
• **HIV Test:** Testing is required for those applying for residence permits (Bavaria only).
• **Vaccinations:** None required.

EMBASSIES/CONSULATES
• **U.S. Embassy:** Neustaedtische Kirchstrasse 4-5, Berlin. Tel: 30-238-5174, 8305.
• **Canadian Embassy:** Internationales Handelszentrum Building, Friedrichstrasse 95, Berlin. Tel: 30-20-31-20; e-mail: brlin-cs@dfait-maeci.gc.ca; Website: www.canada.de.
• **British Embassy:** Wilhelmstrasse 70, 10117 Berlin; Tel: 49-30-20457-0; Fax: 49-30-20457-571; Website: http://www.britischebotschaft.de.

HOSPITALS/DOCTORS
• Medical care in Western Europe is of high quality and many physicians speak English. Travelers are advised to obtain, before departure, supplemental travel health insurance with specific overseas coverage. The policy should provide for direct pay-

ment to the overseas hospital and/or physician at the time of service and include a medical evacuation benefit.

- International SOS: International SOS Emergency Services (Deutschland) GmbH, Hugenottenallee 167 63263 Neu-Isenburg, Germany; Alarm Center Tel: 49-6102-3588-100; Alarm Center Fax: 49-6102-202644

Current Advisories and Health Risks

ACCIDENTS AND ILLNESS: Accidents, especially motor vehicle crashes, are the leading cause of death among travelers less than 55 years of age; cardiovascular diseases cause most fatalities in older travelers; infections cause most illness during travel, but represent less than 1% of the fatalities.

AIDS/HIV: The region's adult prevalence rate was reported at 0.3% during 2004. Heterosexual transmission has increased recently in several Western European countries. Sex between men is still the most common route of infection in Germany. The role of injecting drug use in the transmission of HIV varies among countries of this region.

HEPATITIS: Although the incidence of hepatitis A in western Germany is among the lowest in Europe, vaccination is recommended. The hepatitis B carrier rate in the general population is estimated at less than 1%. Hepatitis B is spread by infected blood, contaminated needles, and unsafe sex. Vaccination is recommended for stays longer than 3 months; for anyone at occupational or social risk; for any traveler desiring maximal protection.

INFLUENZA: Influenza is transmitted from November through March. The flu vaccine is recommended for all travelers.

LYME DISEASE: This disease is reported countrywide, but most cases are reported in the south, primarily in Bavaria, mostly in the spring and summer. Up to 34% of ticks in some endemic areas are infected. The ticks that transmit Lyme disease are found in brushy, wooded areas and broadleaf (mostly oak) forests under 1,000 meters elevation. Travelers are advised to take measures to prevent tick bites.

RABIES: No human cases have been officially reported for several years. Wild foxes are the primary disease reservoir. Travelers should seek immediate medical evaluation and treatment of any wild animal bite.

TICK-BORNE ENCEPHALITIS (TBE): Most cases of this tick-borne viral illness are reported from the southern lowland forested and wooded areas of the Bayern and Baden-Wurttemburg (Black Forest, upper Rhine valley) regions. The valleys of Kinzig, Elz, and Dreisam, as well as the regions around Freiburg and Pforzheim, are endemic areas. Travelers should take protective measures against tick bites. TBE vaccine (available in Canada and Europe) is recommended only for people at high risk (e.g., forestry workers; campers and hikers with extensive exposure time in risk areas). Routine vaccination against TBE is not recommended.

TRAVELERS' DIARRHEA: Low risk. A quinolone antibiotic, combined with loperamide (Imodium), is recommended for the treatment of acute diarrhea. Persistent diarrhea may be due to a parasitic infection such as giardiasis or cryptosporidiosis.

Ghana

CAPITAL:
Accra
EMBASSY (IN U.S.):
202-686-4520
GMT:
+0 hour
TELEPHONE COUNTRY CODE:
233
USADIRECT:
0191
ENTRY REQUIREMENTS*
• **Passport/Visa:** Travelers should contact the Embassy of Ghana for entry information.
• **HIV Test:** Not required.
• **Vaccinations:** A yellow fever vaccination certificate is required from all travelers arriving from all countries, including the United States and Canada.
*Travelers should check with this country's embassy (or a consulate) in the United States, Canada, or the United Kingdom for any changes in these requirements.
EMBASSIES/CONSULATES
• **U.S. Embassy:** Ring Road East, Accra; Tel: 21-775-347,48; Website: usembassy. state.gov/ghana.
• **Canadian Embassy:** 42 Independence Avenue, Accra; Tel: 21-22-85-55, 22-85-66; Fax: 77-37-92; e-mail: accra@dfait-maeci.gc.ca.
• **British High Commission:** Osu Link, off Gamel Abdul Nasser Avenue, (PO Box 296), Accra; Tel: 233-21-7010650, 221665; Fax: 233-21-7010655; e-mail: high. commission.accra@fco.gov.uk; Website: www.britishhighcommission.gov.uk/ghana.
HOSPITALS/DOCTORS:
Medical care in Ghana is generally below Western standards. Travelers are advised to obtain, before departure, supplemental travel health insurance with specific overseas coverage. The policy should provide for direct payment to the overseas hospital and/or physician at the time of service and include a medical evacuation benefit.
• Police Hospital, Accra; used by U.S. Embassy personnel.
• Nyaho Clinic, Accra; used by U.S. Embassy personnel.
• Korle Bu Teaching Hospital, Accra (1,500 beds); general medical/surgical facility and cardiothoracic center.
• Tudu Clinic, Accra.

Current Advisories and Health Risks

AIDS/HIV: Ghana's HIV/AIDS epidemic is spreading more slowly than in the southern and eastern regions of Africa. HIV prevalence is estimated at about 4% of the overall adult population.

AFRICAN SLEEPING SICKNESS (TRYPANOSOMIASIS): Low apparent risk, but cases were reported in Ghana in the early 1980s. Sleeping sickness is currently reported in Ivory Coast, a neighboring country. As a precaution, all travelers to Ghana should take measures to prevent insect (tsetse fly) bites.

CHOLERA: This disease is reported active in this country, but the threat to tourists is very low. Cholera vaccine is recommended primarily for people at high risk (e.g., relief workers) who work and live in highly endemic areas under less than adequate sanitary conditions.

FILARIASIS: Bancroftian filariasis is reported in northeastern areas. Infection rates of 20% have been reported from the Vea and Tono rice irrigation project areas. Travelers should take measures to prevent mosquito bites.

HEPATITIS: All nonimmune travelers should receive hepatitis A vaccine. Hepatitis E is likely endemic, but the levels are unclear. The hepatitis B carrier rate in the general population is estimated to exceed 10%. Hepatitis B is spread by infected blood, contaminated needles and unsafe sex. Vaccination is recommended for stays longer than 3 months; for anyone at occupational or social risk; for any traveler desiring maximal protection. The risk of illness or injury during travel cannot be predicted; *all* travelers should consider receiving hepatitis B vaccine because of the risk of receiving a medical injection with an unsterile needle or syringe.

INFLUENZA: Influenza is transmitted year-round in the tropics. The flu vaccine is recommended for all travelers.

MALARIA: Risk is present throughout this country year-round, including urban areas. Risk may be elevated during and immediately following the rainy seasons, March through June and October through November in the south; March through October in the north. *Plasmodium falciparum* accounts for 85% of cases, followed by *Plasmodium malariae* and *Plasmodium ovale*. Prophylaxis with atovaquone/proguanil (Malarone), mefloquine (Lariam), or doxycycline is recommended. All travelers should take measures to prevent evening and nighttime mosquito bites.

MENINGITIS: Northern Ghana lies within the sub-Saharan meningitis belt, but cases have also been reported from the central regions of this country. Quadrivalent meningitis vaccine is recommended for travelers staying longer than 1 month during the dry season, December to June, and should be considered for shorter stays if extensive contact with the local populace is anticipated.

ONCHOCERCIASIS: Widely distributed along fast-flowing rivers, but incidence has declined due to black fly control programs. Moderate risk remains in central mountainous areas along the Pru River. Travelers should take precautions against insect bites.

POLIO: This disease is endemic. All travelers should be immunized.

RABIES: Rabies is considered a public health problem in many rural and peri-urban areas. There is a high incidence of dog rabies, with frequent human cases reported. All animal bites or scratches, especially from a dog, should be taken seriously, and immediate medical attention should be sought. No one should pet or pick up any stray animals. All children should be warned to avoid contact with unknown animals. Rabies vaccine is recommended for travel longer than 3 months, and for shorter stays for travelers who plan to visit rural areas.

SCHISTOSOMIASIS: Urinary schistosomiasis is widely distributed; swimming or bathing is unsafe in any freshwater lake, pond, or stream. Many cases are reported in the southeast (southern shore of Lake Volta, the area below the Akosombo Dam along the lower Volta River, and the Accra vicinity) and in the northeast. Limited foci of intestinal schistosomiasis are distributed sporadically, occurring predominantly in the extreme north, the southwest (Tarkwa), and the southeast (along the lower Volta River). Acute infection (Katayama fever) has resulted from swimming in the estuary of the Volta River.

TRAVELERS' DIARRHEA: Large urban areas have treated, piped water that is subject to recontamination during distribution. All water sources should be considered potentially contaminated. Travelers should observe safe food and drink precautions. A quinolone antibiotic, combined with loperamide (Imodium), is recommended for the treatment of acute diarrhea. Persistent diarrhea may be due to a parasitic infection such as giardiasis, amebiasis, or cryptosporidiosis.

TUBERCULOSIS: Tuberculosis (TB) is a major health problem in this country. Travelers planning an extended stay should have a pre-departure TB skin test (PPD test) and be retested after returning from this country.

TYPHOID FEVER: Typhoid vaccine is recommended for those traveling off the usual tourist routes, those visiting friends or relatives, and for long-stay visitors. Because the typhoid vaccines are only 60% to 70% effective, safe food and drink selection remains important.

YELLOW FEVER: Sporadic outbreaks of yellow fever occur in Ghana. The CDC recommends vaccination for all travelers. A vaccination certificate is required for entry to this country.

OTHER DISEASES/HAZARDS: African tick typhus (transmitted by dog ticks; often in urban areas, and bush ticks), anthrax (cutaneous; usually from contact with freshly slaughtered, infected animals), brucellosis (from consumption of raw dairy products), dengue fever (risk in both urban and rural areas; daytime mosquito bite protection recommended),

Lassa fever (sporadic and rare; transmission via contact with infected rodents), leishmaniasis (low risk; cutaneous and visceral leishmaniasis have been reported from neighboring countries), leprosy, leptospirosis (40% of agricultural workers show serologic exposure), tuberculosis (a major health problem), and intestinal worms (very common) are reported.

Great Britain

CAPITAL:
London
EMBASSY (IN U.S.):
202-462-1340
GMT:
+0 hours
TELEPHONE COUNTRY CODE:
44
USADIRECT:
0-800-89-0011
0-500-89-0011
ENTRY REQUIREMENTS
- **Passport/Visa:** Visa is not required for U.S. citizens.
- **HIV test:** Not required.
- **Vaccinations:** None required.
EMBASSIES/CONSULATES
- **U.S. Embassy:** 24 Grosvenor Square, London. Tel: 0207-499-9000; from the United States: Tel: 011-44-207-499-9000; Website: www.usembassy.org.uk.
- **Canadian Embassy:** Canada House, Consular Services, Trafalgar Square, London. Tel: 20-7258-6600; e-mail: ldn@dfait-maeci.gc.ca, Website: www.dfait-maeci.gc.ca/london.
HOSPITALS/DOCTORS:
- International SOS: International SOS Assistance (UK) Ltd., Sixth Floor, Landmark House, Hammersmith Bridge Road, London W6 9DP, England; Alarm Center Tel: 44-020-7762-7008; Alarm Center Fax: 44-020-7748-7744

Current Advisories and Health Risks

HEPATITIS: Low risk of hepatitis A, but the vaccine is recommended as routine for non-immune travelers. Vaccination against hepatitis B should be considered for stays longer than 3 months and by short-term travelers desiring maximal protection. Travelers should be aware that hepatitis B can be transmitted by unsafe sex and the use of contaminated needles and syringes.

INFLUENZA: Influenza is transmitted from November through March. The flu vaccine is recommended for all travelers.

LYME DISEASE: Cases of Lyme disease occur rarely throughout the United Kingdom (England, Scotland, Wales, and northern Ireland). The risk is very low—about 10 times less than on the continent of Europe. Transmission occurs from spring to autumn. Recently, the tick that transmits Lyme disease has been found in parks within the City of London.

TRAFFIC ALERT: Pedestrians should look to their right when crossing the street; traffic is left-sided.

TRAVELERS' DIARRHEA: Low risk; tap water is potable throughout the United Kingdom.

Greece

CAPITAL:
Athens
EMBASSY (IN U.S.):
202-939-5800
GMT:
+1 hour
TELEPHONE COUNTRY CODE:
30
USADIRECT:
00-800-1311

ENTRY REQUIREMENTS
- **Passport/Visa:** No visa is required for tourist/business stays up to 3 months.
- **HIV Test:** Testing not required for tourists
- **Vaccinations:** A yellow fever vaccination certificate is required from all travelers older than 6 months of age arriving from infected or endemic areas.

EMBASSIES/CONSULATES
- **U.S. Embassy:** 91 Vasilissis Sophias Boulevard, Athens; Tel: 1-721-2951; e-mail: consul@global.net; Website: www.usembassy.gr.
- **U.S. Consulate:** Plateia Commercial Center, 43 Tsimiski Street, 7th floor, Thessaloniki; Tel: 31-242-905; e-mail: cons@compulink.gr.
- **Canadian Embassy:** 4 Ioannou Gennadiou Street, Athens; Tel: 1-727-3400; Fax: 727-3480; e-mail: athns@dfait-maeci.gc.ca.
- **British Embassy:** 1 Ploutarchou Street, 106 75 Athens; Tel: 30-210-727-2600; e-mail: information.athens@fco.gov.uk; Website: http://www.british-embassy.gr.

HOSPITALS/DOCTORS
- The Diagnostic and Therapeutic Center of Athens, "HYGEIA" (350 beds); well-equipped, modern facility.
- Apostolos Accident Hospital, Athens (1,000 beds); orthopedics; trauma care.

Current Advisories and Health Risks

AIR POLLUTION: Travelers with respiratory diseases should be aware that severe air-quality problems occur in Athens and other urban areas.

HEPATITIS: There is a higher risk of hepatitis A in Greece than in other western European countries. Hepatitis A vaccine is recommended for nonimmune travelers. The hepatitis B carrier rate in the general population of Greece is estimated at 1% to 4%. Vaccination against hepatitis B should be considered for stays longer than 3 months and by short-term travelers desiring maximal protection. Travelers should be aware that hepatitis B can be transmitted by unsafe sex and the use of contaminated needles and syringes.

INFLUENZA: Influenza is transmitted from November through March. The flu vaccine is recommended for all travelers to this country.

LEISHMANIASIS: Risk of transmission is highest between May and October. Cutaneous leishmaniasis occurs sporadically, with the highest prevalence on the Ionian Islands. Visceral leishmaniasis occurs focally on the mainland, including the Athens area, and on the islands, especially Crete. Travelers to these regions should take measures to avoid sand fly bites.

MALARIA: No risk. Greece was declared malaria free in 1986.

RABIES: No cases of human rabies has been reported since 1970. A canine vaccination program, combined with the low prevalence of rabies among wild animals, has resulted in the eradication of rabies from this country. Any animal bite, however, should be medically evaluated.

TICK-BORNE ENCEPHALITIS (TBE): There is a low risk of TBE, April through September, in northern Greece, where sporadic cases are reported. The TBE vaccine (available in Canada and Europe), is recommended only for people at significant risk of exposure to tick bites, e.g., campers and hikers on extended trips, or forestry workers. The risk to the average tourist is very low.

TRAVELERS' DIARRHEA: Low to medium risk for acute diarrheal disease. A quinolone antibiotic, combined with loperamide (Imodium), is recommended for the treatment of acute diarrhea. Persistent diarrhea may be due to a parasitic disease such as giardiasis.

TYPHOID FEVER: Typhoid fever vaccine is recommended for long-term travelers, adventure travelers, and those wishing maximal disease protection. Because the typhoid vaccines are only 60% to 70% effective, safe food and drink selection remains important.

OTHER DISEASES/HAZARDS: Mediterranean spotted fever (tick-borne; highest incidence found in farmers in the prefecture of Trikala in northern Greece who have a seropositivity rate of 20%), brucellosis, echinococcosis, legionellosis (reported sporadically, usually in summer tourists), Q fever (tick-borne), sand fly fever (endemic), tick-borne relapsing fever (risk in rocky, rural livestock areas), helminthic infections (roundworm, hookworm, and whipworm infections reported occasionally from rural areas), and trichinosis.

Grenada

CAPITAL:
St. George's
EMBASSY (IN U.S.):
202-265-2561
GMT:
−4 hours
TELEPHONE COUNTRY CODE:
809
USADIRECT:
1-800-872-2881
ENTRY REQUIREMENTS
- **Passport/Visa:** Passport is recommended, but tourists may enter with a birth certificate and photo ID. Visa not required for tourist who stay up to 3 months; it may be extended to a maximum of 6 months. For additional information consult the Consulate General of Grenada, 1701 New Hampshire Ave., N.W., Washington, DC 20009 (202-265-2561) or Permanent Mission of Grenada to the U.N. (212-599-0301). Grenada has been independent from Britain since 1974.
- **HIV Test:** Not required.
- **Vaccinations:** A yellow fever vaccination certificate is required from all travelers coming from infected areas.
EMBASSIES/CONSULATES
- **U.S. Embassy:** Lance aux Epines in the "Green Building," approximately 15 minutes from the Point Salines International Airport; Tel: 1-473-444-1173/4/5/6; Fax: 1-473-444-4820; e-mail: usemb_gd@caribsurf.com; Website: www.spiceisle.com.
- **Canadian High Commission:** Accredited to the Canadian High Commission in Barbados. Bishop's Court Hill, St. Michael, Barbados; Postal Address: PO Box 404, Bridgetown, Barbados; Tel: 1-246-429-3550; Fax: 1-246-437-7436; e-mail: bdgtn@international.gc.ca; Website: www.bridgetown.gc.ca.
- **British High Commission:** Netherlands Building, Grand Anse, St George's, Grenada; Tel: 1-473-440-3536, 440-3222; Fax: 1-473-440-4939; e-mail: bhcgrenada@caribsurf.com.
HOSPITALS/DOCTORS:
There is a general hospital in St George's and small hospitals in Mirabeau and Carriacou.
- St. George's General Hospital (240 beds); general medical/surgical facility; Tel: 440-2051.

Current Advisories and Health Risks

- Accidents and injuries are the leading cause of death among travelers younger than the age of 55 and are most often caused by motor vehicle and motorcycle crashes; drownings, aircraft crashes, homicides, and burns are less common causes.
- Heart attacks cause most fatalities in older travelers.
- Infections cause only 1% of fatalities in overseas travelers, but, overall, infections are the most common cause of travel-related illness.
- Travelers are advised to obtain, before departure, supplemental travel health insurance with specific overseas coverage. The policy should provide for direct payment to the overseas hospital and/or physician at the time of service and include a medical evacuation benefit. The policy should also provide 24-hour hotline access to a multilingual assistance center that can help arrange and monitor delivery of medical care and determine if medical evacuation or air ambulance services are required.

DENGUE FEVER: This mosquito-transmitted viral disease is prevalent in the Caribbean. Travelers should take measures to prevent daytime insect bites.

FOOD AND WATER SAFETY: Main water supplies are normally chlorinated and relatively safe, but there is still some risk of diarrhea, particularly in rural areas. Bottled water is available. Milk is pasteurized and dairy products are safe for consumption. Local meat, poultry, seafood, fruits, and vegetables are generally considered safe to eat.

HEPATITIS: Hepatitis A is common. All nonimmune travelers should receive hepatitis A vaccine. Vaccination against hepatitis B should be considered for stays longer than 3 months or by those travelers desiring maximal protection. Travelers should be aware that hepatitis B can be transmitted by unsafe sex and the use of contaminated needles and syringes.

INFLUENZA: Influenza is transmitted year-round in the tropics. The flu vaccine is recommended for all travelers older than age 50; all travelers with any chronic disease or weakened immune system; travelers of any age wishing to decrease the risk of this illness; pregnant women after the first trimester.

MALARIA: There is no risk of malaria.

MARINE HAZARDS:

- Swimming related hazards include jellyfish, spiny sea urchins, and corals.
- Ciguatera poisoning is prevalent and can result from eating reef fish such as grouper, snapper, sea bass, jack, and barracuda. The ciguatoxin is not destroyed by cooking.
- Scuba Diving—Hyperbaric Chamber Referral: Divers' Alert Network (DAN) maintains an up-to-date list of all functioning hyperbaric chambers in North America and the Caribbean. DAN does not publish this list because, at any one time, a given chamber may be nonfunctioning, or its operator(s) may be away or otherwise unavailable. Through Duke University, DAN operates a 24-hour emergency phone line for

anyone (members and nonmembers) to call and ask for diving accident assistance. Dive medicine physicians at Duke University Medical Center can make a referral to the closest functioning hyperbaric chamber.

Guadeloupe (French West Indies)

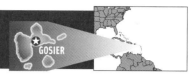

CAPITAL:
Gosier

EMBASSY (FRENCH):
202-944-6000

GMT:
−4 hours

TELEPHONE COUNTRY CODE:
590

USADIRECT:
0-800-99-0011 to place calls from Martinique, St. Martin, St. Barthelemy, or Guadeloupe.

ENTRY REQUIREMENTS
• **Passport/Visa:** Passport required. Visa not required for tourist/business stays of up to 3 months. For further information, consult the Embassy of France (202-944-6200). Internet: www.france-consulat.org. Guadeloupe is a French possession (French Overseas Department).
• **HIV Test:** Not required.
• **Vaccinations:** Not required.

EMBASSIES/CONSULATES
• **U.S. Embassy:** French Caribbean Dept., 14 Rue Blenac, Martinique; Tel: 596-631-303.
• **Canadian Embassy:** Accredited to the Canadian High Commission in Trinidad; Tel: 809-623-4787.

HOSPITALS/DOCTORS
Regional Hospital, Pointe-a-Pitre; general medical/surgical facility; numerous specialties; Tel: 8-910-10. In Gosier: Nicole Duhamel, M.D.; Tel: (84) 3562.

Current Advisories and Health Risks
See Disease Risk Summary for the Caribbean on page 293.

Guatemala

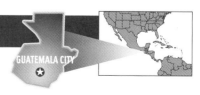

CAPITAL:
Guatemala City

EMBASSY (IN U.S.):
202-745-4952

−6 hours
TELEPHONE COUNTRY CODE:
502
USADIRECT:
138-126
999-9190
ENTRY REQUIREMENTS
- **Passport/Visa:** Passport required for a stay of up to 90 days. For travel by minors and general information, contact the Embassy of Guatemala, 2220 R St., NW, Washington, DC 20008-4081; Tel: 202-745-4952.
- **HIV Test:** Not required.
- **Vaccinations:** A yellow fever vaccination certificate is required from travelers older than 1 year of age coming from infected areas.

EMBASSIES/CONSULATES
- **U.S. Embassy:** Guatemala City. Avenida de la Reforma 7-01 in Zone 10; Tel: 311-1541.
- **Canadian Embassy:** Accredited to the Canadian Embassy in Guatamala. Edyma Plaza Building, 8th Floor, 13 Calle 8-44, Zona 10, Guatemala City, Guatemala; Postal Address: PO Box 400, Guatemala City, Guatemala; Tel: 502-2365-1250, 2363-4348; Fax: 502-2365-1210, 502-2365-1216; e-mail: gtmla@international.gc.ca; Website: www.guatemala.gc.ca.
- **British Embassy:** 16 Calle 00-55, Zona 10, Edificio Torre Internacional, Nivel 11, Guatemala City; Tel: 502-2367-5425-29; Fax: 502-2367-5430; e-mail: embassy @intelnett.com.

HOSPITALS/DOCTORS:
Medical care is below Western standards except in some private clinics. Many doctors may not speak English. Travelers to Guatemala are advised to obtain supplemental travel health insurance with specific overseas coverage. The policy should provide for direct payment to the overseas hospital and/or physician at the time of service and include a medical evacuation benefit.
- Hospital Herrera Llerandi (68 beds); most specialties; Tel: 2-334-5959.
- Hospital Centro Medico (76 beds); Tel: 332-3555.
- Hospital Bella Aurora; Tel: 368-1951/55.
- Hospital Universitario Esperanza; Tel: 339-3244/47.
- Hospital General San Juan De Dios; Tel: 232-3741/44.

Current Advisories and Health Risks

CHOLERA: This disease is reported active in this country, but the threat to tourists is very low. Cholera vaccine is recommended primarily for people at high risk (e.g., relief workers) who work and live in highly endemic areas under less than adequate sanitary conditions.

DENGUE FEVER: Risk occurs year-round countrywide in urban areas at lower elevations; extensive outbreaks occur sporadically. Travelers should take measures to prevent daytime mosquito bites.

HEPATITIS: Hepatitis A vaccine is recommended for all travelers. The hepatitis B carrier rate in the general population is estimated at 1.4% to 3.0%. Hepatitis B is spread by infected blood, contaminated needles, and unsafe sex. Vaccination is recommended for stays longer than 3 months; for anyone at occupational or social risk; for any traveler desiring maximal protection.

LEISHMANIASIS: Cutaneous leishmaniasis is reported occurring in northern departments, especially in the forested areas in Peten Department. Limited risk of visceral leishmaniasis occurs in the semiarid valleys and in the foothills of east-central Guatemala in the Department of El Progresso. Travelers to these areas should take measures to prevent sand fly bites.

MALARIA: Risk exists year-round countrywide below 1,500 meters elevation, except for Guatemala City and the central highland areas, which are risk free. Incidence of vivax malaria is highest in the Pacific lowlands, along the border with El Salvador, and in the north (Peten Department). Chloroquine prophylaxis is recommended for travel to malarious areas.

ONCHOCERCIASIS: Risk occurs near fast-flowing rivers between 300 and 1,600 meters elevation in the Pacific coast foothills and along the border with Mexico in the south. Travelers to these areas should take measures to prevent insect (black fly) bites.

RABIES: Sporadic cases of human rabies are reported countrywide. All animal bites or scratches, especially from a dog, should be treated without delay. Rabies vaccination may be required. Rabies vaccine is recommended for travel longer than 3 months and for shorter stays when travelers plan to venture off the usual tourist routes.

TRAVELERS' DIARRHEA: Travelers should drink only bottled, boiled, or treated water. All food should be thoroughly cooked. A quinolone antibiotic, combined with loperamide (Imodium) is recommended for the treatment of diarrhea. Persistent diarrhea may be due to a parasitic disease such as giardiasis amebiasis, or cryptosporidiosis.

TUBERCULOSIS: Tuberculosis (TB) is a major health problem in this country. Travelers planning an extended stay should have a pre-departure TB skin test (PPD test) and be retested after returning from this country.

TYPHOID FEVER: Typhoid vaccine is recommended for all travelers, with the exception of short-term visitors who restrict their meals to major restaurants and hotels. Because the typhoid vaccines are only 60% to 70% effective, safe food and drink selection remains important.

OTHER DISEASES/HAZARDS: Brucellosis, Chagas disease (endemic in many rural areas), coccidiomycosis, measles, paralytic shellfish poisoning, relapsing fever (tick-borne), syphilis, typhoid fever, tuberculosis, strongyloidiasis and other helminthic infections.

Guinea-Bissau

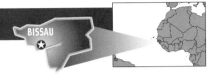

BISSAU ★

CAPITAL:
Bissau

EMBASSY (IN U.S.):
202-872-4222

GMT
+0 hours

TELEPHONE COUNTRY CODE:
245

USADIRECT:
None

ENTRY REQUIREMENTS*

- **Passport/Visa:** Passport, onward/return ticket, and visa required. Visa must be obtained in advance.
- **HIV Test:** Not required.
- **Vaccinations:** A yellow fever vaccination certificate is required from all travelers older than 1 year of age arriving from infected areas and for travelers arriving from: Angola, Benin, Burkina Faso, Burundi, Cape Verde, the Central African Republic, Chad, Congo, Côte d'Ivoire, Democratic Republic of Congo, Djibouti, Equatorial Guinea, Ethiopia, Gabon, The Gambia, Ghana, Guinea, Kenya, Liberia, Madagascar, Mali, Mauritania, Mozambique, Niger, Nigeria, Rwanda, São Tomé and Principe, Senegal, and Sierra Leone.

*Travelers should check with this country's embassy (or a consulate) in the United States, Canada, or the United States for any changes in these requirements.

EMBASSIES/CONSULATES

- **U.S. Embassy:** Bissau. Avenida Domingos Ramos; Tel: 21-2816, 21-3674.
- **Canadian Embassy:** Accredited to the Canadian Embassy in Senegal; Tel: 221-21-0290.
- **British Embassy:** Accredited to the British Embassy in Senegal. 20 Rue du Docteur Guillet, (Boite Postale 6025), Dakar; Tel: 221-823-7392, 823-9971; Fax: 221-823-2766, 823-8415; e-mail: britemb@sentoo.sn.

HOSPITALS/DOCTORS:

Medical care in Guinea-Bissau is below Western standards. Travelers are advised to obtain, before departure, supplemental travel health insurance with specific overseas coverage. The policy should provide for direct payment to the overseas hospital and/or physician at the time of service and include a medical evacuation benefit.

- Simao Mendes National Hospital, Bissau (100 beds); general medical/surgical facility; orthopedics, emergency services.

Current Advisories and Health Risks

AIDS/HIV: The rate of adult HIV infection is 2.8% compared with the average in sub-Saharan Africa of nearly 9%, although there are higher rates in the urban areas and among single women.

AFRICAN SLEEPING SICKNESS (TRYPANOSOMIASIS): Low-level transmission probably occurs in the coastal and northcentral areas. Travelers should take measures to avoid insect (tsetse) fly bites.

HEPATITIS: High risk. All travelers should receive hepatitis A vaccine. The hepatitis B carrier rate in the general population exceeds 10%. Hepatitis B is spread by infected blood, contaminated needles, and unsafe sex. Vaccination is recommended for stays longer than 3 months; for anyone at occupational or social risk; for any traveler desiring maximal protection. The risk of illness or injury during travel cannot be predicted and some experts believe that *all* travelers should be immunized against hepatitis B because of the risk of receiving a medical injection with an unsterile needle or syringe.

MALARIA: Risk is present year-round countrywide, including urban areas. Increased risk occurs during and immediately after the rainy season, June through October. *Plasmodium falciparum* accounts for 90% of cases, the remainder due to *Plasmodium malariae* and *Plasmodium ovale*. Chloroquine-resistant falciparum malaria is reported. Prophylaxis with atovaquone/proguanil (Malarone), mefloquine (Lariam), or doxycycline is recommended.

POLIO: This disease is active in sub-Saharan Africa; all travelers should be fully immunized.

RABIES: Human rabies reported countrywide. Pre-exposure vaccination is recommended for long-term travel to this country, especially for travelers going to remote rural areas.

SCHISTOSOMIASIS: Urinary schistosomiasis occurs in the northern half of Guinea Bissau, extending from the coastal region of Cacheau to the border with Guinea, including the valleys of the Cacheau and Geba River basins. Travelers should avoid swimming, bathing, or wading in freshwater streams, lakes, or ponds.

TRAVELERS' DIARRHEA: High risk. All water sources should be considered potentially contaminated. A quinolone antibiotic is recommended for the treatment of acute diarrhea. Persistent diarrhea may be due to a parasitic infection such as giardiasis, amebiasis, or cryptosporidiosis.

TUBERCULOSIS: Tuberculosis (TB) is a major health problem in this country. Travelers planning an extended stay should have a pre-departure TB skin test (PPD test) and be retested after returning from this country.

TYPHOID FEVER: Typhoid vaccine is recommended for those traveling off the usual tourist routes, those visiting friends or relatives, and for long-stay visitors. Because the typhoid vaccines are only 60% to 70% effective, safe food and drink selection remains important.

YELLOW FEVER: Vaccination is recommended. No cases are recently reported, but yellow fever has been reported in neighboring Guinea.

OTHER DISEASES/HAZARDS: African tick typhus (transmitted by dog ticks, often in urban areas, and bush ticks), brucellosis (from consumption of raw dairy products), lassa fever (risk undetermined), leprosy, onchocerciasis (black fly-transmitted; higher risk near fast-flowing rivers), and intestinal worms (very common).

Guyana

CAPITAL:
Georgetown
EMBASSY (IN U.S.):
202-265-6900
GMT:
−3 hours
TELEPHONE COUNTRY CODE:
592
USADIRECT:
159
ENTRY REQUIREMENTS
- **Passport/Visa:** No visa or tourist card required for stays up to 30 days.
- **HIV Test:** Not required.
- **Vaccinations:** A yellow fever vaccination certificate is required from travelers arriving from infected areas or from any country in the Yellow Fever Endemic Zones of Central and South America and sub-Saharan Africa. Travelers arriving from Belize, Bolivia, Brazil, Colombia, Costa Rica, Ecuador, French Guiana, Guatemala, Honduras, Nicaragua, Panama, Peru, Suriname, and Venezuela are required to have a valid certificate. The *Medical Guide* recommends that any traveler arriving from any country in sub-Saharan Africa be in possession of a valid yellow fever certificate.
EMBASSIES/CONSULATES
- **U.S. Embassy** (Consular Section). 99-100 Young and Duke Streets, Kingston, Georgetown; Tel: 2-54-900. After hours: Tel: 2-57-963.
- **Canadian High Commission:** High and Young Streets, Georgetown, Guyana; Postal Address: PO Box 10880, Georgetown, Guyana; Tel: 592-227-2081/2/3/4/5; Fax: 592-225-8380; e-mail: grgtn@international.gc.ca; Website: www.georgetown.gc.ca.
- **British High Commission:** 44 Main Street, (PO Box 10849), Georgetown; Tel: 592-22-65881/2/3/4; e-mail: firstname.surname@fco.gov.uk.
HOSPITALS/DOCTORS:
- St. Joseph Mercy Hospital, Georgetown: hospital used by embassy personnel.
- Davis Memorial Georgetown; used by embassy personnel.
- Georgetown Hospital (991 beds); government hospital; used for paramedical training.

Current Advisories and Health Risks

CHOLERA: This disease is active in this country. Although cholera vaccination is not re-quired for entry if arriving directly from the United States or Canada, it may be required if arriving from a cholera-infected area, or required for on-going travel to other countries in Latin America, Africa, the Middle East, or Asia. Travelers should consider vaccina-tion (one dose) or a doctor's letter of exemption from vaccination.

FILARIASIS: Bancroftian filariasis is endemic in Georgetown and other cities in the coastal plain,with up to 10% of the population infected. Travelers should take standard precautions to prevent mosquito bites.

HEPATITIS: All nonimmune travelers should receive hepatitis A vaccine. Hepatitis E has not been reported but could occur. The hepatitis B carrier rate in the general population is less than 5%. Vaccination against hepatitis B is recommended for all health-care workers and should be considered by anyone planning an extended visit to this country.

LEISHMANIASIS: Outbreaks of cutaneous leishmaniasis have occurred in military person-nel. Most cases are acquired in the interior forests and savanna areas in the northeast. Visceral leishmaniasis has not been not reported. Travelers to these areas should take measures to prevent insect (sand fly) bites.

MALARIA: Occurs year-round in all regions below 900 meters elevation. The highest risk is in the northwestern areas bordering Venezuela and in rural areas of the southern interior. In the coastal plain, including the outskirts of Georgetown, increased transmis-sion occurs during and just after the rainy seasons (May through mid-August and November through January). There is little if any malaria in a narrow strip of coastal plain in the northeast. Falciparum malaria accounts for 60% of cases, vivax 40%. Prophylaxis with atovaquone/proguanil (Malarone), mefloquine (Lariam), or doxycy-cline is currently recommended in malarious areas.

TRAVELERS' DIARRHEA: High risk outside of first-class hotels and resorts. Travelers are advised to drink only bottled, boiled, filtered, or treated water, and consume only well-cooked food. A quinolone antibiotic is recommended for the treatment of acute diarrhea. Diarrhea not responding to antibiotic treatment may be due to a parasitic disease such as giardiasis or amebiasis or an intestinal virus. Cryptosporidiosis is also reported.

YELLOW FEVER: No recent cases have been reported. There were unconfirmed reports of cases occurring in 1983 in the extreme south near the Brazil border. Vaccination is rec-ommended for travel to this area. This country is in the Yellow Fever Endemic Zone. Although yellow fever vaccination may not be required for entry into this country, it may be required for on-going travel to other countries in Latin America, Africa, the Middle East, or Asia.

OTHER DISEASES/HAZARDS: Chagas disease (very low prevalence in the northwest dis-trict), mansonellosis (black fly-borne), onchocerciasis (regionally endemic), AIDS (HIV infects 25% of prostitutes), paracoccidiomycosis, rabies, schistosomiasis (not reported, but occurs in neighboring Suriname), tuberculosis (incidence increased in the 1980s), typhoid fever, strongyloidiasis and other helminthic infections are reported. Animal hazards include snakes (vipers), centipedes, scorpions, black widow spiders, brown recluse spiders, banana spiders, pruning spiders, and wolf spiders. Electric eels and various carnivorous fish (including piranha) may be found in this country's fresh waters. Portuguese man-of-war, sea wasps, and stingrays are found in the coastal waters and could be a hazard to swimmers.

Haiti

PORT-AU-
PRINCE

CAPITAL:
Port-au-Prince
EMBASSY (IN U.S.):
202-322-4090
GMT:
−5 hours
TELEPHONE COUNTRY CODE:
509
USADIRECT:
183

ENTRY REQUIREMENTS
• **Passport/Visa:** Travelers should possess valid passport. A visa is not required.
• **HIV Test:** Not required.
• **Vaccinations:** A yellow fever vaccination certificate is required from all travelers arriving from infected areas.

EMBASSIES/CONSULATES
• **U.S. Embassy:** Harry Truman Blvd., Port-au-Prince; Tel: 509-22-0200, 22-0354, 23-0955 or 22-0269; Fax: 509-23-1641; Website: usembassy.state.gov/haiti.
• **Canadian Embassy:** Édifice Banque de Nouvelle-écosse (Bank of Nova Scotia), Delmas 18, Port-au-Prince; Tel: 509-298-3050; Fax: 298-3001; e-mail: prnce@dfait-maeci.gc.ca.
• **British Consulate:** Hotel Montana (PO Box 1302), Port-au-Prince; Tel: 509-257-3969; Fax: 509-257-4048; e-mail: britcon@transnethaiti.com.

HOSPITALS/DOCTORS:
• Hopital de l' Universite d'Etat d'Haiti, Rue Monseigneur Guilloux, Port-au-Prince; Tel: 509-222-1221 or 509-223-4254. (Medical school and academic center.)
• Hopital du Canape-Vert, Rue du Canape-Vert, Port-au-Prince; Tel: 509-245-1053 or 509-245-0205; commonly used by U.S. Embassy personnel.
• Further information on hospitals and doctors in Haiti is available online at www.haitimedical.com.
• Medical care in Haiti may be substandard. Travelers are advised to obtain, before departure, supplemental travel health insurance with specific overseas coverage. The pol-

icy should provide for direct payment to the overseas hospital and/or physician at the time of service and include a medical evacuation benefit.

Current Advisories and Health Risks

AIDS/HIV: There is a high incidence of HIV infection in the general population with heterosexual and bisexual contact the predominant mode of transmission. Haiti is one of 15 countries that are home to nearly 50% of HIV infections worldwide. HIV prevalence in female prostitutes is estimated at 70%. Tropical spastic paresis, due to the human T-lymphotropic virus, type 1 (HTLV-1), is endemic. All travelers are cautioned against unsafe sex, unsterile medical injections, IV drug use, and blood transfusions.

DENGUE FEVER: Year-round risk, increasing April through September. Dengue occurs primarily in the coastal-urban areas and is probably under-reported. To prevent dengue, travelers should take protective measures against daytime mosquito bites.

FILARIASIS: Bancroftian filariasis has been reported in coastal areas, primarily in the north and around the Gulf of La Gonave. Another focus is reported near Leogane. To prevent filariasis, travelers to risk areas should take protective measures against mosquito bites.

HEPATITIS: All nonimmune travelers should receive hepatitis A vaccine. The hepatitis B carrier rate in the general population is estimated at 5.5% to 13%. Hepatitis B is transmitted by blood, unsafe sex, and contaminated needles and syringes. Vaccination against hepatitis B should be considered for stays longer than 3 months; by anyone at occupational or social risk; by any traveler desiring maximal protection.

INFLUENZA: Influenza is transmitted year-round in the tropics. The flu vaccine is recommended for all travelers to this country.

MALARIA: Malaria is a major public health problem in Haiti. Risk is present countrywide year-round at elevations under 500 meters. Peak transmission occurs from September through January, with a secondary peak from April through June. There is increased risk of malaria in the northern coastal areas. Falciparum malaria accounts for 99% to 100% of cases. Chloroquine-resistant falciparum malaria has not been reported. Prophylaxis with chloroquine is currently recommended. All travelers should take measures to prevent evening and nighttime mosquito bites.

MARINE HAZARDS: Swimming-related hazards include jellyfish, spiny sea urchins, and sharp coral. Ciguatera poisoning occurs and can result from eating coral reef fish such as grouper, snapper, sea bass, jack, and barracuda. The ciguatoxin is not destroyed by cooking.

SCUBA DIVING: Divers' Alert Network (DAN) maintains an up-to-date list of all hyperbaric chambers in North America and the Caribbean. In association with Duke University Medical Center in North Carolina, DAN operates a 24-hour emergency phone number (919-684-8111) for members and nonmembers to call and their staff is available to answer questions and, if necessary, make referral to the closest functioning hyperbaric chamber.

RABIES: Occasional human cases are reported. All animal bites or scratches, especially from a dog, should be evaluated immediately.

TRAVELERS' DIARRHEA: All travelers should observe strict food and drink precautions, especially outside of resort areas. Tap water should be avoided. A quinolone antibiotic, combined with loperamide (Imodium), is recommended for the treatment of acute diarrhea. Persistent diarrhea may be due to a parasitic disease such as cyclosporiasis (highly endemic) or giardiasis.

TUBERCULOSIS: Tuberculosis (TB) is a major health problem in this country. Travelers planning an extended stay should have a pre-departure TB skin test (PPD test) and be retested after returning from this country.

TYPHOID FEVER: Typhoid vaccine is recommended for those traveling off the usual tourist routes, those visiting friends or relatives, and for long-stay visitors. Because the typhoid vaccines are only 60% to 70% effective, safe food and drink selection remains important.

OTHER DISEASES/HAZARDS: Brucellosis (from consumption of raw dairy products or occupational exposure), helminthic (worm) infections, leptospirosis, relapsing fever (louseborne), toxoplasmosis, and viral encephalitis.

Honduras

★ TEGUCIGALPA

CAPITAL:
Tegucigalpa
EMBASSY (IN U.S.):
202-223-0185
GMT:
−6 hours
TELEPHONE COUNTRY CODE:
504
USADIRECT:
800-0123
ENTRY REQUIREMENTS*
• **Passport/Visa:** A valid passport is required.
• **HIV Test:** Not required.
• **Vaccinations:** A yellow fever vaccination certificate is required from travelers coming from infected or endemic areas.
*Travelers should check with this country's embassy (or a consulate) in the United States, Canada, or the United Kingdom for any changes in these requirements.

478

EMBASSIES/CONSULATES

- **U.S. Embassy:** Avenida La Paz, Tegucigalpa. Tel: 236-9320, 238-5114; Fax: 238-4357; Website: www.usmission.hn.
- **U.S. Consulate:** San Pedro Sula. Tel: 558-1580.
- **Canadian Embassy:** Centro Financiero BANEXPO, 3rd Floor, Boulevard San Juan Bosco, Colonia Payaqui, Tegucigalpa. Tel: 232-4551; Fax: 232-8767; e-mail: tglpa@dfait-maeci.gc.ca.
- **British Embassy:** Accredited to the British Embassy in Guatemala. 16 Calle 00-55, Zona 10, Edificio Torre Internacional, Nivel 11, Guatemala City; Tel: 502-2367-5425-29; Fax: 502-2367-5430; e-mail: embassy@intelnett.com.

HOSPITALS/DOCTORS

- Centro Medico CEMESA, San Pedro Sula; modern treatment and diagnostic facility; CT scanning and MRI capability; new outpatient building located on the hospital grounds.
- Hospital Leonardo Martinez, Tegucigalpa (286 beds); general medical/surgical facility; most specialties.
- Hospital Escuela, Tegucigalpa (400 beds); Most specialties; ER, ICU.

Current Advisories and Health Risks

CHAGAS DISEASE: Very low risk to travelers, but risk is slightly increased in the southern half of the country, especially in the Tegucigalpa area. Transmission occurs primarily in rural-agricultural areas, and is associated with sleeping in adobe-style huts and houses that harbor the night-biting triatomid (assassin) bug.

CHOLERA: This disease is active in this country, but the threat to tourists is very low. Cholera is an extremely rare disease in travelers from developed countries. Cholera vaccine is recommended primarily for people at high risk (e.g., relief workers) who work and live in highly endemic areas under less than adequate sanitary conditions.

DENGUE FEVER: This disease is widespread throughout Central America and the Caribbean. Most outbreaks in Honduras have occurred in the south, but risk of disease also occurs along the northern coast, particularly in the San Pedro Sula area. All travelers should take measures to prevent daytime mosquito bites.

HEPATITIS: A vaccine is recommended for all nonimmune travelers. Hepatitis E has not been reported but could occur. The hepatitis B carrier rate in the population is estimated at 3%. Hepatitis B is spread by infected blood, contaminated needles, and unprotected sex. Vaccination is recommended for stays longer than 3 months; for anyone at occupational or social risk; for any traveler desiring maximal protection.

INFLUENZA: Influenza is transmitted year-round in the tropics. The flu vaccine is recommended for all travelers.

LEISHMANIASIS: Cutaneous and mucocutaneous leishmaniasis is widespread in rural areas, with elevated risk in the northern one half and western one third of the country.

Visceral leishmaniasis has been reported on Tigre Island and in southern rural areas. Travelers should take measures to prevent insect (sand fly) bites. Use of a permethrin-treated bed net is advised to prevent nighttime bites.

MALARIA: Risk of malaria occurs year-round in rural areas below 1,000 meters elevation, including the municipalities of Tegucigalpa and San Pedro Sula. Most cases occur in the coastal lowlands along the border with Nicaragua. *Plasmodium vivax* accounts for 97% of reported cases. Falciparum malaria may occur along the Nicaraguan border and in the Caribbean coastal region, but chloroquine-resistant *Plasmodium falciparum* has not been reported. Chloroquine prophylaxis is recommended in malarious areas, including Ceiba, Tela, and Roatan and other Bay islands. All travelers should take measures to prevent evening and nighttime mosquito bites.

MARINE HAZARDS: Swimming-related hazards include jellyfish, spiny sea urchins, and coral. Ciguatera poisoning is prevalent and can result from eating coral reef fish such as grouper, snapper, sea bass, jack, and barracuda. The ciguatoxin is not destroyed by cooking.

RABIES: Honduras has one of the highest incidences of animal (dog) rabies in Latin America. Sporadic cases of human rabies are reported countrywide. All animal bites or scratches, especially from a dog, should be medically evaluated. Although rabies is rare among tourists, there is risk. No one should pet or pick up any stray animals. All children should be warned to avoid contact with unknown animals. Rabies vaccine is recommended for travel longer than 3 months, and for shorter stays for travelers who plan to travel off the usual tourist routes.

TRAVELERS' DIARRHEA: Honduras is the least-developed country in Central America and has inadequate treatment and distribution systems for piped water. Tap water is not considered potable. A quinolone antibiotic combined with loperamide (Imodium), is recommended for the treatment of acute diarrhea. Persistent diarrhea may be due to a parasitic infection such as giardiasis, amebiasis, or cryptosporidiosis.

TUBERCULOSIS: Tuberculosis a major health problem in this country, with 2% of the population infected. Travelers planning an extended stay should have a pre-departure TB skin test (PPD test) and be retested after returning from this country.

TYPHOID FEVER: Typhoid vaccine is recommended for those traveling off the usual tourist routes, those visiting friends or relatives, and for long-stay visitors. Because the typhoid vaccines are only 60% to 70% effective, safe food and drink selection remains important.

YELLOW FEVER: Yellow fever is not active. Vaccination is required only for travelers coming from infected areas.

OTHER DISEASES/HAZARDS: Brucellosis (limited risk in cattle-raising areas; associated with unpasteurized dairy products), coccidiomycosis, cysticercosis, leptospirosis, measles, myiasis (caused by human bot fly), AIDS (Honduras has the highest incidence of AIDS cases in Central America), typhoid fever, tuberculosis, strongyloidiasis and other helminthic (worm) infections.

Hong Kong (China)

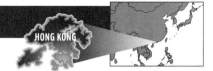

CAPITAL:
Beijing
EMBASSY (IN U.S.):
202-328-2500
GMT:
+8 hours
TELEPHONE COUNTRY CODE:
852
USADIRECT:
800-96-1111
800-93-2266
ENTRY REQUIREMENTS
- **Passport/Visa:** Passport and onward/return transportation by sea/air required. Visa not required for tourist/business stays of up to 90 days. Confirmed hotel and flight reservations recommended during peak travel months. Departure tax 80. Hong Kong dollars (approx. $10.30) and airport security tax 33. Hong Kong dollars (approx. $4.29) paid at airport. Visa required for work or study. For other types of travel, consult the Visa Section of the Embassy of the People's Republic of China (202-338-6688). Internet: www.china-embassy.org
- **HIV Test:** Not required.
- **Vaccinations:** None required.
EMBASSIES/CONSULATES
- **U.S. Embassy:** Hong Kong. 26 Garden Road; Tel: 5-239-011.
- **Consulate General of Canada:** 14th Floor, One Exchange Square, Central, Hong Kong SAR, People's Republic of China; Postal Address: PO Box 11142, Central, Hong Kong SAR, China; Tel: 85-2-2810-4321; Fax: 85-2-2810-6736; e-mail: hkong@international.gc.ca; Website: www.dfait-maeci.gc.ca/hongkong.
- **British Consulate-General:** No. 1 Supreme Court Road, Central, Hong Kong, PO Box 528; Tel: 852-2901-3000; Website: www.britishconsulate.org.hk.
HOSPITALS/DOCTORS:
Medical care in Hong Kong is of high quality and many physicians speak English. Travelers are advised to obtain, before departure, supplemental travel health insurance with specific overseas coverage. The policy should provide for direct payment to the overseas hospital and/or physician at the time of service and include a medical evacuation benefit.
- Hong Kong Adventist Hospital; 24-hour emergency service; Tel: 5-574-6211.
- An extensive listing of hospitals in Hong Kong may be found at http://www.geoexpat.com/resources/hospitals/

Current Advisories and Health Risks

HEPATITIS: Hepatitis A vaccine is recommended for all travelers. The hepatitis B carrier rate in the general population is estimated at 10%. Hepatitis B is spread by infected blood, contaminated needles, and unsafe sex. Vaccination is recommended for stays longer than 3 months; for anyone at occupational or social risk; for any traveler desiring maximal protection.

JAPANESE ENCEPHALITIS (JE): Rare, sporadic cases are reported. JE vaccine is not routinely recommended.

MALARIA: The urban area of Hong Kong is risk free. Malaria has been reported in rural northern border areas. Malaria prophylaxis is not recommended.

Hungary

BUDAPEST

CAPITAL:
Budapest
EMBASSY (IN U.S.):
202-362-6730
GMT:
+1 hour
TELEPHONE COUNTRY CODE:
36
USADIRECT:
06-800-011-11
ENTRY REQUIREMENTS
- **Passport/Visa:** Passport, onward/return ticket and proof of sufficient funds required. Visa not required for stay of up to 90 days. AIDS test required for persons staying longer than 1 year. For longer stays and employment, visas must be obtained before you travel. For more information check with the Embassy of the Republic of Hungary, 3910 Shoemaker St., NW, Washington, DC 20008 (202-362-6730), or the nearest Consulate General: New York (212-752-0661) or Los Angeles (310-473-9344). Internet: www.hungaryemb.org
- **HIV Test:** Not required.
- **Vaccinations:** None required.
EMBASSIES/CONSULATES
- **U.S. Embassy:** Szabadsag Ter 12, Budapest; Tel: 1-475-4400; Fax: 36-1-475-4188/4113; Website: www.usis.hu/consular.htm.
- **Canadian Embassy:** Zugligetti út 51-53, Budakeszi út 32, Budapest; Tel: 1-392-3360; Fax: 36-1-392-3390; e-mail: bpest@dfait-maeci.gc.ca.
- **British Embassy:** Harmincad u. 6., Budapest 1051; Tel: 36-1-266-2888; Fax: 36-1-429-6360; e-mail: info@britemb.hu; Website: http://www.britishembassy.hu.

HOSPITALS/DOCTORS:
Medical care in Hungary is adequate for most problems. Travelers to this country are advised to obtain supplemental travel health insurance with specific overseas coverage. The policy should provide for direct payment to the overseas hospital and/or physician at the time of service and include a medical evacuation benefit.

• **SOS-Hungary:** 24-hour emergency services for foreign nationals and corporations; Tel: 1-24-00-475; Website: www.soshungary.hu

Current Advisories and Health Risks

TICK-BORNE DISEASES: Lyme disease occurs countrywide, with most transmission during the warmer months, April through September. European tick-borne encephalitis (TBE) is endemic, especially in the lowland forests. The highest incidence of TBE in Hungary occurs in forested areas of the three western counties neighboring Austria and Slovenia and in the northern Komarom County bordering Czechoslovakia. Most adult cases occur among male forestry workers. A vaccine is available in Canada and Europe, but is not routinely recommended for tourists.

For additional information, consult the Disease Risk Summary for Europe on page 300.

India

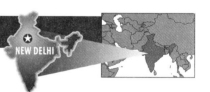

NEW DELHI

CAPITAL:
New Delhi
EMBASSY (IN U.S.):
2536 Massachusetts Ave., NW Washington, DC 20008
202-939-9806/983
Website: www.indiagov.org
GMT
+5 hours
TELEPHONE COUNTRY CODE:
91
USADIRECT:
000-117
ENTRY REQUIREMENTS
• **Passport/Visa:** A valid passport and visa are required.
• **HIV Test:** All students older than age 18; anyone between the ages of 18 and 70 with a visa valid for 1 year or more; and anyone extending a stay to a year or more, excluding accredited journalists and those working in foreign missions. Test must be taken within 30 days of arrival.
• **Vaccinations:** India requires a yellow fever vaccination certificate from all travelers arriving from any country, any part of which is infected, as well as from countries in the Yellow Fever Endemic Zones, including Trinidad and Tobago.

- **U.S. Embassy:** Shanti Path, Chanakyapuri, New Delhi. Tel: 91-11-419-8000; Fax: 91-11-419-0017; Website: usembassy.state.gov/posts/in1/wwwhmain.html.
- **Canadian Embassy:** 7/8 Shantipath, Chanakyapuri, New Delhi. Tel: 91-11-687-6500; Fax: 687-0031; e-mail: delhi@dfait-maeci.gc.ca.
- **British High Commission:** Chanakyapuri, New Delhi 110021; Tel: 91-11-2687-2161; Fax: 91-11-2687-2882; e-mail: postmaster.NEDEL@fco.gov.uk.

HOSPITALS/DOCTORS:

- Dr. Kimberley Chawla, East West Rescue, Indian Air Ambulance & Emergency Medical Assistance; 38 Golf Links, New Delhi, India
- Dr. U. Mohan Rau Memorial Hospital, Madras
- Talwar Medical Centre, Greater Kailash II, New Delhi. Well-equipped medical /surgical facility
- East-West Medical Center, New Delhi
- Irwin Hospital, New Delhi (1,173 beds); most specialties
- Hospital for Orthopaedics, Sports Medicine, Arthritis, Trauma and Hosmat Neurosciences Centre. Major speciality hospital of 100 beds located in central Bangalore
- The Bangalore Hospital, Rashtriya Vidyalaya Road, Bangalore
- Marble City Hospital & Research Center, 21, North Civil Lines, Jabalpur, Madhya Pradesh; cardiothoracic and neurosurgery capability
- J.J. Hospital, Bombay (1,200 beds); most specialties, including orthopedics
- Woodlands Hospital & Medical Center, Calcutta (preferred for private patients)
- Dr. Santanu Chatterjee, Wellesley Medicentre, Calcutta
- International SOS: International SOS Services (India) Pvt. Ltd., 2-B, Second Floor, Berjaya House, New Friends Colonommunity Centre, y CNew Delhi - 110065, India; Admin/AC Tel: 91-11-5189-7800; Admin/AC Fax: 91-11-5189-7801

Current Advisories and Health Risks

AIDS/HIV: With a population nearing one billion and an estimated five to eight million HIV-infected people, India is now considered the country that has the largest number of people infected with HIV in the world. HIV has spread beyond high-risk groups and is now firmly embedded in the Indian population and is fast spreading into rural areas. Commercial sex workers continue to play a key part in the heterosexual spread of HIV, which is the dominant mode of transmission in India except in two regions (Nagaland and Manipur) where intravenous drug use is widespread. Between 30% and 60% of prostitutes and 15% of truck drivers are infected with HIV/AIDS in India. Another important mode of transmission is through contaminated blood and blood products and unsterile needles and syringes.

ANIMAL HAZARDS: Animal hazards include snakes (kraits, cobras, coral snakes, vipers), scorpions, spiders, and leeches (abundant in the streams, marshes, and jungles).

CHOLERA: This disease is reported active in this country. Cholera is an extremely rare disease in travelers from developed countries. The cholera vaccine is recommended primarily for people at high risk (e.g., relief workers) who work and live in highly endemic areas under less than adequate sanitary conditions. Many countries, including Canada, license an oral cholera vaccine. The vaccine is not available in the United States.

DENGUE FEVER: Periodic epidemics of dengue and dengue hemorrhagic fever occur in urban and semirural areas countrywide below 1,000 meters elevation, with most outbreaks occurring in the north-central states. Relatively few cases are reported from the western states. In southern areas, the risk of dengue is year-round. In the northern states, the risk is elevated from April through November. To prevent dengue, travelers should take measures to prevent daytime mosquito bites.

FILARIASIS: Bancroftian filariasis, which is transmitted by mosquitoes, is widespread in southern, central, and northern India, especially in Uttar Pradesh and Bihar States. Malayan filariasis occurs in southern India, especially Kerala State. The risk to tourists is low. All travelers, however, should take measures to prevent insect bites.

HEPATITIS: Hepatitis A vaccine is recommended for all travelers. Hepatitis E accounts for 70% of sporadic, acute viral hepatitis and 95% of "epidemic" hepatitis. Most cases are transmitted by sewage-contaminated water in rural areas. A vaccine against hepatitis E is not available. Travelers can reduce their risk of illness by drinking only boiled, bottled, or chemically treated water. The hepatitis B carrier rate in the general population is estimated at 5%. Hepatitis B is spread by infected blood, contaminated needles, and unprotected sex. Vaccination is recommended for long-stay travelers (>3 months); those who may be at occupational or social risk; anybody desiring maximal protection.

INFLUENZA: Influenza is transmitted from November through March in areas north of the Tropic of Cancer and throughout the year in areas to the south. Vaccination is recommended for all travelers.

JAPANESE ENCEPHALITIS (JE): This disease occurs year-round, except in northern India where the risk is primarily April through November. The risk is low in the western states. Only sporadic cases occur in the southern states. Most cases of Japanese encephalitis occur along the eastern coastal states, the northern states bordering Nepal, the northeastern states, and the southwestern state of Kerala. The disease has spread into Uttar Pradesh, with yearly epidemics reported. The Culex mosquito (a nighttime biter) transmits this disease, mostly in rural areas below 1,000 meters elevation. Vaccination against Japanese encephalitis is recommended for travelers who will be staying more than 3 to 4 weeks in rural-agricultural endemic areas during the peak transmission period. Long-term urban expatriates should also be vaccinated on the assumption that rural travel will occur. In addition, personal protection measures against mosquito bites should be taken, especially in the evening.

LEISHMANIASIS: Cases of visceral leishmaniasis, transmitted by sand flies, occur in large numbers in rural areas, especially in the northeastern states, with Bihar having the greatest incidence. Sporadic cases of cutaneous leishmaniasis have been reported in the western states along the Pakistani-Indian border. Most cases of cutaneous leishmaniasis occur in adults in urban or periurban hutment areas (slums). Travelers should take measures to prevent insect (sand fly) bites.

MALARIA: The risk of malaria is present countrywide year-round, excluding high altitude areas (above 2,000 meters elevation) of the states of Himachal Pradesh, Jammu and Kashmir, and Sikkim. Malaria risk occurs year-round in the tropical cities of Bombay, Calcutta, and Madras. Malaria risk in the more temperate New Delhi is seasonal, with the major risk being from July to November, peaking in September. The incidence of malaria has increased recently in Delhi, Tamil Nadu State, and Haryana State. The most intense malaria transmission in India occurs in the eastern and northeastern states. Large outbreaks of falciparum malaria have occurred in Rajasthan State and in Assam State. Vivax malaria accounts for 60% to 65% of cases countrywide, falciparum malaria accounts for the remainder. Prophylaxis with atovaquone/proguanil (Malarone), mefloquine (Lariam), or doxycycline is recommended. All travelers should take measures to prevent evening and nighttime mosquito bites.

MARINE HAZARDS: Stingrays, sea wasps, cones, jellyfish, sea urchins, and anemones are common in India's coastal waters and are potential hazards to unprotected swimmers.

MENINGITIS: Meningococcal meningitis reported active in Delhi as of June 2005. Although the CDC does not currently recommend routine vaccination for travel to India, travelers to the Delhi region should consult a travel medicine specialist.

POLIOMYELITIS (POLIO): India is one of the few countries where polio remains active. All travelers to India should be fully immunized.

RABIES: India has the highest incidence of rabies in the world, with more than 30,000 human cases occurring annually. Travelers should seek immediate treatment of any animal bite, especially that of a dog. Rabies vaccination is indicated following the unprovoked bite of a dog, cat, bat, or monkey. Bites by other animals should be considered individually. Rabies vaccine is recommended for anyone planning long-term travel to this country, and for short-term travelers desiring extra protection, especially if they are visiting rural areas where the risk of animal bites is higher and where medical care is less readily available.

ROAD SAFETY: Travel by road is dangerous. Outside major cities, main roads and highways are poorly maintained and always congested. Even main roads often have only two lanes, with poor visibility and inadequate warning markers. Heavy traffic, including overloaded trucks and buses, scooters, pedestrians, and livestock, is the norm. Travel at night is particularly hazardous.

TRAVELERS' DIARRHEA: High risk year-round, countrywide. Risk is higher in rural villages. Water supplies are frequently obtained from wells that are commonly contaminated. Untreated sewage, industrial wastes, and agricultural runoffs contaminate most of India's rivers. Piped water supplies throughout the country are quite limited and all water should be considered nonpotable outside of deluxe hotels. A quinolone antibiotic, combined with loperamide (Imodium), is recommended for the treatment of acute diarrhea. Persistent diarrhea may be due to a parasitic disease such as giardiasis, amebiasis, or cryptosporididosis.

TUBERCULOSIS: Tuberculosis is a major health problem in this country, with 2% of the population infected. Travelers planning an extended stay should have a pre-departure TB skin test (PPD test) and be retested after returning from this country. Domestic employees hired by long-term visitors and expatriates should be screened for tuberculosis.

TYPHOID FEVER: High risk of typhoid. Typhoid vaccine is recommended for those traveling off the usual tourist routes, those visiting friends or relatives, and for long-stay visitors. Typhoid vaccines are 60% to 70% effective; safe food and drink precautions should continue to be observed.

YELLOW FEVER: There is no yellow fever risk in India.

OTHER DISEASES/HAZARDS: Anthrax (cutaneous, primarily from contact with infected, freshly slaughtered animals), angiostrongyliasis (human cases from ingesting raw snails, slugs, prawns, fish, land crabs, and vegetables), brucellosis (unpasteurized dairy products are a common source), cysticercosis (neurocysticercosis causes 2% of epileptic seizures in this country), echinococcosis, Kyasanur Forest disease (tick-borne arboviral fever; risk elevated during the dry season), leprosy, leptospirosis, Indian tick typhus (tick-borne hemorrhagic fever has been reported in the forest areas in Karnataka State), helminthic infections (ascariasis, ancylostomiasis, trichuriasis, and strongyloidiasis are prevalent), leptospirosis, melioidosis, paragonimiasis (human cases from ingesting raw crabs), scabies, polio (all travelers should be fully immunized), trachoma (widespread in rural areas), typhus (both murine and scrub typhus occur), and West Nile fever.

Indonesia

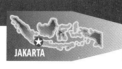

JAKARTA

CAPITAL:
Jakarta
EMBASSY (IN U.S.):
202-775-5200
GMT:
+7 hours
TELEPHONE COUNTRY CODE:
62

001-801-10

ENTRY REQUIREMENTS

- **Passport/Visa:** Passport and onward/return ticket required. Visa not required for tourist stays of up to 2 months.
- **HIV Test:** Not required.
- **Vaccinations:** A yellow fever vaccination certificate is required of all travelers arriving from infected areas or from any country in the Yellow Fever Endemic Zones.

EMBASSIES/CONSULATES

- **U.S. Embassy:** Medan Merdeka Selatan 5, Jakarta. Tel: 62-21-3435-9000; Fax: 62-21-3435-9922; e-mail: jakconsul@state.gov; Website: www.usembassyjakarta.org.
- **Canadian Embassy:** 6th Floor, World Trade Centre, Jl Jend Sudirman, Jakarta. Tel: 62-21-525-0709; Fax: 62-21-571-2251; e-mail: jkrta@dfait-maeci.gc.ca; Website: www.dfait-maeci.gc.ca.
- **British Embassy:** Jalan M H Thamrin 75, Jakarta 10310; Tel: 62-21-315-6264.

HOSPITALS/DOCTORS:

Medical care in Indonesia is generally adequate for most medical problems faced by travelers. Travelers are advised to obtain, before departure, supplemental travel health insurance with specific overseas coverage. The policy should provide for direct payment to the overseas hospital and/or physician at the time of service and include a medical evacuation benefit.

- Bali International Medical Centre; Tel: 361-761-263
- Sanglah Public Hospital, Denspasar, Bali; 361-224-049
- Metropolitan Medical Center, Jakarta; 21-520-3435
- Kediri Baptist Hospital, Kediri, Java; 0354-684-172
- International SOS:
  - Pt. Asih Eka Abadi, Jl Puri Sakti No. 10, Cipete, Jakarta Selatan, Indonesia; Alarm Center Tel: 62-21-750-6001; Alarm Center Fax: 62-21-750-6002; Clinic Tel: 62-21-750-5980; Clinic Fax: 62-21-750-6002
  - SOS Medika Klinik—Kuningan, Ground floor , Setiabudi Building II, Jalan H.R. Rasuna Sais, Kuningan, Jakarta, Indonesia; Clinic Tel: 62-21-520-1034 /-525-5367; Clinic Fax: 62-21-5207524
  - International SOS Clinic Bali, Klinik SOS Medika, Jalan Bypass Ngurah Rai 505 X, Kuta 80361, Bali Indonesia; Alarm Center Tel: 62-361-710-505; Alarm Center Fax: 62-361-710-515; Clinic Tel: 62-361-720-100; Clinic Fax: 62-361-721-919
  - PKT Office, Jalan Pupuk Raya 54, Balikpapan, Indonesia; Admin Tel: 62-542-765966; Admin Fax: 62-542-764237

Current Advisories and Health Risks

AIDS/HIV: In 2001, HIV was present in more than 5% of members of high-risk groups. Since 2001, there are reports of increasing HIV rates among injecting drug users and commercial sex workers. The provinces of DKI Jakarta, Papua, Riau, West Java, East Java, and Bali have the highest prevalences.

ANIMAL HAZARDS: Animal hazards include snakes (kraits, cobras, pit vipers), spiders, scorpions, tarantulas, crocodiles, panthers, bears, wild pigs, and wild cattle. Stingrays, jellyfish, sea wasps, poisonous fish (multiple species), and the Indo-Pacific man-of-war are common in the country's coastal waters and are potential hazards to careless or unprotected swimmers.

CHOLERA: This disease is reported active in this country, but the threat to tourists is very low. Vaccination against cholera is not routinely recommended.

DENGUE FEVER: Year-round risk, elevated during the rainy season from November through April. Risk is higher in densely populated urban areas. Travelers should take measures to prevent daytime mosquito bites.

FILARIASIS: Highly endemic. The Bancroftian and Malayan varieties of this disease are transmitted by mosquitoes in both urban and rural environments. Tourists are usually not affected by this illness.

HEPATITIS: Hepatitis A vaccine is recommended for all travelers. Outbreaks of hepatitis E have been reported in West Kalimantan and the virus is assumed to be widespread. The hepatitis B carrier rate in the general population is estimated at 8% to 10%. Hepatitis B is spread by infected blood, contaminated needles, and unsafe sex. Vaccination is recommended for stays longer than 3 months; for anyone at occupational or social risk; for any traveler desiring maximal protection.

INFLUENZA: Influenza is transmitted year-round in the tropics. The flu vaccine is recommended for all travelers.

JAPANESE ENCEPHALITIS (JE): This viral disease is transmitted by mosquitoes throughout the Indonesian archipelago, but the risk of illness is generally low. Most cases are reported from East Java, Bali, followed by Lombok, Kalimantan, and Sumatra. The peak transmission period is from October through April (the rainy season). Vaccination against Japanese encephalitis is recommended for travelers who will be staying in rural-agricultural endemic areas for 4 weeks or more during the peak transmission season. All travelers should take measures to prevent evening and nighttime mosquito bites.

MALARIA: Although about one half of the population of Indonesia is at risk of exposure to malaria, and the incidence is increasing, especially in Central Java, most travelers are at low risk. There is no risk of malaria in the major metropolitan areas of Jakarta, Medan, Surabaya, and Yogyakarta and the main resort and tourist beach areas of Java and southern Bali. Malaria risk is primarily in rural areas below 1,200 meters elevation. The highest rates of malaria are in Irian Jaya (the western half of the island of New Guinea), Sulawesi, Sumatra, Flores, and the Kokap Subdistrict area of Java. Chloroquine-resistant falciparum malaria is widespread and increasing in incidence. Chloroquine-resistant vivax malaria is reported from Sumatra and Irian Jaya, and probably occurs elsewhere. Prophylaxis with atovaquone/proguanil (Malarone), mefloquine

(Lariam), or doxycycline is recommended for travel to risk areas. All travelers should take measures to prevent evening and nighttime mosquito bites.

RABIES: Significant risk occurs in rural as well as urban areas of this country, except in Bali, which is reported to be free of rabies. All animal bites should be medically evaluated, especially those inflicted by dogs.

SCHISTOSOMIASIS: Risk is present year-round in the Lindu and Napu Valleys of central Sulawesi. Travelers to these areas should avoid swimming, bathing, or wading in freshwater lakes, ponds, or streams.

TRAVELERS' DIARRHEA: Hotels and restaurants generally serve reliable food and potable water. Elsewhere, travelers should strictly observe food and drink safety precautions. A quinolone antibiotic, combined with loperamide (Imodium), is recommended for the treatment of acute diarrhea. Persistent diarrhea may be due to a parasitic infection such as giardiasis, amebiasis, or cryptosporidiosis.

TUBERCULOSIS: Tuberculosis (TB) is a major health problem in this country. Travelers planning an extended stay should have a pre-departure TB skin test (PPD test) and be retested after returning from this country.

TYPHOID FEVER: Typhoid vaccine is recommended for those traveling off the usual tourist routes, those visiting friends or relatives, and for long-stay visitors. Because the typhoid vaccines are only 60% to 70% effective, safe food and drink selection remains important.

OTHER DISEASES/HAZARDS: Angiostrongyliasis (from ingesting raw seafood, snails, or vegetables), brucellosis (primarily from unpasteurized dairy products), capillariasis (from eating raw fish, especially fresh catch, crab, squid), paragonimiasis (associated with eating raw freshwater crabs and crayfish), clonorchiasis (isolated cases reported; associated with eating raw freshwater fish or crayfish), leprosy (highly endemic), relapsing fever (tick-borne), scrub typhus (year-round in grassy, rural areas), and helminthic (worm) infections (ascariasis, trichuriasis, hookworm disease, and strongyloidiasis). Because hookworm is a problem on the beaches, travelers are advised to sit below the 'waterline' (that washes the sand).

Iran

CAPITAL:
Tehran
EMBASSY (IN U.S.):
202-965-4990
GMT:
+3 hours

TELEPHONE COUNTRY CODE:
98

USADIRECT:
None

ENTRY REQUIREMENTS
- **Passport/Visa:** A valid passport and visa are required. The United States does not maintain diplomatic or consular relations with Iran. For visa information, contact the Embassy of Pakistan, Iranian Interests Section, 2209 Wisconsin Ave., NW, Washington, DC 20007 (202-965-4990).
- **HIV Test:** Not required.
- **Vaccinations:** None required.

EMBASSIES/CONSULATES:
The U.S. government does not maintain diplomatic relations with Iran. American interests are represented by the Swedish Embassy; Tel: 675-011 or 675-020.
- **Canadian Embassy:** 57 Shahid Javad-e-Sarfaraz (Darya-E-Noor), Ostad Motahari Avenue, Tehran, Iran; Postal Address: PO Box 11365-4647, Tehran, Iran; Tel: 98-21-873-2623; Fax: 98-21-873-3202; e-mail: teran@international.gc.ca; Website: www.iran.gc.ca.
- **British Embassy:** 198 Ferdowsi Avenue, Tehran 11344, (PO Box No 11365-4474); Tel: 98-21-670-5011-19; Fax: 671-0761; e-mail: BritishEmbassyTehran@fco.gov.uk; Website: www.britishembassy.gov.uk/iran.

HOSPITALS/DOCTORS:
Medical care in Iran can be of high quality and many physicians have trained in Europe and speak English. Travelers are advised to obtain supplemental travel health insurance with specific overseas coverage. The policy should provide for direct payment to the overseas hospital and/or physician at the time of service and include a medical evacuation benefit.
- Khatem Ul-Anbia Specialty Hospital, Tehran; full-service hospital; all specialties; Tel: 21-879-7751-9.
- Milad Hospital, Hemmat Highway, Tehran; full-service hospital; all specialties; Tel: 21-806-2250-2.

Current Advisories and Health Risks

CHOLERA: This disease is reported active, but the risk to travelers is very low; vaccination is not routinely recommended.

FILARIASIS: Reported in the southeastern province of Baluchistan-Sistan where the mosquito vector is present. Travelers to these areas should take measures to prevent mosquito bites.

HEPATITIS: All travelers should receive the hepatitis A vaccine. The hepatitis B carrier rate in the general population is estimated at 4%. Vaccination against hepatitis B is recommended for all health-care workers and should be considered by anyone planning an extended visit to this country.

LEISHMANIASIS: Cutaneous leishmaniasis occurs throughout Iran in the rural and semi-rural areas at the margins of deserts throughout the country. Visceral leishmaniasis (kala-azar) is widespread (except for the arid zones in the southeast and deserts), particularly in Fars, Azarbbayjan-e Khavari, and the northeastern Khorasan provinces. Travelers to these areas should take protective measures against sand fly bites.

MALARIA: Malaria (mainly *Plasmodium vivax*) occurs in areas north of the Zagros Mountains and in the western and southwestern regions, with most transmission occurring between March and November. In rural areas of the provinces of Hormozgan, Kerman, and Sistan-Buluchestan, chloroquine-resistant falciparum malaria is reported. Prophylaxis with atovaquone/proguanil (Malarone), mefloquine (Lariam), or doxycycline is recommended for travel to malarious areas.

RABIES: Animal rabies is common in the wolf and stray dog population. As many as 20 to 50 human rabies cases occur annually, usually in rural villages.

SCHISTOSOMIASIS: Transmission occurs year-round and increases in the spring rainy seasons, March to May. Distribution is focal along a branch of the Rud-e Karun River, between Ahvaz and Dezful, in the western province of Khuzestan. Travelers to these areas should avoid swimming or wading in freshwater ponds, lakes, or streams.

TUBERCULOSIS: Tuberculosis (TB) is a health problem in this country. Travelers planning an extended stay should have a pre-departure TB skin test (PPD test) and be retested after returning from this country.

TYPHOID FEVER: Typhoid vaccine is recommended for all travelers, with the exception of short-term visitors who restrict their meals to major restaurants and hotels. Because the typhoid vaccines are only 60% to 70% effective, safe food and drink selection remains important.

OTHER DISEASES/HAZARDS: Brucellosis (from unpasteurized dairy products), Crimean-Congo hemorrhagic fever (tick-transmitted; most cases reported from East Azerbaijan and areas near the Caspian Sea), echinococcosis, North Asian tick typhus, tick-borne relapsing fever, and helminthic (worm) infections.

Iraq

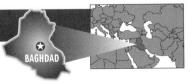

CAPITAL:
Baghdad
EMBASSY (IN U.S.):
202-483-7500
GMT:
+3 hours

TELEPHONE COUNTRY CODE:
964
USADIRECT:
None
ENTRY REQUIREMENTS
• **Passport/Visa:** The Iraqi government is currently reviewing entry requirements. U.S. citizens should consult the Embassy of Iraq in Washington, DC at 202-483-7500. Canadian and UK citizens are advised to consult the Iraqi Diplomatic Mission in their respective countries:
• **Iraqi Diplomatic Mission, Canada:** 215 McLeod St., Ottawa, ON, K2POZ8. Tel: 613-236-9177; Fax: 613-236-9641; e-mail: otaemb@iraqmofamail.net
• **Iraqi Diplomatic Mission, UK:** NOTE: no address available at this time. Tel: 44-2075812264; Fax: 44-2075893356; e-mail: lonemb@iraqmofamail.net
• **HIV test:** Not required
• **Vaccinations:** A yellow fever vaccination certificate is required of travelers arriving from infected areas.
EMBASSIES/CONSULATES
• **British Embassy:** International Zone; Tel: FTN-8280-1000; Fax: FTN-8280-2341.
HOSPITALS/DOCTORS
Travelers are advised to obtain supplemental travel health insurance with specific overseas coverage. The policy should provide for direct payment to the overseas hospital and/or physician at the time of service and include a medical evacuation benefit. At this time, travelers to Iraq should be prepared to pay cash for all medical services.

Current Advisories and Health Risks

IMMUNIZATIONS: All travelers should be fully immunized against tetanus-diphtheria, measles-mumps-rubella, polio, varicella (chickenpox), hepatitis A and B, and typhoid.

MEDICATIONS: Travelers should bring at least a 10-day supply of a quinolone antibiotic (Levaquin, 750 mg once daily) for the self-treatment of an infectious illness, such as pneumonia, or severe diarrhea.

MALARIA: Endemic in northern Iraq. Risk areas include rural and urban areas in the northern provinces of Dahuk, Ninawa, Irbil, Tamin, and As Sulaymaniyah below 1,500 meters elevation. Small, scattered, sporadic outbreaks probably occur in the southern and central areas from the Tigris-Euphrates river basin to the border with Iran. There is no malaria in Baghdad. Nearly all cases of malaria in Iraq are currently of the vivax variety. Chloroquine-resistant falciparum malaria has not been reported. Travelers to malarious areas are advised to take weekly chloroquine and avoid mosquito bites.

SCHISTOSOMIASIS: Risk occurs near the Tigris and Euphrates rivers, especially in the central regions. No transmission occurs south of Basra. Travelers should avoid swimming or wading in freshwater ponds, lakes, or streams in risk areas.

TRAVELERS' DIARRHEA: High risk. There is a high incidence of shigellosis and salmonellosis in this country. Travelers should drink only bottled, boiled, or treated water. All food should be well cooked. A quinolone antibiotic is recommended for the treatment of acute diarrhea. Diarrhea not improving with antibiotic treatment may be due to a parasitic disease such as amebiasis or giardiasis.

OTHER DISEASES/HAZARDS: Brucellosis (usually transmitted by raw goat or camel milk), rabies (transmitted by jackals, foxes, and dogs), relapsing fever (louse-borne; endemic in northern Iraq), sand fly fever (risk may be limited to the southwestern border with Saudi Arabia), tuberculosis, typhus (flea-borne; sporadic cases in southern areas), typhoid fever, and helminthic infections (roundworm, hookworm, and whipworm infections are common).

See Disease Risk Summary for the Middle East on page 310.

Ireland

DUBLIN ★

CAPITAL:
Dublin
EMBASSY (IN U.S.):
202-462-3939
GMT:
+0 hours
TELEPHONE COUNTRY CODE:
353
USADIRECT:
1-800-550-000
ENTRY REQUIREMENTS
• **Passport/Visa:** Passport required.
• **HIV Test:** Not required.
• **Vaccinations:** None required.
EMBASSIES/CONSULATES
• **U.S. Embassy:** Dublin. 42 Elgin Road, Ballsbridge; Tel: 1-688-777.
• **Canadian Embassy:** 65 St. Stephen's Green, Dublin 2, Ireland; Tel: 353-1-417-4100; Fax: 353-1-417-4101; e-mail: dubln@international.gc.ca; Website: www.dublin.gc.ca.
• **British Embassy:** 29 Merrion Road, Ballsbridge, Dublin 4; Tel: 00-353-1-205-3700; Fax: 00-353-1-205-3731; e-mail: chancery.dublx@fco.gov.uk; Website: www.britishembassy.ie.
HOSPITALS/DOCTORS:
• Our Lady's Hospital for Sick Children, Dublin (pediatrics); Tel: 558-511 or 800-365.
• Consultant's Clinic, Dublin (ob/gyn); Tel: 544-506.
• St. Jane's Hospital, Dublin (595 beds); all specialties; 4-bed ICU unit; Tel: 532-867/8.

- W.A. Ryan, M.D., Dublin; Tel: 1-2691-581.
- Blackrock Clinic, Rock Road, Blackrock Co., Dublin; Tel: 883-364.
- Charlemont Clinic, Dublin (Professor Risteard Mulcahy, cardiology); Tel: 784-277.

Current Advisories and Health Risks

HEPATITIS: Low risk. Hepatitis A vaccine is not routinely recommended. The carrier rate of the hepatitis B virus in the general population is less than 0.5 percent. Hepatitis E has not been reported.

LYME DISEASE: Endemic level undetermined but clinical cases reportedly occur among all age groups, usually during the summer months. *Ixodes ricinus* tick population peaks in May and September. Travelers to rural areas should take measures to prevent tick bites, especially in brushy, wooded, and forested areas.

TRAVELERS' DIARRHEA: Low risk. Water throughout Ireland is potable. Cryptosporidiosis and giardiasis are endemic at low levels. Incidence of amebiasis is not known but presumed low.

OTHER DISEASES/HAZARDS: Hemorrhagic fever with renal syndrome (no cases currently reported although virus appears to be circulating in the rodent population of Ireland), leptospirosis (acquired through contact with infective animal urine, often when swimming in polluted water), leptospirosis (human infection from exposure to livestock), and Q fever (rare cases in humans).

Israel

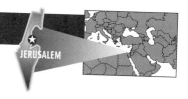

CAPITAL:
Jerusalem
EMBASSY
202-364-5500
GMT:
+2 hours
TELEPHONE COUNTRY CODE:
972
USADIRECT:
1-800-949-4949
ENTRY REQUIREMENTS
- **Passport/Visa:** An onward or return ticket and proof of sufficient funds are required for entry to Israel. A 3-month visa may be issued for no charge on arrival. No visa is required for travel to the Gaza Strip.
- **HIV Test:** The Government of Israel reserves the right to refuse entry to someone suspected of being HIV positive.
- **Vaccinations:** None required.

- **U.S. Embassy:** 71 Hayarkon Street, Tel Aviv; Tel: 3-519-7575; 3-519-7551; Fax: 972-3-516-4390; e-mail: amctelaviv@state.gov; Website: consular.usembassy-israel.org.il.
- **U.S. Consulates:** 27 Nablus Road, Jerusalem; Tel: 2-622-7200; 2-622-7250; Fax: 972-2-627-2233; e-mail: jerusalemacs@state.gov; Website: www.uscongen-jerusalem.org.
- **Canadian Embassy:** 3/5 Nirim Street, Tel Aviv; Tel: 3-636-3300; Fax: 972-3-636-3383; e-mail: taviv@dfait-maeci.gc.ca; Website: www.dfait-aeci.gc.ca/telaviv.
- **British Embassy:** 192 Hayarkon Street, Tel Aviv 63405; Tel: 972-3-725-1222; Fax: 972-3-524-3313; e-mail: webmaster.telaviv@fco.gov.uk; Website: www.britemb.org.il.

HOSPITALS/DOCTORS:

Medical care in Israel is of high quality and many physicians speak English. Travelers are advised to obtain, before departure, supplemental travel health insurance with specific overseas coverage. The policy should provide for direct payment to the overseas hospital and/or physician at the time of service and include a medical evacuation benefit.

- Herzliya Medical Centers, Haifa and Tel Aviv. Official referral hospitals for the Multinational Forces in the Sinai; the Haifa facility can do open-heart procedures; both of these prestigious private hospitals also accept Blue Cross/Blue Shield payments.
- Chaim Sheba Medical Center, Tel Aviv (1,500 beds); all specialties; emergency department.
- Ichilov Municipal Hospital, Tel Aviv (public hospital; 500 beds); all specialties; emergency department.
- Hadassah-Hebrew Medical Center, Jerusalem (680 beds).
- Rothschild Hadassah University Hospital, Jerusalem (680 beds); all specialties.
- Rambam Medical Center, Haifa (850 beds); all specialties.
- Soroka University Hospital, Beer-Sheva (700 beds).

Current Advisories and Health Risks

CHOLERA: Cases of cholera have been reported in the Gaza Strip.

HEPATITIS: Hepatitis A is moderately to highly endemic. All nonimmune travelers should receive the hepatitis A vaccine before visiting this country. Hepatitis E may occur, but levels are unclear. The hepatitis B carrier rate in the general population is estimated at less than 1%. Hepatitis B vaccine is recommended for stays longer than 3 months and for short-term travelers wanting increased protection. Travelers should be aware that the risk of hepatitis B is increased by unsafe sex and the use of unsterile needles and syringes. Hepatitis C is endemic.

INFLUENZA: Influenza is transmitted from November through March. Flu vaccine is recommended for all travelers.

LEISHMANIASIS: Focally distributed countrywide. Cutaneous leishmaniasis is present in the Jordan Valley, particularly from the northern Dead Sea region to Massua; other risk areas include the wadis of the Negev Desert (including Keziot), the Arava Valley, and Samaria. Visceral leishmaniasis is reported in the Judean foothills of central Israel and the

Galilee Region of northern Israel. Peak transmission of leishmaniasis occurs between April and October. Travelers should take measures to prevent insect (sand fly) bites.

MALARIA: There is no risk of malaria in Israel.

MEDITERRANEAN SPOTTED (BOUTONNEUSE) FEVER: Highest risk of transmission is in southern Israel, especially the northwest part of the Negev desert and the coastal plain area. This rickettsial disease (caused by *Rickettsia conorii*) is transmitted by the brown dog tick and has emerged as the most common insect-borne disease in Israel. Travelers, especially to rural areas, should avoid dogs (as well as sheep and goats), which harbor the infective ticks. Infective ticks are also found on grass and around hay stacks, and along wild animal paths.

RABIES: Incidence of rabies in animals, especially foxes, is increasing, but no recent human cases of rabies have been reported. Travelers should seek immediate medical attention for any dog or wild animal bite.

SCHISTOSOMIASIS: This disease is apparently no longer a threat in Israel. Urinary schistosomiasis was once endemic in the Jordan River, but no recent indigenous cases have been reported.

TICK-BORNE RELAPSING FEVER (CAVE FEVER): Cave fever, caused by the spirochete *Borrelia persica*, is transmitted in rural areas by ticks that inhabit animal burrows, cracks in boulders, archeological sites, caves, tombs, and bunkers. Ten percent of the caves in Israel are infested by ticks (55% infested in the lower Galilee). Risk areas include the Negev, the West Bank, the coastal plain, and the northern areas. Treatment, as well as prophylaxis, with tetracycline, are effective.

TRAVELERS' DIARRHEA: Medium risk. Although the risk of bacterial gastroenteritis is lower than in the neighboring Arab countries, it is much higher than in Western Europe. A quinolone antibiotic, combined with loperamide (Imodium), is recommended for the treatment of acute diarrhea. Persistent diarrhea may be due to a parasitic infection such as giardiasis, amebiasis, or cryptosporidiosis.

OTHER DISEASES/HAZARDS: Anthrax (mostly cutaneous; usually from agricultural exposure), brucellosis (usually transmitted by raw goat/sheep milk; common cause of fever in humans), echinococcosis (carried by a small percentage of rural dogs; low incidence in humans; more common in northern areas), leptospirosis (human cases frequently reported), tuberculosis, typhoid fever, and West Nile fever.

Italy

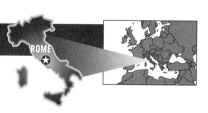

CAPITAL:
Rome
EMBASSY (IN U.S.):
202-612-4400

GMT:

+1 hour

TELEPHONE COUNTRY CODE:

39

USADIRECT:

800-172-444

ENTRY REQUIREMENTS

- **Passport/Visa:** Passport required.
- **HIV Test:** Not required.
- **Vaccinations:** None required.

EMBASSIES/CONSULATES

- **U.S. Embassy:** Rome. Via Veneto 119/A; Tel: 6-46-741.
- **U.S. Consulate:** Florence; Tel: 55-239-8276 or 217-605.
- **Canadian Embassy:** Via Zara 30, Rome, Italy 00198; Tel: 39-06-44-59-81; Fax: 39-06-44-598-29-12; e-mail: rome.citizenservices@international.gc.ca; Website: www.rome.gc.ca.
- **British Embassy:** Via XX Settembre 80a, 00187 Rome; Tel: 39-06-4220-0001; e-mail: info@rome.mail.fco.gov.uk; Website: www.britain.it.

HOSPITALS/DOCTORS:

Two hospitals in Rome that have a large number of English-speaking staff include

- Salvator Mundi International Hospital Viale Mura Gianicolensi 67 (near the Vatican); Tel: 06588961.
- Rome American Hospital, Via E. Longoni 69; Tel: 0622551.

An updated listing of physicians and hospitals in Rome is found at Website: www.usembassy.it/cons/acs/doctors.htm

Medical care in Western Europe is of high quality and many physicians speak English. Travelers are advised to obtain, before departure, supplemental travel health insurance with specific overseas coverage. The policy should provide for direct payment to the overseas hospital and/or physician at the time of service and include a medical evacuation benefit.

Current Advisories and Health Risks

ACCIDENTS AND INJURIES: Accidents, especially motor vehicle crashes, are the leading cause of death among travelers younger than 55 years of age; cardiovascular diseases cause most fatalities in older travelers; infections cause most illness during travel but fewer than 1% of the fatalities.

DIROFILARIASIS: Low risk; human dirofilariasis has been reported from the Monferrato area. Other risk areas include Torino, Allessandria, Vercelli, and Pavia. The parasite is transmitted to humans by mosquito bites.

HEPATITIS: Increased risk of hepatitis A occurs in the south and on the islands of Sicily and Sardinia. All nonimmune travelers should receive hepatitis A vaccine. The overall carrier rate of hepatitis B in the general population is estimated at 2.5%. Hepatitis B is spread by infected blood, contaminated needles, and unsafe sex. Vaccination is recommended for stays longer than 3 months; for anyone at occupational or social risk; for any traveler desiring maximal protection. The risk of illness or injury during travel cannot be predicted and some experts believe that *all* travelers should be immunized against hepatitis B because of the risk of receiving a medical injection with an unsterile needle or syringe.

LEISHMANIASIS: Cutaneous and visceral leishmaniasis occurs in southern rural areas, including the islands of Sardinia and Sicily and along the Mediterranean coast; risk from visceral leishmaniasis is elevated in Sicily and the Campania Region. Transmission occurs May through November, peaking in July through August. Travelers to risk areas should take measures to prevent insect (sand fly) bites.

RABIES: No human cases have recently been reported, but animal rabies occurs in the fox population near the Austrian border.

TICK-BORNE DISEASES: Lyme disease, tick-borne encephalitis (TBE), and boutonneuse fever (Mediterranean spotted fever) are reported. Risk areas for Lyme disease are limited primarily to northern Italy, along the Ligurian coast and the Adriatic coast. TBE has been reported around Florence, near the Swiss border and from the Trento area. Boutonneuse fever occurs countrywide in rural areas but is more common along the Ligurian coast and the islands of Sicily and Sardinia. Travelers to all these regions should take measures to prevent tick bites.

TRAVELERS' DIARRHEA: Low risk in major cities, such as Rome, Milan, and Verona, where the water supplies are adequately treated. Higher risk exists in the south and on the islands of Sicily and Sardinia. A quinolone antibiotic is recommended for the treatment of acute diarrhea. Persistent diarrhea may be due to a parasitic disease such as giardiasis.

Ivory Coast (Côte d'Ivoire)

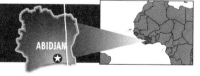

ABIDJAN ★

CAPITAL:
Abidjan
EMBASSY (IN U.S.):
202-797-0300
GMT:
+0 hours
TELEPHONE COUNTRY CODE:
225
USADIRECT:
None

ENTRY REQUIREMENTS

- **Passport/Visa:** Valid passport and visa are required.
- **HIV Test:** Not required.
- **Vaccinations:** A yellow fever vaccination certificate is required from all travelers more than 1 year of age arriving from all countries.

EMBASSIES/CONSULATES

- **U.S. Embassy:** 5 Rue Jesse Owens, Abidjan: Tel: 225-20-21-09-79; Fax: 225-20-22-45-23, 225-20-22-32-59.
- **Canadian Embassy:** Immeuble Trade Centre, 23 Avenue Nogues, Le Plateau, Abidjan. Tel: 225-20-30-07-00; Fax: 225-20-30-07-20; e-mail: abdjn@dfait-maeci.gc.ca; Website: www.dfait-maeci.gc.ca/abidjan
- **British Embassy:** At the time of publication, all activities have been suspended at the British Embassy, Abidjan. Further information may be obtained from Africa Department (Equatorial), FCO London on 44-0-20-7008-3166.

HOSPITALS/DOCTORS

- Treichville University Hospital, Abidjan (1,500 beds); general medical/surgical facility; most specialties
- Polyclinic International St. Ann Marie, Cocody (300 beds); general medical/surgical facility; emergency department; dialysis; heliport.
- Travelers should contact the U.S. Embassy for additional health-care referrals.

Current Advisories and Health Risks

ACCIDENTS, ILLNESS, AND MEDICAL INSURANCE: Accidents and injuries are the leading cause of death among travelers younger than age 55 and are most often caused by motor vehicle and motorcycle crashes; drownings, aircraft crashes, homicides, and burns are less common causes. Important safety rules to follow are (1) Do not drive at night; (2) Do not rent a motorcycle, moped, bicycle, or motorbike, even if you are experienced; and (3) Don't swim alone, at night, or if intoxicated.

- Heart attacks cause most fatalities in older travelers.
- Infections cause only 1% of fatalities in overseas travelers, but, overall, infections are the most common cause of travel-related illness.
- Travelers are advised to obtain, before departure, supplemental travel health insurance with specific overseas coverage. The policy should provide for direct payment to the overseas hospital and/or physician at the time of service and include a medical evacuation benefit. The policy should also provide 24-hour hotline access to a multilingual assistance center that can help arrange and monitor delivery of medical care and determine if medical evacuation or air ambulance services are required.

AFRICAN SLEEPING SICKNESS (TRYPANOSOMIASIS): African trypanosomiasis is highly endemic in focal areas throughout the country. Measures to prevent insect (tsetse fly) bites are recommended.

AFRICAN TICK TYPHUS: This tick-borne illness (which is similar to Mediterranean spotted fever) occurs countrywide. Travelers should take measures to prevent tick bites.

AIDS/HIV: AIDS cases are increasing to near epidemic levels. The reasons include (1) an increase in IV drug abuse; (2) an increase in prostitution and promiscuity; (3) an increase in sexually transmitted diseases; (4) decreased availability of sterile needles and syringes; and (5) little or no education or public health prevention programs.

CHOLERA: This disease is active in this country, but the threat to tourists is very low. Cholera is an extremely rare disease in travelers from developed countries. Cholera vaccine is recommended primarily for people at high risk (e.g., relief workers) who work and live in highly endemic areas under less than adequate sanitary conditions.

- The oral cholera vaccine (Dukoral) provides up to 60% crossover protection against ETEC diarrhea.
- Many countries, including Canada, license an oral cholera vaccine. The oral vaccine is not available in the United States.
- Cholera vaccine is not "officially" required for entry into, or exit from, any country. Despite this, some countries, on occasion, require proof of cholera vaccination from travelers coming from cholera-infected countries. Anticipating such a situation, certain travelers may wish to carry a medical exemption letter from their health-care provider. Travel Medicine, Inc., recommends that travelers use the International Certificate of Vaccination (Yellow Card) for this purpose, having their health-care provider affirm that they are "exempt from cholera vaccine" and validate the exemption with both the provider's signature and the appropriate official stamp (the "Uniform Stamp" in the United States).

HEPATITIS: There is high risk of hepatitis A. All nonimmune travelers should receive the hepatitis A vaccine. Vaccination against hepatitis B should be considered for stays longer than 3 months and by short-term travelers desiring maximal protection. Travelers should be aware that hepatitis B can be transmitted by unsafe sex and the use of contaminated needles and syringes.

INFLUENZA: Influenza is transmitted year-round in the tropics. The flu vaccine is recommended for all travelers older than age 50; all travelers with any chronic disease or weakened immune system; travelers of any age wishing to decrease the risk of this illness; pregnant women after the first trimester.

INSECTS: All travelers should take measures to prevent both daytime and nighttime insect bites. Insect-bite prevention measures include a DEET-containing repellent applied to exposed skin, insecticide (permethrin) spray applied to clothing and gear, and use of a permethrin-treated bed net at night while sleeping.

LEISHMANIASIS: Leishmaniasis (kala-azar variety), transmitted by sand flies, occurs in this country. Insect-bite precautions are recommended.

MALARIA: High risk countrywide throughout the year. Falciparum malaria accounts for 90% of cases. Chloroquine-resistant *Plasmodium falciparum* is widespread.

- Prophylaxis with atovaquone/proguanil (Malarone), mefloquine (Lariam), or doxycycline is recommended.

- All travelers should take measures to prevent evening and nighttime mosquito bites. Insect-bite prevention measures include a DEET-containing repellent applied to exposed skin, insecticide (permethrin) spray applied to clothing and gear, and use of a permethrin-treated bed net at night while sleeping.

MENINGITIS: This country is in Africa's "meningitis belt." Vaccination is recommended for travelers, especially during the dry season, December through June, who anticipate having close contact with the indigenous population.

ONCHOCERCIASIS: Onchocerciasis, transmitted by black flies, is prevalent. Exposure of longer than just 1 week or 2 is generally required for infection. Travelers should take measures to prevent insect (black fly) bites, especially when near the shores of fast-running rivers.

POLIO: This disease is endemic in sub-Saharan Africa. All travelers should be fully immunized.

RABIES: Sporadic cases of human rabies are reported countrywide. All animal bites or scratches, especially from a dog, should be taken seriously, and immediate medical attention should be sought. No one should pet or pick up any stray animals. All children should be warned to avoid contact with unknown animals. Rabies vaccine is recommended for travel longer than 3 months, for shorter stays for travelers who plan to venture off the usual tourist routes where they may be more exposed to the stray dog population, or when travelers desire extra protection.

SCHISTOSOMIASIS: Schistosomiasis occurs countrywide. Travelers should avoid freshwater lakes, streams, and irrigation ditches.

TUBERCULOSIS: Tuberculosis is a major health problem in this country. Travelers planning an extended stay should have a pre-departure TB skin test (PPD test) and be retested after leaving this country.

TYPHOID FEVER: Vaccination against typhoid fever is recommended for travelers venturing outside of tourist areas; long-term travelers; adventure travelers; those wishing maximum disease protection. Because the typhoid vaccines are only 60% to 70% effective, safe food and drink selection remains important.

YELLOW FEVER: Yellow fever is active in this country. In 2001, 20 suspected cases were reported in Abidjan. Yellow fever vaccine is required for entry to the Ivory Coast.

OTHER DISEASES/HAZARDS: African tick typhus (transmitted by dog ticks, often in urban areas, and bush ticks), brucellosis (from consumption of raw dairy products), cutaneous larval migrans, dengue (low risk; human incidence not known), Ebola fever (rare outbreaks), filariasis (presumably endemic; incidence not known), Lassa fever (viral disease, spread by rodents; low risk to tourists), paragonimiasis, toxoplasmosis, typhoid fever, and intestinal worms (very common) are reported.

Jamaica

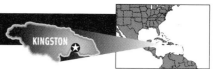

KINGSTON

CAPITAL:
Kingston

EMBASSY (IN U.S.):
202-452-0660

GMT:
−5 hours

TELEPHONE COUNTRY CODE:
876

USADIRECT:
1-800-872-2881

ENTRY REQUIREMENTS

- **Passport/Visa**: If traveling directly from the U.S., Puerto Rico, or the U.S. Virgin Islands, U.S. citizens can enter Jamaica with a certified copy of a U.S. birth certificate or a U.S. passport.
- **HIV Test:** Not required.
- **Vaccinations:** A yellow fever vaccination certificate is required from all travelers arriving from infected areas.

EMBASSIES/CONSULATES

- **U.S. Embassy:** Oxford Manor Building, 1st floor, 16 Oxford Road, Kingston; Tel: 935-6018, 929-4850 through 59.
- **U.S. Consulate:** St. James Place, 2nd Floor, Gloucester Avenue, Montego Bay; Tel: 952-0160.
- **Canadian Embassy:** 3 West Kings House Road, Kingston; Tel: 926-1500; Fax: 1-876-511-3493; e-mail: kngtn@dfait-maeci.gc.ca.
- **British High Commission:** PO Box 575, 28 Trafalgar Road, Kingston 10; Tel: 1-876-510-0700; Fax: 1-876-510-0737; e-mail: bhckingston@cwjamaica.com.

HOSPITALS/DOCTORS:

Medical care in Jamaica is below Western standards. There are 16 public and 6 private hospitals. Travelers are advised to obtain, before departure, supplemental travel health insurance with specific overseas coverage. The policy should provide for direct payment to the overseas hospital and/or physician at the time of service and include a medical evacuation benefit.

- University Hospital, Kingston (504 beds); general medical/surgical facility; ICU; burn unit; emergency services.

Current Advisories and Health Risks

AIDS/HIV: The Caribbean is the second most affected region in the world. Jamaica's HIV/AIDS infection rate is rising and it is the second leading cause of death among children younger than 4 years of age and of women between the ages of 20 and 29. The prevalence rate in adults between the ages of 15 and 49 years in 2002 ranges from 1.5% to 2%.

DENGUE FEVER: This mosquito-transmitted viral disease is prevalent in the Caribbean and occurs year-round, especially in coastal and lowland urban areas. All travelers to Jamaica should take measures to prevent daytime insect bites.

HEPATITIS: Hepatitis A vaccine is recommended. Hepatitis B is spread by infected blood, contaminated needles, and unsafe sex. Vaccination is recommended for stays longer than 3 months; for anyone at occupational or social risk; for any traveler desiring maximal protection. The risk of illness or injury during travel cannot be predicted and some experts believe that *all* travelers should be immunized against hepatitis B because of the risk of receiving a medical injection with an unsterile needle or syringe.

INFLUENZA: Influenza is transmitted year-round in the tropics. The flu vaccine is recommended for all travelers.

LEPTOSPIROSIS: This spirochetal infection is reported from this country, but the incidence is low. Contact with water contaminated with animal urine results in disease transmission.

MALARIA: There is no risk of malaria in Jamaica.

MARINE HAZARDS: Swimming related hazards include jellyfish, spiny sea urchins, and corals. Ciguatera poisoning is prevalent and can result from eating reef fish such as grouper, snapper, sea bass, jack, and barracuda. The ciguatoxin is not destroyed by cooking.

SCUBA DIVING: Divers' Alert Network (DAN) maintains an up-to-date list of all hyperbaric chambers in North America and the Caribbean. In association with Duke University Medical Center in North Carolina, DAN operates a 24-hour emergency phone number (919-684-8111) for members and nonmembers to call. Their staff is available to answer questions and, if necessary, make referral to the closest functioning hyperbaric chamber.

TRAVELERS' DIARRHEA: Low to moderate risk. In urban and resort areas, the hotels and restaurants generally serve reliable food and potable water. A quinolone antibiotic, combined with loperamide (Imodium), is recommended for the treatment of acute diarrhea. Persistent diarrhea may be due to a parasitic infection such as giardiasis, amebiasis, or cryptosporidiosis.

TUBERCULOSIS: Tuberculosis (TB) ia a major health problem in this country. Travelers planning an extended stay should have a pre-departure TB skin test (PPD test) and be retested after returning from this country.

TYPHOID FEVER: Typhoid vaccine is recommended for those traveling off the usual tourist routes, those visiting friends or relatives, and for long-stay visitors. Because the typhoid vaccines are only 60% to 70% effective, safe food and drink selection remains important.

Japan

TOKYO

CAPITAL:
Tokyo

EMBASSY (IN U.S.):
202-939-6700

GMT:
+9 hours

TELEPHONE COUNTRY CODE:
81

USADIRECT:
To place calls using KDD: 00-539-111
To place calls using IDC: 00-665-5111
To place calls using JT: 00-441-1111

ENTRY REQUIREMENTS

- **Passport/Visa:** Passport and onward/return ticket required. Visa not required for tourist/commercial business stays of up to 90 days.
- **HIV Test:** Not required.
- **Vaccinations:** None required.

EMBASSIES/CONSULATES

- **U.S. Embassy:** 1-10-5 Akasaka, Minato-ku, Tokyo; Tel: 81-3-3224-5000; Fax: 81-3-3224-5856; Website: usembassy.state.gov/tokyo, www.csjapan.doc.gov.
- **U.S. Consulates:** 2-11-5 Nishitenma, Kita-ku, Osaka, Osaka-Kobe; Tel: 81-6-6315-5900; 2564 Nishihara, Urasoe, Naha, Okinawa; Tel: 81-98-876-4211; Kita 1-Jo Nishi 28-chome, Chuo-ku; Tel: 81-11-641-1115; 2-5-26; Ohori, Chuo-ku, Fukuoka 810-0052; Tel: 81-92-751-9331; Nishiki SIS Building 6th Floor, Naka-ku, Nagoya; Tel: 81-52-203-4011.
- **Canadian Embassy:** 3-38 Akasaka 7-chome, Minato-ku, Tokyo; Tel: 81-3-5412-6200; Fax: 81-3-5412-6289; e-mail: tokyo@dfait-maeci.gc.ca; Website: www.dfait-maeci.gc.ca/ni-ka.
- **British Embassy:** No 1 Ichiban-cho, Chiyoda-ku, Tokyo 102-8381; Tel: 81-3-5211-1100; Fax: 81-3-5275-3164; e-mail: embassy.tokyo@fco.gov.uk; Website: www.uknow.or.jp.

HOSPITALS/DOCTORS:
Medical care in Japan is of high quality and many physicians may not speak English. Travelers are advised to obtain, before departure, supplemental travel health insurance with specific overseas coverage. The policy should provide for direct payment to the overseas hospital and/or physician at the time of service and include a medical evacuation benefit.

- Tokyo Medical and Surgical Clinic; Tel: 03-3436-3028
- Sakabe International Clinic, Kyoto; Tel: 075-231-1624

- International SOS: International SOS Japan Ltd., 8th Floor, Kudan-minami C&M Bldg., 3-9-14 Kudan-minami, Chiyoda-ku, Tokyo 102-0074, Japan, A/C English Tel: 71-3-5210-4334, A/C Fax: 71-3-5210-2272

Current Advisories and Health Risks

ANISAKIASIS: Raw fish, often consumed as sushi or sashimi, is a potential source of parasitic disease. One such disease, anisakiasis, is transmitted by raw or undercooked saltwater fish, squid, or octopus. Humans are usually infected by eating herring, salmon, cod, mackerel or Pacific red snapper in which infectious larvae are present. Although the sushi bars in Japan are strictly regulated, consumption of raw fish is not without some risk.

HELMINTHIC INFECTIONS (FLUKES AND WORMS):

- Paragonimiasis (lung fluke disease). Transmitted by raw crab or crayfish or the juice of raw crabs or crayfish.
- Clonorchiasis (an infection of the bile ducts by the liver fluke). Transmitted by raw fish and pickled fish in vinegar (sunomono). Thorough cooking or freezing freshwater fish will kill parasites.
- Diphyllobothriasis (fish tapeworm disease). Transmitted by salmon sushi.
- Gnathostomiasis (a fish roundworm disease). Transmitted by raw freshwater fish, as well as raw chicken, eels, and frogs.

HEPATITIS: Hepatitis A vaccine is recommended for all travelers. The hepatitis B carrier rate in the general population is estimated at 2%. Hepatitis B is spread by infected blood, contaminated needles, and unsafe sex. Vaccination is recommended for stays longer than 3 months; for anyone at occupational or social risk; for any traveler desiring maximal protection.

INFLUENZA: Influenza is transmitted from November through March; flu vaccine is recommended for all travelers.

JAPANESE ENCEPHALITIS (JE): Unvaccinated foreigners are at potential risk of illness in rural rice and pig farming areas where the infective mosquitoes are most active, especially during the warmer, rainier months (April through November in Okinawa and July through September elsewhere). The highest risk of infection occurs in southeastern Japan where 80% of cases occur on Kyushu, Shikoku, and Chubu; there is negligible risk in northern Hokkaido. Vaccination against Japanese encephalitis is recommended for travelers who will be staying in endemic rural-agricultural areas for 3 to 4 weeks or longer during the peak transmission periods. Travelers to rural areas should also take measures to prevent mosquito bites, especially in the evening and nighttime when the mosquitoes are most active.

LYME DISEASE: Sporadic cases have been reported from Hokkaido, Honshu, Shikoku, and Kyushu islands. Hikers and forest workers are at most risk. The prevalence of Lyme disease bacteria in ticks is estimated to be as high as 24% in some areas.

MALARIA: There is no risk of malaria in Japan.

SCHISTOSOMIASIS: This disease was officially eradicated in 1996.

SCRUB TYPHUS: Mite-borne; risk is present in grassy rural areas countrywide; incidence is highest in Kanagawa, Chiba, Miyazaki, Kagoshima Prefectures and in the Akita and Niigata regions; greatest risk occurs during May and November.

TRAVELERS' DIARRHEA: Low risk. A quinolone antibiotic, combined with loperamide (Imodium), is recommended for the treatment of diarrhea. Persistent diarrhea may be due to a parasitic infection.

OTHER DISEASES/HAZARDS: Angiostrongyliasis (occurs mostly in the southwestern islands, including Kyushu Ryukyu), fasciolopsiasis (giant intestinal fluke disease; prevented by thoroughly cooking all aquatic plants and vegetables), Japanese spotted fever, and Kawasaki disease. Air pollution is a major problem in Osaka, Tokyo, and Yokohama.

Jordan

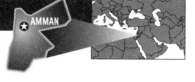

CAPITAL:
Amman
EMBASSY (IN U.S.):
202-966-2664
GMT:
+2 hours
TELEPHONE COUNTRY CODE:
962
USADIRECT:
1-880-0000
ENTRY REQUIREMENTS
- **Passport/Visa:** Travelers can obtain a visa at international ports of entry.
- **HIV Test:** Not required.
- **Vaccinations:** Yellow fever vaccination certificate is required if traveling from an infected area and more than 1 year of age.

EMBASSIES/CONSULATES
- **U.S. Embassy:** Abdoun, Amman; Tel: 6-592-0101; Fax: 962-6-592-4102; Website: www.usembassy-amman.org.jo
- **Canadian Embassy:** Pearl of Shmeisani Building, Amman; Tel: 6-566-6124; Fax: 6-568-9227; e-mail: amman@dfait-maeci.gc.ca
- **British Embassy:** (PO Box 87) Abdoun, 11118 Amman; Fax: 962-6-5909279; e-mail: becommercial@nets.com.jo; Website: www.britain.org.jo

HOSPITALS/DOCTORS

- Ashrifiyah Hospital, Amman (520 beds); most medical specialties; burn unit
- King Hussein Medical Center, Amman (600 beds); all specialties; latest state-of-the-art Western medical and surgical equipment
- University of Jordan Hospital (400 beds); teaching facility; all specialties
- Al Khalidi Medical Center, Amman (170-beds); Tel: 962-6-464-4281; private hospital providing general medical/surgical services; 24-hour emergency services

Current Advisories and Health Risks

ACCIDENTS, ILLNESS, AND MEDICAL INSURANCE:

- Accidents and injuries are the leading cause of death among travelers younger than age 55 and are most often caused by motor vehicle and motorcycle crashes; drownings, aircraft crashes, homicides, and burns are less common causes.
- Heart attacks cause most fatalities in older travelers.
- Infections cause only 1% of fatalities in overseas travelers, but, overall, infections are the most common cause of travel-related illness.
- Travelers are advised to obtain, before departure, supplemental travel health insurance with specific overseas coverage. The policy should provide for direct payment to the overseas hospital and/or physician at the time of service and include a medical evacuation benefit. The policy should also provide 24-hour hotline access to a multilingual assistance center that can help arrange and monitor delivery of medical care and determine if medical evacuation or air ambulance services are required.

HEPATITIS: Hepatitis A vaccine is recommended for all nonimmune travelers. Hepatitis E may occur, but endemic levels are unclear. The hepatitis B carrier rate in the general population is estimated at 7% to 10%. Vaccination against hepatitis B should be considered for stays longer than 3 months and by short-term travelers desiring maximal protection. Travelers should be aware that hepatitis B can be transmitted by unsafe sex and the use of contaminated needles and syringes. Hepatitis C is likely endemic.

LEISHMANIASIS: Cutaneous leishmaniasis is focally distributed countrywide, except in the eastern desert areas. The disease is hyperendemic in the middle and lower Jordan Valley. An outbreak has been reported at Qurayqira in Wadi Araba in southern Jordan. There is a low risk of cutaneous leishmaniasis in northern areas. Historically, visceral leishmaniasis has been reported in the north, but may be more widespread. Travelers to Jordan should take measures to prevent insect (sand fly) bites.

MALARIA: There is no risk of malaria in this country.

SCHISTOSOMIASIS: Level of risk is unclear. In 1991, the Ministry of Health declared Jordan free of schistosomiasis, but there could be continuing transmission, especially from irrigation projects. Possible risk areas include the Jordan River and East Ghor canal, the Zarqa River, Yarmouk River, Lake Tiberius, and Jarash Spring. Travelers should avoid swimming or wading in freshwater rivers, ponds, streams, or irrigated areas.

TRAVELERS' DIARRHEA: High risk. Piped water supplies are unreliable and may be contaminated. Travelers should observe food and drink safety precautions. Bottled mineral water is available locally. A quinolone antibiotic, combined with loperamide (Imodium), is recommended for the treatment of acute diarrhea. Diarrhea not responding to treatment with an antibiotic, or chronic diarrhea, may be due to a parasitic disease such as giardiasis, amebiasis, or cryptosporidiosis.

TYPHOID FEVER: Typhoid vaccine is recommended for long-term travelers, adventure travelers, and those wishing maximal disease protection. Because the typhoid vaccines are only 60% to 70% effective, safe food and drink guidelines should continue to be observed.

OTHER DISEASES/HAZARDS: Cholera (low risk; sporadic cases may occur), Mediterranean spotted fever (boutonneuse fever; occurs regionally), brucellosis (high incidence; transmitted by consumption of unpasteurized dairy products, such as cheese), dengue (historically reported from the Jordan Valley but current data not available), echinococcosis (reported sporadically, especially in northern areas), leptospirosis, rabies (most cases occur in foxes, wolves, and jackals, with spillover into the dog population; rabies occurs sporadically in humans), relapsing fever (tick-borne; caves, rocky shelters, and stone buildings may harbor infected ticks), sand fly fever (foci occur countrywide; transmission highest April through October), tuberculosis, murine typhus (flea-borne), typhoid fever, and helminthic infections (roundworm, hookworm, and whipworm infections are common in rural areas; incidence is estimated at 5%).

Kazakhstan

CAPITAL:
Almaty

EMBASSY (IN U.S.):
202-333-4507

GMT:
+4 hours

TELEPHONE COUNTRY CODE:
7

USADIRECT:
8^800-121-4321; ^ indicates second dial tone.

ENTRY REQUIREMENTS

• **Passport/Visa:** Passport and visa required.

• **Vaccinations:** A yellow fever vaccination certificate is required from travelers coming from infected areas.

• **HIV Test:** Foreign visitors (except nationals of CIS countries) staying in Kazakhstan for longer than 3 months may be required to take an HIV test.

- **U.S. Embassy**: 99/97A Furmanova Street, Almaty; Tel: 7-3272-63-39-21; 7-3272-50-76-27, Fax: 7-3272-50-62-69; e-mail:consularalmaty@state.gov.
- **Canadian Embassy**: 34 Karasai Batir Street (Vinogradov St.), Almaty; Tel: 7-3272-50-11-51; Fax: 7-3272-58-24-93; e-mail: almat@dfait-maeci.gc.ca.
- **British Embassy:** Ul Furmanova 173, Almaty; Tel: 73272-506191, 506192, 506229; Fax: 73272-506260; e-mail: british-embassy@kaznet.kz.

HOSPITALS/DOCTORS

There is a large network of hospitals, emergency centers, and pharmacies. The largest include the Central Hospital, the Maternity and Childhood Institute Clinic, and the Medical Teaching Institute Clinic in Almaty, and the Spinal Centre and Hospital of Rehabilitation Treatment in Karaganda. However, standards within the public health-care system have declined significantly since the Soviet era. It is hard to determine the level of expertise of the doctors, and visitors cannot rely on the availability of Western medicines. Medical insurance is strongly recommended and should include medical evacuation insurance.

- International SOS:
  - International SOS Clinic (Almaty), 11 Luganskogo Street, Almaty 480051, Republic of Kazakhstan; Clinic/Admin Tel: 7-3272-581-911; Clinic/Admin Fax: 7-3272-581-585
  - International SOS Clinic, River Palace Hotel, 55, Aiteke bi Street, Atyrau, 465050, Republic of Kazakhstan; Clinic/Admin Tel: 7-3122-586-911; Clinic/Admin Fax: 7-3122-586-211
  - International SOS (Office), 1B Gornaya Street, Almaty 480051, Republic of Kazakhstan; Tel: 7-3272-581912; Fax: 7-3272-581-909

Current Advisories and Health Risks

ACCIDENTS, ILLNESS, AND MEDICAL INSURANCE

- Accidents and injuries are the leading cause of death among travelers younger than age 55 and are most often caused by motor vehicle and motorcycle crashes; drownings, aircraft crashes, homicides, and burns are less common causes.
- Heart attacks cause most fatalities in older travelers.
- Infections cause only 1% of fatalities in overseas travelers, but, overall, infections are the most common cause of travel-related illness.
- Travelers are advised to obtain, before departure, supplemental travel health insurance with specific overseas coverage. The policy should provide for direct payment to the overseas hospital and/or physician at the time of service and include a medical evacuation benefit. The policy should also provide 24-hour hotline access to a multilingual assistance center that can help arrange and monitor delivery of medical care and determine if medical evacuation or air ambulance services are required.

ARBOVIRAL DISEASES: Tahjna virus fever (mosquito-borne; virus circulates through much of the former USSR), sand fly fever (sand fly-borne; limited to regions of southern central Asia, April through October), dengue fever (mosquito-borne; no recent cases reported), West Nile fever (mosquito-borne; cases have occurred in the Tadzikstan), North Asian tick fever (occurs wherever tick vectors are found).

CHOLERA: This disease is active in this country. The risk of cholera, however, is extremely low in international travelers from developed countries. Cholera vaccine is recommended primarily for travelers at high risk who work and live in highly endemic areas under less than adequate sanitary conditions.
- The oral cholera vaccine (Dukoral) provides up to 60% crossover protection against ETEC diarrhea.

CRIMEAN-CONGO HEMORRHAGIC FEVER: Tick-transmitted viral illness, also known as central Asian hemorrhagic fever. Risk areas are rural steppe, savannah, semi-desert, and foothill/low mountain habitats below 2,000 meters elevation. Outbreaks occurred in south-central Kazakhstan during 1989.

FOOD AND WATER SAFETY: All water should be regarded as being a potential health risk. Water used for drinking, brushing teeth, or making ice should have first been boiled or otherwise sterilized. Milk is pasteurized and dairy products are safe for consumption. Only eat well-cooked meat and fish, preferably served hot. Pork, salad, and mayonnaise may carry increased risk. Vegetables should be cooked and fruit should be peeled.

HEPATITIS: All nonimmune travelers should receive hepatitis A vaccine. The hepatitis B carrier rate in the general population of the countries in these regions is estimated to be as high as 8%. Vaccination against hepatitis B should be considered for stays longer than 3 months and by short-term travelers desiring maximal protection. Travelers should be aware that hepatitis B can be transmitted by unsafe sex and the use of contaminated needles and syringes.

INFLUENZA: Influenza is transmitted from November through March. The flu vaccine is recommended for all travelers older than age 50; all travelers with chronic disease or a weakened immune system; travelers of any age wishing to decrease the risk of this illness; pregnant women after the first trimester.

LEISHMANIASIS: Risk for cutaneous leishmaniasis primarily limited to the Uzbekistan, Kazakhstan, and Turkmenistan. Travelers to these regions should take measures to prevent sand fly bites.

LYME DISEASE: Lyme disease may occur in rural forested areas below 1,500 meters elevation. Travelers are advised to take measures to prevent tick bites during the peak transmission season, March through September. The vaccine available in the United States (Lymerix) does not protect against the strain of Lyme disease found in Europe or Asia.

MALARIA: No malaria is reported in this country at this time.

TICK-BORNE ENCEPHALITIS (TBE): Although the tick vector of tick-borne encephalitis (TBE) is distributed widely in brushy, wooded areas, especially south and east of Lake Balkhash, the chance of contracting TBE is very low. Visitors working or camping in forested areas are those at most risk. Travelers in these areas are advised to take measures to prevent tick bites, especially during the peak transmission season, March through October. The TBE vaccine (available in Canada and Europe), is recommended only for people at significant risk of exposure to tick-bites, e.g., campers and hikers on extended trips, or forestry workers.

- -

TRAVELERS' DIARRHEA: All water supplies are suspect, including municipal tap water, which may be untreated and grossly contaminated. Surface water is often polluted with organic, industrial, and agricultural waste/runoff. All drinking water should preferably be bottled or from a reliable source. A quinolone antibiotic, combined with loperamide (Imodium), is recommended for the treatment of acute diarrhea. Diarrhea not responding to treatment with an antibiotic may be due to a parasitic disease such as giardiasis.

- -

TUBERCULOSIS: Tuberculosis (TB) is a major public health problem in this country. Travelers planning an extended stay should have a pre-departure TB skin test (PPD test) and be retested after leaving this country.

- -

TYPHOID FEVER: Typhoid vaccine is recommended. Because the typhoid vaccines are only 60% to 70% effective, food and drink precautions should continue to be observed.

- -

OTHER DISEASES/HAZARDS: Brucellosis (from unpasteurized dairy products), echinococcosis (dog feces are infective), rabies, rickettsialpox, tick-borne relapsing fever (reported from Kirghizstan, Turkmenistan, and Uzbekistan), typhoid fever, tularemia, tuberculosis, and soil-transmitted and helminthic infections (roundworm, hookworm, and whipworm infections and strongyloidiasis).

Kenya

NAIROBI
★

CAPITAL:
Nairobi
EMBASSY (IN U.S.):
2249 R St., NW
Washington, DC 20008
202-387-6101
Website: www.kenyaembassy.com
GMT:
+3 hours
TELEPHONE COUNTRY CODE:
254
USADIRECT:
None

ENTRY REQUIREMENTS
- **Passport/Visa:** Visa required; airport visas are available.
- **HIV Test:** Not required.
- **Vaccinations:** A yellow fever vaccination certificate is required from all travelers older than 1 year of age arriving from infected areas. However, the CDC recommends yellow fever vaccine for all travelers (from any country) older than 9 months of age who travel outside urban areas.

EMBASSIES/CONSULATES
- **U.S. Embassy:** Mombasa Road, Nairobi. Tel: 254-2-537-800; Fax: 254-2-537-810.
- **Canadian Embassy:** Comcraft House, Haile Selassie Avenue, Nairobi. Tel: 254-2-21-48-04; Fax: 254-2-22-69-87; e-mail: nrobi@dfait-maeci.gc.ca.
- **British High Commission:** Upper Hill Road, Nairobi PO Box 30465-00100 Nairobi; Tel: 254-20-284-4000; Fax: 254-20-284-4033; e-mail: Nairobi-Chancery@fco.gov.uk.

HOSPITALS/DOCTORS
- Nairobi Hospital, Argwings Kodhen Rd; private hospital; most major specialties
- Aga Khan Jubilee Hospital (183 beds); 3rd Parklands Ave., Nairobi; private hospital; most major specialties, including neurosurgery
- Centenary House Hospital, Nairobi; Tel: 2-449-284/449-285/449-286/449-287; e-mail: acheliswest@form-net.com
- Aga Khan Hospital, Vanga Rd, Mombasa; 101-bed general medical/surgical facility with most specialties; Tel: 312-953.
- Aga Khan Hospital, Otieno Oyoo St., Kisumu; Tel: 43516.

Current Advisories and Health Risks

AIDS/HIV: Heterosexual contact is the predominant means of transmission. More than 10% of the general population is HIV infected. HIV prevalence is estimated at up to 85% of the high-risk, sexually active urban population. Unofficial estimates of HIV-infection rates among commercial sex workers in Nairobi and Mombasa have exceeded 90%. All travelers are cautioned against unsafe sex, unsterile medical or dental injections, and blood transfusions.

AFRICAN SLEEPING SICKNESS (TRYPANOSOMIASIS): Sporadic cases are reported, with occasional outbreaks. Disease transmission primarily is restricted to Nyanza Province (with a focus in the Lambwe Valley near Lake Victoria) and Western Province, extending along the Tanzania border into extreme southwestern Rift Valley Province, and the Masai Mara game preserve. Travelers to these areas should take measures to prevent tsetse fly bites.

ALTITUDE SICKNESS (AMS): Climbers ascending Mt. Kilimanjaro and Mt. Kenya are at risk for acute mountain sickness and should consider slow ascent as well as prophylaxis with acetazolamide (Diamox). Immediate descent is the best treatment for moderate to severe AMS.

ANIMAL HAZARDS: Snakes (vipers, cobras, black mambas, puff adders) are primarily found in the large arid regions of northern Kenya. Other animal hazards include centipedes, scorpions, and black widow spiders. Sea cones, sea urchins, and anemones inhabit the shallow coastal waters of Kenya and may pose a threat to swimmers.

CHOLERA: This disease is active in this country. Cholera is an extremely rare disease in travelers from developed countries. Cholera vaccine is recommended primarily for people at high risk (e.g., relief workers) who work and live in highly endemic areas under less than adequate sanitary conditions. Many countries, including Canada, license an oral cholera vaccine. The vaccine is not available in the United States.

DENGUE FEVER: The risk of dengue is considered to be low but outbreaks of disease have been reported in coastal areas. Dengue has been documented in neighboring Somalia.

HEPATITIS: All nonimmune travelers should receive hepatitis A vaccine. The hepatitis B carrier rate in the general population is estimated at 6%. Hepatitis B is spread by infected blood, contaminated needles, and unprotected sex. Vaccination is recommended for long-stay travelers (over 3 months); those who may be at occupational or social risk; anybody desiring maximal protection.

INFLUENZA: Influenza is transmitted year-round in the tropics. Vaccination is recommended for all travelers.

LEISHMANIASIS: Cutaneous leishmaniasis is reported from the highland areas, including the eastern slopes of Mt. Elgon, the Aberdare Range, the Baringo District, and Rift Valley Province. Risk areas for visceral leishmaniasis (kala azar) include Rift Valley Province (Baringo, West Potok, and Turkana districts), Eastern Province (Machakos, Kitue, and Meru districts) and North Eastern Province. All travelers to these areas should take measures to prevent sand fly bites.

MALARIA: Malaria occurs year-round with the highest transmission rates during and just after the semi-annual rainy seasons, March through May and late September through November. Risk is countrywide below 2,500 meters elevation, including urban areas and game parks. There is no risk of malaria in Nairobi and in the highland areas above 2,500 meters elevation (the Aberdare Range, Mt. Kenya, Mt. Elgon).

Primary risk areas include Western Province, Nyanza Province (Lake Victoria Basin), Coast Province (including the Tana River Valley and the coastal areas south of Mombasa and Malindi to the Tanzanian border), and southern Eastern Province. Seasonal malaria occurs in the game parks along the border with Tanzania. Transmission is limited in arid areas of the Rift Valley, northern Eastern, North Eastern, and Coast Provinces. Malaria may occur in the highland areas (above 1,600 meters elevation) during and just after periods of exceptionally heavy rainfall. *Plasomodium falciparum* causes 85% of cases, followed by *Plasmodium malariae* and less frequently by *Plasmodium ovale.* Chloroquine-resistant falciparum malaria is prevalent.

- Prophylaxis with atovaquone/proguanil (Malarone), mefloquine (Lariam), or doxycycline is recommended.
- All travelers should take measures to prevent evening and nighttime mosquito bites.

MENINGITIS: Risk of meningococcal disease is seasonally elevated during June through February in western areas within the sub-Saharan meningitis belt (Western, Nyanza, and western and northern Rift Valley Provinces). Vaccination is recommended for those expecting prolonged, close contact with the indigenous population. There have been no reports of meningitis in travelers.

RABIES: Risk is increasing in urban areas, including Nairobi. Rabies vaccine is recommended for all stays of longer than 3 months; shorter stays at locations more than 24 hours from a reliable source of postexposure rabies vaccine. Consider vaccination for shorter stays in travelers desiring maximal protection. All dog bites or scratches while in this country should be medically evaluated.

RIFT VALLEY FEVER: Cases of this mosquito-transmitted viral illness are reported primarily from the coastal areas of Lake Victoria and the Indian Ocean. The risk to tourists is low.

SCHISTOSOMIASIS: Urinary schistosomiasis is widely distributed, including the areas along the coastal plain and the lower Tana River Valley (Coast Province), in the Taveta region (extreme southwestern Coast Province), in Kitui District (Eastern Province), and bordering Lake Victoria (Nyanza Province). Intestinal schistosomiasis occurs primarily east of Nairobi, in the Taveta region bordering Tanzania, in the Nyanza Province bordering Lake Victoria, and on the islands of Rusinga and Mfangano. Travelers should avoid swimming, wading, or bathing in freshwater lakes, streams, ponds, or irrigation ditches.

TRAVELERS' DIARRHEA: Moderate to high risk aside from deluxe hotels and resorts. The public water supply in Nairobi is considered potable, but bottled water is recommended for consumption. All water sources outside of major hotels and resorts should be considered potentially contaminated. Travelers should observe food and drink safety precautions. A quinolone antibiotic, combined with loperamide (Imodium), is recommended for the treatment of acute diarrhea. Persistent diarrhea may be caused by a parasitic disease such as giardiasis, amebiasis, or cryptosporidiosis.

TUBERCULOSIS: Tuberculosis (TB) is a major public health problem in this country and is related, in part, to the high incidence of AIDS. Travelers planning an extended stay should have a pre-departure TB skin test (PPD test) and be retested after return from this country.

TYPHOID FEVER: Typhoid vaccine is recommended for those traveling off the usual tourist routes, those visiting friends or relatives, and long-stay visitors. Typhoid vaccines are 60% to 70% effective; safe food and drink precautions should continue to be observed.

WEST NILE FEVER: This mosquito-transmitted viral illness is reported from the coastal areas of Lake Victoria and the Indian Ocean. The risk to tourists is very low.

YELLOW FEVER: The first ever outbreak in Kenya occurred in 1992 in three districts in the Rift Valley and occasional sporadic outbreaks have occurred since. Yellow fever vaccination is recommended for anyone older than age 9 months traveling to rural areas.

OTHER DISEASES/HAZARDS: African tick typhus, anthrax, brucellosis, echinococcosis (highest known prevalence in the world occurs in the Turkana population in northwest Kenya), filariasis (mosquito-borne; endemic in the coastal zone and along the Sabaki River), leptospirosis (associated with rodent-infected areas; reportedly widespread around Kisumu and along the coast), onchocerciasis (last remaining focus was located on southwestern slopes of Mt. Elgon), plague (outbreak occurred in 1990 in Nairobi's Embakasi area), toxoplasmosis, syphilis, trachoma, tuberculosis (a major health problem), typhoid fever, and intestinal worms (very common).

Kiribati

★ TARAWA

CAPITAL:
Tarawa

EMBASSY (IN U.S.):
202-638-3800

GMT:
+12 hours

TELEPHONE COUNTRY CODE:
686

USADIRECT:
None

ENTRY REQUIREMENTS
- **Passport/Visa:** Passport is required.
- **HIV Test:** Not required.
- **Vaccinations:** A yellow fever vaccination certificate is required of travelers arriving from infected areas.

EMBASSIES/CONSULATES:
This country consists of 33 atolls and one island scattered over five million square km. Kiribati was formerly the Gilberts of the British Gilbert and Ellice Islands colony.
- **Canadian Embassy:** Accredited to the Consulate General of Canada in Sydney, Australia. Level 5, Quay West, 111 Harrington Street, Sydney, New South Wales 2000, Australia; Tel: 61-2-9364-3000; Fax: 61-2-9364-3098; e-mail: sydny@international.gc.ca.
- **British High Commission Office:** None.

HOSPITALS/DOCTORS:
Medical care is substandard throughout the country including in Tarawa. Adequate evacuation coverage for all travelers is a high priority. In the event of serious medical

conditions, every effort should be made to go to Honolulu. Hospital accommodations are inadequate throughout the country and advanced technology is lacking.

- Tungaru Central Hospital; general medical facility.
- Betio Hospital; general medical facility.

Current Advisories and Health Risks

ACCIDENTS, ILLNESS, AND MEDICAL INSURANCE:

- Accidents and injuries are the leading cause of death among travelers younger than age 55 and are most often caused by motor vehicle and motorcycle crashes; drownings, aircraft crashes, homicides, and burns are less common causes.
- Heart attacks cause most fatalities in older travelers.
- Infections cause only 1% of fatalities in overseas travelers, but, overall, infections are the most common cause of travel-related illness.
- Travelers are advised to obtain, before departure, supplemental travel health insurance with specific overseas coverage. The policy should provide for direct payment to the overseas hospital and/or physician at the time of service and include a medical evacuation benefit. The policy should also provide 24-hour hotline access to a multilingual assistance center that can help arrange and monitor delivery of medical care and determine if medical evacuation or air ambulance services are required.

HEPATITIS: Hepatitis A vaccine is recommended for nonimmune travelers. Vaccination against hepatitis B should be considered for stays longer than 3 months and by short-term travelers desiring maximal protection. Travelers should be aware that hepatitis B can be transmitted by unsafe sex and the use of contaminated needles and syringes.

INFLUENZA: Influenza is transmitted year-round in the tropics. The flu vaccine is recommended for all travelers older than age 50; all travelers with chronic disease or a weakened immune system; travelers of any age wishing to decrease the risk of this illness; pregnant women after the first trimester.

MALARIA: No risk.

MARINE HAZARDS:

- Swimming-related hazards include jellyfish, spiny sea urchins, and coral.
- Ciguatera poisoning is prevalent and can result from eating coral reef fish such as grouper, snapper, sea bass, jack, and barracuda. The ciguatoxin is not destroyed by cooking.

TYPHOID FEVER: Typhoid vaccine is recommended, especially for long-term travelers, adventure travelers, and those wishing maximal disease protection. Because the typhoid vaccines are only 60% to 70% effective, safe food and drink guidelines should be observed.

Kuwait

CAPITAL:

Kuwait City

EMBASSY (IN U.S.):

202-966-0702

GMT:

+3 hours

TELEPHONE COUNTRY CODE:

95

USADIRECT:

None

ENTRY REQUIREMENTS

- **Passport/Visa**: Passport and visa required.
- **HIV Test:** Test required for residency and work permits; U.S. test accepted.
- **Vaccinations:** A yellow fever vaccination certificate is required from travelers arriving from infected areas.

EMBASSIES/CONSULATES

- **U.S. Embassy:** Al-Masjid Al-Aqsa Street, Plot 14, Block 14, Bayan, Safat; Tel: 965-539-5307 or 539-5308; Website: www.usembassy.gov.kw.
- **Canadian Embassy:** 24, Al-Mutawakel Street, Block 4, Da'aiyah, Safat, Kuwait City; Tel: 965-56-3025; Fax: 965-256-0173; e-mail: kwait@dfait-maeci.gc.ca; Website: www.dfait-maeci.gc.ca/kuwait.
- **British Embassy:** Arabian Gulf Street, Postal Address: PO Box 2, Safat 13001, Kuwait, Commercial Section Address: PO Box 300, Safat 13003, Kuwait; Tel: 240-3335; Fax: 965-240-7395; e-mail: britemb@qualitynet.net.

HOSPITALS/DOCTORS

- Medical insurance is essential. Both private and government health services are available.

Current Advisories and Health Risks

ACCIDENTS, ILLNESS, AND MEDICAL INSURANCE

- Accidents and injuries are the leading cause of death among travelers younger than age 55 and are most often caused by motor vehicle and motorcycle crashes; drownings, aircraft crashes, homicides, and burns are less common causes.
- Heart attacks cause most fatalities in older travelers.
- Infections cause only 1% of fatalities in overseas travelers, but, overall, infections are the most common cause of travel-related illness.
- Travelers are advised to obtain, before departure, supplemental travel health insurance with specific overseas coverage. The policy should provide for direct payment to the overseas hospital and/or physician at the time of service and include a medical evacuation benefit. The policy should also provide 24-hour hotline access to a multilingual assistance center that can help arrange and monitor delivery of medical care and determine if medical evacuation or air ambulance services are required.

CHOLERA: This disease is reported active in this country (sporadic cases only), but the threat to tourists is very low. Cholera vaccine is recommended primarily for people at high risk (e.g., relief workers) who work and live in highly endemic areas under less than adequate sanitary conditions.

- The oral cholera vaccine (Dukoral) provides up to 60% crossover protection against ETEC diarrhea.
- Many countries, including Canada, license an oral cholera vaccine. The oral vaccine is not available in the United States.
- Cholera vaccine is not "officially" required for entry into, or exit from, any country. Despite this, some countries, on occasion, require proof of cholera vaccination from travelers coming from cholera-infected countries. Anticipating such a situation, certain travelers may wish to carry a medical exemption letter from their health-care provider. Travel Medicine, Inc., recommends that travelers use the International Certificate of Vaccination (Yellow Card) for this purpose, having their health-care provider affirm that they are "exempt from cholera vaccine" and validate the exemption with both the provider's signature and the appropriate official stamp (the "Uniform Stamp" in the United States).

HEPATITIS: All nonimmune travelers should receive the hepatitis A vaccine. Hepatitis E is endemic, but levels are unclear. The hepatitis B carrier rate is estimated to be 4% of the population. Hepatitis B vaccine is recommended for stays longer than 3 months and for short-term travelers wanting increased protection. Travelers should be aware that the risk of hepatitis B is increased by unsafe sex and the use of unsterile needles and syringes.

INFLUENZA: Influenza is transmitted from November through March. The flu vaccine is recommended for all travelers older than age 50; all travelers with chronic disease or a weakened immune system; travelers of any age wishing to decrease the risk of this illness; pregnant women after the first trimester.

INSECTS: All travelers should take measures to prevent both daytime and nighttime insect bites. Insect-bite prevention measures include a DEET-containing repellent applied to exposed skin, insecticide (permethrin) spray applied to clothing and gear, and use of a permethrin-treated bed net at night while sleeping.

LEISHMANIASIS: Cutaneous and visceral leishmaniasis, transmitted by sand flies, may occur, but levels are unclear. Travelers should take precautions to prevent insect (sand fly) bites.

RABIES: Sporadic cases of human rabies are reported countrywide. All animal bites or scratches, especially from a dog, should be taken seriously, and immediate medical attention sought. Although rabies is rare among tourists, there is risk. No one should pet or pick up any stray animals. All children should be warned to avoid contact with unknown animals.

- Rabies vaccine is recommended for travel longer than 3 months, for shorter stays for travelers who plan to venture off the usual tourist routes where they may be more exposed to the stray dog population, or when travelers desire extra protection.

TRAVELERS' DIARRHEA: Moderate risk outside of first-class hotels. Drinking water outside main towns and cities is likely to be contaminated and sterilization is considered essential. A quinolone antibiotic, combined with loperamide (Imodium), is recommended for the treatment of acute diarrhea.

TUBERCULOSIS: Tuberculosis (TB) is a health problem in this country. Travelers planning an extended stay should have a pre-departure TB skin test (PPD test) and be retested after leaving this country. Travelers should avoid crowded public places and public transportation whenever possible. Domestic help hired by long-stay visitors should be screened for TB.

TYPHOID FEVER: Typhoid vaccine is recommended, especially for long-term travelers, adventure travelers, and those wishing maximal disease protection. Because the typhoid vaccines are only 60% to 70% effective, safe food and drink guidelines should continue to be observed.

Kyrgyzstan

BISHKEK

CAPITAL:
Bishkek
EMBASSY (IN U.S.):
202-338-5141
GMT:
+5 hours
TELEPHONE COUNTRY CODE:
996
USADIRECT:
None
ENTRY REQUIREMENTS
- **Passport/Visa:** Passport and visa required.
- **HIV Test:** HIV testing is required for persons staying longer than 1 month.
- **Vaccinations:** None required.

EMBASSIES/CONSULATES
- **U.S. Embassy:** 171 Prospect Mira, 720016 Bishkek; Tel: 996-312-551-241, Fax: 996-312-551-264.
- **Canadian Embassy:** 189 Moskovskaya Street, Bishkek; Tel: 996-312-65-05-06; Fax: 996-65-01-01; e-mail: canada_honcon@infotel.kg.
- **British Embassy:** Accredited to the British Embassy in Kazakhstan. Ul Furmanova 173, Almaty; Tel: 73272-506191, 506192, 506229; Fax: 73272-506260; e-mail: british-embassy@kaznet.kz.

HOSPITALS/DOCTORS

Due to an unstable economy and other factors, health care in Kyrgyzstan is well below western standards. Shortages of medicines and materials are common, and several sources report that corruption, even extortion, is common, although reform initiatives are underway. Travelers who experience serious health events while traveling in Kyrgyzstan are strongly advised to seek treatment in Western Europe. It is essential, therefore, to purchase adequate evacuation coverage in advance of departure.

Current Advisories and Health Risks

ACCIDENTS, ILLNESS, AND MEDICAL INSURANCE

• Accidents and injuries are the leading cause of death among travelers younger than age 55 and are most often caused by motor vehicle and motorcycle crashes; drownings, aircraft crashes, homicides, and burns are less common causes.

• Heart attacks cause most fatalities in older travelers.

• Infections cause only 1% of fatalities in overseas travelers, but, overall, infections are the most common cause of travel-related illness.

• Travelers are advised to obtain, before departure, supplemental travel health insurance with specific overseas coverage. The policy should provide for direct payment to the overseas hospital and/or physician at the time of service and include a medical evacuation benefit. The policy should also provide 24-hour hotline access to a multilingual assistance center that can help arrange and monitor delivery of medical care and determine if medical evacuation or air ambulance services are required.

ARBOVIRAL DISEASES: Tahjna virus fever (mosquito-borne; virus circulates through much of the former USSR), sand fly fever (sand fly-borne; limited to regions of southern central Asia, April through October), dengue fever (mosquito-borne; no recent cases reported), West Nile fever (mosquito-borne; cases have occurred in the Tadzikstan), North Asian tick fever (occurs wherever tick vectors are found).

CHOLERA: This disease is active in this country. The risk of cholera, however, is extremely low in international travelers from developed countries. Cholera vaccine is recommended only for travelers at high risk who work and live in highly endemic areas under less than adequate sanitary conditions.

• The manufacture and availability of cholera vaccine in the United States ceased in June 2000. Many countries, including Canada, license an oral cholera vaccine.

• Cholera vaccine is not "officially" required for entry into, or exit from, any country.

CRIMEAN-CONGO HEMORRHAGIC FEVER: Also known as central Asian hemorrhagic fever. Risk areas are rural steppe, savannah, semi-desert, and foothill/low mountain habitats below 2,000 meters elevation. Outbreaks occurred in south central Kazakhstan during 1989.

FOOD AND WATER SAFETY: The water in Kyrgyzstan has a high metal content. Milk is pasteurized and dairy products are safe for consumption. Travelers should eat only well-cooked meat and fish, preferably served hot. Pork, salad, and mayonnaise may carry increased risk. Vegetables should be cooked and fruit peeled.

HEPATITIS: All nonimmune travelers should receive hepatitis A vaccine before visiting these regions. The hepatitis B carrier rate in the general population of the countries in these regions is estimated as high as 8%. Vaccination against hepatitis B should be considered for stays longer than 3 months and by short-term travelers desiring maximal protection. Travelers should be aware that hepatitis B can be transmitted by unsafe sex and the use of contaminated needles and syringes.

INFLUENZA: Influenza is transmitted from November through March. The flu vaccine is recommended for all travelers older than age 50; all travelers with chronic disease or a weakened immune system; travelers of any age wishing to decrease the risk of this illness; pregnant women after the first trimester.

LYME DISEASE: May occur in rural forested areas below 1,500 meters elevation.

MALARIA: Limited foci of vivax malaria exist in Kazakhstan and Uzbekistan. Tajikstan has reported an increase in malaria following the civil war (1992 to 1996), with *Plasmodium vivax* identified in 84% of cases and *Plasmodium falciparum* in 16% of cases. Most cases of malaria in Tajikstan are reported from the region of Khatlon Oblast. Information on chloroquine resistance is not available.

TICK-BORNE ENCEPHALITIS (TBE): Peak transmission period is April through June. Risk is present primarily in rural brushy and forested areas below 1,500 meters elevation. TBE is usually known as "Central European tick-borne encephalitis" or "Russian spring-summer encephalitis" west of the Urals.

TRAVELERS' DIARRHEA: All water supplies are suspect, including municipal tap water, which may be untreated and grossly contaminated. A quinolone antibiotic, combined with loperamide (Imodium), is recommended for the treatment of acute diarrhea. Diarrhea not responding to treatment with an antibiotic may be due to a parasitic disease such as giardiasis.

TUBERCULOSIS: Tuberculosis (TB) is a major public health problem in this country. Travelers planning an extended stay should have a pre-departure TB skin test (PPD test) and be retested after leaving this country.

TYPHOID FEVER: Typhoid vaccine is recommended. Because the typhoid vaccines are only 60% to 70% effective, food and drink precautions should continue to be observed.

OTHER DISEASES/HAZARDS: Brucellosis (from unpasteurized dairy products), echinococcosis (dog feces are infective), rabies, rickettsialpox, tick-borne relapsing fever (reported from Kirghizstan, Turkmenistan, and Uzbekistan), typhoid fever, tularemia, tuberculosis, and soil-transmitted and helminthic infections (roundworm, hookworm, and whipworm infections and strongyloidiasis).

Laos

CAPITAL:
Vientiane
EMBASSY (IN U.S.):
202-332-6416
GMT:
+7 hours
TELEPHONE COUNTRY CODE:
856
USADIRECT:
None
ENTRY REQUIREMENTS*
- **Passport/Visa:** A visa, good for 30 days, is required.
- **HIV Test:** Not required.
- **Vaccinations:** A yellow fever vaccination certificate is required from all travelers arriving from infected areas.

EMBASSIES/CONSULATES
- **U.S. Embassy:** Thanon Bartholonie (aka Rue Bartholonie, near Tat Dam), Vientiane; Tel: 856-21-212-581, 212-582, 212-585; Fax: 856-21-512-584; Website: usembassy. state.gov/laos
- **Canadian Embassy:** Accredited to the Australian Embassy. J Nehru Street, Phone Xay, Vientiane, Laos; Postal Address: PO Box 292, Vientiane, Laos; Tel: 856-21-413-600; Fax: 856-21-413-601.
- **British Embassy:** Accredited to the British Embassy in Thailand. Wireless Road, Bangkok, 10330; Tel: 66-2-305-8333; Fax: 66-2-305-8372, 8380; Website: www.britishemb.or.th.

HOSPITALS/DOCTORS:
Medical care in Laos is below Western standards. Those with a serious medical problem should seek evacuation to Bangkok or Singapore. Travelers are advised to obtain, before departure, supplemental travel health insurance with specific overseas coverage. The policy should provide for direct payment to the overseas hospital and/or physician at the time of service and include a medical evacuation benefit.
- Mahosot Hospital, Vientiane (220 beds); capabilities well below Western standards.
- Clinique Diplomatique, Pakse Provincial Hospital (160 beds); capabilities well below Western standards.

Current Advisories and Health Risks

AIDS/HIV: AIDS is endemic, but levels are below those of the surrounding countries, due in part to the geopolitical isolation of Laos.

ANIMAL HAZARDS: Animal hazards include snakes (cobras, vipers), spiders (black and brown widow), tigers, leopards, and large leeches.

CHOLERA: This disease is reported active in this country, but the threat to tourists is very low. Cholera vaccine is recommended primarily for people at high risk (e.g., relief workers) who work and live in highly endemic areas under less than adequate sanitary conditions.

DENGUE FEVER: Risk is countrywide, year-round, but may be elevated in urban areas, especially during the warmer and wetter months, usually May through October. The mosquitoes that transmit dengue fever are more active during the daytime and are present in populous urban areas as well as rural areas. Prevention of dengue consists of taking measures to prevent daytime mosquito bites.

FILARIASIS: Both the Bancroftian and Malayan varieties are highly endemic in rural and urban areas. Travelers should take personal protection measures against mosquito bites.

HELMINTHIC INFECTIONS (FLUKES AND WORMS): Oriental lung fluke disease (paragonimiasis) and liver fluke diseases (clonorchiasis, opisthorchiasis, fascioliasis) are prevalent. Travelers should avoid eating raw freshwater fish; raw, salted, or wine-soaked crustacea (freshwater crabs or crayfish); or undercooked water vegetables and plants, especially watercress. Soil-transmitted infections (caused by hookworms, roundworms, whipworms, strongyloides) are highly prevalent in most rural areas. Travelers should wear shoes (to prevent the hookworm and strongyloides larvae from penetrating the skin) and food should be thoroughly washed/cooked (to destroy roundworm and whipworm eggs).

HEPATITIS: All nonimmune travelers should receive hepatitis A vaccine. Hepatitis E has not been reported, but is likely. The hepatitis B carrier rate in the general population is estimated to exceed 10%. Hepatitis B is spread by infected blood, contaminated needles, and unsafe sex. Vaccination is recommended for stays longer than 3 months; for anyone at occupational or social risk; for any traveler desiring maximal protection. The risk of illness or injury during travel cannot be predicted and some experts believe that *all* travelers should be immunized against hepatitis B because of the risk of receiving a medical injection with an unsterile needle or syringe.

INFLUENZA: Influenza is transmitted year-round in the tropics. The flu vaccine is recommended for all travelers.

INSECTS: All travelers should take measures to prevent both daytime and nighttime insect bites. Insect-bite prevention measures include a DEET-containing repellent applied to exposed skin, insecticide (permethrin) spray applied to clothing and gear, and use of a permethrin-treated bed net at night while sleeping.

JAPANESE ENCEPHALITIS (JE): Risk is elevated in rural and peri-urban areas, especially where mosquito-breeding sites and pig farming coexist. Sporadic cases occur throughout the year, but disease transmission is higher during the warmer and wetter months (usually May through October). Vaccination is recommended for travelers planning an extended stay (more than 3 to 4 weeks) in rural-agricultural areas during the peak transmission season. All travelers should take measures to prevent mosquito bites.

MALARIA: Risk is present countrywide, but is more prevalent in mountainous and rural areas than in the lowland plains or urban areas. There is no risk of malaria in Vientiane. Multidrug-resistant falciparum malaria is reported, especially near the border with Thailand. Prophylaxis with atovaquone/proguanil (Malarone), mefloquine (Lariam), or doxycycline is recommended.

PLANT HAZARDS: Bamboo, rattan, and large palm- or fern-like trees, which can cause serious puncture wounds and slow-healing lacerations, are widespread in the forested areas of the country. Regas are large forest trees whose black resinous sap can cause a potent poison ivy-type skin reaction. Stinging nettles, small thorny trees, and many species of euphorbs can also cause skin reactions.

RABIES: Sporadic cases of human rabies are reported countrywide. All animal bites or scratches, especially from a dog, should be evaluated medically. Rabies vaccine is recommended for travel longer than 3 months, for shorter stays for travelers who plan to venture off the usual tourist routes where they may be more exposed to the stray dog population, or when travelers desire extra protection.

ROAD SAFETY: Travelers planning travel outside urban centers by road or river should contact the U.S. Embassy for current security information.

SCHISTOSOMIASIS: Risk is present year-round. Focal distribution occurs along the Mekong River (including Vientiane), and in the Louangphrabang and Champasak provinces. Travelers should avoid swimming, bathing, or wading in freshwater rivers, lakes, ponds, or streams.

TRAVELERS' DIARRHEA: Piped water supplies countrywide are frequently untreated and may be grossly contaminated. Travelers should observe all food and drink safety precautions. A quinolone antibiotic, combined with loperamide (Imodium), is recommended for the treatment of acute diarrhea. Persistent diarrhea may be due to a parasitic infection such as giardiasis, amebiasis, or cryptosporidiosis.

TUBERCULOSIS: Tuberculosis (TB) is a major health problem in this country. Travelers planning an extended stay should have a pre-departure TB skin test (PPD test) and be retested after returning from this country.

TYPHOID FEVER: Typhoid vaccine is recommended for those traveling off the usual tourist routes, those visiting friends or relatives, and for long-stay visitors. Because the typhoid vaccines are only 60% to 70% effective, safe food and drink selection remains important.

OTHER DISEASES/HAZARDS: Brucellosis (often transmitted by the consumption of unpasteurized dairy products), cholera (endemic; outbreaks occur frequently), echinococcosis, leprosy (highly endemic), leptospirosis, melioidosis, plague, rabies (enzootic at high levels), scrub typhus (mite-borne), and tuberculosis (highly endemic) are reported.

Latvia

RIGA

CAPITAL:
Riga
EMBASSY (IN U.S.):
202-726-8213
GMT:
+2 hours
TELEPHONE COUNTRY CODE:
371
USADIRECT:
800-2288

ENTRY REQUIREMENTS

- **Passport/Visa:** Latvian entry requirements for U.S. citizens: Passport valid for at least 6 months. No visa if remaining up to 90 days in a 1-year period. Any traveler going to Russia, even in transit, will require Russian visa before entry into Latvia. Travelers planning to remain for more than 90 days must apply in-country for temporary residence. Contact the Latvian Embassy 4325 17th St., NW., Washington, DC. 20011; Tel: 202-726-8213. Within Latvia, contact the Ministry of Interior's Citizenship & Immigration Department at Raina Bulvaris 5, Riga LV-1508, 371-721-9424 or 371-721-9427; fax 371-782-0306.
- **HIV Test:** Test required for persons seeking residency permits; U.S. tests results accepted.
- **Vaccinations:** None required.

EMBASSIES/CONSULATES

- **U.S. Embassy:** Raina Boulevard 7, Riga; Tel: 371-703-6200; Fax: 371-782-0047; Website: www.usis.bkc.lv/embassy.
- **Canadian Embassy:** Doma Iaukums 4, 4th Floor; Riga; Tel: 371-783-0141; Fax: 371-783-0140; e-mail: riga@dfait-maeci.gc.ca.
- **British Embassy:** 5 J Alunana Iela, Riga, LV 1010; Tel: 371-777-4700; Fax: 371-777-4707; e-mail: british.embassy@apollo.lv; Website: www.britain.lv.

HOSPITALS/DOCTORS:

Diptheria, hepatitis, and tick-borne encephalitis are widespread. According to the World Health Organization, tuberculosis is a significant problem in Latvia, with 9% of all cases being multidrug resistant. State ambulance service for emergencies is available by dialing 03 anywhere in Latvia. However, quick response is poor in rural areas. Air ambulance service is available for medical evacuations.

- The dental surgery at Stabu iela 9 has an emergency service from 0200-0800 and the reception of the City Clinical Hospital No. 1 at Bruninieku iela 8 is open 24 hours. Health insurance is advised. A full range of medicines is available at pharmacies; however it is advisable to bring any medicines necessary because instructions on the packet are in Latvian, and familiar brands may not be available.

Current Advisories and Health Risks

ACCIDENTS, ILLNESS, AND MEDICAL INSURANCE: Accidents and injuries are the leading cause of death among travelers under the age of 55 and are most often caused by motor vehicle and motorcycle crashes; drownings, aircraft crashes, homicides, and burns are less common causes. Important safety rules to follow are (1) Do not drive at night; (2) Do not rent a motorcycle, moped, bicycle, or motorbike, even if you are experienced; and (3) Don't swim alone, at night, or if intoxicated.

• Heart attacks cause most fatalities in older travelers.

• Infections cause only 1% of fatalities in overseas travelers, but, overall, infections are the most common cause of travel-related illness.

• Travelers are advised to obtain, before departure, supplemental travel health insurance with specific overseas coverage. The policy should provide for direct payment to the overseas hospital and/or physician at the time of service and include a medical evacuation benefit. The policy should also provide 24-hour hotline access to a multilingual assistance center that can help arrange and monitor delivery of medical care and determine if medical evacuation or air ambulance services are required.

AIDS/HIV: Increased cases of AIDS and HIV have been reported in eastern Europe. Infected blood and contaminated needles and syringes are important sources of infection in these countries. Travelers should consider carrying sterile needles and syringes and should avoid, if possible, blood transfusions and medical injections.

DIPHTHERIA: All travelers, especially adults, should be fully immunized against diphtheria.

HEPATITIS: All nonimmune travelers should receive hepatitis A vaccine. The hepatitis B carrier rate is estimated at 4%. Vaccination against hepatitis B should be considered for stays longer than 3 months and by short-term travelers desiring maximal protection. Travelers should be aware that hepatitis B can be transmitted by unsafe sex and the use of contaminated needles and syringes.

INFLUENZA: Influenza is transmitted from November to March. The flu vaccine is recommended for all travelers over age 50; all travelers with any chronic disease or weakened immune system; travelers of any age wishing to decrease the risk of this illness; pregnant women after the first trimester.

LYME DISEASE: Lyme borreliosis presents a risk to travelers throughout the country through the warmer months. Tick-bite precautions are recommended.

MALARIA: There is no risk of malaria in western or eastern Europe.

RABIES: Occurs primarily in wild animals, especially foxes, in many rural areas of Europe. Human cases are infrequent. Any animal bite should be immediately evaluated.

ROAD SAFETY: Highways are slowly being upgraded after years of little or no maintenance, but are treacherous to the unwary. The speed limit in towns is 50 km/hour and 90 km/hour on open roads, unless otherwise marked. Legal alcohol limit for drivers is zero and speed traps are common. U.S. driver's licenses are not valid in Latvia, so travelers should obtain valid international driver's license issued through AAA. After 90 days, Americans in the country must apply for a Latvian license. Contact Latvian Traffic Safety Administration (CSDD), Bauskas Iela 68, Riga LV-1004, 371-627-437.

TICK-BORNE ENCEPHALITIS (TBE): The tick vector for TBE is widely distributed in brushy and forested areas at elevations up to 1,500 meters, especially around Jelgava (both town and region), Ventspils, Limbazi, and Riga regions. Infections can occur in parks within Riga. Risk exists only between April and October. Visitors working or camping in these areas are those most at risk and are advised to take measures to prevent tick bites, especially during the peak transmission season. The TBE vaccine (available in Canada and Europe), is recommended for people at significant risk of exposure to tick bites, for example, campers and hikers on extended trips, or forestry workers.

TRAVELERS' DIARRHEA: Low risk in most western European countries. Higher risk occurs in the Balkans and eastern Europe. Travelers to Latvia should drink only bottled, boiled, or treated water and avoid undercooked food. A quinolone antibiotic, combined with loperamide (Imodium), is recommended for the treatment of diarrhea.

TUBERCULOSIS: Tuberculosis (TB) is a major public health problem in this country. Travelers planning an extended stay should have a pre-departure TB skin test (PPD test) and be retested after leaving this country.

TYPHOID FEVER: Typhoid vaccine is recommended, especially for long-term travelers, adventure travelers, and those wishing maximal disease protection. Because the typhoid vaccines are only 60% to 70% effective, safe food and drink guidelines should continue to be observed.

OTHER DISEASES/HAZARDS: Raw cod ("lutefish") and other fish may contain the fish tapeworm. Travelers should avoid undercooked or raw fish.

Lebanon

CAPITAL:
Beirut
EMBASSY (IN U.S.):
202-939-6300
GMT:
+2 hours
TELEPHONE COUNTRY CODE:
961

USADIRECT:
426-801 to place calls within Beirut; 01-426-801 to place calls outside of Beirut

ENTRY REQUIREMENTS

- **Passport/Visa:** Required. U.S. citizens staying no longer than 1 month (extendible up to 3 months) can obtain their visa on arrival in Lebanon (no fee). For longer stays, visa must be obtained from the Lebanese Embassy or Consulate. Business visa requires company letter stating purpose of travel. Minors need authorization from both parents (a notarized parental consent form/letter) to enter Lebanon. Note: All visa applicants holding an Israeli visa on their passport at the time of applying for visa or arrival in Lebanon will not be granted a visa and/or be admitted to Lebanon without the prior approval of the Lebanese Immigration Authorities. For further visa information, contact the Embassy of Lebanon , 2560 28th St., NW, Washington, DC 20008 202-939-6300.
- **HIV Test:** Required for those seeking residence permits; U.S. test is accepted.
- **Vaccination:** A yellow fever vaccination certificate is required from travelers arriving from infected areas.

EMBASSIES/CONSULATES

- **U.S. Embassy:** Antelias, Beirut; Tel: 961-4-542-600, 543-600, 544-310, 544-130, 544-140; Fax: 961-4-544-209; Website: www.usembassy.com.lb.
- **Canadian Embassy:** 43 Jal El Dib Highway (sea side), 1st Floor, Coolrite Building, Jal El Dib, Beirut; Tel: 961-4-713-900; Fax: 961-4-710-595; e-mail: berut@dfait-maeci. gc.ca, Website: www.canadianembassy-lb.org.
- **British Embassy:** Serail Hill, Beirut Centre-Ville, PO Box 11-471 Beirut; Tel: 961-1-990400; Fax: 961-1-990420; e-mail: britemb@cyberia.net.lb; Website: www.britishembassy.org.lb.

HOSPITALS/DOCTORS:

The majority of hospitals in the region are private and require proof of the patient's ability to pay before providing treatment (even in emergency cases). The two best hospitals in the country are the Hôtel Dieu in Achrafieh, Beirut and the American University/AUB Hospital in Hamra, Beirut.

- American University of Beirut Medical Center, Riad El-Solh, Beirut; 420-bed multi-specialty hospital that is the main health-care center for Lebanon; Riad El-Solh, Beirut; Tel: 1-345325

Current Advisories and Health Risks

See Disease Risk Summary for the Middle East on page 310.

Lesotho

★ MASERU

CAPITAL:
Maseru

EMBASSY (IN U.S.):
202-797-5533

GMT:
+2 hours
TELEPHONE COUNTRY CODE:
266
USADIRECT:
None
ENTRY REQUIREMENTS
- **Passport/Visa:** Travelers should possess valid passport. Visa not required.
- **HIV Test:** Not required.
- **Vaccinations:** A yellow fever vaccination certificate is required from all travelers older than 1 year arriving from infected areas.

EMBASSIES/CONSULATES
- **U.S. Embassy:** Maseru; Tel: 312-666/7
- **Canadian Embassy** (South Africa): Tel: 27-287-062
- **British High Commission:** Accredited to the British High Commission in South Africa. 255 Hill Street, Arcadia 0002, Pretoria; Tel: 27-12-421-7500; Fax: 27-12-421-7555; e-mail: bhc@icon.co.za; Website: http://www.britain.org.za.

HOSPITALS/DOCTORS:
In Lesotho's villages very basic healthcare is provided by volunteer community health workers. Larger clinics/health centers in rural areas are staffed by teams of doctors, nurses, and other workers, but a single clinic may be responsible for serving anywhere from 6,000 to 10,000 individuals, so overcrowding and shortages are not uncommon. The best available care is through the district hospitals at Mokhotlong, Berea and Qacha's Nek, and through Maseru Private Hospital at Thetsane, a modern facility established in 1996 that includes a 24-hour casualty and emergency unit. Despite reports that healthcare overall has improved measurably in Lesotho over the last decade, it is still advised that travelers who experience serious health events seek treatment in Johannesburg, South Africa.

Current Advisories and Health Risks

HEPATITIS: All susceptible travelers should receive immune globulin prophylaxis or hepatitis A vaccine. The hepatitis B carrier rate in the general population is estimated at 8%. Vaccination against hepatitis B is recommended for health-care workers and all long-term visitors to this country.

MALARIA: Transmission of malaria reportedly does not occur in Lesotho. Risk areas in surrounding South Africa are north of this region.

SCHISTOSOMIASIS: No infected areas are reported in Lesotho. Both urinary and intestinal schistosomiasis, however, occur in eastern and northern regions of the neighboring Natal Province of South Africa.

TRAVELERS' DIARRHEA: Travelers should observe all food and drink safety precautions. A quinolone antibiotic (Cipro or Floxin) is recommended for the treatment of acute diarrhea. Diarrhea not responding to treatment with an antibiotic, or chronic diarrhea, may be due to a parasitic disease such as giardiasis or amebiasis, and treatment with metronidazole (Flagyl) or tinidazole (Fasigyn) should be considered. All cases of diarrhea should be treated with adequate fluid replacement.

OTHER DISEASES/HAZARDS: AIDS (low incidence; HIV prevalence estimated at less than 1%), African tick typhus (contracted from dog ticks—often in urban areas and from bush ticks), brucellosis, tuberculosis (a major health problem), typhoid fever, and intestinal worms (uncommon).

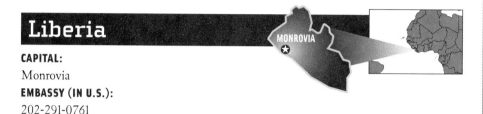

Liberia

CAPITAL:
Monrovia
EMBASSY (IN U.S.):
202-291-0761
GMT:
+0 hours
TELEPHONE COUNTRY CODE:
231
USADIRECT:
None

ENTRY REQUIREMENTS

- **Passport/Visa:** Passport, visa, and evidence of a yellow fever vaccination required. Travelers must obtain visas before arrival. There is a $40 U.S. airport tax on departing passengers. Obtain exit permit from immigration authorities on arrival; one photo required. For specific requirements, call the Embassy of the Republic of Liberia , 5201 16th St., NW, Washington, DC 20011; 202-723-0437; Website: www.liberiaemb.org.
- **HIV Test:** Not required.
- **Vaccinations:** A yellow fever vaccination certificate is required from all travelers older than 1 year arriving from all countries.

EMBASSIES/CONSULATES

- **U.S. Embassy:** Monrovia. 111 United Nations Drive; Tel: 222-991/2/3/4.
- **Canadian Consulate:** Monrovia. EXCHEM Compound; Tel: 223-903.
- **Canadian Embassy:** Accredited to the Canadian Embassy in Côte d'Ivoire. Immeuble Trade Center, 23, avenue Noguès, Le Plateau, Abidjan, Côte d'Ivoire; Postal Address: PO Box 4104, Abidjan 01, Côte d'Ivoire; Tel: 225-20-30-07-00; Fax: 225-20-30-07-20; e-mail: abdjn@international.gc.ca; Website: www.dfait-maeci.gc.ca/abidjan.
- **British High Commission:** Accredited to the British Embassy in Sierra Leone. Spur Road, Freetown; Tel: 232-22-232961, 232362, 232563-5; Fax: 232-22-228169, 232070; e-mail: bhc@sierratel.sl.

HOSPITALS/DOCTORS

- Medical care in Liberia is in a state of near collapse. Travelers are advised to obtain supplemental travel health insurance that includes a medical evacuation benefit.

- ELWA Mission Hospital, Monrovia (45 beds); 24-hour emergency services.
- JFK Memorial Hospital, Monrovia (337 beds); general medical/surgical facility.
- Firestone Plantation Hospital, Monrovia (200 beds); general medical/surgical facility; emergency services.
- Travelers should contact the U.S. Embassy for physician referrals.

Current Advisories and Health Risks

IMMUNIZATIONS: All travelers should be up to date on their routine immunizations: tetanus-diphtheria (Td), measles-mumps-rubella (MMR), polio, influenza, and varicella (chickenpox). Immunizations against hepatitis A, hepatitis B, meningitis, rabies, and typhoid fever are recommended.

MALARIA: All travelers to Liberia including infants, children, and former residents of this country should take one of the following antimalarial drugs: atovaquone/proguanil, doxycycline, mefloquine, or (in special circumstances) primaquine. Travelers should also take measures to prevent evening and nighttime mosquito bites. Insect-bite prevention measures include a DEET-containing repellent applied to exposed skin, insecticide (permethrin) spray applied to clothing, and use of a permethrin-treated bed net at night.

For additional information, consult the Disease Risk Summary for sub-Saharan Africa on page 307.

Libya

TRIPOLI

CAPITAL:
Tripoli
EMBASSY (IN U.S.):
The United States does not maintain an embassy in Libya.
GMT:
+1 hour
TELEPHONE COUNTRY CODE:
218
USADIRECT:
None
ENTRY REQUIREMENTS*
- **Passport/Visa:** Since December 1981, U.S. passports have not been valid for travel into, or through Libya without authorization from the Department of State. Application for exemptions to this restriction should be submitted in writing to Passport Services, U.S. Department of State, 1111 19th St., NW, Washington, DC 20524, Attn: CA/PPT/PAS. Application and inquiries for visas must be made through a country that maintains diplomatic relations with Libya. *Attention:* U.S. citizens need a U.S. Treasury Dept. license in order to engage in any transactions related to travel to and within Libya. *Before planning any travel to Libya, U.S. citizens should contact the*

Licensing Division, Office of Foreign Assets Control, U.S. Department of Treasury (202-622-2480) or www.treas.gov/ofac.

- **HIV Test:** Testing is required for those seeking residence permits.
- **Vaccinations:** A yellow fever vaccination certificate is required for all travelers older than one year arriving from infected areas.

*Travelers should check with this country's embassy (or a consulate) in the United States, Canada, or the United Kingdom for any changes in these requirements.

EMBASSIES/CONSULATES

The United States does not maintain an embassy in Libya.

- **Canadian Embassy:** Great Al-Fateh Tower Building, Tower 1, 7th Floor, Tripoli, Libya; Postal Address: PO Box 93392, Al-Fateh Tower Post Office, Tripoli, Libya; Tel.: 218-21-335-1633; Fax: 218-21-335-1630; e-mail: trpli@international.gc.ca; Website: www.libya.gc.ca.
- **British Embassy:** PO Box 4206; Tripoli; Tel: 218-21-340-3644/5; Fax: 218-21-340-3648.

HOSPITALS/DOCTORS:

Medical care in Libya is below Western standards. Travelers are advised to obtain, before departure, supplemental travel health insurance with specific overseas coverage. The policy should provide for direct payment to the overseas hospital and/or physician at the time of service and include a medical evacuation benefit.

- Medilink International operates an emergency care and family practice clinic in Tripoli for expatriates and for visitors to the country. The emergency clinic is located in Ghirgharesh, Tripoli, close to the main expatriate compounds. Membership plans are available. The Clinic also arranges referrals for hospital care in Tripoli; Tel: 218-213400571.
- Tripoli Central Hospital (1,200 beds); general medical/surgical facility; emergency services; ICU.
- Central Hospital (Benghazi); general medical/surgical facility.

Current Advisories and Health Risks

ACCIDENTS AND ILLNESS: Motor vehicle accidents, injuries and drownings are the leading cause of death among travelers under the age of 55. Cardiovascular disease causes most fatalities in older travelers. Infections cause less than 1% of fatalities in overseas travelers, but, overall, are the most common cause of travel-related illness.

HEPATITIS: Hepatitis A vaccine is recommended for all travelers. Hepatitis E is reported, but the levels are unclear. The hepatitis B carrier rate in the general population is estimated at 5%. Vaccination is recommended for stays longer than 3 months; for anyone at occupational or social risk; for any traveler desiring maximal protection. The risk of illness or injury during travel cannot be predicted and *all* travelers should consider hepatitis B vaccine because of the risk of receiving a medical injection with an unsterile needle or syringe.

LEISHMANIASIS: Low risk of cutaneous leishmaniasis is present. Sporadic cases have been reported from rural villages in the northwest, in the semiarid area extending from

Tripoli to the Tunisian border, and from the coast to the plateau of the Jebel Nefusa. No cases have been reported from Tripoli. Visceral leishmaniasis (kala-azar) has been reported from the Benghazi region and the northeastern coastal areas. Visceral leishmaniasis tends to be associated with settlements, with dogs as the primary reservoir. Travelers to these regions should take measures to prevent sand fly bites.

MALARIA: Very low to absent risk of malaria is present from February to August in the valleys and isolated oases in the southwest (Fezzan). There is no malaria risk in urban areas.

RABIES: Animal rabies occurs throughout this country. Foxes, jackals, and hyenas are the principal animal reservoirs.

SAND FLY FEVER: Potential risk is present. Transmission occurs primarily April through October throughout the coastal regions. Travelers to these regions should take measures to prevent insect (sand fly) bites.

SCHISTOSOMIASIS: Risk is present in widespread areas of the southwest, including valleys in the central Fezzan and the Ghat district on the Algerian border. Transmission also occurs in Darnah on the northeastern coast. Cases also reported from Taourga, an oasis located 240 km east of Tripoli. Travelers should avoid swimming or wading in freshwater lakes, irrigation systems, ponds, or streams.

TRAVELERS' DIARRHEA: Moderate to high risk outside of hotels and resorts. Travelers are advised to drink only bottled, boiled, filtered, or treated water and consume only well-cooked food. A quinolone antibiotic is recommended for the treatment of acute diarrhea. Persistent diarrhea may be due to a parasitic infection such as giardiasis, amebiasis, or cryptosporidiosis.

TUBERCULOSIS: Tuberculosis (TB) is a health problem in this country. Travelers planning an extended stay should have a pre-departure TB skin test (PPD test) and be retested after returning from this country.

TYPHOID FEVER: Typhoid vaccine is recommended for those traveling off the usual tourist routes, those visiting friends or relatives, and for long-stay visitors. Because the typhoid vaccines are only 60% to 70% effective, safe food and drink selection remains important.

OTHER DISEASES/HAZARDS: Boutonneuse fever (occurs primarily in coastal areas; contracted from dog ticks, often in suburban areas), brucellosis (risk from raw goat/sheep milk and cheese), echinococcosis (10% of the children in Benghazi are infected), relapsing fever (tick-borne and louse-borne), toxoplasmosis (infection rates as high as 50%), tuberculosis, typhus, and helminthic infections (roundworm, hookworm disease).

Lithuania

CAPITAL:

Vilnius

EMBASSY (IN U.S.):

202-234-5860

GMT:

+2 hours

TELEPHONE COUNTRY CODE:

370

USADIRECT:

8^800-900-28; ^ indicates second dial tone.

ENTRY REQUIREMENTS

- **Passport/Visa:** U.S. citizens: Passport required. No visa for most stays of 90 days or less.
- **HIV Test:** Required for applicants for permanent residence permits.
- **Vaccinations:** None required.

EMBASSIES/CONSULATES

- **U.S. Embassy:** Akmenu 6, Vilnius; Tel: 370-2-223-031.
- **Canadian Embassy:** Gedimino pr. 64, Vilnius; Tel: 370-2-220-898 and 220-865; Fax: 370-2-22-0884; e-mail: canvno@aiva.lt.
- **British Embassy:** Antakalnio 2, LT-10308 Vilnius; Tel: 370-5-246-2900; Fax: 370-5-246-2901; Website: www.britain.lt.

HOSPITALS/DOCTORS:

Medical facilities are slowly improving. Elderly travelers, those with existing health problems, or those with an emergency medical condition may be at risk because medical facilities do not always meet U.S. standards. Most medical supplies are now widely available, including disposable needles, anesthetics and antibiotics, and other pharmaceuticals. Doctors and hospitals often expect immediate cash payment. U.S. medical insurance is not always valid outside the United States. Supplemental medical insurance with specific overseas coverage, including medical evacuation coverage, is advised.

Current Advisories and Health Risks

ACCIDENTS/ILLNESSES AND MEDICAL INSURANCE

- Accidents and injuries are the leading cause of death among travelers younger than 55 years of age and most often are caused by motor vehicle and motorcycle crashes; drownings, aircraft crashes, homicides, and burns are less common causes. Important safety rules to follow are (1) do not drive at night, (2) do not rent a motorcycle, moped, bicycle, or motorbike, even if you are experienced, and (3) do not swim alone, at night, or if intoxicated.
- Heart attacks cause most fatalities in older travelers.
- Infections cause only 1% of fatalities in overseas travelers, but overall, infections are the most common cause of travel-related illness.

- Travelers are advised to obtain, before departure, supplemental travel health insurance with specific overseas coverage. The policy should provide for direct payment to the overseas hospital and/or physician at the time of service and include a medical evacuation benefit. The policy should also provide 24-hour hotline access to a multilingual assistance center that can help arrange and monitor delivery of medical care and determine if medical evacuation or air ambulance services are required.

AIDS/HIV: Increased cases are reported, especially from Eastern Europe. Travelers should be aware that HIV can be transmitted by unsafe sex and the use of contaminated needles and syringes.

DIPHTHERIA: There is risk of diphtheria. All travelers to the Balkans, including adults, should be fully immunized against diphtheria.

HEPATITIS: All nonimmune travelers should receive hepatitis A vaccine. The hepatitis B carrier rate is estimated at 4%. Vaccination against hepatitis B should be considered for stays longer than 3 months and by short-term travelers desiring maximum protection. Travelers should be aware that hepatitis B can be transmitted by unsafe sex and the use of contaminated needles and syringes.

LYME DISEASE: Risk of transmission exists, especially in forested areas. The ticks that transmit Lyme disease are most abundant and active April through September. The Lyme disease vaccine previously available in the United States is not effective against European strains of *Borrelia*.

RABIES: Occurs primarily in wild animals, especially foxes, in many rural areas of Europe. All animal bites should be medically evaluated.

ROAD SAFETY: Roads range from 2- to 6-lane highways connecting major cities to small dirt roads. Lanes are not always clearly marked; lighting often is poor. Be alert to visible and hidden dangers. Winter driving is especially hazardous because roads are rarely plowed.

TRAVELERS' DIARRHEA: Low to moderate risk. Tap water should be avoided. A quinolone antibiotic, combined with loperamide (Imodium), is recommended for the treatment of diarrhea.

TUBERCULOSIS: Tuberculosis (TB) is a major public health problem in this country. Travelers planning an extended stay should have a pre-departure TB skin test (PPD test) and be retested after leaving this country.

TYPHOID FEVER: Typhoid vaccine is recommended, especially for long-term travelers, adventure travelers, and those wishing maximum disease protection. Because the typhoid vaccines are only 60% to 70% effective, safe food and drink guidelines should continue to be observed.

OTHER DISEASES/HAZARDS: Raw cod ("lutefish") in the Balkans may contain the fish tapeworm. Travelers are advised to avoid raw or undercooked fish.

Luxembourg

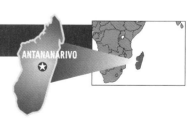

CAPITAL:
Luxembourg
EMBASSY (IN U.S.):
202-265-4171 or 4172
GMT:
+1 hour
TELEPHONE COUNTRY CODE:
35
USADIRECT:
800-2-0111
ENTRY REQUIREMENTS
- **Passport/Visa:** Passport required. Visa not required for tourist/business stay of up to 90 days.
- **HIV Test:** Not required.
- **Vaccinations:** None required.

EMBASSIES/CONSULATES
- **U.S. Embassy:** 22 Boulevard Emmanuel Servais, Luxembourg City; Tel: 352-460123; Fax: 352-461401; Website: www.amembassy.lu.
- **Canadian Embassy:** Price Waterhouse Coopers, 400 Route d'Esch, Luxembourg; Tel: 352-448-481.
- **British Embassy:** 14 Boulevard Roosevelt, L-2450 Luxembourg; Tel: 352-22-98-64/65/66; Fax: 352-22-98-67; e-mail: britemb@pt.lu; Website: webplaza.pt.lu/public/britemb.

HOSPITALS/DOCTORS:
Medical care in Luxembourg is of high quality, and many physicians speak English. Travelers are advised to obtain, before departure, supplemental travel health insurance with specific overseas coverage. The policy should provide for direct payment to the overseas hospital and/or physician at the time of service and include a medical evacuation benefit.

Current Advisories and Health Risks

See the Disease Risk Summary for Europe on page 300.

Madagascar

CAPITAL:
Antananarivo
EMBASSY (IN U.S.):
202-265-5525

+3 hours

TELEPHONE COUNTRY CODE:

261

USADIRECT:

None

ENTRY REQUIREMENTS

- **Passport/Visa:** A visa is required. Travelers should contact the Embassy of Madagascar.
- **HIV Test:** Not required.
- **Vaccinations:** A yellow fever vaccination certificate is required for all travelers arriving from, or transiting, infected areas.

EMBASSIES/CONSULATES

- **U.S. Embassy:** Antananarivo. 14 & 16 Rue Rainitovo, Antsahavola; Tel: 2-212-57-200-89 or 207-18.
- **Consulate of Canada:** c/o QIT Madagascar Minerals Ltd., Villa 3H, Lot II J 169, Ivandry, Antananarivo Madagascar; Postal Address: PO Box 4003, Antananarivo, 101, Madagascar; Tel: 261-20-22-425-59, 22-423-22; Fax: 261-20-22-425-06; e-mail: consulat.canada@wanadoo.mg.
- **British Embassy:** Lot II 164 Ter, Alarobia–Amboniloha, BP 167, Antananarivo 101; Tel: 261-20-22-49378/79/80; Fax: 261-20-22-49381; e-mail: ukembant@simicro.mg.

HOSPITALS/DOCTORS:

Hospital Befelatnana, Antananarivo (1,300 beds); general medical/surgical facility. Fort Dauphin Hospital, Faradofay (80 beds).

Current Advisories and Health Risks

AIDS/HIV: HIV prevalence appears to be low, even in the high-risk urban population.

CHOLERA: This disease is active in this country. The risk of cholera, however, is extremely low among international travelers from developed countries, such as the United States and Canada. Cholera vaccine (no longer available in the United States) is recommended only for travelers at high risk who work and live in highly endemic areas under less than adequate sanitary conditions.

HEPATITIS: All nonimmune travelers should receive hepatitis A vaccine. Hepatitis E presumably occurs, but incidence is not known. The hepatitis B carrier rate in the general population is estimated at 5% to 10%. Vaccination against hepatitis B is recommended for all long-term visitors to this country.

LEISHMANIASIS: Low risk. Incidence status undetermined.

MALARIA: Risk is present year-round in the coastal areas, but transmission is more seasonal in the central highland plateau, occurring primarily in November through May. There is minimal risk of malaria in Antananarivo and in the towns of Antsirabe,

Manjakandriana, and Andramasina. The highest risk of malaria occurs in the eastern coastal areas. Malaria occurs on the high plateau, formerly risk free. Prophylaxis with atovaquone/proguanil (Malarone), mefloquine (Lariam), or doxycycline is currently recommended before travel to malarious areas.

ANIMAL HAZARDS: Centipedes, scorpions, and black widow spiders. Portuguese man-of-war, sea nettles, sea wasps, stingrays, and several species of poisonous fish are common in the country's coastal waters and are potential hazards to unprotected swimmers.

PLAGUE: Human cases are reported annually. Travelers should avoid contact with wild rodents (and their fleas) or patients with the pneumonic form of the disease. Doxycycline or tetracycline can be used prophylactically if exposure occurs.

SCHISTOSOMIASIS: Widely distributed. Urinary schistosomiasis predominates on the west coast and in the northern regions, whereas intestinal schistosomiasis predominates in the central and southern coastal zones of Toamasina Province; the coastal zone of Fianarantsoa Province; and inland, in areas at moderate elevations to the south of the central highlands. Risk-free areas include the vicinities of Antsiranana and Antananarivo and the Presquile Peninsula, including Maroantsetra and Antalaha.

TRAVELERS' DIARRHEA: High risk. Water distribution systems are found only in major urban areas and are old and in poor repair. Piped water supplies frequently are contaminated. Travelers should observe all food and drink safety precautions. A quinolone antibiotic is recommended for the treatment of acute diarrhea. Diarrhea not responding to treatment with an antibiotic, or chronic diarrhea, may be due to a parasitic disease such as giardiasis or amebiasis.

OTHER DISEASES/HAZARDS: Brucellosis, filariasis (mosquito-borne; endemic, primarily along the eastern border), leprosy, rabies (dogs are the main source of human infection), tuberculosis (a major health problem in lower socioeconomic groups), trachoma, typhoid fever, and intestinal worms (very common).

Malawi

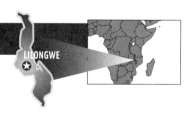

CAPITAL:
Lilongwe
EMBASSY (IN U.S.):
202-797-1103
GMT:
+2 hours
TELEPHONE COUNTRY CODE:
265
USADIRECT:
None

- **Passport/Visa:** Passport required. Visa not required for stay of up to 6 months.
- **HIV Test:** Not required.
- **Vaccinations:** A yellow fever valid vaccination certificate is required from all travelers older than 1 year arriving from infected areas.

EMBASSIES/CONSULATES

- **U.S. Embassy:** Area 40, City Center, Lilongwe; Tel: 773-166, 773-342, and 773-367; Fax: 770-471.
- **Canadian Embassy:** Accord Centre, M. Chipembere Highway, Blantyre-Limbe; Tel: 645-441; Fax: 645-004 or 643-446; e-mail: kokhai@malawibiz.com.
- **British High Commission:** PO Box 30042, Lilongwe 3; Tel: 265-1-772-400; Fax: 265-1-772-657; e-mail: bhclilongwe@fco.gov.uk.

HOSPITALS/DOCTORS:

Medical care in Malawi is below Western standards, even in the best private facilities. Travelers are advised to obtain, before departure, supplemental travel health insurance with specific overseas coverage. The policy should provide for direct payment to the overseas hospital and/or physician at the time of service and include a medical evacuation benefit.

- Queen Elizabeth Central Hospital, Blantyre (640 beds); Tel: 63-0333; general medical/surgical facility.
- Likuni Hospital, Lilongwe; Tel: 72-1400; recommended as the best local hospital.
- Blantyre Adventist Hospital, Kabula Hill Road; Tel: 62-0488.
- Adventist Health Centre, Presidential Way, Lilongwe; Tel: 73-1819.

Current Advisories and Health Risks

AFRICAN SLEEPING SICKNESS (TRYPANOSOMIASIS): Sleeping sickness is endemic throughout the country, including the Kasungu and Vwaza game reserves, near the Luangwa Valley of Zambia. Travelers should take precautions against insect (tsetse fly) bites.

AIDS/HIV: Greater than 10% of the adult population of this country are affected. Travelers are advised against unsafe sex, medical and dental injections, and blood transfusions.

ANIMAL HAZARDS: Animal hazards include snakes (vipers, cobras), centipedes, scorpions, and black widow spiders.

CHOLERA: This disease is reported active in this country, but the threat to tourists is deemed low. Cholera vaccination is not routinely recommended.

HEPATITIS: High risk. All travelers should receive hepatitis A vaccine. The hepatitis B carrier rate in the general population is estimated at 8%. Hepatitis B is spread by infected blood, contaminated needles, and unsafe sex. Vaccination is recommended for stays longer than 3 months; for persons at occupational or social risk; and for any traveler desiring maximum protection. Because the risk of illness or injury during travel cannot be predicted, some experts believe that *all* travelers should be immunized against hepatitis B because of the risk of receiving a medical injection with an unsterile needle or syringe.

INFLUENZA: Influenza is transmitted year-round in the tropics; flu vaccine is recommended for all travelers.

MALARIA: Risk is present year-round throughout this country, including urban areas. Highest malaria transmission rates occur along the shores of Lake Malawi, especially during the rainy season, November to April. Falciparum malaria accounts for approximately 90% of cases. Prophylaxis with atovaquone/proguanil (Malarone), mefloquine (Lariam), or doxycycline is recommended. All travelers should take measures to prevent evening and nighttime mosquito bites.

PLAGUE: An outbreak of bubonic plague occurred in 1997 in southern Malawi, with eight cases identified.

RABIES: Sporadic cases of human rabies are reported countrywide. Immediate medical attention should be sought for all animal bites or scratches, especially from a dog. Although rabies is rare among tourists, there is risk. Rabies vaccine is recommended for travel longer than 3 months, for adventure travelers, or when travelers desire extra protection.

SCHISTOSOMIASIS: Risk areas are distributed countrywide, with an intense focus along the shores of Lake Malawi, as well as the Shire River. Travelers should avoid swimming, bathing, or wading in any freshwater lake, pond, or stream.

TRAVELERS' DIARRHEA: High risk. Travelers should observe all food and drink safety precautions. A quinolone antibiotic, combined with loperamide (Imodium), is recommended for the treatment of acute diarrhea. Persistent diarrhea may be due to a parasitic disease such as giardiasis, amebiasis, or cryptosporidiosis.

TUBERCULOSIS: Tuberculosis (TB) is a major health problem in this country. Travelers planning an extended stay should have a pre-departure TB skin test (PPD test) and be retested after returning from this country.

TYPHOID FEVER: Typhoid vaccine is recommended for all travelers, with the exception of short-term visitors who restrict their meals to major restaurants and hotels, such as business travelers and cruise passengers. Because the typhoid vaccines are only 60% to 70% effective, safe food and drink selection remains important.

YELLOW FEVER: Vaccination is recommended for travel outside urban areas. This country is in the Yellow Fever Endemic Zone. A valid vaccination certificate may be required for ongoing travel to other countries.

OTHER DISEASES/HAZARDS: African tick typhus, brucellosis (from consumption of raw dairy products), echinococcosis, filariasis (may occur along the lower Shire River and along the shores of Lake Malawi), leptospirosis, meningitis, toxoplasmosis, trypanoso-miasis (reported from the Kasungu and Vwaza game reserves, near the Luangwa Valley of Zambia), trachoma, and intestinal helminths (very common).

Malaysia

KUALA LUMPUR

CAPITAL:
Kuala Lumpur
EMBASSY (IN U.S.):
202-328-2700
GMT:
+8 hours
TELEPHONE COUNTRY CODE:
60
USADIRECT:
1-800-80-0011
ENTRY REQUIREMENTS
- **Passport/Visa:** Passport required. Visa not required for stay of up to 3 months.
- **HIV Test:** Medical exam required for work permits. U.S. test result may be accepted.
- **Vaccinations:** A yellow fever vaccination certificate is required for all travelers older than 1 year arriving from infected areas. A certificate also required for travelers who have, within the preceding 6 days, transited any country within the Yellow Fever Endemic Zone.
EMBASSIES/CONSULATES
- **U.S. Embassy:** 376 Jalan Tun Razak, Kuala Lumpur; Tel: 3-2168-5000; Fax: 60-3-242-2207; Website: usembassymalaysia.org.my; e-mail: klconsular@state.gov.
- **Canadian Embassy:** 7th Floor, Plaza OSK, 172 Jalan Ampang; Tel: 32718-3333; Fax: 6-03-2718-3399; e-mail: klmpr@dfait-maeci.gc.ca; Website: www.dfait-maeci. gc.ca/kualalumpur.
- **British High Commission:** 185 Jalan Ampang, 50450 Kuala Lumpur (PO Box 11030), 50732 Kuala Lumpur; Tel: 60-3-2170-2200; Fax: 60-3-2170-2370; Website: www.britain.org.my, www.i-uk.com/malaysia.
HOSPITALS/DOCTORS:
Medical care in Malaysia is of high quality, and many physicians speak English. Travelers are advised to obtain, before departure, supplemental travel health insurance with specific overseas coverage. The policy should provide for direct payment to the overseas hospital and/or physician at the time of service and include a medical evacuation benefit.
- Gleneagles Intan Medical Centre, Jalan Ampang, Kuala Lumpur; Tel: 03-4257-1300. Many specialties; 24-hour emergency services; advanced 16-slice CT scanner.
- Bukit Mertajam Specialist Hospital, Pulau Penang; Tel: 04-538-7577. Most special-ties, including ob/gyn, renal dialysis.

• International SOS: International SOS (Malaysia) Sdn Bhd, Level 10, Menara Chan, 138 Jalan Ampang, 50450 Kuala Lumpur, Malaysia; Alarm Center Tel: 603-2716-3033; Alarm Center Fax: 603-2716-3040.

Current Advisories and Health Risks

ANIMAL HAZARDS: Animal hazards include snakes (kraits, vipers, cobras), centipedes, scorpions, and black widow spiders. Other possible hazards include tigers, bears, and wild pigs.

CHOLERA: This disease is reported active in this country, but the threat to tourists is very low. Cholera vaccine is recommended primarily for people at high risk (e.g., relief workers) who work and live in highly endemic areas under less than adequate sanitary conditions.

DENGUE FEVER: Occurs countrywide, with increased risk in urban and periurban areas. Peak infection rates occur in the late monsoon season (October through February in east peninsular Malaysia, Sabah, and Sarawak; July through August in west peninsular Malaysia.) All travelers should take measures to prevent daytime insect bites.

FILARIASIS: Very low risk for tourists; higher risk for expatriates and long-term residents (e.g., missionaries). Filariasis is endemic countrywide in freshwater swampy areas and inland hilly forested areas. Moderate risk exists in rural areas. Travelers should take measures to prevent mosquito bites.

HEPATITIS: All travelers should receive hepatitis A vaccine. Hepatitis E is endemic, but levels are unclear. The hepatitis B carrier rate in the general population is estimated at 5%. Hepatitis B is spread by infected blood, contaminated needles, and unprotected sex. Vaccination is recommended for stays longer than 3 months; for persons at occupational or social risk, and for anyone desiring maximum protection.

INFLUENZA: Influenza is transmitted year-round in the tropics. The flu vaccine is recommended for all travelers at risk.

JAPANESE ENCEPHALITIS: Sporadic cases of Japanese encephalitis (JE) occur year-round, especially in Sarawak, Penang, Perak, Selangor, and Johore. Risk occurs primarily in areas with rice growing and pig farming. JE vaccine is recommended for travelers staying longer than 3 to 4 weeks in rural endemic areas.

MALARIA: Risk exists in remote areas of peninsular Malaysia that are off usual tourist routes, and in Sarawak (Northwest Borneo). Urban and coastal areas are risk-free, and persons making day trips to rural tourist areas are not at risk. Prophylaxis with atovaquone/proguanil (Malarone), mefloquine (Lariam), or doxycycline is recommended for travel to risk areas. All travelers should take measures to prevent evening and nighttime mosquito bites.

MARINE HAZARDS: Stingrays, sea wasps, sea cones, jellyfish, the Indo-Pacific man-of-war, spiny sea urchins, and anemones are common in the country's coastal waters and are potentially hazardous to unprotected or careless swimmers.

SCHISTOSOMIASIS: Slight risk of infection (from *S. malayensisis*) is present in Perak and Pahang states. The human health significance of the presence of this parasite is unclear. It may not be pathogenic. Travelers to these areas should avoid exposure to freshwater lakes, ponds, and streams.

TRAVELERS' DIARRHEA: A quinolone antibiotic, combined with loperamide (Imodium), is recommended for the treatment of acute diarrhea. Persistent diarrhea may be due to a parasitic disease such as giardiasis, amebiasis, or cryptosporidiosis.

TUBERCULOSIS: Tuberculosis (TB) is a major health problem in this country. Travelers planning an extended stay should have a pre-departure TB skin test (PPD test) and be retested after returning from this country.

TYPHOID FEVER: Typhoid vaccine is recommended for all travelers, with the exception of short-term visitors who restrict their meals to major restaurants and hotels. Because the typhoid vaccines are only 60% to 70% effective, safe food and drink selection remains important.

OTHER DISEASES/HAZARDS: Angiostrongyliasis, intestinal helminthic infections (ascariasis, hookworm infection, strongyloidiasis, trichuriasis), other helminths (clonorchiasis, paragonimiasis), leptospirosis (countrywide risk, except in urban areas), leprosy (moderate to high prevalence), rabies (low risk; last case reported in 1985), and scrub typhus (mite-borne; risk elevated in grassy rural areas).

Mali

CAPITAL:
Bamako
EMBASSY (IN U.S.):
202-332-2249
GMT:
+0 hours
TELEPHONE COUNTRY CODE:
223
USADIRECT:
None
ENTRY REQUIREMENTS
• **Passport/Visa:** A valid passport and visa are required.
• **HIV Test:** Not required.

- **Vaccinations:** A yellow fever vaccination certificate is required for all travelers older than 1 year of age arriving from *all* countries.

EMBASSIES/CONSULATES

- **U.S. Embassy:** Rue Rochester NY and Rue Mohamed V, Bamako; Tel: 223-22-38-33; Fax: 223-22-37-12.
- **Canadian Embassy:** Immeuble Séméga, route de Koulikoro, Bamako; Tel: 223-21-22-36; Fax: 223-21-43-62; e-mail: bmako@dfait-maeci.gc.ca.
- **British Embassy:** Accredited to the British Embassy in Senegal. 20 Rue du Docteur Guillet, (Boite Postale 6025), Dakar; Tel: 221-823-7392, 823-9971; Fax: 221-823-2766, 823-8415; e-mail: britemb@sentoo.sn.

HOSPITALS/DOCTORS:

Medical facilities are very limited and inadequate for dealing with emergencies. Health insurance (including adequate medical evacuation coverage) is therefore essential. Many medicines are unavailable, and doctors and hospitals expect immediate cash payment for health-care services.

- Point G Hospital, Bamako (550 beds); general medical/surgical facility.
- Centre Medical Interentreprise, Bamako.

Current Advisories and Health Risks

ACCIDENTS/ILLNESSES AND MEDICAL INSURANCE

- Accidents and injuries are the leading cause of death among travelers younger than 55 years of age and most often are caused by motor vehicle and motorcycle crashes; drownings, aircraft crashes, homicides, and burns are less common causes.
- Heart attacks cause most fatalities in older travelers.
- Infections cause only 1% of fatalities in overseas travelers, but overall, infections are the most common cause of travel-related illness.
- Travelers are advised to obtain, before departure, supplemental travel health insurance with specific overseas coverage. The policy should provide for direct payment to the overseas hospital and/or physician at the time of service and include a medical evacuation benefit. The policy should also provide 24-hour hotline access to a multilingual assistance center that can help arrange and monitor delivery of medical care and determine if medical evacuation or air ambulance services are required.

AFRICAN SLEEPING SICKNESS (TRYPANOSOMIASIS): There is a low risk of trypanosomiasis in Mali, primarily in the Koulikoro and Sikasso regions. Travelers to these regions should take precautions to prevent tsetse fly bites.

AIDS/HIV: HIV prevalence is apparently low in the general population, but as many as 40% of surveyed prostitutes are infected.

ANIMAL HAZARDS: Animal hazards include snakes (vipers, cobras), centipedes, scorpions, and black widow spiders; crocodiles and hippopotamuses inhabit the rivers of Mali; lions and panthers are the major terrestrial hazards.

CHOLERA: This disease is reported active in this country, but the threat to tourists is very low. Cholera vaccine is recommended primarily for people at high risk (e.g., relief workers) who work and live in highly endemic areas under less than adequate sanitary conditions.

- The oral cholera vaccine (Dukoral) provides up to 60% crossover protection against ETEC diarrhea.
- Many countries, including Canada, license an oral cholera vaccine. The oral vaccine is not available in the United States.
- Cholera vaccine is not "officially" required for entry into, or exit from, any country. Despite this, some countries, on occasion, require proof of cholera vaccination from travelers coming from cholera-infected countries. Anticipating such a situation, certain travelers may wish to carry a medical exemption letter from their health-care provider. Travel Medicine, Inc., recommends that travelers use the International Certificate of Vaccination (Yellow Card) for this purpose, having their health-care provider affirm that they are "exempt from cholera vaccine" and validate the exemption with both the provider's signature and the appropriate official stamp (the "Uniform Stamp" in the United States).

FILARIASIS: Bancroftian filariasis is reported in southern areas. Travelers should take measures to prevent insect (mosquito) bites.

FOOD AND WATER SAFETY: All water should be regarded as being potentially contaminated. Water used for drinking, brushing teeth, or making ice should have first been boiled or otherwise sterilized. Milk is unpasteurized and should be boiled. Powdered or tinned milk is available and preferred; reconstitution must be with pure water. Avoid dairy products, which are likely to have been made from unboiled milk. Only well-cooked meat and fish, preferably served hot, should be consumed. Pork, salad, and mayonnaise may carry increased risk. Vegetables should be cooked and fruit peeled.

HEPATITIS: All nonimmune travelers should receive hepatitis A vaccine. Hepatitis E presumably occurs, but endemic levels are unclear. The hepatitis B carrier rate in the general population is estimated at 9% to 18%. Vaccination against hepatitis B should be considered for stays longer than 3 months and by short-term travelers desiring maximum protection. Travelers should be aware that hepatitis B can be transmitted by unsafe sex and the use of contaminated needles and syringes.

INFLUENZA: Influenza is transmitted year-round in the tropics. The flu vaccine is recommended for all travelers older than 50; all travelers with chronic disease or a weakened immune system; travelers of any age wishing to decrease the risk of this illness; and pregnant women after the first trimester.

INSECTS: All travelers should take measures to prevent both daytime and nighttime insect bites. Insect bite prevention measures include a DEET-containing repellent applied to exposed skin, insecticide (permethrin) spray applied to clothing and gear, and use of a permethrin-treated bed net at night while sleeping.

LEISHMANIASIS: Risk of cutaneous leishmaniasis exists primarily in rural areas of the southern and central Sahel. Current incidence and distribution data are not available, but sporadic cases have been reported from semi-desert regions, with a major focus in the Nioro District of Kayes Region. Visceral leishmaniasis (kala-azar) is currently not reported. All travelers to these regions should take measures to prevent sand fly bites.

MALARIA: Risk is present year-round countrywide, including urban areas. Risk is increased during and immediately following the rainy season (June to October). The highest risk of malaria occurs in southern Mali, particularly in the southern savanna and central Sahel zones. There is less risk in the northern Saharan region. Falciparum malaria accounts for approximately 85% of cases; *P. malariae* causes most other cases. Chloroquine-resistant falciparum malaria is prevalent, and mefloquine resistance has recently been reported.

• Prophylaxis with atovaquone/proguanil (Malarone), mefloquine (Lariam), or doxycycline is recommended.

• All travelers should take measures to prevent evening and nighttime mosquito bites. Insect bite prevention measures include a DEET-containing repellent applied to exposed skin, insecticide (permethrin) spray applied to clothing and gear, and use of a permethrin-treated bed net at night while sleeping.

MENINGITIS: The southern half of Mali lies within the sub-Saharan meningitis belt. Periodic epidemics occur within this country. Most infections are caused by serogroup A organisms, but serogroup C disease also occurs.

• Meningitis vaccine is recommended for all travelers staying longer than 1 month during the dry season, December to June, and should be considered for shorter stays during the dry season if prolonged contact with the local populace is anticipated. The vaccine is also recommended for all health-care workers and all travelers into epidemic regions at any time of year.

ONCHOCERCIASIS: Highly endemic foci are found in the Sikasso and Kayes regions along rivers where black flies breed. Travelers should take measures to prevent insect (black fly) bites.

RABIES: Human rabies is reported countrywide. Although rabies is rare among tourists, there is risk. No one should pet or pick up any stray animals. All children should be warned to avoid contact with unknown animals. All animal bites or scratches, especially from a dog, should be taken seriously and immediate medical attention sought.

• Rabies vaccine is recommended for travel longer than 3 months; for shorter stays for travelers who plan to venture off the usual tourist routes, where they may be more exposed to the stray dog population; or when travelers desire extra protection.

SCHISTOSOMIASIS: Prevalence is particularly high in irrigated areas. Urinary schistosomiasis occurs throughout southern Mali, primarily in the upper reaches of the Niger River and the upper basin of the Senegal River. Intestinal schistosomiasis is almost as extensively distributed. A new focus of disease has recently been reported from the

Bandiagara and Bankas districts, where the Dogon tribe is located. To prevent schistosomiasis, travelers should avoid swimming, bathing, or wading in freshwater lakes, ponds, or streams.

TRAVELERS' DIARRHEA: High risk. Surface water is almost always contaminated and ground water from deep wells commonly brackish. Piped water supplies are either untreated and often contaminated. Travelers should observe all food and drink precautions. A quinolone antibiotic is recommended for the treatment of acute diarrhea. Diarrhea not responding to treatment with an antibiotic may be due to a parasitic disease.

TUBERCULOSIS: Tuberculosis (TB) is a major public health problem in this country. Travelers planning an extended stay should have a pre-departure TB skin test (PPD test) and be retested after leaving this country.

TYPHOID FEVER: Typhoid vaccine is recommended. Because the typhoid vaccines are only 60% to 70% effective, safe food and drink guidelines should continue to be observed.

YELLOW FEVER: The Southwestern region is considered no longer infected by the World Health Organization. The most recent outbreak of yellow fever occurred during late 1987 in the regions of Kayes and Koulikoro. Vaccination is currently required for entry to this country. Southern Mali is in the Yellow Fever Endemic Zone.

OTHER DISEASES/HAZARDS: Anthrax (reported from Kati and Koulikoro provinces), brucellosis (from consumption of raw dairy products), dracunculiasis (endemic at low levels), dengue (no apparent activity), ehrlichiosis (tick-borne; a single case was reported in 1992 in a Canadian traveler), echinococcosis, hemorrhagic fever with renal syndrome (level of risk unclear; no human cases reported), Lassa fever, leprosy (4 to 7 cases/1,000 population in Bamako), relapsing fever (tick-borne and louse-borne), Rift Valley fever, toxoplasmosis, tuberculosis (a major health problem), typhoid fever, and intestinal worms (very common).

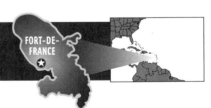

Martinique (French West Indies)

CAPITAL:
Fort-de-France
EMBASSY (IN U.S.):
202-944-6000
GMT:
−4 hours
TELEPHONE COUNTRY CODE:
596

USADIRECT:
0800-99-0011 to place calls from Martinique, St. Martin, St. Barthelemy, or Guadeloupe

ENTRY REQUIREMENTS
- **Passport/Visa:** French West Indies: includes the islands of Guadeloupe, Isles des Saintes, La Desirade, Marie Galante, Saint Barthelemy, St. Martin, and Martinique. Passport required. Visa not required for tourist/business stay of up to 3 months. For further information, consult the Embassy of France; Tel: 202-944-6200; Website: www.france-consulat.org.
- **HIV Test:** Not required.
- **Vaccinations:** None required.

EMBASSIES/CONSULATES
- **U.S. Embassy**: French Caribbean Dept. 14 Rue Blenac, Martinique; Tel: 596-631-303.

HOSPITALS/DOCTORS:
La Maynard Hospital, Fort-de-France Regional Hospital Center (764 beds); general medical/surgical facility; trauma and 24-hour emergency services.

Current Advisories and Health Risks

For additional information, consult the Disease Risk Summary for the Caribbean on page 293.

Mauritania

NOUAKCHOTT

CAPITAL:
Nouakchott

EMBASSY (IN U.S.):
202-232-5700

GMT:
+0 hours

TELEPHONE COUNTRY CODE:
222

USADIRECT:
None

ENTRY REQUIREMENTS
- **Passport/Visa:** Passport, proof of yellow fever vaccination, and visa are required.
- **HIV Test:** Not required.
- **Vaccinations:** A yellow fever vaccination certificate is required from all travelers older than 1 year arriving from *all* countries. *Exception*: Not required for travelers from a noninfected area who stay for less than 2 weeks.

EMBASSIES/CONSULATES
- **U.S. Embassy:** Nouakchott; Tel: 52660.
- **Canadian Embassy:** Senegal; Tel: 221-210-290.

- **British Embassy:** Accredited to the British Embassy in Morocco. 17 Boulevard de la Tour Hassan (BP 45), Rabat; Tel: 212-37-72-96-96; Fax: 212-37-70-45-31; e-mail: consular.rabat@fco.gov.uk; Website: www.britain.org.ma.

HOSPITALS/DOCTORS:

Medical care in Mauritania is below Western standards. Hospital facilities are not suitable for inpatient care but can provide emergency services. Travelers are advised to obtain, before departure, supplemental travel health insurance with specific overseas coverage. The policy should provide for direct payment to the overseas hospital and/or physician at the time of service and include a medical evacuation benefit.

- **National Hospital, Nouakchott** (460 beds); general medical/surgical facility; limited specialties.

Current Advisories and Health Risks

ACCIDENTS AND INJURIES: Automobile accidents can be catastrophic because of a lack of adequate facilities to care for acute trauma cases.

AIDS/HIV: HIV prevalence appears to be low, but AIDS/HIV infection constitutes a growing public health problem.

DENGUE FEVER: Undetermined risk, but probably low. Dengue virus is present in neighboring Senegal.

HEPATITIS: High risk. All travelers should receive hepatitis A vaccine. Hepatitis E likely occurs, but data are not available. The hepatitis B carrier rate in the general population is estimated to be as high as 22%. Vaccination against hepatitis B is recommended for health-care workers and all long-term visitors to this country.

LEISHMANIASIS: Sporadic cases of cutaneous leishmaniasis have been reported along the border with Senegal and near the southern border with Mali. Travelers should take measures to prevent insect (sandfly) bites.

MALARIA: Except for the northern areas of Dakhlet-Nouadhibou and Tiris-Zemmour, risk is countrywide, including urban areas, year-round, particularly along the Senegal River Basin, where the risk may be elevated during and immediately after the rainy season, July to September. Prophylaxis with atovaquone/proguanil (Malarone), mefloquine (Lariam), or doxycycline is recommended for travel to malarious regions of this country.

MENINGITIS: Mauritania lies partly within the "meningitis belt" of Africa. Quadrivalent meningococcal vaccine is recommended for travelers staying longer than 1 month during the dry season, December to June, and should be considered for shorter stays at any time of the year if extensive, close contact with the local populace is anticipated.

POLIOMYELITIS: Because of the persistence of polio in sub-Saharan Africa, polio immunization is recommended for all travelers.

RABIES: Vaccination recommended for all long-term visitors, or any traveler wanting maximum protection. All animal bites, especially dog bites, should be medically evaluated for the potential for rabies transmission.

SCHISTOSOMIASIS: Risk is greatest in the south along the Senegal River and extending into the southeast, and a smaller area further north, around the Adrar mountain range in the vicinity of Atar, in central western Mauritania. Infection rates of urinary schistosomiasis are highest in the south central border regions of Gorgol, Guidimaka, and Hodh el Gharbi. Travelers should avoid swimming, bathing, or wading in freshwater lakes, ponds, or streams.

TRAVELERS' DIARRHEA: High incidence. Drinking water in this country is widely contaminated. A quinolone antibiotic, combined with loperamide (Imodium), is recommended for the treatment of acute diarrhea. Persistent diarrhea may be due to a parasitic disease such as giardiasis, amebiasis, or cryptosporidiosis.

TUBERCULOSIS: Tuberculosis (TB) is a major health problem in this country. Travelers planning an extended stay should have a pre-departure TB skin test (PPD test) and be retested after returning from this country.

TYPHOID FEVER: Typhoid vaccine is recommended for all travelers to this country. Because the typhoid vaccines are only 60% to 70% effective, safe food and drink selection remains important.

YELLOW FEVER: Vaccination is recommended by the CDC for all travelers older than 9 months of age arriving from any country.

OTHER DISEASES/HAZARDS: African tick typhus (may occur), brucellosis (from consumption of raw dairy products), Crimean-Congo hemorrhagic fever (tick-borne; outbreak was reported in 2003), Rift Valley fever (outbreak in 1998), and intestinal worms (very common). Animal hazards include snakes (vipers, cobras, adders), centipedes, scorpions, and black widow spiders. Marine hazards include poisonous fishes (weever, scorpion fish, and toadfish) and venomous marine invertebrates such as the Portuguese man-of-war, stinging corals, feather hydroids, and sea nettles, sea anemones, sea urchins, and sea cucumbers.

Mauritius

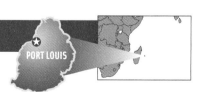

CAPITAL:
Port Louis
EMBASSY (IN U.S.):
202-244-1491
GMT:
+4 hours

TELEPHONE COUNTRY CODE:
230
USADIRECT:
01-120

ENTRY REQUIREMENTS

- **Passport/Visa:** Visa not required for visits for up to 6 months.
- **HIV Test:** Required for foreigners seeking work or permanent residence.
- **Vaccinations:** Required for travelers coming from infected or endemic countries. *Note:* Many travelers to Mauritius transit through Kenya. A yellow fever vaccination certificate is required of all travelers from Kenya including transit passengers.

EMBASSIES/CONSULATES

- **U.S. Embassy:** Rogers House (fourth floor) on John F. Kennedy Street, Port Louis; Tel: 230-208-2347 or 202-4400; Fax: 230-208-9534; e-mail: usembass@intnet.mu; Website: www.usembassymauritius.com.
- **Canadian Embassy:** 18 Jules Koenig Street, c/o Blanche Birger Co. Ltd., Port Louis; Tel: 230-212-5500; Fax: 230-208-3391; e-mail: canada@intnet.mu.
- **British High Commission:** Les Cascades Building, Edith Cavell Street, Port Louis, PO Box 1063; Tel: 230-202-9400; Fax: 230-202-9408; e-mail: bhc@intnet.mu.

HOSPITALS/DOCTORS:

Public medical facilities are numerous and of a high standard, and there are several private clinics. All treatment at state-run hospitals is free for Mauritians, but foreign visitors have to pay. There is no reciprocal health agreement with the United Kingdom; health insurance is advised.

- Service Aide Medicale Urgence (SAMU) is a government organization that provides assistance to anyone who calls 114 (Volcy Pougnet Street, Port Louis).
- MegaCare is a private organization that provides assistance to subscribers only (99 Draper Avenue, Quatre Bornes; Tel: 230-212-6270).

Current Advisories and Health Risks

ACCIDENTS/ILLNESSES AND MEDICAL INSURANCE

- Accidents and injuries are the leading cause of death among travelers younger than 55 years of age and most often are caused by motor vehicle and motorcycle crashes; drownings, aircraft crashes, homicides, and burns are less common causes.
- Heart attacks cause most fatalities in older travelers.
- Infections cause only 1% of fatalities in overseas travelers, but overall, infections are the most common cause of travel-related illness.
- Travelers are advised to obtain, before departure, supplemental travel health insurance with specific overseas coverage. The policy should provide for direct payment to the overseas hospital and/or physician at the time of service and include a medical evacuation benefit. The policy should also provide 24-hour hotline access to a multilingual assistance center that can help arrange and monitor delivery of medical care and determine if medical evacuation or air ambulance services are required.

ANIMAL HAZARDS: Animal hazards include snakes (cobras, vipers), spiders (black and brown widow), crocodiles, and leeches.

DENGUE FEVER: Dengue fever occurs in urban and rural areas. Protection against daytime mosquito bites is recommended.

FILARIASIS: Risk is present throughout this country. Travelers should take measures to prevent insect (mosquito) bites.

FOOD AND WATER SAFETY: Except for tap water available in resorts, water used for drinking should first be boiled or otherwise sterilized. Bottled water is readily available. Milk is unpasteurized and should be boiled. Powdered or tinned milk is available and preferred; reconstitution must be with pure water. Avoid dairy products, which are likely to have been made from unboiled milk. Vegetables should be cooked and fruit peeled.

HEPATITIS: All nonimmune travelers should receive hepatitis A vaccine. The hepatitis B carrier rate in the general population is estimated to exceed 10%. Vaccination against hepatitis B should be considered for stays longer than 3 months and by short-term travelers desiring maximum protection. Travelers should be aware that hepatitis B can be transmitted by unsafe sex and the use of contaminated needles and syringes.

INFLUENZA: Influenza is transmitted year-round in the tropics. The flu vaccine is recommended for all travelers older than 50 years of age; all travelers with chronic disease or a weakened immune system; travelers of any age wishing to decrease the risk of this illness; and pregnant women after the first trimester.

LEISHMANIASIS: Both cutaneous and visceral leishmaniasis are reported. Travelers should take measures to prevent insect (sand fly) bites.

MALARIA: Risk (predominantly from *P. vivax*) is present between January and May in rural areas of Pamplemousses, Plaines Wilhelms, Riviere de Rampart, and Grand Port. There is no risk in Port Louis or in coastal resorts and their immediate surroundings.
- Chloroquine prophylaxis is recommended in risk areas.
- All travelers should take measures to prevent evening and nighttime mosquito bites. Insect bite prevention measures include a DEET-containing repellent applied to exposed skin, insecticide (permethrin) spray applied to clothing and gear, and use of a permethrin-treated bed net at night while sleeping.

MARINE HAZARDS
- Stingrays, jellyfish, and several species of poisonous fish are common in the country's coastal waters and are potential hazards to unprotected swimmers.
- Ciguatera poisoning is prevalent and can result from eating coral reef fish such as grouper, snapper, sea bass, jack, and barracuda. The ciguatoxin is not destroyed by cooking.

SCHISTOSOMIASIS: Risk is present throughout this country, including urban areas. Travelers should avoid swimming, bathing, or wading in freshwater lakes, ponds, or streams.

- -

TRAVELERS' DIARRHEA: Moderate risk. A quinolone antibiotic, combined with loperamide (Imodium), is recommended for the treatment of acute diarrhea. Diarrhea not responding to treatment with an antibiotic, or chronic diarrhea, may be due to a parasitic disease such as giardiasis, amebiasis, or cryptosporidiosis.

- -

TYPHOID FEVER: Typhoid vaccine is recommended for long-term travelers, adventure travelers, and those wishing maximum disease protection. Because the typhoid vaccines are only 60% to 70% effective, safe food and drink guidelines should continue to be observed.

- -

OTHER DISEASES/HAZARDS: Echinococcosis, leprosy (highly endemic), rabies, tick-borne typhus, tuberculosis (highly endemic), and soil-transmitted helminthic disease (ascariasis, hookworm disease, strongyloidiasis) are reported.

Mexico

CAPITAL:
Mexico City
EMBASSY (IN U.S.):
202-736-1000
GMT:
−6 hours
TELEPHONE COUNTRY CODE:
52
USADIRECT:
01-800-288-2872
001-800-462-4240
ENTRY REQUIREMENTS
- **Passport/Visa:** Photo identification and proof of citizenship are required for entry by all U.S. citizens. A passport is the best document. A visa is required only for stays exceeding 180 days.
- **HIV Test:** Not required.
- **Vaccinations:** None required.
EMBASSIES/CONSULATES
- **U.S. Embassy:** Paseo de la Reforma 305, Colonia Cuauhtemoc, Mexico City; Tel: 5-209-9100; within Mexico, 01-5-209-9100; e-mail: ccs@usembassy.net.mx.
- **Canadian Embassy:** Calle Schiller No. 529, Rincón del Bosque, Colonia Bosque de Chapultepec Mexico City; Tel: 5724-7900 (within Mexico, the toll-free telephone number is 01-800-706-290); e-mail: mxico@dfait-maeci.gc.ca or embassy@canada.org.mx.
- **British Embassy:** Rio Lerma 71, Col. Cuauhtemoc, 06500 Mexico City; Tel: 52-55-5242-8500; Fax: 52-55-5242-8517; e-mail: ukinmex@att.net.mx; Website: www.embajadabritannica.com.mx.

HOSPITALS/DOCTORS

- The British-American Hospital (160 beds); private hospital; most of the staff are U.S. or British board-certified; specialties include cardiology, ob/gyn, emergency medicine, neurology.
- In Monterrey: Hospital Jose A. Muguerza; private hospital; most specialties, including cardiology, ob/gyn, kidney dialysis.
- In Guadalajara: Civil Hospital (1,000 beds); some specialties; English-speaking, U.S.-trained physicians on staff.

Current Advisories and Health Risks

ALTITUDE SICKNESS (AMS): Risk of altitude sickness, or acute mountain sickness (AMS), is present with travel to high-altitude destinations above 8,000 feet. Azetazolamide (Diamox) prophylaxis should be considered. The best treatment for AMS is descent.

AMEBIASIS: There is a high incidence of amebiasis in Mexico, especially in the southern areas, where up to 8% to 10% of the population tests positive for harboring parasites. Travelers should follow safe food and drink precautions.

CHAGAS DISEASE: Risk occurs below 1,500 meters elevation in the rural areas of the southern and western states. Most risk occurs in those rural-agricultural areas where there are adobe-style huts and houses that potentially harbor the night-biting triatomid (assassin) bugs. Travelers sleeping in such structures should take precautions against nighttime bites. Unscreened blood transfusions are also a source of infection and should be avoided.

CHOLERA: This disease is reported active in this country, but the threat to tourists is very low. Vaccination is not routinely recommended.

DENGUE FEVER: Dengue occurs in most areas below 1,200 meters elevation, especially in the southern and central Pacific urban coastal areas and in extreme northeastern Mexico. Increased risk may occur during the rainy season, from July through October. All travelers are advised to take precautions against daytime mosquito bites.

ENVIRONMENTAL POLLUTION: Acute respiratory infections are a common cause of illness in Mexico, often aggravated by air pollution. Extreme conditions can occur in Mexico City and Guadalajara, especially December to May. Travelers with heart disease, emphysema, and asthma may need to limit or avoid travel to regions with poor air quality. Lead is found in drinking water in some areas; in polluted air, paints, and some canned foods and beverages; and leached into beverages stored in lead-glazed pottery.

GNATHOSTOMIASIS: This food-borne disease is acquired through ingesting a parasite found in raw or undercooked freshwater fish (usually eaten in the form of tilapia, or ceviche, a famous Mexican raw fish dish). Most exposure occurs in northwestern Mexico, particularly in the states of Sinaloa, Oaxaca, Veracruz, Tamaulipas, Naryarit, and Guerrero, which includes the city of Acapulco. All travelers to these regions should avoid eating raw freshwater fish.

HELMINTHIC INFECTIONS: Hookworm, roundworm, and whipworm infections, and also strongyloidiasis, are highly prevalent in most rural areas. (Hookworm disease infects up to 90% of some rural villagers.) Travelers should wear shoes to prevent the hookworm and *Strongyloides* larvae from penetrating the skin. All food should be thoroughly cooked to destroy roundworm, whipworm, and pork tapeworm eggs.

- -

HEPATITIS: All nonimmune travelers should receive hepatitis A vaccine. Hepatitis E infections have been reported. To prevent hepatitis E, travelers, especially pregnant women, should avoid unsafe water, especially well water. The hepatitis B carrier rate in the adult population ranges from 0.3% to 1.6%. Carrier rates up to 4% have been reported from Chiapas State. Hepatitis B is spread by infected blood, contaminated needles, and unprotected sex. Vaccination is recommended for long-stay (longer than 3 months) travelers; persons who may be at occupational or social risk; and anybody desiring maximum protection.

- -

INFLUENZA: Risk extends from November to March in areas north of the Tropic of Cancer and throughout the year in areas south of that. Vaccination is recommended.

- -

INSECTS: All travelers should take measures to prevent both daytime and nighttime insect bites. Insect bite prevention measures include a DEET-containing repellent applied to exposed skin, insecticide (permethrin) spray applied to clothing and gear, and use of a permethrin-treated bed net at night.

- -

LEISHMANIASIS: Cutaneous leishmaniasis is endemic in rural areas in the southern territory of Quintana Roo, eastern Yucatan, Campeche, eastern Tabasco, Chiapas, Oaxaca, and eastern Veracruz. Mucocutaneous leishmaniasis (espundia) has occurred in Jalisco State, and visceral leishmaniasis (kala-azar) has occurred in Guerrero and Morelos states. Diffuse cutaneous leishmaniasis occurs in both the northeast and southeast regions. Mucocutaneous leishmaniasis has occurred in Jalisco State. This disease is transmitted by sand flies, which are most active between sunset and dawn. All travelers should take measures to prevent insect bites, especially in forested areas. Slow-healing or nonhealing skin infections should alert travelers to this possible diagnosis.

- -

MALARIA: Malaria is endemic in rural areas below 1,000 meters elevation and is more widespread than most travelers realize. The disease, however, has been eliminated from large urban areas and the major resorts. Risk occurs in rural areas of the following states: Campeche, Chiapas, Guerrero, Michoacán, Nayarit, Oaxaca, Quintana Roo, Sinaloa, and Tabasco. In addition, risk exists in the state of Jalisco (in mountainous northern area only). Risk also exists in parts of Sonora, Chihuahua, and Durango. No risk along the United States–Mexico border. There is no risk in the major resorts along the Pacific and Gulf coasts.

- -

MARINE HAZARDS

- Swimming-related hazards include jellyfish, spiny sea urchins, and coral.
- Ciguatera poisoning is prevalent and can result from eating coral reef fish such as grouper, snapper, sea bass, jack, and barracuda. The ciguatoxin is not destroyed by cooking.

• For scuba diving hyperbaric chamber referral, the Divers' Alert Network (DAN) maintains an up-to-date list of all hyperbaric chambers in North America and the Caribbean. In association with Duke University Medical Center in North Carolina, DAN operates a 24-hour emergency phone number (919-684-8111) for members and nonmembers to call, and DAN staff is available to answer questions and, if necessary, make referral to the closest functioning hyperbaric chamber.

ONCHOCERCIASIS: This black fly-transmitted disease is limited to areas along rivers between 600 and 1,500 meters elevation in Chiapas and Oaxaca states. The highest risk is during October through April. Travelers should take measures to prevent insect (black fly) bites.

RABIES: Several dozen or more human cases are reported annually. Ninety percent of cases are acquired from contact with rabid dogs, usually in rural areas. Rabid vampire bats reportedly are a problem in Sinaloa State. Travelers should especially avoid stray dogs and seek immediate treatment of any animal bite. Rabies vaccination is especially indicated following the unprovoked bite of a dog, cat, bat, or monkey.

SEABATHER'S ERUPTION: Reported in and near Cancun. This condition is caused by sea anemone larvae trapped under the bathing suit, causing skin irritation, rash, and fever.

TRAVELERS' DIARRHEA: High risk countrywide outside of major resorts and deluxe hotels. More diarrhea occurs during the rainy season, May through October. Bacterial organisms, mostly *E. coli* and *Campylobacter*, account for 80% of cases. A quinolone antibiotic, plus loperamide (Imodium), is recommended for the treatment of acute diarrhea. Persistent diarrhea may be due to a parasitic infection such as giardiasis, amebiasis, or cryptosporidiosis.

TUBERCULOSIS: Tuberculosis (TB) is an important public health problem, particularly among the native Indian populations in southern Mexico and Baja California; drug-resistant strains of the causative organism (*M. tuberculosis*) are common. Travelers planning an extended stay should have a pre-departure TB skin test (PPD test) and be retested after leaving this country or returning home.

TYPHOID FEVER: This disease is common, and more cases of typhoid fever are reported in travelers returning from Mexico than from any other Latin American country. There is increased risk of typhoid from June through October, countrywide. Vaccination against typhoid fever is recommended for travelers venturing outside of tourist areas; long-term travelers; adventure travelers; those wishing maximum disease protection; and those visiting friends and relatives. Because the typhoid vaccines are only 60% to 70% effective, safe food and drink selection remains important.

VIRAL ENCEPHALITIS: Rare cases of St. Louis encephalitis, Venezuelan equine encephalitis, and eastern and western encephalitis are reported. Mosquito bite prevention is recommended.

OTHER DISEASES/HAZARDS: Anthrax (small outbreaks reported in Zacatecas, central Mexico), brucellosis (90% of cases associated with contact with goats; greatest risk occurs in the northern and central states), coccidiomycosis (fungal respiratory infection ["valley fever"] is endemic in the dry north of Baja California Norte, in Sonora and Chihuahua states, and along the Pacific Coast; outbreaks have occurred in church groups from the United States doing construction work; cough and fever are main symptoms), cysticercosis and neurocysticercosis (caused by the ingestion of pork tapeworm eggs; common, especially in Guanajuato and Michocan states), histoplasmosis (contact with bat guano transmits this fungal disease), leptospirosis, Lyme disease (presumably occurs), relapsing fever (tick-borne; endemic in northern and central Mexico), typhus (both louse- and flea-borne; reported in Chiapas State), and tick-borne rickettsioses (spotted fever group; reported in some rural areas; one case of human monocytic ehrlichiosis was reported in Yucatan).

Micronesia

★PALIKIR

CAPITAL:
Palikir
EMBASSY (IN U.S.):
202-223-4383
GMT:
+10 hours
TELEPHONE COUNTRY CODE:
691
USADIRECT:
288
ENTRY REQUIREMENTS
- **Passport/Visa:** Passport required. Micronesia is self-governing in free association with the United States. The 600 islands and atolls were formerly part of the U.S. Trust Territory of the Pacific. Micronesia comprises four archipelagos: the Federated States of Micronesia (Caroline Islands), the Republic of the Marshall Islands, the Northern Mariana Islands, and the Republic of Palau.
- **HIV Test:** Anyone applying for a permit needs to obtain a medical clearance, which may include an HIV test.
- **Vaccinations:** None required.
EMBASSIES/CONSULATES
- **U.S. Embassy:** Kasalehlie Street, Kolonia, Pohnpei; Tel: 691-320-2187; Fax: 691-320-2186.
- **Canadian Embassy:** Accredited to the Australian Embassy. H&E Enterprises Building, Kolonia, Pohnpei, Micronesia; Tel: 691-320-5448; Fax: 691-320-5449.
- **British High Commission:** Accredited to the British High Commission in Fiji. Victoria House, Gladstone Road, Suva (PO Box 1355); Tel: 679-3229100; Fax: 679-3229132; Website: http://www.britishhighcommission.gov.uk/fiji.

HOSPITALS/DOCTORS:
There are hospitals on each of the four major islands and a few scattered clinics. The quality of health care is variable. Health insurance with a medical evacuation benefit is recommended.

Current Advisories and Health Risks

ACCIDENTS/ILLNESSES AND MEDICAL INSURANCE
- Accidents and injuries are the leading cause of death among travelers younger than 55 years of age and most often are caused by motor vehicle and motorcycle crashes; drownings, aircraft crashes, homicides, and burns are less common causes. Important safety rules to follow are (1) do not drive at night, (2) do not rent a motorcycle, moped, bicycle, or motorbike, even if you are experienced, and (3) do not swim alone, at night, or if intoxicated.
- Heart attacks cause most fatalities in older travelers.
- Infections cause only 1% of fatalities in overseas travelers, but overall, infections are the most common cause of travel-related illness.
- Travelers are advised to obtain, before departure, supplemental travel health insurance with specific overseas coverage. The policy should provide for direct payment to the overseas hospital and/or physician at the time of service and include a medical evacuation benefit. The policy should also provide 24-hour hotline access to a multilingual assistance center that can help arrange and monitor delivery of medical care and determine if medical evacuation or air ambulance services are required.

CHOLERA: Cholera is an extremely rare disease in travelers from developed countries. Cholera vaccine is recommended primarily for people at high risk (e.g., relief workers) who work and live in highly endemic areas under less than adequate sanitary conditions.
- The oral cholera vaccine (Dukoral) provides up to 60% crossover protection against ETEC diarrhea.
- Many countries, including Canada, license an oral cholera vaccine. The oral vaccine is not available in the United States.
- Cholera vaccine is not "officially" required for entry into, or exit from, any country. Despite this, some countries, on occasion, require proof of cholera vaccination from travelers coming from cholera-infected countries. Anticipating such a situation, certain travelers may wish to carry a medical exemption letter from their health-care provider. Travel Medicine, Inc., recommends that travelers use the International Certificate of Vaccination (Yellow Card) for this purpose, having their health-care provider affirm that they are "exempt from cholera vaccine" and validate the exemption with both the provider's signature and the appropriate official stamp (the "Uniform Stamp" in the United States).

DENGUE FEVER: Sporadic cases and outbreaks are reported. A dengue fever/dengue hemorrhagic fever outbreak occurred in Yap State in 1995. Travelers should take protective measures against daytime mosquito bites.

FILARIASIS: Sporadic cases are reported. Travelers should take measures to prevent mosquito bites.

HEPATITIS: Hepatitis A vaccine is recommended for all nonimmune travelers. The hepatitis B carrier rate in parts of Oceania is as high as 15%. Vaccination against hepatitis B should be considered for stays longer than 3 months and by short-term travelers desiring maximum protection. Travelers should be aware that hepatitis B can be transmitted by unsafe sex and the use of contaminated needles and syringes.

INFLUENZA: Influenza is transmitted year-round in the tropics. The flu vaccine is recommended for all travelers over age 50; all travelers with any chronic disease or weakened immune system; travelers of any age wishing to decrease the risk of this illness; pregnant women after the first trimester.

INSECTS: All travelers should take measures to prevent both daytime and nighttime insect bites. Insect bite prevention measures include a DEET-containing repellent applied to exposed skin, insecticide (permethrin) spray applied to clothing and gear, and use of a permethrin-treated bed net at night while sleeping.

JAPANESE ENCEPHALITIS: There is no apparent risk of Japanese encephalitis (JE).

MALARIA: There is no malaria in Micronesia.

MARINE HAZARDS
- Swimming-related hazards include jellyfish, spiny sea urchins, and coral.
- Ciguatera poisoning is prevalent and can result from eating coral reef fish such as grouper, snapper, sea bass, jack, and barracuda. The ciguatoxin is not destroyed by cooking.

TRAVELERS' DIARRHEA: Low to moderate risk. In urban and resort areas, the hotels and restaurants generally serve reliable food and potable water. Elsewhere, travelers should observe all food and drink safety precautions. A quinolone antibiotic, combined with loperamide (Imodium), is recommended for the treatment of acute diarrhea.

TYPHOID FEVER: Vaccination against typhoid fever is recommended for: travelers venturing outside of tourist areas; long-term travelers; adventure travelers; and those wishing maximum disease protection. Because the typhoid vaccines are only 60% to 70% effective, safe food and drink selection remains important.

Moldova

CAPITAL:
Chisinau
EMBASSY (IN U.S.):
202-667-1130/31

GMT:
+2 hours
TELEPHONE COUNTRY CODE:
373
USADIRECT:
None

ENTRY REQUIREMENTS

Passport required. Visa applicants are advised to contact the Moldovan embassy for current requirements. An HIV test is required for persons staying more than 3 months.

- **Vaccinations:** (recommended, depending on length of stay, itinerary and personal risk factors) hepatitis A and B, influenza, rabies, tick-borne encephalitis, and typhoid. Routine immunizations, including for tetanus/diphtheria and childhood diseases should be reviewed and updated as necessary.

EMBASSIES/CONSULATES

- **U.S. Embassy:** Strada Alexei Mateevici 103, Chisinau; Tel: 373-22-23-37-72; Fax: 373-22-24-25-00; e-mail: enquiries.chisinau@fco.gov.uk; Website: www.britishembassy. gov.uk/moldova.
- **Canadian Embassy:** Accredited to the Canadian Embassy in Romania. 36 Nicolae Iorga, 010436 Bucharest, Romania; Postal Address: PO Box 2966, Post Office No. 22, Bucharest, Romania; Tel: 40-21-307-5000; Fax: 40-21-307-5010; e-mail: bucst@international.gc.ca; Website: www.bucharest.gc.ca.
- **British Embassy:** Str. Nicolae Iorga 18, Chisinau 2005; Tel: 37322-22-59-02; Fax: 37322-25-18-59; e-mail: enquiries.chisinau@fco.gov.uk; Website: www. britishembassy.md.

HOSPITALS/DOCTORS:

Medical care in Moldova is well below Western standards. In hospitals, even in Chisinau, technology is lacking and overcrowding is common. It may be difficult to obtain even basic medications and supplies. Travelers are advised to purchase adequate medical evacuation coverage. Also, travelers are advised to contact the U.S. or U.K. embassies for hospital and doctor referrals. If a serious health event occurs, every effort should be made to get treatment in Western Europe.

Current Advisories and Health Risks

CRIMEAN-CONGO HEMORRHAGIC FEVER: Cases have been reported, but risk is not high. Travelers spending extended periods in wooded areas should take appropriate precautions.

FOOD AND WATER-BORNE ILLNESSES: These pose the highest risk. Contaminated water and unsanitary food preparation conditions are common. Outside of first-class hotels in Chisinau, water should be boiled or purified, or travelers should drink bottled water.

MALARIA: No risk.

TICK-BORNE ENCEPHALITIS: As with Crimean-Congo hemorrhagic fever, cases have been reported, but travelers are not at serious risk. Appropriate precautions should be taken in wooded areas.

TUBERCULOSIS: Moldova is in the highest WHO risk category for TB. An estimated 100 persons per 100,000 are infected with the disease.

Mongolia

ULAANBAATAR ★

CAPITAL:

Ulaanbaatar

EMBASSY (IN U.S.):

202-333-7117

GMT:

+8 hours

TELEPHONE COUNTRY CODE:

976

USADIRECT:

None

ENTRY REQUIREMENTS

- **Passport/Visa:** Passport and visa required.
- **HIV Test:** Required for students and anyone staying longer than 3 months; U.S. test result accepted.
- **Vaccinations:** None required.

EMBASSIES/CONSULATES

- **U.S. Embassy:** Micro Region 11, Big Ring Road, Ulaanbaatar; Tel: 976-1-329-095; Website: www.us-mongolia.com.
- **Canadian Embassy:** Diplomatic Services Building, Suite 56, Ulaanbaatar; Tel: 976-11-328-285; Fax: 976-11-328-289.
- **British Embassy:** 30 Enkh Taivny Gudamzh (PO Box 703), Ulaanbaatar 13; Tel: 976-11-458133; Fax: 976-11-458036; e-mail: britemb@magicnet.mn.

HOSPITALS/DOCTORS:

Medical care is substandard throughout the country. Adequate medical evacuation coverage for all travelers is a high priority. For serious medical conditions, every effort should be made to go to Japan. Hospital accommodations are inadequate throughout the country, and advanced technology is lacking. Shortages of routine medications and supplies may be encountered.

- International SOS: SOS Medica Mongolia Clinic, Gutal Corporation Building, Chinggis Khan Avenue, Ulaanbaatar, Mongolia, Tel. (976) (11) 345526; Fax: 976-11-342550; e-mail: contactus@sosmedica.mn

Current Advisories and Health Risks

ACCIDENTS/ILLNESS AND MEDICAL INSURANCE

- Accidents and injuries are the leading cause of death among travelers younger than 55 years of age and most often are caused by motor vehicle and motorcycle crashes; drownings, aircraft crashes, homicides, and burns are less common causes.
- Heart attacks cause most fatalities in older travelers.
- Infections cause only 1% of fatalities in overseas travelers, but overall, infections are the most common cause of travel-related illness.
- Travelers are advised to obtain, before departure, supplemental travel health insurance with specific overseas coverage. The policy should provide for direct payment to the overseas hospital and/or physician at the time of service and include a medical evacuation benefit. The policy should also provide 24-hour hotline access to a multilingual assistance center that can help arrange and monitor delivery of medical care and determine if medical evacuation or air ambulance services are required.

CHOLERA: Sporadic cases may occur. Cholera is an extremely rare disease in travelers from developed countries. Cholera vaccine is recommended primarily for people at high risk (e.g., relief workers) who work and live in highly endemic areas under less than adequate sanitary conditions.

- The oral cholera vaccine (Dukoral) provides up to 60% crossover protection against ETEC diarrhea.
- Many countries, including Canada, license an oral cholera vaccine. The oral vaccine is not available in the United States.
- Cholera vaccine is not "officially" required for entry into, or exit from, any country. Despite this, some countries, on occasion, require proof of cholera vaccination from travelers coming from cholera-infected countries. Anticipating such a situation, certain travelers may wish to carry a medical exemption letter from their health-care provider. Travel Medicine, Inc., recommends that travelers use the International Certificate of Vaccination (Yellow Card) for this purpose, having their health-care provider affirm that they are "exempt from cholera vaccine" and validate the exemption with both the provider's signature and the appropriate official stamp (the "Uniform Stamp" in the United States).

HEPATITIS: All nonimmune travelers should receive hepatitis A vaccine. Hepatitis B vaccine is recommended for stays longer than 3 months or frequent short stays; for adventure travelers; for all health-care workers; with the possibility of acupuncture, dental work, or tattooing, or of a new sexual partner, during stay; and with expected exposure to blood and body fluids. Consider for shorter stays in risk-averse travelers desiring maximum pre-travel preparation, or if extensive travel by road or extensive use of public transportation is anticipated. Increased awareness is recommended regarding safe sex and body fluid and blood precautions.

INFLUENZA: Influenza is transmitted from November through March. The flu vaccine is recommended for all travelers older than 50 years of age; all travelers with chronic disease or a weakened immune system; travelers of any age wishing to decrease the risk of this illness; and pregnant women after the first trimester.

MENINGITIS: Epidemics of serogroup A and C disease have been reported from Mongolia. With the emergence of the W-135 strain of meningococcal disease, the quadrivalent vaccine, rather than the bivalent vaccine, is recommended.

RABIES: Sporadic cases of human rabies are reported countrywide. All animal bites or scratches, especially from a dog, should be taken seriously, and immediate medical attention sought. Although rabies is rare among tourists, there is risk. No one should pet or pick up any stray animals. All children should be warned to avoid contact with unknown animals.

- Rabies vaccine is recommended for travel longer than 3 months; for shorter stays for travelers who plan to venture off the usual tourist routes, where they may be more exposed to the stray dog population; or when travelers desire extra protection.

TRAVELERS' DIARRHEA: High risk. Travelers should follow safe food and drink guidelines. A quinolone antibiotic, combined with loperamide (Imodium), is recommended for the treatment of acute diarrhea.

TUBERCULOSIS: Tuberculosis (TB) is a major public health problem in this country. Travelers planning an extended stay should have a pre-departure TB skin test (PPD test) and be retested after leaving this country.

TYPHOID FEVER: Typhoid vaccine is recommended. Because the typhoid vaccines are only 60% to 70% effective, safe food and drink guidelines should continue to be observed.

Morocco

RABAT

CAPITAL:
Rabat
EMBASSY (IN U.S.):
202-462-7979
GMT:
+0 hours
TELEPHONE COUNTRY CODE:
212
USADIRECT:
002-11-0011
ENTRY REQUIREMENTS

- **Passport/Visa:** Passport valid for 6 months. No visa required for stays less than 90 days. Contact the Embassy of Morocco, 1601 21st St. NW, Washington, DC 20009; Tel: 202-462-7979/82; or Moroccan consulate, 10 E. 40th St., New York, NY 10016; Tel: 212-758-2625.

- **HIV Test:** Not required.
- **Vaccinations:** None required.

EMBASSIES/CONSULATES

- **U.S. Embassy:** 2 Avenue de Marrakech, Rabat; Tel: 37-76-2265; Website: www.usembassy-morocco.org.ma.
- **Canadian Embassy:** 13 bis, rue Jaafar Assadik, Agdal-Rabat; Tel: 37-68-7400; Fax: 37-68-7430; e-mail: rabat@dfait-maeci.gc.ca.
- **British Embassy:** 17 Boulevard de la Tour Hassan (BP 45), Rabat; Tel: 212-37-72-96-96; Fax: 212-37-70-45-31; e-mail: consular.rabat@fco.gov.uk; Website: www.britain.org.ma.

HOSPITALS/DOCTORS:

Not all facilities meet high-quality standards, and specialized treatment may not be available. Medical facilities generally adequate for nonemergency matters in urban areas, but medical staff are seldom able to communicate in English. Travelers driving in the mountains and remote areas should carry a medical kit and a Moroccan phone card for emergencies. In event of car accidents involving injuries, immediate ambulance service is not guaranteed or provided. Doctors and hospitals often expect immediate cash payment. Supplemental medical insurance with specific overseas coverage, including medical evacuation, is recommended.

Current Advisories and Health Risks

ACCIDENTS/ILLNESSES: Motor vehicle accidents, injuries and drownings are the leading cause of death among travelers younger than 55 years of age. Cardiovascular disease causes most fatalities in older travelers. Infections cause less than 1% of fatalities in overseas travelers but overall are the most common cause of travel-related illness.

AFRICAN TICK TYPHUS: Widespread, primarily in rural and suburban coastal areas. Travelers to rural areas should take measures to avoid tick bites.

HEPATITIS: Hepatitis A vaccine is recommended for nonimmune travelers. Hepatitis E is endemic at a high level. The hepatitis B carrier rate in the population is estimated to be as high as 6%. Hepatitis B is spread by infected blood, contaminated needles, and unsafe sex. Vaccination is recommended for stays longer than 3 months; for persons at occupational or social risk; and for any traveler desiring maximum protection. Because the risk of illness or injury during travel cannot be predicted, some experts believe that *all* travelers should be immunized against hepatitis B because of the risk of receiving a medical injection with an unsterile needle or syringe.

LEISHMANIASIS

- Cutaneous leishmaniasis (CL) is widespread in semiarid rural areas, with increased vector activity June through September, particularly in Er Rachidia, Ouarzazate, and Tata provinces. CL due to *L. tropica* apparently is distributed countrywide in rural areas, including the Haut Atlas mountain region (Azilal and Essaouira Provinces),

Marrakech Province, and Agadir and Tiznit provinces. *L. infantum* is focally distributed in urban areas throughout the country.

- Visceral leishmaniasis (kala-azar) is focally distributed throughout Morocco, including Fes, Marrakech, and the southwest Atlas region.
- All travelers should take precautions against sand fly bites in these areas.

MALARIA: Year-round but very limited risk in rural areas of Khouribga Province. The risk of malaria (caused exclusively by *P. vivax*) is highest from May to October. Prophylaxis is not routinely recommended. All travelers in rural areas should take measures to prevent evening and nighttime mosquito bites. Insect-bite prevention measures include a DEET-containing repellent applied to exposed skin, insecticide (permethrin) spray applied to clothing and gear, and use of a permethrin-treated bed net at night while sleeping.

RABIES: Sporadic cases of human rabies, usually transmitted by rabid dogs, have been reported, primarily from the populated northern urban and rural areas. Rabies vaccine is recommended for those persons anticipating an extended stay, those whose work or activities may bring them into contact with animals, or when extra protection is desired. Prompt medical evaluation and treatment of any animal bite is essential, regardless of vaccination status.

SCHISTOSOMIASIS: Year-round risk, with highest incidence in the summer. Urinary schistosomiasis is widespread, particularly along the wadis and slopes of the Anti- and Haut Atlas Mountains and the Atlantic and Mediterranean coasts, and in oases and irrigated agricultural areas. Recognized foci occur in central and southern areas, including Agadir, Beni Mellal, El Kelaa des Srarhna, Er Rachidia, Marrakech, Ouarzazate, Taroudannt, Tata, and Tiznit provinces. Activity also reported in northern areas, including Kenitra, Nador, and Tanger provinces. Travelers should avoid freshwater exposure.

TRAVELERS' DIARRHEA: Water sources in Morocco should be considered potentially contaminated. In urban and resort areas, the first-class hotels and restaurants generally serve reliable food and potable water. A quinolone antibiotic, combined with loperamide (Imodium), is recommended for the treatment of acute diarrhea. Persistent diarrhea may be due to a parasitic disease such as giardiasis or amebiasis.

TUBERCULOSIS: Tuberculosis (TB) is is considered a public health problem in this country. Travelers planning an extended stay should have a pre-departure TB skin test (PPD test) and be retested after leaving this country.

TYPHOID FEVER: Typhoid vaccine is recommended for long-term travelers, adventure travelers, and those wishing maximum disease protection. Because the typhoid vaccines are only 60% to 70% effective, safe food and drink guidelines should continue to be observed.

OTHER DISEASES/HAZARDS: AIDS/HIV (endemic at low levels), brucellosis (risk from unpasteurized goat/sheep milk and cheese), cholera, echinococcosis (highly prevalent countrywide), leprosy, leptospirosis, relapsing fever (tick-borne), sand fly fever (primarily in the northern half of the country), toxoplasmosis (infection rates as high as 52%), tuberculosis (a major public health problem), typhoid fever, and intestinal helminthic infections (especially roundworm infections) are common in rural areas.

Mozambique

CAPITAL:
Maputo

EMBASSY (IN U.S.):
202-293-7146

GMT:
+2 hours

TELEPHONE COUNTRY CODE:
258

USADIRECT:
None

ENTRY REQUIREMENTS
- **Passport/Visa:** A visa, valid for 30 days, is required.
- **HIV Test:** Not required.
- **Vaccinations:** A yellow fever vaccination certificate is required from all travelers older than 1 year arriving from infected areas.

EMBASSIES/CONSULATES
- **U.S. Embassy:** 193 Avenida Kenneth Kaunda, Maputo; Tel: 258-1-49-2797, 49-0723; Fax: 258-1-49-0114; e-mail: consularmaputo@state.gov.
- **Canadian Embassy:** 1128 Julius Nyerere Avenue, Maputo; Tel: 258-1-492-623; Fax: 258-1-492-667; e-mail: mputo@dfait-maeci.gc.ca.
- **British High Commission:** Av Vladimir I Lenine 310, Caixa Postal 55, Maputo; Tel: 258-1-356-000; Fax: 258-1-356-060.

HOSPITALS/DOCTORS
- Travelers should contact their country's embassy or consulate for physician referrals.

Current Advisories and Health Risks

ACCIDENTS/ILLNESSES AND MEDICAL INSURANCE
- Accidents and injuries are the leading cause of death among travelers younger than 55 years of age and most often are caused by motor vehicle and motorcycle crashes; drownings, aircraft crashes, homicides, and burns are less common causes.
- Heart attacks cause most fatalities in older travelers.
- Infections cause only 1% of fatalities in overseas travelers, but overall, infections are the most common cause of travel-related illness.
- Travelers are advised to obtain, before departure, supplemental travel health insurance with specific overseas coverage. The policy should provide for direct payment to the

overseas hospital and/or physician at the time of service and include a medical evacuation benefit. The policy should also provide 24-hour hotline access to a multilingual assistance center that can help arrange and monitor delivery of medical care and determine if medical evacuation or air ambulance services are required.

AFRICAN SLEEPING SICKNESS (TRYPANOSOMIASIS): Approximately 75 cases are reported annually, mostly from Tete Province. All travelers should take precautions against insect (tsetse fly) bites.

AIDS/HIV: Heterosexual contact is the predominant mode of transmission. Lower risk compared with that in other countries in sub-Saharan Africa. HIV-1 prevalence estimated at 2.6% of the high-risk urban population. All travelers are cautioned against unsafe sex, unsterile medical or dental injections, and unnecessary blood transfusions.

ANIMAL HAZARDS: Animal hazards include snakes (vipers, cobras, mambas), centipedes, scorpions, and black widow spiders.

CHOLERA: This disease is active in this country. Cholera is an extremely rare disease in travelers from developed countries. Cholera vaccine is recommended primarily for people at high risk (e.g., relief workers) who work and live in highly endemic areas under less than adequate sanitary conditions.
- The oral cholera vaccine (Dukoral) provides up to 60% crossover protection against ETEC diarrhea.
- Many countries, including Canada, license an oral cholera vaccine. The oral vaccine is not available in the United States.
- Cholera vaccine is not "officially" required for entry into, or exit from, any country. Despite this, some countries, on occasion, require proof of cholera vaccination from travelers coming from cholera-infected countries. Anticipating such a situation, certain travelers may wish to carry a medical exemption letter from their health-care provider. Travel Medicine, Inc., recommends that travelers use the International Certificate of Vaccination (Yellow Card) for this purpose, having their health-care provider affirm that they are "exempt from cholera vaccine" and validate the exemption with both the provider's signature and the appropriate official stamp (the "Uniform Stamp" in the United States).

HEPATITIS: All nonimmune travelers should receive hepatitis A vaccine. Hepatitis E presumably occurs, but endemic levels are unclear. The hepatitis B carrier rate in the general population is estimated at 11%. Vaccination against hepatitis B should be considered for stays longer than 3 months and by short-term travelers desiring maximum protection. Travelers should be aware that hepatitis B can be transmitted by unsafe sex and the use of contaminated needles and syringes.

MALARIA: High risk is present throughout this country, including urban areas. There is increased malaria risk along the coast and in the lower Zambezi Valley. Outbreaks are reported in Xai-Xai and Maputo. Falciparum malaria accounts for up to 95% of cases.

Other cases of malaria are due to the *P. malariae* species, rarely to *P. ovale* and *P. vivax*. Chloroquine-resistant falciparum malaria occurs.

• Prophylaxis with atovaquone/proguanil (Malarone), mefloquine (Lariam), or doxycycline is recommended.
• All travelers should take measures to prevent evening and nighttime mosquito bites. Insect bite prevention measures include a DEET-containing repellent applied to exposed skin, insecticide (permethrin) spray applied to clothing and gear, and use of a permethrin-treated bed net at night while sleeping.

MARINE HAZARDS: Stingrays, jellyfish, moon jelly, sea wasps, blue cones, octopi, bat rays and eagle rays, and several species of poisonous fish are common in the country's coastal waters and are potential hazards to unprotected swimmers.

MENINGITIS: Group C meningococcal meningitis outbreaks have been reported. Vaccination is recommended for those travelers who will have close, prolonged contact with the indigenous population.

RABIES: Sporadic cases of human rabies are reported countrywide, including in Maputo. All animal bites or scratches, especially from a dog, should be taken seriously, and immediate medical attention sought. Rabies vaccination may be required. This may require medical evacuation to another country if rabies vaccine and rabies immune globulin are not available locally. Although rabies is rare among tourists, there is risk. No one should pet or pick up any stray animals. All children should be warned to avoid contact with unknown animals.

• Rabies vaccine is recommended for travel longer than 3 months; for shorter stays for travelers who plan to venture off the usual tourist routes, where they may be more exposed to the stray dog population; or when travelers desire extra protection.

SCHISTOSOMIASIS: Risk of urinary schistosomiasis is reported from all provinces, with infection rates up to 60% in some areas. Intestinal schistosomiasis appears almost as widely distributed, with major risk areas along the southern coastal plain, the Zambezi River Valley and the vicinity of Lake Malawi. All travelers should avoid swimming, bathing, or wading in freshwater lakes, ponds, or streams.

TRAVELERS' DIARRHEA: High risk. Potable water is often in critically short supply. Piped water supplies in urban areas may be grossly contaminated. Travelers should observe all food and drink safety precautions. A quinolone antibiotic, combined with loperamide (Imodium), is recommended for the treatment of acute diarrhea.

TUBERCULOSIS: Tuberculosis (TB) is a major public health problem in this country. Travelers planning an extended stay should have a pre-departure TB skin test (PPD test) and be retested after leaving this country.

TYPHOID FEVER: Typhoid vaccine is recommended. Because the typhoid vaccines are only 60% to 70% effective, safe food and drink guidelines should continue to be observed.

YELLOW FEVER: Vaccination recommended. No cases are currently reported.

OTHER DISEASES/HAZARDS: African tick typhus (contracted from dog ticks—often in urban areas—and from bush ticks), brucellosis, filariasis (mosquito-borne; occurs in northern coastal areas and along the Zambezi River), leishmaniasis (endemic levels unclear; may occur), leprosy, plague (no human cases reported since 1978), Rift Valley fever, tuberculosis (a major health problem), trachoma, typhoid fever, and intestinal worms.

Myanmar (Burma)

CAPITAL:
Rangoon
EMBASSY (IN U.S.):
202-332-9044
GMT:
+6 hours
TELEPHONE COUNTRY CODE:
95
USADIRECT:
None

ENTRY REQUIREMENTS
- **Passport/Visa:** Passport and visa required. Single-entry tourist visas (valid for 3 months), issued for stay of up to 28 days. Tourist visas are issued for package or group tours as well as Foreign Independent Travelers (FITs).
- **HIV Test:** Not required.
- **Vaccinations:** A yellow fever vaccination certificate is required of all travelers arriving from infected areas. A certificate is also required of nationals and residents of Myanmar departing for an infected area.

EMBASSIES/CONSULATES
- **U.S. Embassy:** Rangoon, 581 Merchant Street; Tel: 1-282-055 or 282-182.
- **British Embassy:** 80 Strand Road (PO Box 638), Rangoon; Tel: 95-1-256918, 380322, 370863-5, 370867, 371852-3, 256438; Fax: 95-1-370866.
- **Canadian Embassy:** Accredited to the Australian Embassy. 88 Strand Road, Rangoon, Myanmar; Tel: 95-1-251797/8, 251810; Fax: 95-1-246159, 246160.

HOSPITALS/DOCTORS:
Medical care is substandard throughout the country including in Yangon (Rangoon). Adequate medical evacuation coverage for all travelers is a high priority. For serious medical conditions, every effort should be made to go to Bangkok or Singapore. Adequate medical care is available in Yangon at one or more internationally staffed outpatient clinics. Travelers are advised to obtain, before departure, supplemental travel health insurance with specific overseas coverage. The policy should provide for direct

payment to the overseas hospital and/or physician at the time of service and include a medical evacuation benefit.

- Asia Royal Cardiac and Medical Care, Yangon; Tel: 532-802 or 531-003.
- Shwe Gon Dine Specialist Centre, Yangon; Tel: 544-128.
- Bahosi Medical Center (Pioneer Services International Co., Ltd.), War Dan Street, Yangoon; Tel: 212-933 or 211-704.
- International SOS: Myanmar International SOS Limited, The New World Inya Lake Hotel, 37 Kaba Aye Pagoda Road, Yangon, Union of Myanmar; Alarm Center Tel: 95-1-667-777; Alarm Center Fax: 95-1-667-766; Clinic Tel: 95-1-667-779; Clinic Fax: 95-1-667-766

Current Advisories and Health Risks

ANIMAL HAZARDS: Animal hazards include snakes (vipers, cobras), centipedes, scorpions, and black widow spiders. Other possible hazards include crocodiles, pythons, and large, aggressive lizards, all abundant in and near Burma's swamps and rivers, and leopards, wildcats, and bears, all found in the hilly regions of the country.

CHOLERA: This disease is reported active in this country, but the threat to tourists is very low. Cholera vaccine is not routinely recommended.

DENGUE FEVER: Mosquito-borne; highly endemic, countrywide, with peak transmission May through October, especially in urban areas. Prevention consists of taking personal protection measures against daytime insect bites.

FILARIASIS: Bancroftian and Malayan filariasis (mosquito-borne) are highly endemic in rural and urban areas. All travelers should take measures to prevent insect (mosquito) bites.

HEPATITIS: All travelers should receive the hepatitis A vaccine. The hepatitis B carrier rate in the general population is estimated at 10%. Hepatitis B is spread by infected blood, contaminated needles, and unprotected sex. Vaccination is recommended for stays longer than 3 months; for persons at occupational or social risk; and for anyone desiring maximum protection.

INFLUENZA: Influenza is transmitted year-round in the tropics. The flu vaccine is recommended for all travelers at risk.

JAPANESE ENCEPHALITIS: Both rural and urban areas may experience epidemics of Japanese encephalitis (JE), with sporadic cases occurring year-round, countrywide. Peak transmission occurs during the monsoon season, May through December. Vaccination against JE is recommended for travelers who will be staying in rural-agricultural areas longer than 3 to 4 weeks.

MALARIA: Occurs countrywide with the greatest risk of transmission May through December. Malaria is most prevalent in forested foothill areas below 1,000 meters elevation; lower incidences in the plains and urban areas. Rangoon and Mandalay are risk-free. Mefloquine-resistant falciparum malaria is reported along the Thai-Burmese border. Prophylaxis with atovaquone/proguanil (Malarone) or doxycycline is recommended.

MARINE HAZARDS: Stingrays, sea wasps, sea cones, jellyfish, spiny sea urchins, and anemones are common in the country's coastal waters and are potentially hazardous to unprotected or careless swimmers.

POLIOMYELITIS (POLIO): Polio transmission still occurs in Myanmar near the border with Bangladesh, where polio is endemic. All travelers should be fully immunized. Adult travelers should receive a polio booster, as necessary.

RABIES: Sporadic cases of human rabies are reported countrywide. All animal bites or scratches, especially from a dog, should be immediately evaluated for the risk of rabies.

TRAVELERS' DIARRHEA: Potable drinking water is almost nonexistent in Burma. Rural water supplies usually are grossly contaminated, and urban water supplies invariably are subject to contamination. Travelers should observe all food and drink safety precautions. A quinolone antibiotic, combined with loperamide (Imodium), is recommended for the treatment of acute diarrhea. Persistent diarrhea may be due to a parasitic disease such as giardiasis or amebiasis.

TUBERCULOSIS: Tuberculosis (TB) is a major health problem in this country. Travelers planning an extended stay should have a pre-departure TB skin test (PPD test) and be retested after leaving this country. Travelers should avoid crowded public places and public transportation whenever possible. Domestic help hired by long-stay visitors should be screened for TB.

TYPHOID FEVER: Typhoid vaccine is recommended, especially for long-term travelers, adventure travelers, and those wishing maximum disease protection. Because the typhoid vaccines are only 60% to 70% effective, safe food and drink guidelines must be observed.

OTHER DISEASES/HAZARDS: Brucellosis (usually from consumption of unpasteurized dairy products), helminthic infections (ascariasis and hookworm disease are highly endemic in urban and rural areas), echinococcosis, leprosy (highly endemic), rabies (dogs are the primary source of infection), murine typhus (flea-borne), scrub typhus (mite-borne; risk elevated in grassy rural areas), tuberculosis (highly endemic), and typhoid.

Namibia

WINDHOEK
★

CAPITAL:
Windhoek
EMBASSY (IN U.S.):
202-986-0540

GMT:
+2 hours
TELEPHONE COUNTRY CODE:
264
USADIRECT:
None
ENTRY REQUIREMENTS
- **Passport/Visa:** Passport, onward/return ticket and proof of sufficient funds are required. Visa not required for tourist or business stay up to 90 days. Passport and visa required for U.S. travelers; all others should contact the Embassy of Namibia.
- **HIV Test:** Not required.
- **Vaccinations:** Yellow fever vaccine required for persons traveling from a country any part of which is infected and for those older than 1 year of age. Yellow fever vaccine required also for travelers arriving from countries in the endemic zones and for travelers on unscheduled flights who have transited an infected area.

EMBASSIES/CONSULATES
- **U.S. Embassy:** 14 Lossen Street, Ausspannplatz, Private Bag 12029, Windhoek; Tel: 264-61-22-1061; Fax: 264-61-22-9792.
- **Canadian Embassy:** 8th Floor, Metje-Behnsen Building, Independence Avenue, Windhoek; Tel: 264-61-227-417; Fax: 222-859.
- **British High Commission:** 116 Robert Mugabe Avenue, Windhoek (PO Box 22202), Windhoek; Tel: 264-61-274800; Fax: 264-61-228895; e-mail: bhc@mweb.com.na.

HOSPITALS/DOCTORS:
Medical care in Namibia is below Western standards. Travelers should contact the U.S. or Canadian embassy for physican referrals. Travelers are advised to obtain, before departure, supplemental travel health insurance with specific overseas coverage. The policy should provide for direct payment to the overseas hospital and/or physician at the time of service and include a medical evacuation benefit.
- State Hospital, Windhoek (440 beds); general medical/surgical facility.
- Aeromed, Windhoek; Tel: 61-231-236 or 258-108.
- International SOS: International SOS Namibia, 2 Newton Avenue, Pioneers Park, Windhoek, Namibia; Alarm Center/Admin Tel: 264-61-230-505; Alarm Center/Admin Fax: 264-61-248114

Current Advisories and Health Risks

AFRICAN SLEEPING SICKNESS (TRYPANOSOMIASIS): Sporadic cases are reported. Travelers should take personal protection measures against insect (tsetse fly) bites, especially in the Okavango Delta of the Caprivi Strip.

ANIMAL HAZARDS: Animal hazards include snakes (mambas, adders, vipers, cobras, coral snakes), scorpions, sac spiders, and brown widow and black widow spiders.

CHOLERA: This disease is reported active in this country, but the threat to tourists is very low. Cholera vaccine is recommended primarily for people at high risk (e.g., relief workers) who work and live in highly endemic areas under less than adequate sanitary conditions.

HEPATITIS: Hepatitis A vaccine is recommended for all travelers. Hepatitis E is endemic, but the levels are unclear. The hepatitis B carrier rate in the general population is estimated to be as high as 15%. Hepatitis B is spread by infected blood, contaminated needles, and unsafe sex. Vaccination is recommended for stays longer than 3 months; for persons at occupational or social risk; and for any traveler desiring maximum protection.

INFLUENZA: Influenza is transmitted year-round in the tropics. The flu vaccine is recommended for all travelers.

LEISHMANIASIS: Sporadic cases of cutaneous leishmaniasis have been reported, primarily from the southern Keetmanshoop-Karasburg-Bethanie vicinity, and also from the central and more northern areas of the inland plateau and escarpment. Travelers should take measures to prevent sand fly bites. Visceral leishmaniasis is not reported.

MALARIA: Risk occurs primarily from November to May or June, during and just after the rainy season, in the north-central and northeastern rural regions along the borders with Angola, Zambia, and Botswana, including Angola, and the Caprivi strip. Malaria risk has recently extended somewhat into the central plateau and eastern semi-arid areas, but not the coastal desert. Chloroquine-resistant falciparum malaria is widespread. Prophylaxis with atovaquone/proguanil (Malarone), mefloquine (Lariam), or doxycycline is recommended. All travelers should take measures to prevent evening and nighttime mosquito bites.

PLAGUE: Flea-borne; many cases were reported in the late 1990s, mostly from the northern areas, particularly the Oshakati/Onandjokwe vicinity of Owambo District.

POLIOMYELITIS (POLIO): Polio has been reported active in sub-Saharan Africa, including neighboring Botswana. All travelers should be fully immunized against this disease.

RABIES: Most cases are transmitted by dogs, many in urban areas. Jackals may also transmit this disease. All animal bites or scratches should be evaluated medically. Rabies vaccine and rabies immune globulin may be indicated.

SCHISTOSOMIASIS: Risk is present in the northeast along the Angolan border, extending into the Caprivi Strip. Travelers should avoid swimming, bathing, or wading in freshwater lakes, ponds, or streams.

TRAVELERS' DIARRHEA: The water in major urban areas is treated, and in Swakopund, Walvis Bay, and Windhoek, the major hotels and restaurants serve generally safe food and drink. A quinolone antibiotic, combined with loperamide (Imodium), is recommended for the treatment of acute diarrhea. Persistent diarrhea may be due to a parasitic infection such as giardiasis, amebiasis, or cryptosporidiosis.

TUBERCULOSIS: Tuberculosis (TB) is a major health problem in this country. Travelers planning an extended stay should have a pre-departure TB skin test (PPD test) and be retested after returning from this country.

TYPHOID FEVER: Typhoid vaccine is recommended for those traveling off the usual tourist routes, for those visiting friends or relatives, and for long-stay visitors. Because the typhoid vaccines are only 60% to 70% effective, safe food and drink selection remains important.

OTHER DISEASES/HAZARDS: African tick typhus, brucellosis, relapsing fever (tick-borne; sandy floors of village mud huts provide favorable habitat for these ticks), trachoma, typhus, and intestinal worms (very common).

Nepal

KATHMANDU

CAPITAL:
Kathmandu
EMBASSY (IN U.S.):
202-667-4550
GMT:
+5 hours
TELEPHONE COUNTRY CODE:
977
USADIRECT:
0-800-77-001
ENTRY REQUIREMENTS
- **Passport/Visa:** Required. Tourist visas can be purchased on arrival at Tribhuvan International Airport in Kathmandu and at all other ports of entry. For additional information about "trekking permits" and entry requirements, contact the Royal Nepalese Embassy.
- **HIV Test:** Not required.
- **Vaccinations:** A yellow fever vaccination certificate is required from all travelers older than 1 year arriving from infected areas.

EMBASSIES/CONSULATES
- **U.S. Embassy:** Pani Pokhari, Kathmandu; Tel: 1-411-179; Website: www.south-asia. com/USA.
- **Canadian Embassy:** Lazimpat, Kathmandu; Tel: 1-415-193,389,391; e-mail: cco@cco.org.np.
- **British Embassy:** Lainchaur, Kathmandu (PO Box 106); Tel: 977-1-4410583, 4411281, 4414588, 4411590; Fax: 977-1-4411789, 4416723; e-mail: britemb@wlink.com.np.

HOSPITALS/DOCTORS
- CIWEC Clinic Travel Medicine Center, Kathmandu; e-mail: advice@ciwec-clinic. com; Website: http://www.ciwec-clinic.com. The CIWEC Clinic provides inoculations and emergency treatment for travelers; rabies and JE vaccines are available.

- Kalimati Clinic, Kathmandu. This facility can supply Japanese encephalitis (JE) vaccine.
- Patan Hospital, Kathmandu. This is the third largest hospital in the Kathmandu Valley. It provides the most consistent inpatient care in Nepal, but foreigners should be aware that the care and the facilities are not on par with Western expectations. The hospital is located 20 minutes by car from the airport, local tourist spots, and major hotels.
- Baidya & Bansam Hospital (B&B Hospital), Lalitpur. This is a 100-bed private hospital. Emergency services are available 24 hours a day; attending physician on site. The facility is unable to handle neurosurgical or cardiothoracic trauma. B&B Hospital can handle other major trauma cases, multiple trauma cases, and mass casualties.
- Bir Hospital (300 beds); general medical and surgical facility; blood bank.
- United Mission Hospital (100 beds); general medical and surgical facility.

Current Advisories and Health Risks

ALTITUDE SICKNESS (AMS): Risk of altitude sickness, or acute mountain sickness (AMS), increases above 2,200 meters elevation (8,000 feet). Trekkers should follow precautions (e.g., gradual ascent) to reduce the risk of altitude illness and consider prophylaxis with acetazolamide (Diamox). The best treatment for AMS is descent.

CHOLERA: This disease is active in this country, but cholera is an extremely rare disease in travelers from developed countries. Cholera vaccine is not routinely recommended.

DENGUE FEVER: Dengue is not currently reported in Nepal.

HEPATITIS: Hepatitis A is highly endemic, and vaccination is recommended for all nonimmune travelers. Hepatitis E accounts for a majority of cases of acute viral hepatitis in adults in Nepal. To reduce the risk of disease, travelers should drink only boiled, bottled, or chemically treated water. The carrier rate of the hepatitis B virus in the general population is 1% to 6%. Hepatitis B is spread by infected blood, contaminated needles, and unprotected sex. Vaccination is recommended for long-stay (longer than 3 months) travelers; persons who may be at occupational or social risk; and anybody desiring maximum protection.

INFLUENZA: Influenza is transmitted from November through March. Flu vaccine is recommended.

JAPANESE ENCEPHALITIS: Japanese encephalitis (JE) is highly endemic in rural areas of the Terai plain and Inner Terai zone, including hills, mountains, and the Kathmandu Valley, especially in the southern agricultural areas bordering India, at elevations below 1,000 meters. JE is reported year-round, but transmission increases between June and October, declining in late September. Travelers who will be living in known JE-endemic areas, such as most of the Terai, and long-term expatriates who live in Kathmandu, particularly in the rural areas of the valley, should receive JE vaccine. The vaccine is available at most travel clinics in the United States and Canada, and also at the Kalimati Clinic in Kathmandu.

LEISHMANIASIS: Visceral leishmaniasis (kala-azar) occurs year-round, primarily in rural areas in districts of the southeastern Terai region at elevations below 1,000 meters. Districts include Bara, Dhanukha, Jhapa, Mahottari, Makwanpur, Morang, Parsa, Rautahat, Saptari, Sarlahi, Siraha, Sunsari, and Udaipur, adjoining the Indian state of Bihar. Travelers to these districts should take measures to prevent insect (sand fly) bites.

MALARIA: Kathmandu and the northern Himalayan districts are malaria free. Trekkers do not need prophylaxis. Risk does occur along the Indian border in lowland areas of Nepal below 1,200 meters elevation in the plains districts of Bara, Dhanukha, Kapilvastu, Mahotari, Parsa, Rautahat, Rupandehi, and Sarlahi. Malaria occurs year-round in endemic areas; transmission increases during the monsoon season, usually July through October. Chloroquine-resistant falciparum malaria has been reported. Atovaquone/proguanil (Malarone), mefloquine (Lariam), or doxycycline prophylaxis is recommended for travel to malarious areas.

MENINGITIS: Outbreaks of meningococcal disease occur sporadically. Vaccination is not currently recommended for travel to this country.

POLIO: All travelers should be fully immunized against this disease.

RABIES: This disease is prevalent, especially in the Dang district, western Nepal. Human rabies is usually transmitted by dog bites, but bites by monkeys should also be considered dangerous. Pre-travel rabies vaccine should be considered for stays longer than 3 months, for shorter stays involving travel to locations more than 24 hours away from a reliable source of post-exposure rabies vaccine, and for travelers wanting maximum protection. All animal bites or scratches should be medically evaluated. Rabies vaccine and rabies immune globulin are available at the CIWEC Clinic in Kathmandu. All animal bites should be examined as soon as possible by a physician who can administer rabies vaccine, if indicated.

TRAVELERS' DIARRHEA: The food and drink in first-class restaurants and hotels in Kathmandu are generally considered safe. There is a high risk of diarrhea associated with reheated food and blended fruit and yogurt drinks. Potentially contaminated water should be boiled or filtered, especially to remove parasites, such as cryptosporidia, which are not killed by chlorine. The three most common causes of diarrhea in Nepal are *E. coli*, *Campylobacter*, and *Shigella* bacteria. A quinolone antibiotic, combined with loperamide (Imodium), is recommended for the treatment of acute diarrhea. Persistent diarrhea may be due to a parasitic disease such as giardiasis, amebiasis, or cryptosporidiosis.

TUBERCULOSIS: Tuberculosis (TB) is a major health problem in this country. Travelers planning an extended stay should have a pre-departure TB skin test (PPD test) and be retested after leaving this country or returning home.

TYPHOID FEVER: Typhoid vaccine is recommended for those traveling off the usual tourist routes, for those visiting friends or relatives, and for long-stay visitors. Typhoid vaccines are only 60% to 70% effective; safe food and drink precautions should continue to be observed.

OTHER DISEASES/HAZARDS: Cutaneous myiasis (one dose of ivermectin may be curative), cysticercosis, filariasis (occurs primarily in the southern Terai), leprosy (highly prevalent), hookworm disease, AIDS (low incidence; reported primarily in commercial sex workers), scabies, trachoma (a leading cause of blindness in Nepal), and tuberculosis (highly prevalent; a serious public health problem).

Netherlands

CAPITAL:
The Hague
EMBASSY (IN U.S.):
202-483-3176
GMT:
+1 hour
TELEPHONE COUNTRY CODE:
31
USADIRECT:
0-800-022-9111
ENTRY REQUIREMENTS
• **Passport/Visa:** Passport required.
• **HIV Test:** Not required.
• **Vaccinations:** None required.
EMBASSIES/CONSULATES
• **U.S. Embassy:** Lange Voorhout 102, The Hague; Tel: 70-624-911.
• **Canadian Embassy:** Sophialaan 7, The Hague; Tel: 70-614-111.
• **British Embassy:** Lange Voorhout 10, 2514 ED, The Hague; Tel: 31-70-427-0427; Fax: 31-70-427-0347; Website: www.britain.nl.
HOSPITALS/DOCTORS
• Wilhelmina Gasthuis/Zinnan Gasthuis, Amsterdam (923 beds); coronary care; ICU; emergency unit; first aid.
• I.C.C. Academish Ziekenhuis, Rotterdam (1,004 beds); general medical/surgical facility; all major medical specialties.
• Academish Zeikenhuis, Utrecht (1,074 beds); all medical specialties including ob/gyn; pediatrics; emergency unit; hemodialysis; trauma team.
• Bronovo Hospital, The Hague.
• International SOS: SOS (Netherlands) B.V., Physical Location, Beurs-World Trade Center, Beursplein 37, 3011 AA Rotterdam, The Netherlands; Admin Tel: 31-10-206-6188; Admin Fax: 31-10-206-6189.

Current Advisories and Health Risks

EHRLICHIOSIS: Lyme disease occurs in the southern and eastern parts of the Netherlands. A case of human granulocyctic ehrlichiosis was reported in 1998 from the Gelderland region. Travelers to these areas should take precautions to prevent tick bites.

HEPATITIS: Low risk. Hepatitis B accounts for about 20% of all cases of acute viral hepatitis.

LYME DISEASE: Lyme disease occurs in the southern and eastern parts of the Netherlands. A case of human granulocyctic ehrlichiosis was reported in 1998 from the Gelderland region. Travelers to these areas should take precautions to prevent tick bites.

SWIMMER'S EAR (OTITIS EXTERNA): Large outbreaks occurred in 1994 associated with swimming in recreational freshwater lakes during hot summer months. Infection caused by *Pseudomonas* bacteria in the external ear canal. Prevent/treat with acetic acid solution (VōSol Otic ear drops).

TRAVELERS' DIARRHEA: Low risk. Water is safe throughout the Netherlands.

New Caledonia

CAPITAL:
Nouméa
EMBASSY (IN U.S.):
202-944-6000
GMT:
+11 hours
TELEPHONE COUNTRY CODE:
687
USADIRECT:
None
ENTRY REQUIREMENTS
- **Passport/Visa:** No visa required for stays of less than 30 days. New Caledonia is a French Overseas Territory. It is an island group approximately 1,500 km (930 miles) off the northeast coast of Australia. It consists of the island of New Caledonia along with a number of other smaller islands. The Loyalty Group lies to the east of New Caledonia, the main islands being Ouvéa, Lifou, and Maré. The remaining islands are the Chesterfield Group, Hinter, Huon Group, Matthew, and Walpole.
- **Vaccinations:** A yellow fever vaccination certificate is required for travelers older than 1 year of age arriving from infected areas.
- **HIV Test:** Not required.
EMBASSIES/CONSULATES
- **U.S. Embassy:** There is no U.S. Embassy in New Caledonia.

- **Canadian/Australian Embassy:** Immeuble Foch, 7th Floor, 19 rue du Marechal Foch, Nouméa; Tel: 687-272-414; Fax: 687-278-001.
- **British Embassy:** Accredited to the British Embassy in France. 35 Rue Du Faubourg St. Honoré, 75383 Paris Cedex 08; Tel: 33-1-44-51-31-00; Fax: 33-1-44-51-34-83.

HOSPITALS/DOCTORS

- Nouméa has one public hospital, three private clinics, and an adequate selection of pharmacies. Hotels can generally recommend an English-speaking doctor or dentist.
- Although adequate medical care is available in Noumea or Kouma, it is not up to the standards of industrialized countries. Medical care is substandard in the rest of the country. For serious medical conditions, travelers should be evacuated to Australia.
- International SOS: International SOS Nouvelle Caledonie, 32 rue A. Benebig-Vallee des Colons, B.P. 4640-98847 Noumea Cedex, Nouvelle Caledonie; Admin Tel/Fax: 687-261090

Current Advisories and Health Risks

For additional information, consult the Disease Risk Summary for Australia on p. 315.

New Zealand

CAPITAL:
Wellington

EMBASSY (IN U.S.):
202-328-4800

GMT:
+12 hours

TELEPHONE COUNTRY CODE:
64

USADIRECT:
000-911

ENTRY REQUIREMENTS

- **Passport/Visa:** A visa is not required for stays up to 3 months.
- **HIV Test:** Not required.
- **Vaccinations:** None required.

EMBASSIES/CONSULATES

- **U.S. Embassy:** Yorkshire General Building, 4th floor, Corner of Shortland and O'Connell Sts., Auckland; Tel: 64-9-303-2724; Fax: 64-9-366-0870; Website: homepages.ihug.co.nz/~amcongen.
- **Canadian Embassy:** 3rd Floor, 61 Molesworth St., Thorndon, Wellington; Tel: 64-4-473-9577; Fax: 64-4-471-2082; e-mail: wlgtn@dfait-maeci.gc.ca; Website: www.dfait-maeci.gc.ca/newzealand.
- **British High Commission:** 44 Hill Street, Wellington 1 (PO Box 1812), Wellington; Tel: 64-4-924-2888; Fax: 64-4-473-4982; e-mail: PPAMailbox@fco.gov.uk; Website: www.britain.org.nz.

HOSPITALS/DOCTORS:
Medical facilities, both public and private, are of a high standard. Telephone numbers for doctors and hospitals are listed at the front of the white pages of local telephone directories. Should visitors need drugs or pharmaceutical supplies outside normal shopping hours, they should refer to "Urgent Pharmacies" in the local telephone directory for the location of the nearest pharmacy or check with their hotel. Many hotels have doctors on call.

- Wellington Hospital (959 beds); Tel: 4-385-5999.
- Greenlane Hospital (565 beds), Auckland; Tel: 9-604-106.
- Epsom Medical Center, Auckland; Tel: 9-794-540.
- Public Health Service Health Link South, Ltd., 10 Oxford TCE, Christchurch, South Island; Tel: 03-3799-480.
- Lake District Hospital, Frankton, Queenstown (20 beds); Tel: 64-03-442-3053; private hospital that can provide basic emergency services.
- International SOS: International SOS (New Zealand) Ltd., Level 21, 151 Queen Street, PO Box 105- 783, Auckland, New Zealand; Alarm Center Tel: 64-9-359-1635; Alarm Center Fax: 64-9-359-1648.

Current Advisories and Health Risks

ACCIDENTS/ILLNESSES AND MEDICAL INSURANCE
- Accidents and injuries are the leading cause of death among travelers younger than 55 years of age and most often are caused by motor vehicle and motorcycle crashes; drownings, aircraft crashes, homicides, and burns are less common causes.
- Heart attacks cause most fatalities in older travelers.
- Infections cause only 1% of fatalities in overseas travelers, but overall, infections are the most common cause of travel-related illness.
- Travelers are advised to obtain, before departure, supplemental travel health insurance with specific overseas coverage. The policy should provide for direct payment to the overseas hospital and/or physician at the time of service and include a medical evacuation benefit. The policy should also provide 24-hour hotline access to a multilingual assistance center that can help arrange and monitor delivery of medical care and determine if medical evacuation or air ambulance services are required.

HEPATITIS: Nonimmune travelers should consider hepatitis A vaccination. Hepatitis E has not been reported. The carrier rate for hepatitis B virus among the general population is 3%, and up to 10% among the Maori tribe and Asian/Polynesian residents. Vaccination against hepatitis B should be considered for stays longer than 3 months and by short-term travelers desiring maximum protection. Travelers should be aware that hepatitis B can be transmitted by unsafe sex and the use of contaminated needles and syringes. Hepatitis C is endemic.

INFLUENZA: Influenza is transmitted from April through September in the Southern Hemisphere. The flu vaccine is recommended for all travelers older than 50 years of age; all travelers with chronic disease or a weakened immune system; travelers of any age wishing to decrease the risk of this illness; and pregnant women after the first trimester.

TRAVELERS' DIARRHEA: Low risk. Tap water is considered potable countrywide. A quinolone antibiotic, combined with loperamide (Imodium), is recommended for the treatment of acute diarrhea. Diarrhea not responding to antibiotic treatment may be due to a parasitic disease such as giardiasis, or to an intestinal virus.

• Spring/summer outbreaks of *Cryptosporidium* diarrhea have occurred since 1996. Close contact with calves and lambs may increase risk.

Nicaragua

MANAGUA

CAPITAL:
Managua
EMBASSY (IN U.S.):
202-939-6570
GMT:
−6 hours
TELEPHONE COUNTRY CODE:
505
USADIRECT:
174
ENTRY REQUIREMENTS
• **Passport/Visa:** Passport, onward/return ticket and entry fee required for a stay of up to 30 days. For more information, travelers may contact the Consulate of Nicaragua, 1627 New Hampshire Ave. NW, Washington, DC 20009; Tel: 202-939-6531 or 6532.
• **HIV Test:** Not required.
• **Vaccinations:** A yellow fever vaccination certificate is required for travelers older than 1 year of age coming from infected countries.
EMBASSIES/CONSULATES
• **U.S. Embassy:** Kilometer 4½ Carretera Sur, Managua; Tel: 2-666-010.
• **Office of the Canadian Embassy:** De los Pipitos, 2 blocks west 25, Nogal Street, Bolonia, Managua, Nicaragua; Postal Address: PO Box 25, Managua, Nicaragua; Tel: 505-2-68-0433,3323; Fax: 505-2-68-0437; e-mail: mngua@ international.gc.ca.
• **British Embassy:** Accredited to the British Embassy in Costa Rica. Apartado 815, Edificio Centro Colon (11th Floor), San José 1007; Tel: 506-258-2025; Fax: 506-233-9938; e-mail: britemb@racsa.co.cr; Website: www.britishembassycr.com.
HOSPITALS/DOCTORS:
Except in the capital, Managua, medical care is below Western standards, especially in rural areas. Travelers to Nicaragua are advised to obtain, before departure, supplemental travel health insurance with specific overseas coverage. The policy should provide for

direct payment to the overseas hospital and/or physician at the time of service and include a medical evacuation benefit.

- Hospital Manolo Morales, Managua (300 beds); general medical/surgical facility; emergency services.
- Clinica Tiscapa. Hospital Bautista (30 beds); private hospital; 24-hour emergency services; patients must arrange for their own physicians.

Current Advisories and Health Risks

CHAGAS DISEASE: Reported in Atlantic coastal, western, and central regions below 1,500 meters elevation. Travelers sleeping in adobe-style huts and houses should take precautions against nighttime insect bites.

CHOLERA: This disease is active in this country. Cholera vaccine (no longer available in the United States) is recommended primarily for people at high risk (e.g., health-care workers) who work and live in highly endemic areas under less than adequate sanitary conditions.

DENGUE FEVER: Outbreaks of dengue occurs sporadically. The *Aedes* mosquitoes, which transmit dengue fever, bite during the daytime and are present in populous urban areas, as well as resort and rural areas.

HEPATITIS: Hepatitis A vaccine is recommended for all travelers. The hepatitis B carrier rate in the general population is estimated at 1.1%. Hepatitis B is spread by infected blood, contaminated needles, and unprotected sex. Vaccination is recommended for stays longer than 3 months; for persons at occupational or social risk; and for anyone desiring maximum protection.

LEISHMANIASIS: Cutaneous leishmaniasis is reported, primarily from the northern, central, and eastern regions, especially around forested areas. Travelers should take measures to prevent insect (sand fly) bites.

MALARIA: Risk is present countrywide below 1,000 meters elevation, including the outskirts of Managua. *P. vivax* accounts for 95% of cases. Chloroquine prophylaxis is recommended in all rural areas.

RABIES: Low risk; all animal bites, however, should be evaluated without delay.

TRAVELERS' DIARRHEA: All travelers are advised to consume only bottled, boiled, or treated water unless they are assured of the safety of municipal water supplies. A quinolone antibiotic is recommended for the treatment of acute diarrhea. Persistent diarrhea may be due to a parasitic disease such as giardiasis or amebiasis.

TYPHOID FEVER: Typhoid vaccine is recommended for all travelers, with the exception of short-term visitors who restrict their meals to major restaurants and hotels. Because the typhoid vaccines are only 60% to 70% effective, safe food and drink selection remains important.

OTHER DISEASES/HAZARDS: Brucellosis, coccidiomycosis, filariasis (possible risk near Lake Managua), measles, syphilis, AIDS (low incidence), tuberculosis, and strongyloidiasis and other helminthic infections.

Niger

CAPITAL:
Niamey

EMBASSY (IN U.S.):
202-483-4224

GMT:
+1 hour

TELEPHONE COUNTRY CODE:
227

USADIRECT:
None

ENTRY REQUIREMENTS

- **Passport/Visa:** Passport and visa required. Visa must be used within 3 months of issuance. Transit visas required for travelers continuing through Niger. For a tourist visa, the general requirements apply, as well as two copies of a bank statement certifying the traveler has at least $500 in his/her bank account. For further information and fees, contact the Embassy of the Republic of Niger, 2204 R St. NW, Washington, DC 20008; Tel: 202-483-4224.
- **HIV Test:** Not required.
- **Vaccinations:** A yellow fever vaccination certificate is required for all travelers older than 1 year arriving from all countries.

EMBASSIES/CONSULATES

- **U.S. Embassy:** Rue des Ambassades, Niamey; Tel: 227-72-26-61 through 72-26-64; Fax: 227-73-31-67 or 72-31-46; e-mail: usemb@intnet.ne.
- **Canadian Embassy:** Boulevard Mali Béro, B.P. 362, Niamey; Tel: 227-75-36-86/87, Fax: 75-31-07; e-mail: niamy@dfait-maeci.gc.ca.
- **British High Commission:** Accredited to the British High Commission in Ghana. Osu Link, off Gamel Abdul Nasser Avenue, (PO Box 296), Accra; Tel: 233-21-7010650, 221665; Fax: 233-21-7010655; e-mail: high.commission.accra@fco.gov.uk; Website: www.britishhighcommission.gov.uk/ghana.

HOSPITALS/DOCTORS:

Health care in Niger is below Western standards. Travelers are advised to obtain, before departure, supplemental travel health insurance with specific overseas coverage. The policy should provide for direct payment to the overseas hospital and/or physician at the time of service and include a medical evacuation benefit. Only the main hospital centers have reasonable capability. The two main hospitals are:

- Niamey Central Hospital (790 beds); general medical/surgical facility; some specialties.
- Gamkalley Hospital, Niamey (20 beds); basic emergency services only.

Current Advisories and Health Risks

AFRICAN SLEEPING SICKNESS (TRYPANOSOMIASIS): No cases have been reported since 1980.

AIDS/HIV: Heterosexual contact is the predominant mode of transmission. HIV prevalence in the general population is estimated to be low, but up to 10% of surveyed commercial sex workers are HIV positive. All travelers are cautioned against unsafe sex, unsterile medical or dental injections, and unnecessary blood transfusions.

ANIMAL HAZARDS: Animal hazards include snakes (vipers, cobras, puff adders), scorpions, and black widow spiders; hippopotamuses and crocodiles are found along the banks of the Niger River.

CHOLERA: This disease is reported active in this country, but the threat to tourists is very low. Cholera vaccine is recommended primarily for people at high risk (e.g., relief workers) who work and live in highly endemic areas under less than adequate sanitary conditions.

HEPATITIS: All travelers should receive hepatitis A vaccine. Hepatitis E presumably occurs, but endemic levels are unclear. The hepatitis B carrier rate in the general population is estimated at 16% to 21%. Hepatitis B is spread by infected blood, contaminated needles, and unsafe sex. Vaccination is recommended for stays longer than 3 months; for persons at occupational or social risk; and for any traveler desiring maximum protection.

INFLUENZA: Influenza is transmitted year-round in the tropics. The flu vaccine is recommended for all travelers at risk.

LEISHMANIASIS: Foci of cutaneous leishmaniasis have been reported in southern, central, and western (including the Niamey vicinity) areas but probably occur throughout Niger. Visceral leishmaniasis has been reported from the Air Mountains, northwestern Agadez Department; isolated cases have been reported from the Zinder Department. Travelers should take measures to prevent insect (sand fly) bites.

MALARIA: Risk is present year-round countrywide, including major cities. Prophylaxis with atovaquone/proguanil (Malarone), mefloquine (Lariam), or doxycycline is recommended.

MENINGITIS: Southwestern and southern Niger lie within the sub-Saharan "meningitis belt." Quadrivalent meningococcal vaccine is recommended for all travelers during the dry season, December through June, especially if prolonged contact with the local populace is anticipated.

POLIOMYELITIS (POLIO): This disease is active. All travelers should be fully immunized.

RABIES: Rabies vaccine is recommended for all stays longer than 3 months. All animal bites, especially from a dog, should be evaluated without delay.

SCHISTOSOMIASIS: Urinary schistosomiasis is widely distributed in the Niger River valley in the southwest, with foci in south-central Niger along the Nigerian border. Travelers should avoid swimming, bathing, or wading in freshwater lakes, ponds, or streams.

TRAVELERS' DIARRHEA: Niger River water is bacterially contaminated. The water in Lake Chad is highly saline. Travelers should observe all food and drink safety precautions. A quinolone antibiotic, combined with loperamide (Imodium), is recommended for the treatment of acute diarrhea. Persistent diarrhea may be due to a parasitic disease such as giardiasis, amebiasis, or cryptosporidiosis.

TUBERCULOSIS: Tuberculosis (TB) is a major health problem in this country. Travelers planning an extended stay should have a pre-departure TB skin test (PPD test) and be retested after returning home.

TYPHOID FEVER: Typhoid vaccine is recommended for all travelers, with the exception of short-term visitors who restrict their meals to major restaurants and hotels. Because the typhoid vaccines are only 60% to 70% effective, safe food and drink selection remains important.

YELLOW FEVER: A yellow fever vaccination certificate is required for entry to this country.

OTHER DISEASES/HAZARDS: African tick typhus, brucellosis (from consumption of raw dairy products), dracunculiasis, filariasis (mosquito-borne; risk occurs in the rural southwest), leprosy, leptospirosis, onchocerciasis (black fly-borne; endemic foci along rivers in the southwest), tuberculosis (a major health problem), and intestinal worms (very common) are reported.

Nigeria

CAPITAL:
Lagos
EMBASSY (IN U.S.):
202-822-1500
GMT:
+1 hour
TELEPHONE COUNTRY CODE:
234
USADIRECT:
None

ENTRY REQUIREMENTS

- **Passport/Visa:** Passport, proof of sufficient funds, hotel confirmation, and visa are required.
- **HIV Test:** Not required.
- **Vaccinations:** A yellow fever vaccination certificate is required for all travelers older than 1 year arriving from infected areas.

EMBASSIES/CONSULATES

- **U.S. Embassy:** 9 Mambilla, Maitama District, Abuja; Tel: 9-523-0916; e-mail: Lagoscons2@state.gov.
- **Canadian Embassy:** 4 Anifowoshe Street, Victoria Island, Lagos; Tel: 1-262-2512 or 262-2513 or 262-2515; Fax: 262-2516.
- **British High Commission:** Shehu Shangari Way (North), Maitama, Abuja; Tel: 234-9-413-2010, 2011, 2796, 2880, 2883, 2887, 9817; Fax: 234-9-413-3552.

HOSPITALS/DOCTORS:

The quality of government medical facilities in Nigeria is unacceptable by Western standards. Better medical care is available only in private and nonprofit facilities, some of which meet U.S. standards. Travelers are advised to obtain, before departure, supplemental travel health insurance with specific overseas coverage. The policy should provide for direct payment to the overseas hospital and/or physician at the time of service and include a medical evacuation benefit.

- Saint Nicholas Hospital, 57 Campbell St., Lagos Island, Lagos; Tel: 635576 or 631739. Private facility with 57 beds; English-speaking staff; general internal medicine; general surgery; orthopedics; ob/gyn. Ancillary services include laboratory, 24-hour emergency unit. *Comment*: Ultrasound with CT scanner is available 8 kilometers away. No blood bank. Rudimentary facility but recommended by U.S. Embassy personnel.
- Heritage Hospital/The Cardiac Centre Lagos, Victoria Island, Lagos; new facility with 10-bed ICU capability, two ICU ward beds; emergency unit; outpatient noninvasive cardiac evaluations. Facility maintains a high standard of cleanliness, staffing, and equipment.
- International SOS:
  - IMC (International Medical Clinic) Lagos, No 10, Plot 296 Ozumba Mbadiwe Avenue, (Next to Tribes, the same compound with the German Culture Center or GOETHE Institute), Victoria Island, Lagos; Clinic Tel/Fax: 234-1-461-7710/ 261-6026, Medical Emergency: 234-1-775-6080
  - SMI (Service Medical International) Port Harcourt, Intels Camp, Km 12, Aba Expressway, Port Harcourt; Clinic Tel/Fax: 234-74-611436, Medical Emergency: 234-803-4070006; Admin Tel: 234-703-407-0005
  - IEC (Industrial Emergency Clinic) Onne, Prodeco Onne Camp, Onne Road, Onne, medical emergency only: 234-0-803-408-5715; Admin: 234-0-803-740-1949
  - IMC (International Medical Clinic) Warri, House 13A, 2nd Edewor Estate, Effurun, Warri; Clinic Tel/Fax (234) (53) 255023, Medical Emergency: (234) (802) 290-6364

Current Advisories and Health Risks

AFRICAN SLEEPING SICKNESS (TRYPANOSOMIASIS): Sleeping sickness occurs in scattered areas countrywide. There is a higher risk in the Gboko vicinity of Benue State (south-eastern areas confluent with endemic areas of Cameroon) and the southwestern states of Edo and Delta. Extreme northern areas are tsetse-fly free. Travelers should take measures to prevent insect bites.

AIDS/HIV: The disease is already taking hold in the general population, not only among the middle classes—key personnel in government, industry, and the military are now also at substantial risk, and their loss could further devastate this country's economy. Heterosexual activity is driving the AIDS epidemic, and HIV prevalence is estimated at greater than 10% of the sexually active urban population. The current 4 million to 6 million AIDS/HIV cases are expected to increase to 10 million to 15 million by 2010, impacting one fourth of the adults in the country.

ANIMAL HAZARDS: Animal hazards include snakes (vipers, cobras, puff adders, mambas), scorpions, brown recluse spider, and black widow spiders; potentially harmful marine animals which occur in the coastal waters of Nigeria include sea wasps, Portuguese man-of-war, rosy anemones, sea urchins, weevers, eagle rays, and sea nettles.

ARBOVIRAL FEVERS: Dengue fever (low risk; serologic evidence only), West Nile fever and Sindbis fever (moderate risk to highly endemic), chikungunya fever (may occur in cyclic outbreaks). Travelers should take insect bite precautions.

CHOLERA: Although this disease is active in this country, the threat to tourists is very low. Cholera vaccination is recommended primarily for health-care or relief workers.

FILARIASIS: There is transmission of bancroftian filariasis in the south, including the Igwun Basin of Imo State, and the Niger Delta. Travelers should take measures to prevent mosquito bites.

HEPATITIS: Hepatitis A vaccine is recommended. Hepatitis E is likely endemic, but the levels are unclear. The hepatitis B carrier rate is estimated at 8% to 11% in the general population and 15% in more sexually active, high-risk groups. Hepatitis B is spread by infected blood, contaminated needles, and unprotected sex. Vaccination is recommended for stays longer than 3 months; for persons at occupational or social risk; and for any traveler desiring maximum protection. Because the risk of illness or injury during travel cannot be predicted, some experts believe that all travelers should be immunized against hepatitis B because of the risk of receiving a medical injection with an unsterile needle or syringe.

INFLUENZA: Influenza is transmitted year-round in the tropics. The flu vaccine is recommended for all travelers.

588

LEISHMANIASIS: Cutaneous leishmaniasis is reported, with a higher incidence in the north. Visceral leishmaniasis may occur in the northeast. Travelers should take precautions to prevent insect (sand fly) bites.

LOIASIS: Loiasis (loa-loa) is prevalent in the forested areas of the southeast. Travelers should takes measures to prevent insect (fly) bites.

MALARIA: Malaria occurs year-round, countrywide, including urban areas. Risk is elevated during and just after the rainy seasons. Chloroquine-resistant *P. falciparum* malaria is widespread. Prophylaxis with atovaquone/proguanil (Malarone), mefloquine (Lariam), or doxycycline is recommended. All travelers should take measures to prevent evening and nighttime mosquito bites.

MENINGITIS: Nigeria lies within the sub-Saharan "meningitis belt." Quadrivalent meningococcal vaccine is recommended for travelers staying longer than 1 month during the dry season, December to June, and should be considered for shorter stays, any time of the year, if close contact with the local populace is anticipated.

ONCHOCERCIASIS: Widespread along fast-flowing rivers in both savanna and forest zones in parts of all states. Travelers should take measures to prevent insect (black fly) bites.

POLIOMYELITIS (POLIO): This disease is active; there has been little or no polio immunization in Nigeria's northern states for more than a year as a result of a breakdown in the vaccination program. All travelers to Nigeria should be fully immunized against this disease.

RABIES: Rabies is a public health problem in many rural and urban areas, including Lagos. Rabies vaccine is recommended for travel longer than 3 months; for shorter stays for travelers who plan to venture off the usual tourist routes, where they may be more exposed to the stray dog population; and where rabies vaccine may not be available.

SCHISTOSOMIASIS: High risk areas include the Niger River Basin and Ogun-Oshun River Basin, the southwest (including the vicinities of Lagos and Ibadan), the central and northern highlands, and around Lake Chad. Travelers should avoid swimming, bathing, or wading in freshwater lakes, ponds, or streams.

TRAVELERS' DIARRHEA: High incidence. Most of Nigeria's water sources are man-made lakes, rivers, streams, and wells, most of which are contaminated. Travelers should observe all food and drink safety precautions. A quinolone antibiotic, combined with loperamide (Imodium), is recommended for the treatment of acute diarrhea. Persistent diarrhea may be due to a parasitic infection, such as giardiasis, amebiasis, or cryptosporidiosis.

TUBERCULOSIS: Tuberculosis (TB) is a major health problem in this country. Travelers planning an extended stay should have a pre-departure TB skin test (PPD test) and be retested after returning from this country.

TYPHOID FEVER: Typhoid vaccine is recommended for all travelers, with the exception of short-term visitors who restrict their meals to major restaurants and hotels. Because the typhoid vaccines are only 60% to 70% effective, safe food and drink selection remains important.

YELLOW FEVER: The last outbreak of yellow fever was reported in 2000. Vaccination is recommended for all travelers, especially those going outside of urban areas.

OTHER DISEASES/HAZARDS: African tick typhus, brucellosis (often from consumption of unpasteurized dairy products), dracunculiasis (focally endemic), Lassa fever (sporadic outbreaks reported), leprosy, leptospirosis, loiasis (deer fly-borne; occurs in southern rain forests and swamp forests), paragonimiasis (20% infection rate in the Igwun River Basin), relapsing fever (louse-borne), and intestinal worms (very common).

North Korea

PYONGYANG

CAPITAL:
Pyongyang
EMBASSY (IN U.S.):
None
GMT:
+9 hours
TELEPHONE COUNTRY CODE:
850
USADIRECT:
None
ENTRY REQUIREMENTS
Travel to North Korea is severely restricted and further complicated by ongoing tensions between North Korea and the West. U.S. citizens are advised to contact the Department of State regarding travel to North Korea.
EMBASSIES/CONSULATES
The United States does not maintain diplomatic relations with North Korea. Information on travel to North Korea may in some cases be obtained through the North Korea mission to the United Nations. Tel: 212-972-3106.
- •**Canadian Embassy:** Accredited to the Swedish Embassy. Munsudong, Daehak Street, Taedonggang District, Pyongyang, Democratic People's Republic of Korea; Tel: 850-2-381-7908; Fax: 850-2-381-7663; e-mail: ambassaden.pyongyang@foreign.ministry.se; Website: www.sweden.gov.se/sb/d/4189/l/en/pd/4189/e/3647.
- •**British Embassy:** Munsudong Diplomatic Compound, Pyongyang, Democratic People's Republic of Korea; Tel: 850-2-381-7980; Fax: 850-2-381-7985; e-mail: postmaster.PYONX@fco.gov.uk.

HOSPITALS/DOCTORS:
Medical care throughout North Korea is well below western standards. All travelers are advised to carry adequate medical evacuation coverage. If a serious health event occurs, travelers should seek treatment in Japan if possible.

Current Advisories and Health Risks

DENGUE FEVER: No apparent risk.

HELMINTHIC INFECTIONS: Low risk of ascariasis and hookworm disease. Anisakiasis, fascioliasis, fasciolopsiasis, paragonimiasis, and clonorchiasis are endemic. Travelers should avoid eating uncooked water plants and raw or undercooked seafood and shellfish, including Ke Jang (raw crab in soy sauce).

HEMORRHAGIC FEVER WITH RENAL SYNDROME: Risk of hemorrhagic fever with renal syndrome (HFRS) exists year-round, countrywide. Elevated risk is associated with dusty, dry conditions and peak rodent populations. The virus (hantavirus) that causes HFRS is transmitted by infected rodent secretions (e.g., excreta) and virus-carrying dust particles. Most cases occur from October through December, associated with peak human activity in rodent-infected areas during harvest.

HEPATITIS: All nonimmune travelers should receive hepatitis A vaccine before visiting this country. The hepatitis B carrier rate in the general population is estimated at 6% to 9%. Vaccination against hepatitis B is recommended for anyone planning an extended visit to this country. Hepatitis C is endemic.

JAPANESE ENCEPHALITIS: Risk of Japanese encephalitis (JE) is present, but at low levels. Cases of JE have been reported in the southwest during the transmission season, June through October. Vaccination is recommended for travelers who will be staying in rural-agricultural endemic areas longer than 2 to 3 weeks during the peak transmission season. All travelers to rural areas should take measures to prevent mosquito bites.

MALARIA: Low risk. The U.S. military has reported cases of vivax malaria in soldiers stationed near the DMZ. Malaria is not considered a threat to tourists, and prophylaxis is not currently recommended for travelers.

TRAVELERS' DIARRHEA: Medium to high risk outside of first-class hotels and resorts. Travelers are advised to drink only bottled, boiled, filtered, or treated water and to consume only well-cooked food. All fruit should be peeled before consumption. A quinolone antibiotic is recommended for the treatment of acute diarrhea. Diarrhea not responding to antibiotic treatment may be due to a parasitic disease such as giardiasis, amebiasis, or cryptosporidiosis.

OTHER DISEASES/HAZARDS: Filariasis (low risk occurs in southern coastal provinces, especially Chejudo), leptospirosis (elevated risk associated with areas of stagnant water and muddy soils), rabies (extremely rare), murine typhus (flea-borne), scrub typhus (mite-borne; risk elevated in grassy rural areas; 90% of cases occur in October through December), tuberculosis (highly endemic), typhoid fever, and acute hemorrhagic conjunctivitis. Animal hazards include centipedes and black widow spiders. Lynxes, bears, and wild boars may be encountered in remote areas.

Norway

CAPITAL:
Oslo

EMBASSY (IN U.S.):
202-333-6000

GMT:
+1 hour

TELEPHONE COUNTRY CODE:
47

USADIRECT:
800-190-11
800-199-11 (military)

ENTRY REQUIREMENTS
- **Passport/Visa:** Tourist visa not required.
- **HIV Test:** Not required.
- **Vaccinations:** None required.

EMBASSIES/CONSULATES
- **U.S. Embassy:** Drammensveien 18, Oslo; Tel: 22-44-85-50; Fax: 22-56-27-51; Website: www.usa.no.
- **Canadian Embassy:** Wergelandsveien 7, Oslo; Tel: 22-99-53-00; Fax: 22-99-53-01; e-mail: oslo@dfait-maeci.gc.ca.
- **British Embassy:** Thomas Heftyesgate 8, 0244 Oslo; Tel: 47-23-13-27-00; Fax: 47-23-13-27-41; Website: www.britain.no.

HOSPITALS/DOCTORS
- Riks Hospital, Oslo (1,185 beds); Tel: 2-867-010. All specialties.
- Ullevaal Hospital, Oslo; Tel: 2-118-080. All specialties.

Current Advisories and Health Risks

ACCIDENTS/ILLNESSES AND MEDICAL INSURANCE
- Accidents and injuries are the leading cause of death among travelers younger than 55 years of age and most often are caused by motor vehicle and motorcycle crashes; drownings, aircraft crashes, homicides, and burns are less common causes.
- Heart attacks cause most fatalities in older travelers.
- Infections cause only 1% of fatalities in overseas travelers, but overall, infections are the most common cause of travel-related illness.

- Travelers are advised to obtain, before departure, supplemental travel health insurance with specific overseas coverage. The policy should provide for direct payment to the overseas hospital and/or physician at the time of service and include a medical evacuation benefit. The policy should also provide 24-hour hotline access to a multilingual assistance center that can help arrange and monitor delivery of medical care and determine if medical evacuation or air ambulance services are required.

HEPATITIS: There is very low risk of hepatitis A. The hepatitis A vaccine should be considered by nonimmune travelers desiring maximum disease protection. Vaccination against hepatitis B should be considered for stays longer than 3 months and by short-term travelers desiring maximum protection. Travelers should be aware that hepatitis B can be transmitted by unsafe sex and the use of contaminated needles and syringes.

INFLUENZA: Influenza is transmitted from November through March. The flu vaccine is recommended for all travelers older than 50; all travelers with chronic disease or a weakened immune system; travelers of any age wishing to decrease the risk of this illness; and pregnant women after the first trimester.

LYME DISEASE: Lyme disease is transmitted April through September by ticks in brushy areas and forests in the southern coastal areas at elevations below 1,500 meters. Travelers with outdoor exposure in risk areas should take measures to prevent tick bites.

TICK-BORNE ENCEPHALITIS: Risk of tick-borne encephalitis (TBE) exists in rural wooded areas, April through September, along the south and southwest coast. Risk may be present in other areas, but endemic levels are unclear. TBE vaccine, which is available in Europe and Canada, is recommended only for travelers such as hikers and campers, or forestry workers, anticipating extensive outdoor exposure in endemic areas.

TRAVELERS' DIARRHEA: There is a very low risk of bacterial or parasitic diarrhea in this country. Tap water is potable throughout Norway. A quinolone antibiotic, combined with loperamide (Imodium), is recommended for the treatment of acute diarrhea. Diarrhea not responding to treatment with an antibiotic may be due to a parasitic disease such as giardiasis.

Oman

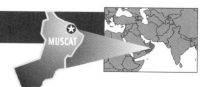

CAPITAL:
Muscat
EMBASSY (IN U.S.):
202-387-1980
GMT:
+4 hours

968
None

ENTRY REQUIREMENTS

- **Passport/Visa:** A 6-month, multiple-entry tourist visa is available, valid for 2 years.
- **HIV Test:** Required for persons newly employed by private sector companies and on renewal of work permit. U.S. test result not accepted.
- **Vaccinations:** A yellow fever and cholera vaccination certificate is required for all travelers older than 1 year arriving from infected areas.

EMBASSIES/CONSULATES

- **U.S. Embassy:** Jameat A'Duwal Al Arabiya Street, Al Khuwair area, Medinat Al Sultan Qaboos 115 Muscat; Tel: 698-989; Fax: 699-189; e-mail: aemctcns@omantel.net.om; Website: www.usa.gov.om.
- **Canadian Embassy:** Flat No. 310, Building 477, Way 2907, Moosa Abdul Rahman Hassan Building, A'Noor Street, Ruwi; Tel: 791-738; Fax: 791-740; e-mail: canada_consulate_oman@hotmail.com.
- **British Embassy:** PO Box 185, Mina Al Fahal, Postal Code 116; Tel: 968-24609000; Fax: 968-24609010; e-mail: Enquiries.Muscat@fco.gov.uk; Website: www. britishembassy.gov.uk/oman.

HOSPITALS/DOCTORS:

Local medical treatment varies in quality and can be inadequate. There is no ambulance service in this country.

Current Advisories and Health Risks

ACCIDENTS/ILLNESSES AND MEDICAL INSURANCE

- Accidents and injuries are the leading cause of death among travelers younger than 55 years of age and most often are caused by motor vehicle and motorcycle crashes; drownings, aircraft crashes, homicides, and burns are less common causes.
- Heart attacks cause most fatalities in older travelers.
- Infections cause only 1% of fatalities in overseas travelers, but overall, infections are the most common cause of travel-related illness.
- Travelers are advised to obtain, before departure, supplemental travel health insurance with specific overseas coverage. The policy should provide for direct payment to the overseas hospital and/or physician at the time of service and include a medical evacuation benefit. The policy should also provide 24-hour hotline access to a multilingual assistance center that can help arrange and monitor delivery of medical care and determine if medical evacuation or air ambulance services are required.

ANIMAL HAZARDS: Centipedes, scorpions, and black widow spiders inhabit the dry interior regions of Oman.

HEPATITIS: Hepatitis A vaccine is recommended for all nonimmune travelers. Hepatitis E has not been reported but likely occurs. Hepatitis B is moderately endemic. Vaccination against hepatitis B should be considered for stays longer than 3 months and by short-term travelers desiring maximum protection. Travelers should be aware that hepatitis B can be transmitted by unsafe sex and the use of contaminated needles and syringes.

INFLUENZA: Influenza is transmitted year-round in the tropics. The flu vaccine is recommended for all travelers older than 50; all travelers with chronic disease or a weakened immune system; travelers of any age wishing to decrease the risk of this illness; and pregnant women after the first trimester.

LEISHMANIASIS: Presumably widespread and focally distributed countrywide. Transmission presumably occurs during April through October, peaking during July through September. Both cutaneous and visceral forms of leishmaniasis may be present in endemic areas. Visceral leishmaniasis is known to occur in focal rural foothill and mountainous areas in the Sharqiyah and Dhahirah regions. Travelers should take protective measures against insect (sand fly) bites.

MALARIA: The risk of malaria is low and is confined to very remote areas of Musandam Province. The capital area around Muscat and the southern Dhofar region are risk-free. Countrywide, *P. falciparum* causes approximately 96% of cases of malaria, *P. vivax* the remainder. Chloroquine-resistant falciparum malaria may be present.
- Malaria chemoprophylaxis is currently not recommended for travel to this country.
- Visitors should take measures to prevent insect bites.
- A travel medicine specialist should be consulted for specific recommendations if extended travel to risk areas is anticipated.

MARINE HAZARDS: Sea urchins and marine rays inhabit the coastal waters of Oman and could pose a hazard to swimmers.

PLAGUE: Plague may be transmitted in some rural areas of this country. Most travelers will not come in contact with the infected fleas or rodents, or with humans with plague pneumonia. People at most risk include anthropologists, geologists, and some medical or missionary personnel.

RABIES: Rabies occurs sporadically in stray dogs and is rarely reported in humans. Rabies vaccine is recommended for persons anticipating an extended stay, for those whose work or activities may bring them into contact with animals, or when extra protection is desired. Prompt medical evaluation and treatment of any animal bite are essential, regardless of vaccination status.

SCHISTOSOMIASIS: Risk for intestinal schistosomiasis exists in southern coastal areas of the Dhofar (Zufar) Governate (near Arazat, Mirbat, Taqah, and Salalah). "Swimmer's itch" (cercarial dermatitis), due probably to noninvasive animal schistosomes, is reported after exposure in freshwater pools in Wadi Darbat. Travelers should avoid swimming or wading in freshwater rivers, ponds, streams, or irrigated areas.

TRAVELERS' DIARRHEA: First-class hotels and restaurants in Muscat generally serve reliable food and potable water. Travelers are advised, however, to drink only bottled, boiled, or treated water and to consume only well-cooked food. A quinolone antibiotic, combined with loperamide (Imodium), is recommended for the treatment of acute diarrhea. Diarrhea not responding to antibiotic treatment may be due to a parasitic disease such as giardiasis, cryptosporidiosis, or amebiasis.

- -

TUBERCULOSIS: Tuberculosis (TB) is a major public health problem in this country. Travelers planning an extended stay should have a pre-departure TB skin test (PPD test) and be retested after leaving this country.

- -

TYPHOID FEVER: Typhoid fever is recommended for long-term travelers, adventure travelers, and those wishing maximum disease protection. Because the typhoid vaccines are only 60% to 70% effective, safe food and drink selection remains important.

- -

OTHER DISEASES/HAZARDS: Boutonneuse fever, brucellosis (usually transmitted by raw goat/sheep milk, especially in the southern Dhofar region), dengue (endemic status unclear; probably not active), echinococcosis (carried by stray dogs; reported sporadically, especially in northern areas), filariasis (cases of bancroftian filariasis are reported annually), leptospirosis, myiasis (due to larvae of the sheep nasal bot fly; a case of ophthalmic myiasis has been reported, with fly maggots infecting the superficial periocular tissue), onchocerciasis (historically reported from southern areas; may occur), rabies (foxes are the main reservoir, with spillover into the dog population), relapsing fever (tick-borne), sandfly fever (viral; mosquito-borne), typhus (flea-borne and louse-borne), and helminthic infections (roundworm, hookworm, and whipworm infections are common in rural areas; incidence is estimated at 5%).

Pakistan

CAPITAL:
Islamabad
EMBASSY (IN U.S.):
203-939-6200
GMT:
+5 hours
TELEPHONE COUNTRY CODE:
92
USADIRECT:
00-800-01001
ENTRY REQUIREMENTS
- **Passport/Visa:** Passport and visa are required. Obtain visa before arrival. Business visa requires company letter, invitation, and fee. Include prepaid envelope for return of passport by registered mail. For applications and inquiries in the Washington, DC

area, contact the Consular Section of the Embassy of Pakistan, 3517 International Court NW, Washington, DC 20008; Tel: 202-243-6500.

- **HIV Test:** Test required if visitors staying more than 1 year.
- **Vaccinations:** A yellow fever vaccination certificate is required for all travelers older than 1 year arriving from any country any part of which is infected. A certificate is also required from those arriving from any country in the Yellow Fever Endemic Zone. *Cholera:* A vaccination certificate is required from travelers arriving from any country any part of which is infected.

EMBASSIES/CONSULATES

- **U.S. Embassy:** Diplomatic Enclave, Ramna 5, Islamabad; Tel: 51-826-161. The Consular Section is located separately in the USAID building, 18 Sixth Ave., Ramna 5; Tel: 51-824-071.
- **Canadian Embassy:** Diplomatic Enclave, Sector G-5, Islamabad; Tel: 92-51-227-91-00; Fax: 92-51-227-91-10; e-mail: isbad@dfait-maeci.gc.ca; Website: www.dfait-maeci.gc.ca/islamabad.
- **British High Commission:** Diplomatic Enclave, Ramna 5, PO Box 1122, Islamabad; Tel: 92-51-201-2000; Fax: 92-51-2012063-Chancery; e-mail: bhc-ukti@dsl.net.pk.

HOSPITALS/DOCTORS:

Travelers are advised to obtain, before departure, supplemental travel health insurance with specific overseas coverage. The policy should provide for direct payment to the overseas hospital and/or physician at the time of service and include a medical evacuation benefit.

- Jinnah Central Hospital, Karachi (800 beds); government hospital; all specialties.
- Seventh Day Adventist Hospital, Karachi (150 beds); Tel: 92-21-721-8021 to 8024. Private hospital; most specialties; emergency services 24 hours a day. The facility has limited trauma capability.
- United Christian Hospital, Lahore.
- Khyber Medical Center, Peshawar.
- Pakistan Institute of Medical Sciences (PIMS), Islamabad; Tel: 92-51-6-1170. This is a 600-bed hospital with emergency services available 24 hours a day. The hospital is a major trauma center and a tertiary care center, capable of handling major trauma cases.

Current Advisories and Health Risks

CHOLERA: This disease is not officially reported as active in this country. Cases do occur, but the threat to travelers is very low.

DENGUE FEVER: Outbreaks of this mosquito-transmitted disease, including dengue hemorrhagic fever, occur in both urban and rural areas. Travelers should take measures to prevent daytime insect bites.

HEPATITIS: All travelers should receive hepatitis A vaccine. There is a very high incidence of hepatitis E in this country. All travelers should avoid drinking water that may be virus-contaminated (e.g., untreated well water, tap water, ground water). The hepatitis B carrier rate in the general population is estimated at 5% to 10%. Hepatitis B is spread by infected blood, contaminated needles, and unsafe sex. Vaccination is recommended for stays longer than 3 months; for persons at occupational or social risk; and for any traveler desiring maximum protection.

INFLUENZA: Influenza is transmitted from November through March. Flu vaccine is recommended for travelers at risk.

JAPANESE ENCEPHALITIS: Risk of Japanese encephalitis (JE) is low and mostly confined to areas near Karachi and the Indus Delta, June through January. Vaccination against JE is recommended for travelers who will be staying more than 3 to 4 weeks in rural-agricultural endemic areas during the peak transmission period.

LEISHMANIASIS: Cutaneous leishmaniasis occurs sporadically in the urban and semirural areas at the margin of the deserts, especially in the west, in Baluchistan. Visceral leishmaniasis occurs primarily in northern areas (northern Punjab Province and the Northwest Frontier Province) at elevations between 2,000 and 6,000 meters. Travelers to these regions should protect themselves against sand fly bites.

MALARIA: Malaria is endemic countrywide at elevations below 6,500 feet (2,000 meters) including the cities. The greatest risk of malaria is in the Punjab, especially after the rainy season, July through August. Prophylaxis with atovaquone/proguanil (Malarone), mefloquine (Lariam), or doxycycline is recommended.

POLIOMYELITIS (POLIO): This disease is active in the Indian subcontinent. All travelers should be fully immunized.

RABIES: Rabies is considered a public health problem in many rural and periurban areas. All animal bites or scratches, especially from a dog, should be evaluated without delay. Rabies vaccine may be required. Although rabies is rare among travelers, there is risk. No one should pet or pick up any stray animals. All children should be warned to avoid contact with unknown animals. Rabies vaccine is recommended for travel longer than 3 months, and for shorter stays for travelers who plan to visit rural areas.

TRAVELERS' DIARRHEA: High risk. Although urban areas usually have water treatment facilities, central distribution systems, and public taps, none of the water in Pakistan should be considered potable. A quinolone antibiotic, combined with loperamide (Imodium), is recommended for the treatment of acute diarrhea. Persistent diarrhea may be due to a parasitic disease such as giardiasis, amebiasis, or cryptosporidiosis.

TUBERCULOSIS: Tuberculosis (TB) is a major health problem in this country. Travelers planning an extended stay should have a pre-departure TB skin test (PPD test) and be retested after leaving this country.

TYPHOID FEVER: Highly endemic. Typhoid vaccine is recommended, although it is only 60% to 70% effective. Food and drink precautions should continue to be observed.

OTHER DISEASES: Brucellosis (human cases associated with occupational exposure to livestock and consumption of unpasteurized dairy products), dracunculiasis (focally endemic in NW Frontier, Punjab, Sind provinces), echinococcosis, filariasis (bancroftian filariasis occurs in the southern Indus Delta), leprosy (widespread among lower socioeconomic groups), Indian tick typhus (boutonneuse fever, reported sporadically), melioidosis (sporadic cases), sand fly fever (highly endemic below 1,800 meters elevation; risk is higher in nondesert areas of Pakistan), West Nile fever (mosquito-transmitted; absent during winter), soil-transmitted intestinal worms (ascariasis and hookworm disease widespread, especially in rural areas), trachoma (widespread in western rural areas), tuberculosis (highly endemic in rural areas), typhoid fever, and typhus (both murine and scrub typhus occur).

Palau

KOROR

CAPITAL:
Koror
EMBASSY (IN U.S.):
202-624-7793
GMT:
+9 hours
TELEPHONE COUNTRY CODE:
680
USADIRECT:
None
ENTRY REQUIREMENTS
• **Passport/Visa:** Not required of U.S. citizens.
• **HIV Test:** Not required.
• **Vaccinations:** None required.
EMBASSIES/CONSULATES
• **U.S. Embassy:** Koror 96940; Tel: 680-488-2920; Fax: 680-488-2911.
• **Canadian Embassy:** Accredited to the Australian Embassy in Micronesia. H&E Enterprises Building, Kolonia, Pohnpei, Micronesia; Postal Address: PO Box S, Kolonia, Pohnpei, Micronesia; Tel: 691-320-5448; Fax: 691-320-5449.
• **British High Commission:** Accredited to the British High Commission in Fiji. Victoria House, Gladstone Road, Suva (PO Box 1355); Tel: 679-3229100; Fax: 679-3229132; Website: http://www.britishhighcommission.gov.uk/fiji.
HOSPITALS/DOCTORS:
Travelers should contact their embassy or consulate for physician referrals.

Current Advisories and Health Risks

ACCIDENTS/ILLNESSES AND MEDICAL INSURANCE
• Accidents and injuries are the leading cause of death among travelers younger than 55 years of age and most often are caused by motor vehicle and motorcycle crashes; drownings, aircraft crashes, homicides, and burns are less common causes.

- Heart attacks cause most fatalities in older travelers.
- Infections cause only 1% of fatalities in overseas travelers, but overall, infections are the most common cause of travel-related illness.
- Travelers are advised to obtain, before departure, supplemental travel health insurance with specific overseas coverage. The policy should provide for direct payment to the overseas hospital and/or physician at the time of service and include a medical evacuation benefit. The policy should also provide 24-hour hotline access to a multilingual assistance center that can help arrange and monitor delivery of medical care and determine if medical evacuation or air ambulance services are required.

DENGUE FEVER: Sporadic cases and outbreaks of dengue fever are reported. Travelers should take protective measures against mosquito bites.

FILARIASIS: Sporadic cases and outbreaks are reported. Travelers should take protective measures against mosquito bites.

HEPATITIS: All nonimmune travelers should receive hepatitis A vaccine. The hepatitis B carrier rate in the general population is approximately 15%. Vaccination against hepatitis B should be considered for stays longer than 3 months and by short-term travelers desiring maximum protection. Travelers should be aware that hepatitis B can be transmitted by unsafe sex and the use of contaminated needles and syringes.

INFLUENZA: Influenza is transmitted year-round in the tropics. The flu vaccine is recommended for all travelers older than age 50; all travelers with chronic disease or a weakened immune system; travelers of any age wishing to decrease the risk of this illness; and pregnant women after the first trimester.

JAPANESE ENCEPHALITIS: Sporadic cases and outbreaks of Japanese encephalitis (JE) are reported. Travelers should take protective measures against mosquito bites.

MALARIA: There is no risk of malaria in this country.

MARINE HAZARDS: Swimming-related hazards include corals, jellyfish, sharks, sea urchins, and sea snakes. Ciguatera poisoning is prevalent and can result from eating coral reef fish such as grouper, snapper, sea bass, jack, and barracuda. The ciguatoxin is not destroyed by cooking.

ROAD SAFETY: Main roads in Koror are in good condition; side roads are in poor condition. Roads on the island of Babelthaob are under construction, with completion scheduled for 2004. The maximum speed limit is 25 miles per hour, but the speed limit is slower in congested areas. Passing slow-moving vehicles is prohibited.

TRAVELERS' DIARRHEA: Medium risk. A quinolone antibiotic, combined with loperamide (Imodium), is recommended for the treatment of diarrhea.

Panama

CAPITAL:
Panama City
EMBASSY (IN U.S.):
202-483-1407
GMT:
−5 hours
TELEPHONE COUNTRY CODE:
507
USADIRECT:
800-0109
ENTRY REQUIREMENTS
- **Passport/Visa:** U.S. citizens must have a passport or proof of citizenship. A tourist card or visa is required.
- **HIV Test:** Test required for persons adjusting visa status while in Panama.
- **Vaccinations:** None required, but Panama recommends yellow fever vaccination for all travelers who are destined for Chepo, Darien, or San Blas. *Routine immunizations:* All travelers should be up to date on tetanus-diphtheria, measles-mumps-rubella, polio, and varicella immunizations.

EMBASSIES/CONSULATES
- **U.S. Embassy:** 40th St. and Balboa Ave., Consular Section, Panama City; Tel: 225-6988.
- **Canadian Embassy:** World Trade Center, Calle 53E, Marbella, Galería Comercial, Piso 1, Panama City, Panama; Tel: 507-264-9731, 7115; Fax: 507-263-8083; e-mail: panam@international.gc.ca; Website: www.panama.gc.ca.
- **British Embassy:** Swiss Tower, Calle 53, PO Box 0816-07946 Panama City; Tel: 507-269-0866; Fax: 507-223-0730; e-mail: britemb@cwpanama.net.

HOSPITALS/DOCTORS:
High-quality medical care is available in Panama, and most physicians speak English. Travelers are advised to obtain, before departure, supplemental travel health insurance with specific overseas coverage. The policy should provide for direct payment to the overseas hospital and/or physician at the time of service and include a medical evacuation benefit.
- Policlinica General y Especializada de Rio Abajo, Rio Abajo, Panama City; Tel: 224-4767.
- Centro Especializado San Fernando, Panama City; Tel: 229-2299.

Current Advisories and Health Risks

AIDS/HIV: Adult HIV prevalence in 2005 reported at 0.9%. Panama has joined Costa Rica and seven other Central American nations in providing antiretroviral therapy to all people who have AIDS.

CHAGAS DISEASE: Chagas disease occurs at low levels in most rural areas of Panama, including the former Canal Zone.

CHOLERA: This disease is active in this country, but the risk to travelers is extremely low; cholera vaccination is not routinely recommended.

DENGUE FEVER: Endemic year-round, countrywide, with risk elevated May through December. All travelers should take measures to prevent mosquito bites.

HEPATITIS: Hepatitis A vaccine is recommended for all travelers. The hepatitis B carrier rate in the general population is estimated at 0.7% to 1.4%. Hepatitis B is spread by infected blood, contaminated needles, and unsafe sex. Vaccination is recommended for stays longer than 3 months; for persons at occupational or social risk; and for any traveler desiring maximum protection.

LEISHMANIASIS: Scattered cases of cutaneous leishmaniasis occur countrywide in rural areas, but most cases are reported from the western or west-central areas. Visceral leishmaniasis is not reported. All travelers should take measures to prevent sand fly bites.

MALARIA: Low-level risk exists year-round in the rural areas of eastern (Darien and San Blas) and western (Bocas Del Toro, Chiriqui, and Veraguas) provinces. Areas immediately adjacent to the Panama Canal and all major urban areas are probably risk-free. Travelers to Darién Province, San Blas Province, and the San Blas Islands (where chloroquine-resistant falciparum malaria is reported) should take one of the following antimalarial drugs: atovaquone/proguanil (Malarone), doxycycline, mefloquine, or primaquine (in special circumstances). Chloroquine is the recommended drug in Bocas Del Toro Province of Panama. All travelers should take measures to prevent mosquito bites.

TRAVELERS' DIARRHEA: Variable risk. All water sources outside major hotels should be considered potentially contaminated. A quinolone antibiotic is recommended for the treatment of diarrhea. Persistent diarrhea may be due to a parasitic infection such as giardiasis, amebiasis, or cryptosporidiosis.

TYPHOID FEVER: Typhoid vaccine is recommended for those traveling off the usual tourist routes, for those visiting friends or relatives, and for long-stay visitors. Because the typhoid vaccines are only 60% to 70% effective, safe food and drink selection remains important.

YELLOW FEVER: This country is in the Yellow Fever Endemic Zone. Yellow fever vaccination is recommended for all travelers older than 9 months of age. No cases of yellow fever have been reported since the 1940s.

OTHER DISEASES/HAZARDS: Cysticercosis, histoplasmosis (from exposure to bat guano), leptospirosis, paragonimiasis (from raw freshwater crabs or crayfish), rabies (currently a minor threat to humans; dogs account for most human exposure), tick-borne rickettsioses (spotted fever group), tuberculosis (the incidence is declining), and intestinal helminth infections, including strongyloidiasis.

Papua New Guinea

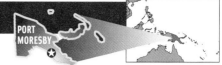

CAPITAL:
Port Moresby

EMBASSY (IN U.S.):
202-745-3680

GMT:
+10 hours

TELEPHONE COUNTRY CODE:
675

USADIRECT:
0-507-128-80

ENTRY REQUIREMENTS

- **Passport/Visa:** Passport, visa, onward/return ticket, and proof of sufficient funds are required.
- **HIV Test:** Test required to obtain a work permit or for anyone seeking residency.
- **Vaccinations:** A yellow fever vaccination certificate is required for all travelers older than 1 year arriving from infected areas.

EMBASSIES/CONSULATES

- **U.S. Embassy:** Armit St., Port Moresby; Tel. 211-445-594 or 054.
- **Canadian Embassy:** Accredited to the Australian High Commission. Godwit Road, Waigani, NCD, Port Moresby, Papua New Guinea; Tel: 675-325-9333; Fax: 675-325-9239.
- **British High Commission:** Locked Mail Bag 212, Waigani NCD 131, Port Moresby; Tel: 675-325-1643, 3251-645, 325-1659, 325-1677; Fax: 675-325-3547; e-mail: bhcpng@ datec.net.pg.

HOSPITALS/DOCTORS:
Medical care in Papua New Guinea is variable. Medical facilities range from a large tertiary care center in Port Moresby to missionary hospitals and clinics in rural and remote areas. Travelers are advised to obtain, before departure, supplemental travel health insurance with specific overseas coverage. The policy should provide for direct payment to the overseas hospital and/or physician at the time of service and include a medical evacuation benefit.

- University of Papua New Guinea-Port Moresby General Hospital; Tel: 324-8200. Busy teaching hospital and tertiary care center.
- Jacobi Medical Center, Port Moresby; Tel: 325-5355.
- International SOS: Niugini Air Rescue, Suite #E, 3rd Floor, Pacific Place, Boroko NCD, Port Moresby, Papua New Guinea; Tel: 675-323-2033; Fax: 675-323-5244

Current Advisories and Health Risks

ANIMAL HAZARDS: Animal hazards include snakes, centipedes, scorpions, red back spiders, mouse spiders. Bites by taipans (the world's deadliest snake) are responsible for 80% of snake bites in the Central Province and the National Capital District of Papua

New Guinea. Other possible hazards include crocodiles, tigers, panthers, bears, wild pigs, and wild cattle. Large leeches, which are not poisonous but inflict slow-healing, easily infected bites, are abundant in the swamps and streams of this country.

CRIME/PERSONAL SECURITY: Crime and personal security are serious concerns. All travelers should obtain a Papua New Guinea Consular Information Sheet from the U.S. State Department before departure.

DENGUE FEVER: Countrywide risk, except for the deep mountain interior above 1,000 meters elevation. Urban areas and low-lying rural areas are considered at higher risk during the monsoon seasons, December through February and May through September. Travelers should take measures to prevent dayime mosquito bites.

FILARIASIS: Bancroftian filariasis is highly endemic in coastal and low-lying regions and some islands off the mainland. All travelers should take measures to avoid mosquito bites.

HEPATITIS: Hepatitis A vaccine is recommended for all travelers. The hepatitis B carrier rate in the general population varies, ranging from 5% to 25%. Hepatitis B is spread by infected blood, contaminated needles, and unsafe sex. Vaccination is recommended for stays longer than 3 months; for persons at occupational or social risk; and for any traveler desiring maximum protection.

INFLUENZA: Influenza is transmitted year-round in the tropics; flu vaccine is recommended for all travelers.

JAPANESE ENCEPHALITIS: Low risk. Endemic status uncertain, but Japanese encephalitis (JE) occurs in neighboring Irian Jaya. Vaccination against this disease is recommended for travelers who will be staying in rural-agricultural endemic areas longer than several weeks. All travelers should take protective measures against mosquito bites, especially in the evening.

MALARIA: Highly endemic. Risk occurs countrywide (including urban areas) year-round at elevations below 1,800 meters; elevated risk is present along coastal areas and in the lowlands, especially during the monsoon, December through February. Chloroquine-resistant falciparum malaria is widespread, and mefloquine-resistant *P. falciparum* has been reported. *P. vivax* strains resistant to chloroquine and primaquine have also been reported. Malaria prophylaxis with atovaquone/proguanil (Malarone), mefloquine (Lariam), or doxycycline prophylaxis is recommended.

MARINE HAZARDS: Stingrays, sea wasps, the Indo-Pacific man-of-war, and poisonous sea cones are common in the country's coastal waters and are potentially hazardous to unprotected or careless swimmers. Fatal tetrodotoxin poisoning has occurred after the consumption of porcupine fish. Ciguatera poisoning may occur and can result from eating coral reef fish such as grouper, snapper, sea bass, jack, and barracuda. The ciguatoxin is not destroyed by cooking.

RABIES: There is no rabies reported from Papua New Guinea.

TRAVELERS' DIARRHEA: Medium to high risk outside of first-class hotels and resorts. A quinolone antibiotic, combined with loperamide (Imodium), is recommended for the treatment of acute diarrhea. Persistent diarrhea may be due to a parasitic infection such as giardiasis, amebiasis, or cryptosporidiosis.

TUBERCULOSIS: Tuberculosis (TB) is a major health problem in this country. Travelers planning an extended stay should have a pre-departure TB skin test (PPD test) and be retested after returning from this country.

TYPHOID FEVER: Typhoid vaccine is recommended for all travelers, with the exception of short-term visitors who restrict their meals to major restaurants and hotels, such as business travelers and cruise passengers. Because the typhoid vaccines are only 60% to 70% effective, safe food and drink selection remains important.

OTHER DISEASES/HAZARDS: Angiostrongyliasis, brucellosis (low incidence), helminthic infections (ascariasis, hookworm disease, and strongyloidiasis are highly endemic in urban and rural areas), paragonimiasis, leprosy (highly endemic), leptospirosis, melioidosis, scrub typhus, tuberculosis (highly endemic), and typhoid fever.

Paraguay

ASUNCIÓN

CAPITAL:
Asunción
EMBASSY (IN U.S.):
202-483-6960
GMT:
−4 hours
TELEPHONE COUNTRY CODE:
595
USADIRECT:
00-811-800
ENTRY REQUIREMENTS
• **Passport/Visa:** A valid passport is required. No visa is required for a 3-month stay.
• **HIV Test:** Not required.
• **Vaccinations:** A yellow fever vaccination certificate is required of travelers arriving from an infected area. The certificate is also required of those arriving from countries in the Yellow Fever Endemic Zones.
EMBASSIES/CONSULATES
• **U.S. Embassy:** 1776 Mariscal Lopez Avenue, Asunción; Tel: 21-213-715; e-mail: usconsulasuncion@hotmail.com.
• **Canadian Embassy:** Prof. Ramírez No. 3 at Juan de Salazar, Asunción; Tel: 21-227-207; Fax: 227-208; e-mail: jsperat@conexion.com.py.

- British Embassy: Accredited to the British Embassy in Argentina. Dr. Luis Agote 2412/52, 1425 Capital Federal, Buenos Aires; Tel: 54-11-4808-2200.

HOSPITALS/DOCTORS:
Medical care in Paraguay is adequate for most needs. Travelers are advised to obtain, before departure, supplemental travel health insurance with specific overseas coverage. The policy should provide for direct payment to the overseas hospital and/or physician at the time of service and include a medical evacuation benefit.

- Medical School: Universidad Nacional de Asunción, Facultad de Ciencias Médicas, Avenida Dr Montero, Asunción; Tel: 21-481-549; Website: www.una.py.
- Adventist Hospital, Asunción (35 beds); missionary hospital; general medical/surgical facility; physicians on 24-hour call.
- Centro Médico Bautista/Baptist Medical Center, Asunción.

Current Advisories and Health Risks

AIDS/HIV: There is relatively low prevalence of HIV/AIDS in the general population.

ANIMAL HAZARDS: Animal hazards include snakes (vipers, coral snakes), centipedes, scorpions, black widow spiders, brown recluse spiders, banana spiders, and wolf spiders. Species of carnivorous fish are present in the fresh waters of Paraguay.

CHAGAS DISEASE: Widely distributed in nearly all rural areas. Risk exists primarily in the Conception, San Pedro, Cordillera, and Paraguari departments in areas where there are adobe-style huts and houses. These structures often harbor the night-biting triatomid (assassin) bugs that transmit this disease. Travelers residing in such structures should spray the sleeping areas with a permethrin insecticide.

DENGUE FEVER: Endemic, but levels are unclear. Risk exists primarily during the warmer months (November through April), especially in urban areas. Precautions against daytime mosquito bites are advised.

HEPATITIS: All travelers should receive hepatitis A vaccine. The hepatitis B carrier rate in the general population is estimated at less than 1%. Hepatitis B is spread by infected blood, contaminated needles, and unprotected sex. Vaccination is recommended for stays longer than 3 months; for persons at occupational or social risk; and for anyone desiring maximum protection.

INFLUENZA: Influenza is transmitted from April through September in the southern hemisphere; flu vaccine is recommended for all travelers.

LEISHMANIASIS: Cutaneous and mucocutaneous leishmaniasis are highly endemic in rural areas in the departments of Alto Parana, Amambay, Caaguazu, Caazapa, Canendiyu, Guaira, and San Pedro. The highest incidence occurs in Caaguazu Department. Travelers should take measures to prevent insect (sand fly) bites.

MALARIA: Malaria risk is present in rural areas on Alto Parana (90% of cases), Amambay, and Canandiyu Departments along the southeastern border with Brazil, and in the central departments of Caaguazu and San Pedro. Urban areas and Iguassu Falls vicinity are risk-free. Vivax malaria accounts for 94% to 99% of cases. Chloroquine prophylaxis is recommended for travel to malarious areas. All travelers should take measures to prevent evening and nighttime mosquito bites. Insect-bite prevention measures include a DEET-containing repellent applied to exposed skin, insecticide (permethrin) spray applied to clothing and gear, and use of a permethrin-treated bed net at night.

SCHISTOSOMIASIS: This disease is not reported in Paraguay but exists in adjacent areas of Brazil along the Parana River.

TRAVELERS' DIARRHEA: Low to moderate risk. A quinolone antibiotic, combined with loperamide (Imodium), is recommended for the treatment of diarrhea. Persistent diarrhea may be due to a parasitic infection such as giardiasis, amebiasis, or cryptosporidiosis.

YELLOW FEVER: There is currently no yellow fever in Paraguay. The CDC recommends yellow fever vaccination for all travelers older than 9 months.

OTHER DISEASES/HAZARDS: Brucellosis (usually from unpasteurized dairy products), coccidiomycosis, leptospirosis, measles, rabies (a relatively minor public health problem), tuberculosis (relatively high incidence, especially among Amerindian children), Venezuelan equine encephalitis, and strongyloidiasis and other helminthic infections.

Peru

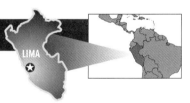

CAPITAL:
Lima
EMBASSY (IN U.S.):
202-833-9860
GMT:
−5 hours
TELEPHONE COUNTRY CODE:
51
USADIRECT:
0-8-50-288
ENTRY REQUIREMENTS
• **Passport/Visa:** No visa is required for tourist visits up to 90 days.
• **HIV Test:** Not required.
• **Vaccinations:** A yellow fever vaccination certificate is required of travelers 6 months or older arriving from infected areas. Peru recommends vaccination for those who intend to visit any rural area of the country.

- **U.S. Embassy:** Avenida Encalada, Block Seventeen, Lima; Tel: 51-1-434-3000, 51-1-434-3032; Fax: 51-1-434-3065, 434-3037; Website: www.rcp.net.pe/usa.
- **U.S. Consulate:** Binational Center (ICPNA), Avenida Tullumayo 125, Cuzco; Tel: 51-8-24-51-02; Fax: 51-8-23-35-41; e-mail: icpnacus@telser.com.pe.
- **Canadian Embassy:** Calle Libertad 130, Miraflores, Lima; Tel: 51-1-444-4015; Fax: 242-4050; e-mail: lima@dfait-maeci.gc.ca.
- **British Embassy:** Torre Parque Mar (Piso 22), Avenida Jose Larco, 1301 Miraflores. Lima; Tel: 51-1-617-3000; Fax: 51-1-617-3100; e-mail: belima@fco.gov.uk.

HOSPITALS/DOCTORS:

Medical care in Peru is below Western standards. Travelers are advised to obtain, before departure, supplemental travel health insurance with specific overseas coverage. The policy should provide for direct payment to the overseas hospital and/or physician at the time of service and include a medical evacuation benefit.
- Clínica Anglo Americana, Avenida Alfredo Salazar, Lima. Emergency. Private 52-bed hospital with medical/surgical capability.
- Clínica Ricardo Palma, Ave. Javier Prado Este 1038, Lima; recommended for travelers/ expatriates.
- Clínica Pardo, Avenue De la Cultura 710, Cuzco; small private hospital with 24-hour emergency services.

Current Advisories and Health Risks

AIDS/HIV: Incidence is lower than in other Latin American countries, such as Brazil. Prevalence of HIV in the blood donor population is 0.1% to 1.2%. An increasing number of HIV infections are associated with heterosexual activity.

ALTITUDE SICKNESS (AMS): Risk of altitude sickness, or acute mountain sickness (AMS), is present in the Sierra region of central Peru, where the Andes mountain ranges (average elevations 2,743 to 5,791 meters) are located. Cuzco, a popular destination, is at 3,500 meters elevation. Travelers to high elevations should consider acetazolamide (Diamox) prophylaxis to reduce their risk of AMS. Travelers arriving at high altitudes should spend several days acclimatizing and restricting strenuous activity. Descent is the best treatment for moderate to severe AMS.

ANIMAL HAZARDS: Animal hazards include snakes, centipedes, scorpions, black widow spiders, brown recluse spiders, banana spiders, and wolf spiders. Nearly all snakes in Peru are found in the Montana region. Fatal bushmaster envenomations have occurred, and ecotourists (e.g., birders) should have access to antivenin and air ambulance evacuation to Lima. Electric eels and piranha may be found in the country's fresh waters. Crocodiles and alligators are abundant.

CHAGAS DISEASE: Widely distributed in rural areas, mostly in the southern one half and northern one fourth of the country. Forty percent of Peruvians are considered at risk. Chagas disease occurs primarily in rural-agricultural areas where there are adobe-style huts and houses. These structures often harbor the night-biting triatomid (assassin) bugs that are responsible for transmitting Chagas disease. Travelers sleeping in such structures should take precautions against nighttime bites. Unscreened blood transfusions are also a source of infection and should be avoided.

CHOLERA: This disease is active in this country, but the threat to tourists is very low. Vaccination is not routinely recommended.

DENGUE FEVER: Presumably occurs year-round in northern coastal and eastern lowland urban areas. Scattered outbreaks have been reported. All travelers are advised to take measures to prevent daytime mosquito bites.

HEPATITIS: All travelers should receive hepatitis A vaccine. Hepatitis E is endemic, but the levels are unclear. The hepatitis B carrier rate in the general population is approximately 1.4%. Risk of hepatitis B is increased in the Amazon Basin and the southern Andes, where the carrier rate of the virus is as high as 20%. Hepatitis B is spread by infected blood, contaminated needles, and unprotected sex. Vaccination is recommended for stays longer than 3 months; for persons at occupational or social risk; and for anyone desiring maximum protection.

INFLUENZA: Influenza is transmitted from March through September in the southern hemisphere. The flu vaccine is recommended for all travelers during this time.

LEISHMANIASIS: This disease is a major public health problem in Peru. Cutaneous leishmaniasis is endemic in Andean and inter-Andean valleys and foothills of Peru between the northern border of the country and latitude of 13 degrees S (approximate latitude of Cuzco) within an altitude range up to 3,000 meters above sea level. Mucosal leishmaniasis is endemic in the tropical rain forests at lower altitudes. Visceral leishmaniasis (kala-azar) does not occur. All travelers to endemic areas in the Andes mountains and the tropical rain forests should take measures to prevent sand fly bites.

MALARIA: There is risk in all departments except Arequipa, Moquegua, Puno, and Tacna. There is no risk of malaria in the urban center of Lima, the coastal areas south of Lima, or the highland tourist areas of Cuzco, Machu Picchu, and Lake Titacaca. *Note*: Sporadic cases of vivax malaria have occurred in the southeastern and northern suburbs of Lima, and there is risk in Puerto Maldonado. Chloroquine-resistant *P. falciparum* is endemic in the regions bordering Brazil. Prophylaxis with atovaquone/proguanil (Malarone), mefloquine (Lariam), or doxycycline is recommended in al malarious areas All travelers should take measures to prevent evening and nighttime mosquito bites.

MARINE HAZARDS: Portuguese man-of-war, sea wasps, and stingrays are found in the coastal waters of Peru and could be a hazard to swimmers.

RABIES: There is a higher risk of rabies in Peru than in other South American countries. Cases of human rabies, usually transmitted by dogs, have increased, but the exact incidence of human rabies is not known. All animal bites or scratches, especially from a dog, require immediate medical evaluation. Rabies vaccine is recommended for travel longer than 3 months and for shorter stays for travelers who plan to venture off the usual tourist routes, where they may be at increased risk.

TRAVELERS' DIARRHEA: Prevention of diarrhea consists primarily in following strict adherence to safe food and drink guidelines. A quinolone antibiotic, combined with loperamide, is recommended for treating acute diarrhea. Persistent diarrhea may be due to a parasitic disease such as giardiasis or amebiasis.

TUBERCULOSIS: Tuberculosis (TB) is a major health problem in this country. Travelers planning an extended stay should have a pre-departure TB skin test (PPD test) and be retested after returning home.

TYPHOID FEVER: Typhoid vaccine is recommended for all travelers, with the exception of short-term visitors who restrict their meals to major restaurants and hotels. Because the typhoid vaccines are only 60% to 70% effective, safe food and drink selection remains important.

YELLOW FEVER: The CDC recommends yellow fever vaccination for all travelers older than 9 months of age.

OTHER DISEASES/HAZARDS: Anthrax (cutaneous; usually transmitted by contact with freshly slaughtered, infected cattle), brucellosis (from ingestion of unpasteurized dairy products, especially goat cheese), bartonellosis (Oroyo fever; focally endemic in Andean valleys), coccidiomycosis (endemic in the Amazonian lowlands), cysticercosis (residents of rural, endemic areas of Peru have a disease prevalence of 8%), cyclosporiasis, diphyllobothriasis (tapeworm infection from raw marine fish), echinococcosis (major health problem in central Andean areas), fascioliasis (liver fluke disease; acquired by consumption of raw aquatic plants; risk elevated in Amazonian lowlands), leptospirosis, paragonimiasis (from ingestion of raw freshwater crabs and crayfish), tuberculosis (a serious public health problem), strongyloidiasis and other helminthic infections, and tick-borne relapsing fever.

Philippines

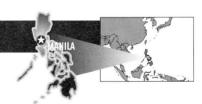

CAPITAL:
Manila
EMBASSY (IN U.S.):
202-467-9300
GMT:
+8 hours
TELEPHONE COUNTRY CODE:
63

USADIRECT:

105-11

ENTRY REQUIREMENTS

Travelers should check with this country's embassy (or a consulate) in the United States, Canada, or the United Kingdom for any changes in these requirements.

- **Passport/Visa:** Travelers should contact the Embassy of the Philippines for entry information.
- **HIV Test:** Applicants for permanent residence must be tested.
- **Vaccinations:** A yellow fever vaccination certificate is required for all travelers older than 1 year arriving from infected areas.

EMBASSIES/CONSULATES

- **U.S. Embassy:** 1201 Roxas Boulevard, Manila City; Tel: 2-523-1001; Fax: 63-2-522-3242; Website: usembassy.state.gov/posts/rp1/wwwh3004.html.
- **Canadian Embassy:** Allied Bank Centre, 6754 Ayala Avenue, Makati City; Tel: 2-867-0001; Fax: 810-4299; e-mail: manil@dfait-maeci.gc.ca; Website: www.dfait-maeci.gc.ca/manila.
- **British Embassy:** 15th–17th Floors LV Locsin Building, 6752 Ayala Avenue cor Makati Avenue, 1226 Makati, (PO Box 2927 MCPO); Tel: 63-2-816-7116–switchboard; Fax: 63-2-813-775–Chancery; e-mail: uk@info.com.ph Information Section.

HOSPITALS/DOCTORS

- Makati Medical Center, Manila (700 beds); multiple-specialty clinic; 24-hour ambulance and emergency services; ICU.
- University of Santo Tomas Hospital, Espana, Manila.
- Calamba Medical Center, Calamba (110 beds); most specialties; 24-hour ambulance and emergency services.
- International SOS: International SOS (Phils.), Inc, Suite 1205/6 One Magnificent Mile Bldg, San Miguel Avenue, Ortigas Center, Pasig City, 1600 Metro Manila, Philippines; Alarm Center Tel: 63-2-637-0707; Alarm Center Fax: 63-2-637-4872

Current Advisories and Health Risks

ANIMAL HAZARDS: Animal hazards include snakes (cobras), centipedes, scorpions, and black widow spiders. Monkey bites are not uncommon, and can transmit rabies and herpes B virus. Stingrays, jellyfish, nettles, sea cucumbers, sea wasps (potentially fatal), sea urchins, sea anemones, and the Indo-Pacific man-of-war are common in the country's coastal waters and are potentially hazardous to unprotected or careless swimmers.

CHOLERA: This disease is reported active in this country, but the threat to tourists is very low. Cholera is an extremely rare disease in travelers from developed countries. Cholera vaccine is recommended primarily for people at high risk who work and live in highly endemic areas under less than adequate sanitary conditions.

DENGUE FEVER: Dengue fever occurs countrywide, including urban and periurban areas, year-round. Peak infection rates occur during the rainy season, May through

November. Prevention of dengue consists in taking daytime protective measures against daytime mosquito bites.

FILARIASIS: Bancroftian and Malayan forms of the disease are transmitted by mosquitoes in rural areas. Filariasis is endemic on Luzon, Leyte, Marinduque, Mindanao, Mindoro, Palawan, Samar, and Sulu. Travelers to these islands should take measures to prevent insect bites.

HELMINTHIC INFECTIONS: Clonorchiasis and and fascioliasis (liver fluke diseases), paragnonimiasis (lung fluke disease), and gnathostomiasis are prevalent in rural areas. Capillariasis and opisthorchiasis are endemic. Anisikiasis is reported (occurs from consuming raw, infected tuna and mackerel). Angiostongyliasis is endemic and is transmitted from raw prawns, fish, land crabs, or shellfish. To prevent these diseases, travelers should avoid eating raw freshwater or saltwater fish and shellfish, wild watercress, and aquatic plants.
- Soil-transmitted helminthic infections (hookworm, roundworm, *Strongyloides*) are prevalent in most rural areas.
- Travelers should wear shoes (to prevent the hookworm and *Strongyloides* larvae from penetrating the skin), and food should be thoroughly washed/cooked (to remove/destroy roundworm eggs).

HEPATITIS: Hepatitis A vaccine is recommended for all nonimmune travelers. Hepatitis E is endemic at moderate levels. The hepatitis B carrier rate in the general population is estimated at 13%. Hepatitis B is spread by infected blood, contaminated needles, and unprotected sex. Vaccination is recommended for stays longer than 3 months; for persons at occupational or social risk; and for any traveler desiring maximum protection. Because the risk of illness or injury during travel cannot be predicted, some experts believe that *all* travelers should be immunized against hepatitis B because of the risk of receiving a medical injection with an unsterile needle or syringe.

INFLUENZA: Influenza is transmitted year-round in the tropics. The flu vaccine is recommended for all travelers.

JAPANESE ENCEPHALITIS: There is year-round risk of Japanese encephalitis (JE) in rural agricultural areas, with peak transmission during the monsoon season, usually May through November. Highest risk of JE occurs on Luzon and Mindanao, with a high incidence in extreme southern Luzon, Negros, Cebu, and the Catanduanes Island. JE vaccine is recommended for stays of more than 3 to 4 weeks in rural agricultural areas (with rice growing or pig farming), or for repeated shorter visits to endemic areas, especially during the peak transmission season. Travelers should take measures to prevent evening and nighttime mosquito bites.

MALARIA: There is year-round risk, countrywide, excluding the islands of Bohol, Catanduanes, Cebu, and Leyte; the plains of the islands of Negros and Panay; and the city of Manila and other urban centers. Risk exists primarily in the forested foothills and rolling terrain below 1,000 meters elevation in those rural areas rarely visited by tourists. Most malaria transmission occurs during and just after the monsoon season, May through November. Chloroquine-resistant falciparum malaria is common. Atovaquone/proguanil (Malarone), mefloquine (Lariam), or doxycycline prophylaxis is advised for travelers going to malaria risk areas.

MENINGITIS: Outbreaks of meningococcal disease were reported in 2005 in Baguio City and in the Cordillera Region. Quadrivalent meningococcal vaccine (groups A, C, Y, W-135) should be considered for travelers staying longer than 1 month in outbreak areas if extensive, close contact with the local populace is anticipated.

POLIOMYELITIS (POLIO): Three cases of paralytic polio from circulating vaccine-derived poliovirus occurred in 2001. The Philippines is now considered free of wild poliovirus. All travelers, however, should be fully immunized against this diseae.

RABIES: Sporadic cases (about 200 cases per year) of human rabies are reported countrywide.
- All animal bites or scratches, especially from a dog, should be taken seriously and immediate medical attention sought. Although rabies is rare among tourists, there is risk. No one should pet or pick up any stray animals. All children should be warned to avoid contact with unknown animals.
- Rabies vaccine is recommended for travel longer than 3 months; for shorter stays for travelers who plan to venture off the usual tourist routes, where they may be more exposed to the stray dog population; or when travelers desire extra protection.

SCHISTOSOMIASIS: Risk exists year-round, primarily in southern Luzon, Leyte, Samar, and Mindanao and on the east coast of Mindoro and Bohol Islands. All travelers to these areas should avoid swimming in freshwater lakes, ponds, or streams.

TRAVELERS' DIARRHEA: There is high risk of travelers' diarrhea outside of first-class hotels and resorts. A quinolone antibiotic, combined with loperamide (Imodium), is recommended for the treatment of acute diarrhea. Persistent diarrhea may be due to a parasitic infection such as giardiasis, amebiasis, or cryptosporidiosis.

TUBERCULOSIS: Tuberculosis (TB) is a major health problem in this country. Travelers planning an extended stay should have a pre-departure TB skin test (PPD test) and be retested after returning from this country.

TYPHOID FEVER: Typhoid vaccine is recommended for those traveling off the usual tourist routes, for those visiting friends or relatives, and for long-stay visitors. Because the typhoid vaccines are only 60% to 70% effective, safe food and drink selection remains important.

OTHER DISEASES/HAZARDS: AIDS/HIV (incidence probably higher than officially reported), chikungunya fever (year-round; reported from urban and village areas of central and southern islands), leptospirosis (risk elevated near end of monsoon season, peaking in early dry season), murine typhus (flea-borne), scrub typhus (mite-borne; risk elevated in grassy rural areas below 3,000 meters elevation on Leyte, Samar, Mindoro, Luzon, Negros, Panay, Palawan, Cebu, and Mindanao), tuberculosis (highly endemic), and typhoid fever.

Poland

WARSAW
★

CAPITAL:
Warsaw
EMBASSY (IN U.S.):
202-232-4517
GMT:
+1 hour
TELEPHONE COUNTRY CODE:
48
USADIRECT:
00-800-111-1111

ENTRY REQUIREMENTS
- **Passport/Visa:** No visa required for stays up to 90 days.
- **HIV Test:** Testing required for foreign students intending to remain in Poland longer than a few weeks; U.S. test result not accepted.
- **Vaccinations:** None required.

EMBASSIES/CONSULATES
- **U.S. Embassy:** Aleje Ujazdowskie 29/31, Warsaw; Tel: 22-628-3041 or 625-0055; Fax: 48-22-625-0289.
- **U.S. Consulates:** Ulica Stolarska 9, Krakow; Tel: 12-429-6655; Fax: 48-12-421-8292. Ulica Paderewskiego 7, Poznan; Tel: 61-851-8516; Fax: 48-61-851-8966.
- **Canadian Embassy:** Reform Plaza, 10th floor, Aleje Jerozolimskie 123, Warsaw; Tel: 22-584-3340; Fax: 584-3192; e-mail: wsaw@dfait-maeci.gc.ca.
- **British Embassy:** Aleje Róz No 1, 00-556 Warsaw; Tel: 48-22-311-0000; Fax: 48-22-311-0311; e-mail: info@britishembassy.pl.

HOSPITALS/DOCTORS
- State Hospital #1, Warsaw (1,500 beds); most major specialties; emergency unit, ICU.
- Medical Academy, Gdansk (1,000 beds); most specialties; ICU.
- Institute of Maritime and Tropical Medicine, Gdynia-Redlowo (90 beds); Tel: 48-58-622-51-63. Emergency services are available 24 hours a day. English-speaking physicians on staff.
- Note: Adequate medical care is available in Poland, but it generally does not meet Western standards.

Current Advisories and Health Risks

ACCIDENTS/ILLNESSES AND MEDICAL INSURANCE

- Accidents and injuries are the leading cause of death among travelers younger than 55 years of age and most often are caused by motor vehicle and motorcycle crashes; drownings, aircraft crashes, homicides, and burns are less common causes.
- Heart attacks cause most fatalities in older travelers.
- Infections cause only 1% of fatalities in overseas travelers, but, overall, infections are the most common cause of travel-related illness.
- Travelers are advised to obtain, before departure, supplemental travel health insurance with specific overseas coverage. The policy should provide for direct payment to the overseas hospital and/or physician at the time of service and include a medical evacuation benefit. The policy should also provide 24-hour hotline access to a multilingual assistance center that can help arrange and monitor delivery of medical care and determine if medical evacuation or air ambulance services are required.

AIR POLLUTION: Travelers with respiratory diseases should be aware that there is severe air pollution in most of the industrial areas of Poland.

HEPATITIS: Hepatitis A vaccine is recommended for all travelers. Hepatitis E may occur but has not been reported. The hepatitis B carrier rate in the general population is estimated at 0.2% to 1.2%. Vaccination against hepatitis B should be considered for stays longer than 3 months and by short-term travelers desiring maximum protection. Travelers should be aware that hepatitis B can be transmitted by unsafe sex and the use of contaminated needles and syringes.

INFLUENZA: Influenza is transmitted from November through March. The flu vaccine is recommended for all travelers older than 50; all travelers with chronic disease or a weakened immune system; travelers of any age wishing to decrease the risk of this illness; and pregnant women after the first trimester.

LYME DISEASE: Lyme disease is reported sporadically. Risk is elevated in the Warmia and the Mazury Lake Region, Western Pomerania, the Bialowieza National Forest, and the Carpathian Mountain Forest. Travelers are advised to take measures to prevent tick bites during the peak transmission season, March through September.

TICK-BORNE ENCEPHALITIS: Although the tick vector of tick-borne encephalitis (TBE) is distributed widely in brushy, wooded areas throughout most of Poland, the chance of contracting TBE is very low. Visitors working or camping in forested areas are those most at risk. There is increased transmission of TBE in the northern forested areas around Gdansk south and eastward to the Russian border, including the areas around Bialystock; the forested lands around Warsaw, Lodz, and Lukow; and along the border with Czechoslovakia south of Wroclaw. Travelers in these areas are advised to take measures to prevent tick bites, especially during the peak transmission season, March through September. The TBE vaccine (available in Canada and Europe) is recommended only for people at significant risk of exposure to tick bites—for example, campers and hikers on extended trips or forestry workers.

- -

TRAVELERS' DIARRHEA: Surface water in Poland is often polluted with organic, industrial, and agricultural waste/runoff. All drinking water should preferably be bottled or from a reliable source. A quinolone antibiotic, combined with loperamide (Imodium), is recommended for the treatment of acute diarrhea. Diarrhea not responding to treatment with an antibiotic may be due to a parasitic disease such as giardiasis.

- -

TYPHOID FEVER: Typhoid vaccine is recommended, especially for long-term travelers, adventure travelers, and those wishing maximum disease protection. Because the typhoid vaccines are only 60% to 70% effective, safe food and drink guidelines should continue to be observed.

- -

OTHER DISEASES/HAZARDS: Brucellosis, cysticercosis (regionally enzootic), echinococcosis (regionally enzootic), hemorrhagic fever with renal syndrome, leptospirosis, rabies (enzootic in foxes; rare in humans), trichinosis (elevated risk in eastern Poland), and typhoid fever.

Portugal

CAPITAL:
Lisbon
EMBASSY (IN U.S.):
202-332-3007
GMT:
+0 hours
TELEPHONE COUNTRY CODE:
351
USADIRECT:
800-800-128
ENTRY REQUIREMENTS
- **Passport/Visa:** A valid passport is required.
- **HIV Test:** Not required.
- **Vaccinations:** A yellow fever vaccination certificate is required for travelers older than 1 year of age coming from infected areas; this requirement applies only to travelers arriving in or destined for the Azores or Madeira Islands. However, no certificate is required for transit passengers on the islands of Funchal, Porto Santo, and Santa Maria.

EMBASSIES/CONSULATES
- **U.S. Embassy:** Avenida das Forças Armadas, Sete Rios, Lisbon; Tel: 351-21-727-3300; Fax: 351-21-726-9109; Website: www.american-embassy.pt.
- **U.S. Consulates:** On the island of San Miguel in the Azores, Avenida D. Henrique, Ponta Delgada; Tel: 351-96-282216/7/8/9. Rua Tentente Coronel Sarmento, Ed.

Infante, Bloco b-4 Andar, Apt. B, 9000 Funchal, Madeira; Tel: 351-29-174-3429, Fax: 351-29-174-3808.

- **Canadian Embassy:** Avenida da Liberdade 196-200, 3rd Floor, Lisbon; Tel: 351-213-16-4600; Fax: 351-213-16-4693; e-mail: lsbon@dfait-maeci.gc.ca; Website: www.dfait-maeci.gc.ca/lisbon.
- **British Embassy:** Rua de São Bernardo 33, 1249-082 Lisbon; Tel: 351-21-392-4000; Fax: 351-21-392-4178; e-mail: Chancery@Lisbon.mail.fco.gov.uk; Website: www.uk-embassy.pt.

HOSPITALS/DOCTORS

- Santa Maria Hospital, Lisbon (1,384 beds); Tel: 1-797-5171 or 797-8035. Most medical specialties, including eye surgery and ENT.
- The British Hospital, Lisbon; Tel: 1-602-020 or 678-161.
- Clínica Médica Internacional de Lisboa (CMIL), Lisbon and Cascais; Tel: 351-1-353-0817 (Lisbon); 351-1-486-5946/7/8 (Cascais). Private clinic with outpatient medical centers serving the Portuguese and international communities in the greater Lisbon area.

Current Advisories and Health Risks

ACCIDENTS/ILLNESSES AND MEDICAL INSURANCE

- Accidents and injuries are the leading cause of death among travelers younger than 55 years of age and most often are caused by motor vehicle and motorcycle crashes; drownings, aircraft crashes, homicides, and burns are less common causes.
- Heart attacks cause most fatalities in older travelers.
- Infections cause only 1% of fatalities in overseas travelers, but overall, infections are the most common cause of travel-related illness.
- Travelers are advised to obtain, before departure, supplemental travel health insurance with specific overseas coverage. The policy should provide for direct payment to the overseas hospital and/or physician at the time of service and include a medical evacuation benefit. The policy should also provide 24-hour hotline access to a multilingual assistance center that can help arrange and monitor delivery of medical care and determine if medical evacuation or air ambulance services are required.

HEPATITIS: All nonimmune travelers should receive hepatitis A vaccine. The carrier rate for the hepatitis B virus in the general population is estimated at 1.3%—high for western Europe. Hepatitis B vaccine is recommended for stays longer than 3 months and for short-term travelers wanting increased protection. Travelers should be aware that the risk of hepatitis B is increased by unsafe sex and the use of unsterile needles and syringes.

INFLUENZA: Influenza is transmitted from November through March. The flu vaccine is recommended for all travelers older than 50; all travelers with chronic disease or a weakened immune system; travelers of any age wishing to decrease the risk of this illness; and pregnant women after the first trimester.

LEISHMANIASIS: Cases of cutaneous leishmaniasis are rare but reported sporadically. Visceral leishmaniasis is said to be increasing. Eighty percent of cases of visceral leishmaniasis occur in the Douro River Basin in the districts of Real, Braganca, Viseau, and Gaurda. Travelers should take measures to prevent sand fly bites.

MALARIA: There is no risk of malaria in Portugal.

MEDITERRANEAN SPOTTED (BOUTONNEUSE) FEVER: Countrywide incidence below 1,000 meters elevation, especially in the Mediterranean coastal areas. Travelers should avoid close contact with dogs, which are carriers of the infective brown dog tick.

RABIES: No risk; Portugal is currently rabie free.

TRAVELERS' DIARRHEA: Medium risk; most sections of major cities have piped, potable water. In rural areas, water supplies may be contaminated. A quinolone antibiotic, combined with loperamide (Imodium), is recommended for the treatment of acute diarrhea.

TYPHOID FEVER: Typhoid vaccine is recommended, especially for long-term travelers, adventure travelers, and those wishing maximum disease protection. Because the typhoid vaccines are only 60% to 70% effective, safe food and drink guidelines should continue to be observed.

OTHER DISEASES/HAZARDS: Amebiasis and giardiasis (endemic), schistosomiasis (may occur in the Algarve Province in the extreme south), ehrlichiosis, echinococcosis, fascioliasis (infection rates of 2% to 7% reported from northern rural communities), leptospirosis, tick-borne relapsing fever, and typhoid fever.

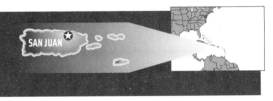

Puerto Rico and U.S. Virgin Islands

CAPITAL:
San Juan

EMBASSY (IN U.S.):
Not applicable.

GMT:
−4 hours

TELEPHONE COUNTRY CODE:
787

USADIRECT:
1-800-CALL-ATT

ENTRY REQUIREMENTS

- **Passport/Visa:** A passport is recommended for U.S. travelers.
- **HIV Test:** Not required.
- **Vaccinations:** None required.

HOSPITALS/DOCTORS:
Ashford Presbyterian Hospital, San Juan; Tel: 721-2160.

Current Advisories and Health Risks

See also the Disease Risk Summary for the Caribbean on page 293.

HEPATITIS: Low to moderate risk. Nonimmune travelers should receive hepatitis A vaccine.

DENGUE FEVER: Risk is present year-round. Highest incidence reported in the vicinity of Yanes. All travelers to Puerto Rico should take measures to prevent insect (mosquito) bites.

SCHISTOSOMIASIS: Risk of intestinal schistosomiasis is focally present throughout Puerto Rico. Seventeen of 79 municipalities tested have seroprevalence rates averaging 10%. The highest exposure (seroprevalence) rates occur around Jayuya (38.5%) and Naguabo (36.4%). Travelers should avoid swimming or wading in freshwater ponds, lakes, or streams.

TRAVELERS' DIARRHEA: Low to moderate risk. In urban and resort areas, the hotels and restaurants generally serve reliable food and potable water.

OTHER DISEASES/HEALTH HAZARDS: Bancroftian filariasis (mosquito-borne; minimal risk to travelers), intestinal helminthic infections (ancylostomiasis, ascariasis, strongyloidiasis, and trichuriasis), rabies (low risk), sexually transmitted diseases, typhoid fever, ciguatera fish toxin poisoning, and swimming-related hazards (jellyfish, spiny sea urchins, and coral).

Qatar

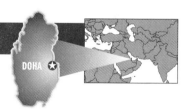

CAPITAL:
Doha
EMBASSY (IN U.S.):
202-274-1600
GMT:
+3 hours
TELEPHONE COUNTRY CODE:
974
USADIRECT:
None
ENTRY REQUIREMENTS

- **Passport/Visa:** A 10-year, multiple-entry visa is available. Travelers should contact the Qatar Embassy in Washington for further details.

- **HIV Test:** Required for work permit or student visa.
- **Vaccinations:** A yellow fever vaccination certificate is required for all travelers arriving from infected areas.

EMBASSIES/CONSULATES

- **U.S. Embassy:** Al-Luqta District on 22nd February St., Doha; Tel: 974-488-4176, Website: www.usembassy.org.qa.
- **Canadian Embassy:** Accredited to the Canadian Embassy in Kuwait. 24, Al Mutawakel Street, Block 4, Da'aiyah, Kuwait City, Kuwait; Tel: 965-256-3025; Fax: 965-256-0173; e-mail: kwait@international.gc.ca; Website: www.kuwait.gc.ca.
- **British Embassy:** PO Box 3, Doha; Tel: 974-4421991; Fax: 974-4438692; e-mail: consular_qatar@fco.gov.uk.

HOSPITALS/DOCTORS:

Hamad Hospital, Doha (600 beds); major referral center; all specialties; well-equipped and staffed.

Current Advisories and Health Risks

ACCIDENTS/ILLNESSES AND MEDICAL INSURANCE

- Accidents and injuries are the leading cause of death among travelers younger than 55 years of age and most often are caused by motor vehicle and motorcycle crashes; drownings, aircraft crashes, homicides, and burns are less common causes.
- Heart attacks cause most fatalities in older travelers.
- Infections cause only 1% of fatalities in overseas travelers, but overall, infections are the most common cause of travel-related illness.
- Travelers are advised to obtain, before departure, supplemental travel health insurance with specific overseas coverage. The policy should provide for direct payment to the overseas hospital and/or physician at the time of service and include a medical evacuation benefit. The policy should also provide 24-hour hotline access to a multilingual assistance center that can help arrange and monitor delivery of medical care and determine if medical evacuation or air ambulance services are required.

ENVIRONMENTAL POLLUTION: Raw sewage is pumped directly into the Persian Gulf, and beaches are considered contaminated.

HEPATITIS: Hepatitis A vaccine is recommended for all nonimmune travelers. Hepatitis E has not been reported, but may occur. The hepatitis B carrier rate in the general population is estimated at 2%. Hepatitis B vaccine is recommended for stays longer than 3 months and for short-term travelers wanting increased protection. Travelers should be aware that the risk of hepatitis B is increased by unsafe sex and the use of unsterile needles and syringes.

INFLUENZA: Influenza is transmitted from November through March. The flu vaccine is recommended for all travelers older than 50; all travelers with chronic disease or a weakened immune system; travelers of any age wishing to decrease the risk of this illness; and pregnant women after the first trimester.

LEISHMANIASIS: Both cutaneous and visceral forms of leishmaniasis may be present in endemic areas. Visitors should take measures to prevent insect (sand fly) bites.

MALARIA: There is no risk of malaria in this country.

TRAVELERS' DIARRHEA: Water is obtained almost exclusively from desalination plants. The high mineral content of underground water makes it unsuitable for drinking. A quinolone antibiotic, combined with loperamide (Imodium), is recommended for the treatment of acute diarrhea. Diarrhea not responding to antibiotic treatment may be due to a parasitic disease such as giardiasis or amebiasis.

TYPHOID FEVER: Typhoid vaccine is recommended, especially for long-term travelers, adventure travelers, and those wishing maximum disease protection. Because the typhoid vaccines are only 60% to 70% effective, safe food and drink guidelines should continue to be observed.

OTHER DISEASES/HAZARDS: Brucellosis (usually transmitted by raw dairy products), rabies (occurs rarely in stray dogs), trachoma, tuberculosis (low incidence), typhoid fever, soil-transmitted helminthic infections (roundworm, hookworm, and whipworm infections are common in rural areas; incidence is estimated at less than 5%).

Romania

CAPITAL:
Bucharest
EMBASSY (IN U.S.):
202-232-4747
GMT:
+2 hours
TELEPHONE COUNTRY CODE:
40
USADIRECT:
021-800-4288
021-801-0151
ENTRY REQUIREMENTS
- **Passport/Visa:** A visa is required for stays longer than 30 days. Travelers should call the Romanian Embassy for further information.
- **HIV Test:** Not required.
- **Vaccinations:** None required.
EMBASSIES/CONSULATES
- **U.S. Embassy:** Strada Tudor Arghezi 7-9, Bucharest; Tel: 401-210-40-42; Website: www.usembassy.ro.
- **U.S. Consulate:** Universitatii 7-9, Etage 1, Cluj-Napoca; Tel: 40-95-19-38-15.

- **Canadian Embassy:** 36 Nicolae Iorga, Bucharest; Tel: 40-1-307-5000; Fax: 40-1-307-5010; e-mail: bucst@dfait-maeci.gc.ca.
- **British Embassy:** 24 Strada Jules Michelet, 70154 Bucharest; Tel: 40-21-201-7200; Fax: 40-21-201-7299.

HOSPITALS/DOCTORS

- Cantacuzina Hospital, Bucharest (1,200 beds); most specialties.
- For physician referrals, travelers should contact the Consular Section of the U.S. Embassy at Strada Filipescu No. 26; Tel: 210-4042.

Current Advisories and Health Risks

ACCIDENTS/ILLNESSES AND MEDICAL INSURANCE

- Accidents and injuries are the leading cause of death among travelers younger than 55 years of age and most often are caused by motor vehicle and motorcycle crashes; drownings, aircraft crashes, homicides, and burns are less common causes.
- Heart attacks cause most fatalities in older travelers.
- Infections cause only 1% of fatalities in overseas travelers, but overall, infections are the most common cause of travel-related illness.
- Travelers are advised to obtain, before departure, supplemental travel health insurance with specific overseas coverage. The policy should provide for direct payment to the overseas hospital and/or physician at the time of service and include a medical evacuation benefit. The policy should also provide 24-hour hotline access to a multilingual assistance center that can help arrange and monitor delivery of medical care and determine if medical evacuation or air ambulance services are required.

AIDS/HIV: High incidence reported, especially in children and newborns—more cases, in fact, than have been reported cumulatively in all other European countries. Most cases occur in the Bucharest and Constanta areas. There is risk of transmission of HIV from unclean needles and syringes, as well as from contaminated blood transfusions. All travelers are cautioned against receiving unnecessary medical or dental injections and blood transfusions, and travelers are advised to carry their own sterile needles and syringes in case a medical injection is necessary.

CHOLERA: Sporadic cases are reported, especially from Tulcea, Braila, and Constanta counties and along the Danube River. Infections associated with the consumption of raw seafood have been reported along the Black Sea coast, but the threat to tourists is very low. Cholera vaccine is recommended primarily for people at high risk (e.g., relief workers) who work and live in highly endemic areas under less than adequate sanitary conditions.

- The oral cholera vaccine (Dukoral) provides up to 60% crossover protection against ETEC diarrhea.
- Many countries, including Canada, license an oral cholera vaccine. The oral vaccine is not available in the United States.
- Cholera vaccine is not "officially" required for entry into, or exit from, any country. Despite this, some countries, on occasion, require proof of cholera vaccination from trav-

elers coming from cholera-infected countries. Anticipating such a situation, certain travelers may wish to carry a medical exemption letter from their health-care provider. Travel Medicine, Inc., recommends that travelers use the International Certificate of Vaccination (Yellow Card) for this purpose, having their health-care provider affirm that they are "exempt from cholera vaccine" and validate the exemption with both the provider's signature and the appropriate official stamp (the "Uniform Stamp" in the United States).

HEPATITIS: All nonimmune travelers should receive hepatitis A vaccine. The hepatitis B carrier rate in the general population is estimated at up to 9%—the highest in Europe. Vaccination against hepatitis B is recommended for anyone planning an extended visit to this country. There is also increased risk of transmission of hepatitis B from medical injections that are administered with unclean needles and syringes.

INFLUENZA: Influenza is transmitted from November through March. The flu vaccine is recommended for all travelers older than 50 years of age; all travelers with chronic disease or a weakened immune system; travelers of any age wishing to decrease the risk of this illness; and pregnant women after the first trimester.

RABIES: Sporadic cases of human rabies are reported countrywide. All animal bites or scratches, especially from a dog, should be taken seriously, and immediate medical attention sought. Access to rabies vaccine or rabies immune globulin may require emergency travel to Western Europe. Although rabies is very rare among tourists, there is risk. No one should pet or pick up any stray animals. All children should be warned to avoid contact with unknown animals. Rabies vaccine is recommended for travel longer than 3 months; for shorter stays for travelers who plan to venture off the usual tourist routes, where they may be more exposed to the stray dog population; or when travelers desire extra protection.

TICK-BORNE DISEASES: Lyme disease, Central European tick-borne encephalitis (TBE), and boutonneuse fever are reported. The ticks that transmit these diseases are found in brushy, wooded areas throughout the country. There is higher risk of TBE in the Tulcea District and in Transylvania at the base of the Carpathian Mountains and Transylvanian Alps. Boutonneuse fever (also known as Mediterranean spotted fever) is endemic along the Black Sea coast.
- A vaccine against TBE is available in Canada and Europe but is recommended only for persons who will have intense outdoor exposure in risk areas from April through October. Travelers to endemic areas should take measures to prevent tick bites.

TRAVELERS' DIARRHEA: High risk outside of first-class hotels and resorts. Water in the larger cities, but not rural areas, is generally potable. Travelers are advised to drink only bottled, boiled, filtered, or treated water and to consume only well-cooked food. All fruit should be peeled before consumption. A quinolone antibiotic, combined with loperamide (Imodium), is recommended for the treatment of acute diarrhea. Diarrhea not responding to antibiotic treatment may be due to a parasitic disease such as giardiasis, amebiasis, or cryptosporidiosis.

TUBERCULOSIS: Tuberculosis (TB) is a major health problem in this country. Travelers planning an extended stay should have a pre-departure TB skin test (PPD test) and be retested after leaving this country. Travelers should avoid crowded public places and public transportation whenever possible. Domestic help hired by long-stay visitors should be screened for TB.

TYPHOID FEVER: Typhoid vaccine is recommended, especially for long-term travelers, adventure travelers, and those wishing maximum disease protection. Because the typhoid vaccines are only 60% to 70% effective, safe food and drink guidelines should continue to be observed.

VIRAL ENCEPHALITIS: An outbreak of mosquito-transmitted West Nile encephalitis occurred in 1996 in the lower Danube valley and Bucharest.

OTHER DISEASES/HAZARDS: Anthrax (sporadic human cases occur, usually cutaneous, related to the slaughter of livestock in rural areas, especially southern areas), brucellosis (enzootic at low levels, particularly in sheep, goats, and cattle; human cases usually due to consumption of unpasteurized milk or milk products), echinococcosis (stray dogs in urban and rural areas commonly infected; human cases reported sporadically), hemorrhagic fever with renal syndrome (similar to hantavirus syndrome; disease transmitted by rodent excreta), leptospirosis, rabies (enzootic in foxes, wolves, and wild canids; rare in humans), trichinosis (from raw or undercooked pork), tuberculosis (highest reported incidence in Europe), typhoid fever, typhus (murine and louse-borne), and helminthic infections (roundworm, hookworm, and whipworm infections and strongyloidiasis).

Russia

CAPITAL:
Moscow
EMBASSY (IN U.S.):
202-939-8918
GMT:
+3 hours
TELEPHONE COUNTRY CODE:
7
USADIRECT:
755-5042 to place calls from within Moscow; 325-5042 to place calls from within St. Petersburg
ENTRY REQUIREMENTS
Travelers should check with this country's embassy (or nearest consulate) in the United States, Canada, or the United Kingdom for any changes in requirements.
- **Passport/Visa:** Tourist visa requires application form, photo, confirmation and voucher from travel agency and/or hotel in Russia, cover letter from travel agency, and a processing fee.

- **HIV Test:** Required for foreigners staying longer than 3 months. U.S. test result acceptable.
- **Vaccinations:** None required.

EMBASSIES/CONSULATES

- **U.S. Embassy:** Novinskiy Bulvar 19/23, Moscow; Tel: 7-095-728-5000; e-mail: uscgyekat@gin.ru.
- **Canadian Embassy:** 23 Starokonyushenny Pereulok, Moscow; Tel: 7-095-956-6666; e-mail: mosco@dfait-maeci.gc.ca.
- **British Embassy:** Smolenskaya Naberezhnaya 10, Moscow 121099; Tel: 7-095-956-7200; Fax: 7-095-956-7201; e-mail: consular.moscow@fco.gov.uk.

HOSPITALS/DOCTORS:

Health care in Russia is often deficient by Western standards. Well-trained doctors and nurses are available in some of the major cities, and there are a growing number of Western-style (and expensive) medical clinics serving foreign travelers and expatriates. U.S. and Canadian embassies and consulates maintain lists of English-speaking physicians. All travelers should consider purchasing a travel insurance policy with telephone assistance and medical evacuation capabilities.

- Emergency medical and ambulance services: Dial 03 countrywide.
- European Medical Centre, 2-OY Tverskoy-Yamskoy Per. 10, Moscow; Tel: 095-787-7000; Website: www.emcmos.ru. Open 24 hours.
- Canadian Family Clinic, Michurinsky Prospekt, #56 (southwest Moscow); Tel: 095-931-5018 or 5318; Fax: 095-932-8653; Website: http://www.mediclub.ru: e-mail: mediclub@cityline.ru.
- American Medical Centers, Grokholsky pereulok, #1 (northeast center of Moscow, metro Prospekt Mira—circle line); Tel: 095-933-7700, Fax: 095-933-7701: Website: http://www.amcenters.com. Offers pre-adoption consulations, provides AIDS test for $30 in English, which is useful for those who need to renew their long-term Russian visa. Open 24 hours.
- Kremlin Hospital, Moscow; all specialties; reportedly among the best medical facilities in Russia; serves the medical needs of the Russian political establishment.
- The British American Family Practice & Urgent Care, St. Petersburg, Grafsky pereulok, #7, St. Petersburg 191002; Tel: 7-812-327-6030.
- American Medical Center, Serpukhovskaya ul., #10, St. Petersburg; Tel: 292-62-72; Website: www.amcenters.com. American and American-trained doctors.
- Euromed, Suvorovski pr., #60, St. Petersburg; Tel/Fax: 327-0301; Website: www. euromed.ru. 24-hour emergency medical and dentistry services. Works with the major European and Asian insurance companies. Discounts.
- The International Clinic, Dostoevskogo ul., #19/21, St. Petersburg; Tel: 320-3870. Offers 24-hour emergency service, medical care; evacuation.
- International SOS:
  - ASSIST 24, 16/1 Dokukina str., 4th floor, 129226 Moscow, Russia; Alarm Center Tel: 7-095-937-6477; Alarm Center Fax: 7-095-937-6472.

- ZAO International Medical Clinic Moscow, Polyclinic No 1, 10th Floor, 31 Grokholsky Pereulok, 129010 Moscow, Russia; Clinic Tel: 7-095-937-5760; Clinic Fax: 7-095-937-5977.
- International SOS Clinic, Sakhincentr, Ground Floor, Office #19, 32 Kommunisticheskyi Prospect, 693000 Yuzhno-Sakhalinsk, Russia; Clinic/Admin Tel: 7-4242-727550; Clinic/ Admin Fax: 7-4242-728671, Mobile: 7-4242-473650.

Current Advisories and Health Risks

ACCIDENTS/ILLNESSES: Accidents, especially motor vehicle crashes, are the leading cause of death among travelers younger than 55 years of age; cardiovascular disease causes most fatalities in older travelers; infections cause most illness during travel but less than 1% of the fatalities.

AIDS/HIV: The epidemic of new cases of HIV and AIDS in Russia is spreading rapidly. The reasons include (1) an increase in IV drug abuse, (2) an increase in commercial sex and sexual promiscuity, (3) an increase in sexually transmitted diseases, (4) decreased availability of sterile needles and syringes, and (5) little or no education or prevention programs (e.g., public service ads on TV).

ARBOVIRAL DISEASES: These insect-borne viral diseases include Karelian fever (most cases occur in July through September), sand fly fever (limited to Moldova and the Crimea), dengue fever, West Nile fever (mosquito-borne; circulates in the Volga Delta region from May through September) and Sindbis fever (detected in the Volga Delta, in July and August).

CHOLERA: This disease is active in parts of this country, but the threat to tourists is very low. Vaccination is not routinely recommended.

DIPHTHERIA: Outbreaks have been reported during the last decade. All travelers, especially adults, should be up to date on their immunizations. (The CDC estimates that 20% to 60% of Americans older than 20 years lack sufficient immunity to diphtheria.) Diphtheria vaccine in the United States is widely available and is administered in combination with the tetanus vaccine (Td vaccine).

HEPATITIS: All nonimmune travelers should receive hepatitis A vaccine. Hepatitis E, transmitted by unsafe drinking water, accounts for about 20% of cases of acute hepatitis in the south. The hepatitis B carrier rate in the general population of Russia is estimated at 4%. Hepatitis B is spread by infected blood, contaminated needles, and unprotected sex. Vaccination is recommended for long-stay (longer than 3 months) travelers; for persons who may be at occupational or social risk; and for anybody desiring maximum protection.

INFLUENZA: Influenza is transmitted from November through March. Vaccination is recommended for travel during the flu season.

JAPANESE ENCEPHALITIS: There has been increased prevalence of Japanese encephalitis (JE) in eastern Russia in the past several years.

LEISHMANIASIS: The risk for cutaneous leishmaniasis is limited primarily to southern regions, including portions of Georgia Republic and the southern Ukraine, below 1,300 meters elevation. Visceral leishmaniasis (kala-azar) is confined to areas along the southeastern coast of the Black Sea, the southeastern and southwestern coasts of the Caspian Sea and the border areas of Georgia and Azerbaijan. Travelers to these regions should take measures to prevent sand fly bites.

LYME DISEASE: Lyme disease occurs focally in rural forested areas, with the highest incidence in the Ural Mountains region. Risk presumably also occurs in the northwest and central areas. Travelers are advised to take measures to prevent tick bites.

MEDITERRANEAN SPOTTED (BOUTONNEUSE) FEVER: Tick-borne; reported most commonly in the Black Sea coastal areas of the Caucasus, Transcaucasus, and Crimea, and along the Caspian Sea coastline.

RABIES: Sporadic cases of human rabies are reported countrywide. All animal bites or scratches, especially from a dog, should be taken seriously, and immediate medical attention sought.

TICK-BORNE ENCEPHALITIS: Tick-borne encephalitis (TBE) is a viral disease that is transmitted in regions from the Baltics to the Crimea and eastward. Peak transmission occurs from April through October. Risk is present primarily in rural brushy and forested areas below 1,500 meters elevation. The greatest number of cases is reported from the regions between Moscow and St. Petersburg, the lower Amur River area in Eastern Siberia, the area around Vladivostok, and southern Kamchatka Island, and in southern Siberia from the Urals to Lake Baikal. A vaccine against TBE is available in Canada and Europe, as well as Russia, but is recommended only for persons who will have intense outdoor exposure in risk areas from April through October. Travelers to endemic areas should take measures to prevent tick bites.

TRAVELERS' DIARRHEA: Medium to high risk outside of the better hotels and resorts. All water supplies in Russia are suspect, including municipal tap water, which may be untreated. Travelers should consume only bottled water or boiled or chemically treated water and observe safe food and drink precautions. A quinolone antibiotic, combined with loperamide (Imodium), is recommended for the treatment of acute diarrhea. Persistent diarrhea may be due to a parasitic infection such as giardiasis, amebiasis, or cryptosporidiosis.

TUBERCULOSIS: Tuberculosis (TB) is a major health problem in this country. Travelers planning an extended stay should have a pre-departure TB skin test (PPD test) and be retested after leaving this country or returning home.

TYPHOID FEVER: Typhoid vaccine is recommended for those traveling off the usual tourist routes, for those visiting friends or relatives, and for long-stay visitors. Because the typhoid vaccines are only 60% to 70% effective, safe food and drink selection remains important.

Rwanda

KIGALI

CAPITAL:
Kigali
EMBASSY (IN U.S.):
202-232-2882
GMT:
+2 hours
TELEPHONE COUNTRY CODE:
250
USADIRECT:
None
ENTRY REQUIREMENTS
• **Passport/Visa:** Valid passport and visa are required.
• **HIV Test:** Not required.
• **Vaccinations:** A yellow fever vaccination certificate is required for all travelers older than 1 year of age arriving from all countries. *Cholera*: Vaccination is not officially required but is advised.
EMBASSIES/CONSULATES
• **U.S. Embassy:** Boulevard de la Revolution, Kigali; Tel: 75601 or 72126.
• **Canadian Embassy:** 1534 Akagera Street, Kigali, Rwanda; Tel: 250-5-73210; Fax: 250-5-72719; e-mail: kgali@international.gc.ca.
• **British Embassy:** Parcelle No 1131, Boulevard de l'Umuganda, Kacyiru Sud, BP 576 Kigali; Tel: 250-585771, 585773, 584098, 586072; Fax: 250-582044, 511586
HOSPITALS/DOCTORS:
Kigali Central Hospital (450 beds); general medical services.

Current Advisories and Health Risks

AFRICAN SLEEPING SICKNESS (TRYPANOSOMIASIS): Sporadic cases occur; risk areas include Akagera Game Park, in the northeast, and Nasho Lake vicinity (east of Kigali).

CHOLERA: This disease is active in this country. The risk of cholera, however, is extremely low in international travelers from developed countries, such as the United States and Canada. Cholera vaccine (no longer available in the United States) is recommended only for persons at high risk who work and live in highly endemic areas under less than adequate sanitary conditions.
• The oral cholera vaccine (Dukoral) provides up to 60% crossover protection against ETEC diarrhea.
• Cholera vaccine is not "officially" required for entry into, or exit from, any country. Despite this, some countries, on occasion, require proof of cholera immunization from

travelers coming from cholera-infected countries. Anticipating such a situation, travelers wish to carry a medical exemption letter from their health-care provider. If possible, it is advisable to contact the embassy or consulate at the destination country to confirm the requirement for cholera vaccination (if any) and the acceptability of a medical exemption letter.

HEPATITIS: High risk. All susceptible travelers should receive hepatitis A vaccine. The hepatitis B carrier rate in the general population is estimated to exceed 10%. Vaccination is recommended for health-care and relief workers.

MALARIA: Risk is present throughout this country, including urban areas. Risk may be less in the northwest prefecture of Ruhengeri. *P. falciparum* accounts for approximately 90% of cases. The remainder of cases are due to the *P. ovale* and *P. malariae* species, rarely to *P. vivax*. Chloroquine-resistant falciparum malaria is reported. Prophylaxis with atovaquone/proguanil (Malarone), mefloquine (Lariam), or doxycycline is recommended.

SCHISTOSOMIASIS: Intestinal schistosomiasis occurs along Lake Kivu and in the northwest around Lakes Bulera and Ruhondu, with risk also in Byumba, Kigali, and Butare prefectures. Travelers to these regions should avoid swimming, bathing, or wading in freshwater lakes, ponds, or streams.

TRAVELERS' DIARRHEA: High risk. Water supplies, even in Kigali, may be contaminated. Travelers should observe all food and drink safety precautions. A quinolone antibiotic is recommended for the treatment of acute diarrhea.

YELLOW FEVER: Vaccination is required for entry. This disease is not currently active.

OTHER DISEASES/HAZARDS: AIDS (HIV seropositivity prevalence is 24.4% to 30% among pregnant women in Kigali), African tick typhus, brucellosis, echinococcosis, filariasis, leishmaniasis (transmission occurs year-round), meningitis, plague, rabies (transmitted primarily by dogs), louse-borne relapsing fever and typhus fever (primarily in the highlands), Rift Valley fever, tuberculosis (a major health problem), trachoma, typhoid fever, and intestinal worms.

Saint Barthélemy

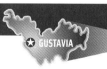

CAPITAL:
Gustavia
EMBASSY (IN U.S.):
202-944-6200
GMT:
−4 hours
TELEPHONE COUNTRY CODE:
590

0800-99-0011

ENTRY REQUIREMENTS

(For French West Indies; islands include Guadeloupe, Isles des Saintes, La Desirade, Marie Galante, Saint Barthélemy, St. Martin, and Martinique.)

- **Passport/Visa:** Passport required. Visa not required for tourist/business stays of up to 3 months. For further information, consult the Embassy of France; Tel: 202-944-6200; Website: http://www.france-consulat.org.
- **Vaccination:** A yellow fever vaccination certificate is required for travelers older than 1 year of age arriving from an infected or endemic zone within 6 days.

EMBASSIES/CONSULATES:

Neither the United States nor Canada has an embassy in St. Barthélemy.

HOSPITALS/DOCTORS:

Health care is of a good standard, but travel health insurance is advisable.

- Gustavia Clinic; Tel. 27-60-35. Staffed by 5 physicians and 3 dentists.

Current Advisories and Health Risks

ACCIDENTS/ILLNESSES AND MEDICAL INSURANCE

- Accidents and injuries are the leading cause of death among travelers younger than 55 years of age and most often are caused by motor vehicle and motorcycle crashes; drownings, aircraft crashes, homicides, and burns are less common causes.
- Heart attacks cause most fatalities in older travelers.
- Infections cause only 1% of fatalities in overseas travelers, but overall, infections are the most common cause of travel-related illness.
- Travelers are advised to obtain, before departure, supplemental travel health insurance with specific overseas coverage. The policy should provide for direct payment to the overseas hospital and/or physician at the time of service and include a medical evacuation benefit. The policy should also provide 24-hour hotline access to a multilingual assistance center that can help arrange and monitor delivery of medical care and determine if medical evacuation or air ambulance services are required.

DENGUE FEVER: This mosquito-transmitted viral disease is widespread in the Caribbean. In Saint Barthélemy, as on all the other islands, risk is present in both urban and rural areas. Travelers should take measures to prevent daytime insect bites.

FOOD AND WATER SAFETY: The water supply is chlorinated and, although relatively safe, may cause mild abdominal upsets. Bottled water is available and is advised for the first few weeks of stay. The drinking water outside main cities and towns may be contaminated, and sterilization is advised. Milk is pasteurized, and dairy products are safe for consumption. Local meat, poultry, seafoods, and fruit are generally considered safe to eat.

HEPATITIS: Nonimmune travelers should receive the hepatitis A vaccine. Vaccination against hepatitis B should be considered for stays longer than 3 months or by those travelers desiring maximum protection. Travelers should be aware that hepatitis B can be transmitted by unsafe sex and the use of contaminated needles and syringes.

INFLUENZA: Influenza is transmitted year-round in the tropics. The flu vaccine is recommended for all travelers older than 50; all travelers with any chronic disease or weakened immune system; travelers of any age wishing to decrease the risk of this illness; and pregnant women after the first trimester.

MALARIA: There is no risk of malaria on St. Barthélemy.

MARINE HAZARDS

- Swimming-related hazards include jellyfish, spiny sea urchins, and corals.
- Ciguatera poisoning is prevalent and can result from eating reef fish such as grouper, snapper, sea bass, jack, and barracuda. The ciguatoxin is not destroyed by cooking.
- For scuba diving hyperbaric chamber referral: The Divers' Alert Network (DAN) maintains an up-to-date list of all functioning hyperbaric chambers in North America and the Caribbean. DAN does not publish this list, becaause at any one time a given chamber may be nonfunctioning, or its operator(s) may be away or otherwise unavailable. Through Duke University, DAN operates a 24-hour emergency phone line for anyone (members and nonmembers) to call and ask for diving accident assistance. Dive medicine physicians at Duke University Medical Center carry beepers, so someone is always on call to answer questions and, if necessary, make referrals to the closest functioning hyperbaric chamber. In a diving emergency, or for the location of the nearest decompression chamber, call 919-684-8111.

SCHISTOSOMIASIS: Disease due to intestinal schistosomiasis is present on this island, but the risk is deemed to be low. Most snail-infested freshwater foci have been identified and can be avoided. Travelers should avoid swimming, bathing, or wading in freshwater ponds, lakes, or streams unless advised they are safe. Chlorinated swimming pools are considered safe.

TRAVELERS' DIARRHEA: Low to moderate risk. In urban and resort areas, the hotels and restaurants generally serve reliable food and potable water. A quinolone antibiotic, combined with loperamide (Imodium), is recommended for the treatment of acute diarrhea.

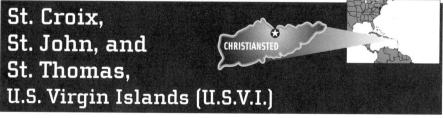

St. Croix, St. John, and St. Thomas, U.S. Virgin Islands (U.S.V.I.)

CHRISTIANSTED

CAPITAL:
Christiansted
EMBASSY (IN U.S.):
Not applicable

GMT:

−4 hours

TELEPHONE COUNTRY CODE:

340

USADIRECT:

None

ENTRY REQUIREMENTS

- **Passport/Visa:** *U.S. citizens:* Proof of identity and/or citizenship—particularly for resident aliens. *All other nationals:* Same as for entry into the United States. Because of the location of the U.S.V.I., pre-clearance inspection process for all flights from territory to destinations in Puerto Rico and continental United States. All travelers must present proof of citizenship to immigration on arrival. Proof of citizenship is one of following: passport issued under competent authority; Alien Registration Card (green card); certified copy of birth certificate with government-issued photo ID (Canadian and U.S. citizens only); or Certificate of Naturalization issued by the U.S. INS.
- **HIV Test:** Not required.
- **Vaccinations:** None required.

EMBASSIES/CONSULATES

Neither Canada, nor the United Kingdom has an embassy in the Virgin Islands.

HOSPITALS/DOCTORS:

Medical care in St. Croix and St. John is adequate for most problems. Travelers are advised to obtain, before departure, supplemental travel health insurance with specific overseas coverage. The policy should provide for direct payment to the overseas hospital and/or physician at the time of service and include a medical evacuation benefit.
- Juan F. Luis Hospital, Diamond, St. Croix; Tel: 1-778-6311.
- Roy L. Scheider Hospital, St. Thomas, U.S.V.I., Tel: 1-773-1311.

Current Advisories and Health Risks

See the Disease Risk Summary for the Caribbean on page 293.

St. Kitts and Nevis

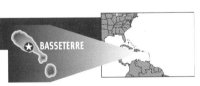

CAPITAL:

Basseterre

EMBASSY (IN U.S.):

202-833-355

GMT:

−4 hours

TELEPHONE COUNTRY CODE:

80

USADIRECT:

1-800-872-2881

ENTRY REQUIREMENTS

- **Passport/Visa:** Visa not required. These islands have been independent of Britain since 1983.
- **HIV Test:** Not required for tourists. An HIV test is required for students, intending immigrants, and anyone seeking employment.
- **Vaccinations:** A yellow fever vaccination certificate is required for travelers older than 6 months of age coming from infected or endemic areas.

EMBASSIES/CONSULATES:

Neither the United States or Canada has an embassy in St. Kitts and Nevis.

- **British High Commission:** PO Box 483, Price Waterhouse Coopers Centre, 11 Old Parham Rd. St John's, Antigua; Tel: 1-268-462-0008/9, 463-0010.

HOSPITALS/DOCTORS

- Joseph N. France Hospital, Basseterre (164 beds); general medical/surgical facility; emergency unit.

Current Advisories and Health Risks

See the Disease Risk Summary for the Caribbean on page 293.

Saint Lucia

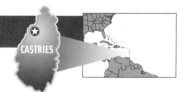

CAPITAL:

Castries

EMBASSY (IN U.S.):

202-463-3550

GMT:

−4 hours

TELEPHONE COUNTRY CODE:

809

USADIRECT:

1-800-872-2881

ENTRY REQUIREMENTS

- **Passport/Visa:** A passport is required for entry.
- **HIV Test:** Not required.
- **Vaccinations:** A yellow fever vaccination certificate is required of all travelers older than 1 year arriving from infected areas.

EMBASSIES/CONSULATES

- **U.S. Embassy:** Accredited to the U.S. Embassy in Barbados. Canadian Imperial Bank of Commerce Building, Broad Street; Tel: 246-436-4950.
- **Canadian High Commission:** (Barbados) Tel: 809-429-3550.
- **British High Commission:** Francis Compton Building, 2nd Floor (PO Box 227), Waterfront. Castries; Tel: 1-758-45-22484/5; Fax: 1-758-45-31543; e-mail: britishhc@candw.lc.

HOSPITALS/DOCTORS:
Victoria Hospital, Castries (211 beds); general medical/surgical facility.

Current Advisories and Health Risks

DENGUE FEVER: This mosquito-transmitted viral disease is prevalent in the Caribbean. Travelers should take measures to prevent insect bites.

HEPATITIS: Low risk to tourists. All nonimmune travelers should receive hepatitis A vaccine.

SCHISTOSOMIASIS: Disease caused by intestinal schistosomiasis (caused by *S. mansoni*) is present on this island but is of limited risk. Most snail-infested freshwater foci have been identified and can be avoided. Risk areas include Cul de Sac River Valley (south of Castries), the Roseau Valley, and around Soufriere and Riche Fond. Travelers should avoid swimming or wading in freshwater ponds, lakes, or streams in these areas.

TRAVELERS' DIARRHEA: Low to moderate risk. In urban and resort areas, the hotels and restaurants generally serve reliable food and potable water. Elsewhere, travelers should observe all food and drink safety precautions. A quinolone antibiotic (Floxin or Cipro) is recommended for the treatment of acute diarrhea. Diarrhea not responding to antibiotic treatment may be due to a parasitic disease such as giardiasis or amebiasis.

OTHER DISEASES/HAZARDS: Brucellosis, filariasis (mosquito-borne; low apparent risk; may occur in the Lesser Antilles from Trinidad north to Guadeloupe), Chagas disease (low apparent risk; reduviid bug vectors have been detected on several other islands), histoplasmosis, helminthic infections (ancylostomiasis, ascariasis, strongyloidiasis, and trichuriasis), leptospirosis (skin contact with water or moist soil contaminated with the urine of infected animals), syphilis, AIDS, tuberculosis, typhoid fever (St. Lucia had the highest incidence reported in the Caribbean in 1987—36 cases per 100,000 population), viral encephalitis, ciguatera fish toxin poisoning, and swimming-related hazards (jellyfish, spiny sea urchins, and coral).

Saint Martin

CAPITAL:
Marigot
EMBASSY (IN U.S.):
202-944-6000
GMT:
−4 hours
TELEPHONE COUNTRY CODE:
590

USADIRECT:

0800-99-0011

ENTRY REQUIREMENTS

• **Passport/Visa:** Visa not required. Saint Martin is a French Dependent Territory.

• **HIV Test:** Not required.

• **Vaccinations:** None required.

EMBASSIES/CONSULATES

• **U.S. Embassy:** Accredited to the U.S. Embassy in Curaçao. J.B. Gorsiraweg #1, Willemstad, Curaçao; Tel: 599-9-461-3066; Fax: 599-9-461-6489.

• **Consulate of Canada:** Lot 95, Terres Basses, St. Martin 97150; Tel: 599-544-2168; Fax: 599-544-2268.

• **British Consulate:** Jan Sofat 38, Willemstad, Curaçao; Tel: 599-9-747-3322; Fax: 599-9-747-3330.

HOSPITALS/DOCTORS:

Hopital de Marigot (55 beds); general medical/surgical facility; physicians on call 24 hours.

Current Advisories and Health Risks

DENGUE FEVER: This mosquito-transmitted viral disease is prevalent in the Caribbean. Travelers should take measures to prevent insect bites.

HEPATITIS: Low risk to tourists. All nonimmune travelers should receive hepatitis A vaccine.

MALARIA: No risk.

TRAVELERS' DIARRHEA: Low to moderate risk. In urban and resort areas, the hotels and restaurants generally serve reliable food and potable water. Elsewhere, travelers should observe all food and drink safety precautions. A quinolone antibiotic (Floxin or Cipro) is recommended for the treatment of acute diarrhea.

OTHER DISEASES/HAZARDS: Typhoid fever, viral encephalitis, ciguatera fish toxin poisoning (outbreaks have occurred), and swimming-related hazards (jellyfish, spiny sea urchins, and coral).

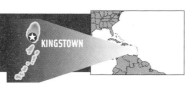

St. Vincent and the Grenadines

CAPITAL:

Kingstown

EMBASSY (IN U.S.):

202-462-7806

GMT:
−4 hours
TELEPHONE COUNTRY CODE:
809
USADIRECT:
1-800-872-2881
ENTRY REQUIREMENTS
- **Passport/Visa:** Visa not required.
- **HIV Test:** Not required for tourists. Test required for applicants seeking temporary and permanent residency visas.
- **Vaccinations:** A vaccination certificate is required of all travelers older than 1 year arriving from infected areas.

EMBASSIES/CONSULATES
- **U.S. Embassy:** Accredited to the U.S. Embassy in Barbados. Canadian Imperial Bank of Commerce Building, Broad Street; Tel: 246-436-4950.
- **Canadian High Commission:** Accredited to the Canadian High Commission in Barbados. Bishop's Court Hill, St. Michael, Barbados; Postal Address: PO Box 404, Bridgetown, Barbados; Tel: 1-246-429-3550; Fax: 1-246-437-7436; e-mail: bdgtn@international.gc.ca; Website: www.bridgetown.gc.ca.
- **British High Commission:** Granby Street (PO Box 132), Kingstown; Tel: 1-784-457-1701; Fax: 1-784-456-2750.

HOSPITALS/DOCTORS
- General Hospital, Kingstown (204 beds); Tel: 456-1185. General medical/surgical facility.

Current Advisories and Health Risks

See the Disease Risk Summary for the Caribbean on page 293.

Samoa (Western)

APIA

CAPITAL:
Apia
EMBASSY (IN U.S.):
212-599-6196
GMT:
−11 hours
TELEPHONE COUNTRY CODE:
685
USADIRECT:
None
ENTRY REQUIREMENTS
- **Passport/Visa:** Passport required.

- **HIV Test:** Not required.
- **Vaccinations:** A yellow fever vaccination certificate is required for travelers older than 6 months of age coming from infected or endemic areas.

EMBASSIES/CONSULATES

- **U.S. Embassy:** Apia; Tel: 21631.
- **Canadian Embassy:** Accredited to the Australian High Commission. Fen Gai Ma Leata Building, Beach Road, Tamaligi, Apia, Samoa; Tel: 68-5-234-11; Fax: 68-5-231-59.
- **Office of the Honorary British Consul:** c/o Kruse Enari & Barlow, Barristers & Solicitors, PO Box 2029, 2nd Floor, NPF Building, Beach Rd, Central Apia; Tel: 685-21895; Fax: 685-21407; e-mail: barlowlaw@keblegal.ws.

HOSPITALS/DOCTORS:

Adequate medical care is available in Apia but does not meet the quality of care in industrialized countries. Medical care is substandard in the rest of the country. Adequate medical evacuation coverage for all travelers is a high priority. For serious medical conditions, every effort should be made to go to New Zealand or Australia. Hospital accommodations are inadequate throughout the country, and advanced technology is lacking.

- National Hospital (335 beds); general medical facility; emergency unit.

Current Advisories and Health Risks

ACCIDENTS/ILLNESSES AND MEDICAL INSURANCE

- Accidents and injuries are the leading cause of death among travelers younger than 55 years of age and most often are caused by motor vehicle and motorcycle crashes; drownings, aircraft crashes, homicides, and burns are less common causes.
- Heart attacks cause most fatalities in older travelers.
- Infections cause only 1% of fatalities in overseas travelers, but overall, infections are the most common cause of travel-related illness.
- Travelers are advised to obtain, before departure, supplemental travel health insurance with specific overseas coverage. The policy should provide for direct payment to the overseas hospital and/or physician at the time of service and include a medical evacuation benefit. The policy should also provide 24-hour hotline access to a multilingual assistance center that can help arrange and monitor delivery of medical care and determine if medical evacuation or air ambulance services are required.

DENGUE FEVER: Most risk of dengue occurs during rainy season months countrywide. Travelers should take protective measures against mosquito bites. Insect bite prevention measures include a DEET-containing repellent applied to exposed skin, insecticide (permethrin) spray applied to clothing and gear, and use of a permethrin-treated bed net at night while sleeping.

FILARIASIS: Malayan filariasis occurs in this country. Travelers should take protective measures against mosquito bites.

HEPATITIS: Hepatitis A vaccine is recommended for all nonimmune travelers. The hepatitis B carrier rate in the general population is estimated at 10%. Vaccination against hepatitis B should be considered for stays longer than 3 months and by short-term travelers desiring maximum protection. Travelers should be aware that hepatitis B can be transmitted by unsafe sex and the use of contaminated needles and syringes.

INFLUENZA: Influenza is transmitted year-round in the tropics. The flu vaccine is recommended for all travelers older than 50 years of age; all travelers with chronic disease or a weakened immune system; travelers of any age wishing to decrease the risk of this illness; and pregnant women after the first trimester.

MALARIA: No risk.

MARINE HAZARDS
• Swimming-related hazards include jellyfish, spiny sea urchins, and coral.
• Ciguatera poisoning is prevalent and can result from eating coral reef fish such as grouper, snapper, sea bass, jack, and barracuda. The ciguatoxin is not destroyed by cooking.

TRAVELERS' DIARRHEA: Moderate risk outside of first-class hotels and resorts. Travelers should drink only bottled, boiled, or treated water. Food should be eaten well cooked. A quinolone antibiotic, combined with loperamide (Imodium), is recommended for the treatment of acute diarrhea. Diarrhea not responding to antibiotic treatment may be due to a parasitic disease such as giardiasis or amebiasis or an intestinal virus.

TYPHOID FEVER: Typhoid vaccine is recommended, especially for long-term travelers, adventure travelers, and those wishing maximum disease protection. Because the typhoid vaccines are only 60% to 70% effective, safe food and drink guidelines should continue to be observed.

São Tomé and Principe

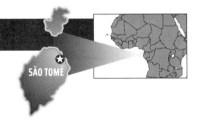

CAPITAL:
São Tomé
EMBASSY (IN U.S.):
212-697-4211
GMT:
+0 hours
TELEPHONE COUNTRY CODE:
239
USADIRECT:
None
ENTRY REQUIREMENTS
• **Passport/Visa:** Valid passport and visa are required.
• **HIV Test:** Not required.

- **Vaccinations:** A yellow fever vaccination certificate is required for all travelers older than 1 year arriving from all countries.

EMBASSIES/CONSULATES

The U.S. Ambassador based in Gabon is attached to São Tomé on a nonresident basis.

- **Canadian Embassy:** Accredited to the Canadian Embassy in Gabon. Quartier Batterie IV, Libreville; Gabon; Tel: 73-73-54; Fax: 73-73-88.
- **British Embassy:** Accredited to the British Embassy in Angola. Rua Diogo Cao, 4, Caixa Postal 1244, Luanda; Tel: 244-2-334582, 334583, 392991, 387681; Fax: 244-2-333331; e-mail: postmaster@luanda.fco.gov.uk.

HOSPITALS/DOCTORS:

Medical care in São Tomé is well below western standards. The main medical facility is the Ayres Menezes Hospital on São Tomé, which is run by the French medical charity Medecins du Monde. Travelers who experience serious health events are advised to seek treatment in Lisbon, Portugal or Johannesburg, South Africa, both of which are linked to São Tomé by regular flights. It is essential, therefore, that travelers purchase adequate medical evacuation coverage prior to departure.

Current Advisories and Health Risks

AIDS/HIV: Incidence is presumed low, but widespread surveys have not been done.

ARBOVIRAL FEVERS: Data are not available to indicate if arboviral fevers such as chikungunya, West Nile fever, Crimean-Congo hemorrhagic fever, and dengue are transmitted on the islands.

CHOLERA: This disease is active in this country. The risk of cholera, however, is extremely low in international travelers from developed countries, such as the United States and Canada. Cholera vaccine (no longer available in the United States) is recommended only for persons at high risk who work and live in highly endemic areas under less than adequate sanitary conditions.

- The oral cholera vaccine (Dukoral) provides up to 60% crossover protection against ETEC diarrhea.
- Cholera vaccine is not "officially" required for entry into, or exit from, any country. Despite this, some countries, on occasion, require proof of cholera immunization from travelers coming from cholera-infected countries. Anticipating such a situation, travelers may wish to carry a medical exemption letter from their health-care provider. If possible, it is advisable to contact the embassy or consulate at the destination country to confirm the requirement for cholera vaccination (if any) and the acceptability of a medical exemption letter.

HEPATITIS: High risk. All susceptible travelers should receive hepatitis A vaccine or immune globulin prophylaxis. The hepatitis B carrier rate in the general population is estimated to exceed 10%. Vaccination against hepatitis B is recommended for health-care workers and all long-term visitors to this country. No data on hepatitis E are currently available.

MALARIA: Risk is present year-round throughout this country, including urban areas. Falciparum malaria accounts for 87% of cases. Chloroquine-resistant falciparum malaria is reported. Prophylaxis with atovaquone/proguanil (Malarone), mefloquine (Lariam), or doxycycline is currently recommended for travel to malarious areas of this country.

SCHISTOSOMIASIS: Widely distributed throughout the island of São Tomé. The major risk area is in the northeast between the Rio Grande and Manuel Jorge rivers, including the capital and environs, the surrounding Agua Grande District, and the adjacent part of Mezoxi District. Travelers should avoid swimming, bathing, or wading in freshwater lakes, ponds, or streams.

TRAVELERS' DIARRHEA: High risk. Piped water supplies should be considered potentially contaminated. Travelers should observe all food and drink safety precautions. A quinolone antibiotic is recommended for the treatment of acute diarrhea. Diarrhea not responding to treatment with an antibiotic, or chronic diarrhea, may be due to a parasitic disease such as giardiasis, amebiasis, or cryptosporidiosis.

YELLOW FEVER: Vaccination is required for entry. No recent yellow fever cases have been reported. This country is in the Yellow Fever Endemic Zone. A valid yellow fever vaccination certificate may be required for travel to other countries in South America, Africa, the Middle East, or Asia.

OTHER DISEASES/HAZARDS: Data on filariasis, loiasis, onchocerciasis, leishmaniasis, intestinal helminthic diseases, and rabies are not available, but these diseases are presumed to occur. Tuberculosis and typhoid fever are considered to be endemic.

Saudi Arabia

CAPITAL:
Riyadh
EMBASSY (IN U.S.):
202-342-3800
GMT:
+3 hours
TELEPHONE COUNTRY CODE:
966
USADIRECT:
1-800-10
ENTRY REQUIREMENTS
- **Passport/Visa:** A valid passport and visa are required. No tourist visas are issued. Regulations and requirements may be subject to change at short notice, and visitors are advised to contact the appropriate diplomatic or consular authority before finalizing travel arrangements.

- **HIV Test:** Required for applicants for residency/work permits.
- **Vaccinations:** A yellow fever vaccination certificate is required for all travelers arriving from, or transiting through, any country any part of which is infected with yellow fever. *Meningococcal vaccine*: Pilgrims for the Hajj or Umrah are required by the government of Saudi Arabia to have a valid certificate of vaccination against meningococcal serogroups A, C, Y, and W-135 before they are issued a visa. During the Hajj (annual pilgrimage to Mecca), Saudi Arabia requires vaccination of pilgrims older than 6 months against meningococcal meningitis. The quadrivalent vaccine protecting against serogroups A, C, Y, and W-135 should be used to immunize travelers.

EMBASSIES/CONSULATES

- **U.S. Embassy:** Collector Road M, Diplomatic Quarter, Riyadh; Tel: 1-488-3800.
- **U.S. Consulate:** Dhahran; Tel: 3-891-3200.
- **U.S. Consulate:** Jeddah; Tel: 2-667-0080.
- **Canadian Embassy:** Diplomatic Quarter, Riyadh, Saudi Arabia; Tel: 966-1-488-2288; Fax: 966-1-488-1997.
- **British Embassy:** PO Box 94351, Riyadh 11693; Tel: 966-1-488-0077; Fax: 966-1-488-2373, 488-0623.

HOSPITALS/DOCTORS:

Medical care in Saudi Arabia is of high quality, and most physicians speak English. There are numerous facilities that provide medical care for foreign expatriates. Travelers are advised to obtain, before departure, supplemental travel health insurance with specific overseas coverage. The policy should provide for direct payment to the overseas hospital and/or physician at the time of service and include a medical evacuation benefit.

- Dr. M. Fakhry and A. Al Mouhawis Hospital (200 beds), Al Khobar, Saudi Arabia; Tel: 3-864-1107.
- King Faisal Specialist Hospital, Riyadh (400 beds); all specialties; ambulance service and helipad; rated best medical facility in Saudi Arabia.
- Aramco Hospital, Dhahran (361 beds); private accredited hospital; most specialties; one of the best medical facilities in the country.

Current Advisories and Health Risks

ANIMAL HAZARDS: There is the risk of carpet viper bites (usually nonfatal in adults) in lowland areas of the Asir region in southern Saudi Arabia.

DENGUE FEVER: There is a very low risk of disease in the eastern coastal areas, where the mosquito vector is found. No current data about disease incidence are available. Travelers to the eastern coastal area should take measures to prevent daytime mosquito bites.

HEPATITIS: Hepatitis A vaccine is recommended for all travelers. Hepatitis E is likely endemic, but no data are currently available. The hepatitis B carrier rate in the general population is estimated at 8% to 10%. Vaccination against hepatitis B should be considered for stays longer than 3 months and by short-term travelers desiring maximum protection.

INFLUENZA: Influenza is transmitted during November through March. The flu vaccine is recommended for all travelers.

LEISHMANIASIS: Transmission of cutaneous leishmaniasis occurs year-round (peaking from July through September) in the oases of the eastern and central emirates. A hyperendemic focus may exist near the Al-Hofuf oasis. Cutaneous leishmaniasis also occurs in the mountains of the western emirates. Visceral leishmaniasis (kala-azar) occurs year-round and is restricted to the southwestern Asir region. Travelers should take measures to prevent sand fly bites.

MALARIA: Transmission of this disease occurs year-round in the hill regions close to Yemen, with increased risk October through April. *P. falciparum* accounts for 85% of the cases; chloroquine-resistant falciparum malaria has been reported in the southwest. There is no malaria in the urban areas of Jedda, Mecca, Medina, and Taif. All travelers to malarious regions should take one of the following antimalarial drugs: atovaquone/proguanil, doxycycline, mefloquine, or (in special circumstances) primaquine.

MENINGITIS: Pilgrims for Hajj or Umrah are required by the Government of Saudi Arabia to have a valid certificate of vaccination against meningococcal disease before they are issued a visa. The CDC recommends that all travelers to Saudi Arabia be vaccinated with the quadrivalent vaccine, which protects against meningococcal serogroups A, C, Y, and W-135. Travelers should receive a certificate of vaccination, issued at least 10 days before arrival, to verify immunization.

POLIO: This disease is active. All travelers should be fully immunized.

RABIES: Human cases occur very sporadically, usually in northern and eastern rural areas. Most animal rabies is in foxes, with spillover into the stray dog population. Travelers should seek immediate treatment of any animal bite. Rabies vaccination is indicated following the unprovoked bite of a dog or fox. Bites by other animals should be considered on an individual basis.

SAND FLY FEVER: This viral disease is endemic. Foci may occur throughout the country, with elevated risk (April through October) in village and periurban areas. All travelers should take precautions against sand fly bites, which occur between dusk and dawn.

SCHISTOSOMIASIS: Risk is present in the western (in wadis and cisterns) and central (in oases) emirates. Intestinal schistosomiasis foci occur in the central (Hail, Riyadh), northern (Al Jawf), northwestern (Tabuk, Medina), and midwestern (Makkah, Al Bahah) emirates and the highlands of the southwestern (Jiazan) and midwestern (Makkah) emirates. In these areas, all travelers should avoid swimming or wading in freshwater ponds, lakes, streams, cisterns, aqueducts, or irrigated areas.

TRAVELERS' DIARRHEA: Water is supplied via potable water distribution systems in all major urban areas of Saudi Arabia and is safe for drinking. Outside of major urban areas, all travelers should drink only boiled, bottled, or treated/filtered water. A quinolone antibiotic, combined with loperamide (Imodium), should be used to treat acute diarrhea.

OTHER DISEASES/HAZARDS: AIDS (very low prevalence; cases are officially attributed to blood transfusions); brucellosis, echinococcosis (carried by stray dogs, especially in rural and agricultural areas); onchocerciasis (black fly-borne; confined to the southwestern Arabian peninsula in focally endemic areas), Q fever, sand fly fever (transmission primarily April through October), trachoma (highly endemic); tuberculosis (moderate prevalence in rural areas among lower socioeconomic groups); typhoid fever; and soil-transmitted helminthic infections (roundworm, hookworm, and whipworm infections).

Senegal

★ DAKAR

CAPITAL:
Dakar
EMBASSY (IN U.S.):
202-234-0540
GMT:
+0 hours
TELEPHONE COUNTRY CODE:
221
USADIRECT:
3072
ENTRY REQUIREMENTS
Travelers should check with this country's embassy (or a consulate) in the United States, Canada, or the United Kingdom for any changes in these requirements.
• **Passport/Visa:** Passport and onward/return ticket required. Visa not needed for stay of up to 90 days.
• **HIV Test:** Not required.
• **Vaccinations:** A yellow fever vaccination certificate is required for all travelers older than 1 year of age arriving from infected areas.
EMBASSIES/CONSULATES
• **U.S. Embassy:** Avenue Jean XXIII, Dakar; Tel: 221-822-4599 or 221-823-4296.
• **Canadian Embassy:** 45, Avenue de la République, Dakar; Tel: 221-823-92-90; Fax: 823-87-49; e-mail: dakar-cs@dfait-maeci.gc.ca or dakar@dfait-maeci.gc.ca; Website: www.dfait-maeci.gc.ca/dakar.
• **British Embassy:** 20 Rue du Docteur Guillet, (Boite Postale 6025), Dakar; Tel: 221-823-7392, 823-9971; Fax: 221-823-2766, 823-8415; e-mail: britemb@sentoo.sn.
HOSPITALS/DOCTORS:
Medical care in Senegal is below Western standards, but several private clinics are at the level of small European hospital or U.S. community hospital standards. The U.S. Embassy maintains a listing of physicians and other health-care providers. Travelers are advised to obtain, before departure, supplemental travel health insurance with specific

overseas coverage. The policy should provide for direct payment to the overseas hospital and/or physician at the time of service and include a medical evacuation benefit.

- CTO Trauma Care Facility, Dakar; general medical/surgical facility; trauma; orthopedics.
- Dantec Hospital, Dakar; general medical/surgical facility; trauma.
- Hospitale Principale, Dakar (650 beds); cardiothoracic surgery; orthopedics.

Current Advisories and Health Risks

AFRICAN SLEEPING SICKNESS (TRYPANOSOMIASIS): Acquiring African trypanosomiasis is a low but potential risk in scattered areas throughout the country. Travelers should take measures to prevent insect (tsetse fly) bites.

AIDS/HIV: Senegal has maintained one of the lowest HIV prevalence levels in sub-Saharan Africa, and HIV rates have stabilized since 1997. USAID reports a 1% prevalence (HIV-1 and HIV-2) for 2002. Senegal's comparatively low HIV/AIDS prevalence in relation to other African countries has been attributed to public health measures that encourage condom use, screening commercial sex workers, and promote public health education.

CHOLERA: This disease is active in this country, but the threat to tourists is very low. Cholera is an extremely rare disease in travelers from developed countries. Cholera vaccine is recommended primarily for people at high risk (e.g., relief workers) who work and live in highly endemic areas under less than adequate sanitary conditions.

HEPATITIS: Hepatitis A vaccine is recommended for all travelers. Hepatitis E is endemic, but the level is unclear. The hepatitis B carrier rate in the general population is estimated to be as high as 18%. Vaccination is recommended for stays longer than 3 months; for persons at occupational or social risk; and for any traveler desiring maximum protection. Because the risk of illness or injury during travel cannot be predicted, all travelers should consider hepatitis B vaccine because of the risk of receiving a medical injection with an unsterile needle or syringe.

INFLUENZA: Influenza is transmitted year-round in the tropics. The flu vaccine is recommended for all travelers.

LASSA FEVER: Cases of Lassa fever occur sporadically, but rarely. Transmission is through contact with the infected urine or dried feces of rodents, especially in rural areas.

LEISHMANIASIS: Risk of cutaneous leishmaniasis occurs in the northwest (Keur Moussa in the Theis Region) and has been reported in the northeast along the Mauritanian border. Sporadic cases occur annually among Peace Corps volunteers stationed countrywide. Visceral leishmaniasis has not been reported. Travelers are advised to take measures to prevent insect (sand fly) bites.

MALARIA: Risk is present year-round throughout this country, including in Dakar and other urban areas. There is less risk in the Cap Vert vicinity and northern Sahel regions from January through July. Risk is elevated during and immediately after the rainy season (May through October in the south and July through September in the north). *P. falciparum* accounts for 90% of malaria cases. Prophylaxis with atovaquone/proguanil (Malarone), mefloquine (Lariam), or doxycycline is recommended. All travelers should take measures to prevent evening and nighttime mosquito bites.

MENINGITIS: Quadrivalent meningococcal meningitis vaccine is recommended for all travelers staying longer than 1 month during dry season, December through June, and should be considered for shorter stays if close contact with the local populace is anticipated.

RABIES: Sporadic cases of human rabies are reported countrywide. All animal bites or scratches, especially from a dog, should be taken seriously, and immediate medical attention sought. Although rabies is rare among tourists, there is risk. No one should pet or pick up any stray animals. All children should be warned to avoid contact with unknown animals. Rabies vaccine is recommended for travel longer than 3 months; for shorter stays for travelers who plan to venture off the usual tourist routes, where they may be more exposed to the stray dog population; or when travelers desire extra protection.

SCHISTOSOMIASIS: Risk of urinary schistosomiasis is present in the Senegal River valley along the Mauritanian border; in the west-central regions of Dakar, Thies, Diourbel, and Fatick; and in the southwestern and south-central areas. Intestinal schistosomiasis occurs in scattered areas. Travelers should avoid swimming, bathing, or wading in freshwater lakes, ponds, or streams.

TRAVELERS' DIARRHEA: The cities of Dakar, Saint-Louis, Kaolack, Thies, and Ziguinchor have municipal water systems and public taps, but these systems may be contaminated. A quinolone antibiotic, combined with loperamide (Imodium), is recommended for the treatment of acute diarrhea. Persistent diarrhea may be due to a parasitic infection such as giardiasis, amebiasis, or cryptosporidiosis.

TUBERCULOSIS: Tuberculosis (TB) is a major health problem in this country. Travelers planning an extended stay should have a pre-departure TB skin test (PPD test) and be retested after returning from this country.

TYPHOID FEVER: Typhoid vaccine is recommended for persons traveling off the usual tourist routes, for those visiting friends or relatives, and for long-stay visitors. Because the typhoid vaccines are only 60% to 70% effective, safe food and drink selection remains important.

YELLOW FEVER: Sporadic outbreaks are reported. The CDC recommends yellow fever vaccination for all travelers older than 9 months of age. Yellow fever vaccination is required for all travelers arriving from infected areas.

OTHER DISEASES/HAZARDS: African tick typhus, brucellosis (from consumption of unpasteurized dairy products), West Nile fever, Rift Valley fever, filariasis (mosquito-borne), Lassa fever (slight risk may occur in the southeast near the border with Mali), leprosy, leptospirosis, murine typhus (flea-borne), onchocerciasis (black fly-borne; contracted near fast-flowing rivers), rabies, tick-borne relapsing fever, tuberculosis (a major health problem), and intestinal worms.

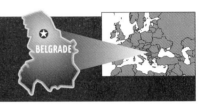

Serbia and Montenegro (former Yugoslavia)

CAPITAL:
Belgrade
EMBASSY (IN U.S.):
202-332-0333
GMT:
+1 hour
TELEPHONE COUNTRY CODE:
38
USADIRECT:
Operator assistance required
ENTRY REQUIREMENTS
- **Passport/Visa:** Visas are not required for entry and stays in Serbia and Montenegro up to 90 days for the citizens of selected countries, including the United States. This covers bearers of all types of U.S. passports—tourist, official, diplomatic. American citizens planning to stay longer than 90 days should leave the country and return visa free; they can do this repeatedly. This does not apply to students, or American citizens who come to work; they can enter the country visa free, but they are required to apply for either a student or work visa within 3 days of arrival.
- **HIV Test:** Not required.
- **Vaccinations:** None required.
EMBASSIES/CONSULATES
- **U.S. Embassy:** Kneza Milosa 50, Belgrade; Tel: 11-645-655.
- **Canadian Embassy:** Kneza Milosa 75, 11000 Belgrade, Serbia and Montenegro; Tel: 381-11-306-3000; Fax: 381-11-306-3042; e-mail: bgrad@international.gc.ca; Website: www.dfait-maeci.gc.ca/canadaeuropa/serbia-montenegro.
- **British Embassy:** Resavska 46, 11000 Belgrade; Tel: 381-11-2645-055, 3060-900, 3615-660; Fax: 381-11-659-651; e-mail: britemb@eunet.yu; Website: www.britemb.org.yu.
HOSPITALS/DOCTORS:
Medical care in Serbia and Montenegro is adequate for most conditions. For treatment of serious or life-threatening illness or accident, travelers should consider transfer to Vienna, Austria, or another European center with more advanced medical facilities. Travelers are advised to obtain, before departure, supplemental travel health insurance with specific overseas coverage. The policy should provide for direct payment to the

overseas hospital and/or physician at the time of service and include a medical evacuation benefit.
- Travelers should contact the U.S. Embassy for physician referrals and telephone numbers.

Current Advisories and Health Risks

See the Disease Risk Summary for Europe on page 300.

Sierra Leone

★ FREETOWN

CAPITAL:
Freetown
EMBASSY (IN U.S.):
202-939-9261
GMT:
+0 hours
TELEPHONE COUNTRY CODE:
232
USADIRECT:
1100
ENTRY REQUIREMENTS
- **Passport/Visa:** Valid passport and visa are required.
- **HIV Test:** Not required.
- **Vaccinations:** A yellow fever vaccination certificate is required of all travelers older than 1 year of age arriving from infected areas.

EMBASSIES/CONSULATES
- **U.S. Embassy:** Corner of Walpole and Siaka Stevens Sts., Freetown; Tel: 22-226-481; Fax: 22-225-471.
- **Canadian Embassy:** Corniche Sud, Conakry, Guinea; Tel: 224-46-23-95; Fax: 224-46-42-35; e-mail: cnaky@dfait-maeci.gc.ca.
- **British High Commission:** Spur Road, Freetown; Tel: 232-22-232961, 232362, 232563-5; Fax: 232-22-228169, 232070; e-mail: bhc@sierratel.sl.

HOSPITALS/DOCTORS:
Medical care in Sierra Leone is below Western standards and in a state of near-collapse. Travelers are advised to obtain, before departure, supplemental travel health insurance that includes a medical evacuation benefit. In case of any serious illness or accident, medical evacuation to another country for treatment is indicated.
- Connaught Hospital, Freetown (240 beds); overcrowded, understaffed facility lacking modern equipment.

Current Advisories and Health Risks

IMMUNIZATIONS: All travelers should be up to date on their routine immunizations: tetanus-diphtheria (Td), measles-mumps-rubella (MMR), polio, influenza, and varicella (chickenpox). Immunizations against hepatitis A, hepatitis B, meningitis, rabies, and typhoid fever are recommended.

MALARIA: All travelers to Sierra Leone including infants, children, and former residents of this country should take one of the following antimalarial drugs: atovaquone/proguanil, doxycycline, mefloquine, or (in special circumstances) primaquine. Travelers should also take measures to prevent evening and nighttime mosquito bites. Insect bite prevention measures include a DEET-containing repellent applied to exposed skin, insecticide (permethrin) spray applied to clothing, and use of a permethrin-treated bed net at night.

For additional information, consult the Disease Risk Summary for Sub-Saharan Africa on page 307.

Singapore

CAPITAL:
Singapore
EMBASSY (IN U.S.):
202-537-3100
GMT:
+8 hours
TELEPHONE COUNTRY CODE:
65
USADIRECT:
800-011-1111 or 800-001-0001
ENTRY REQUIREMENTS
- **Passport/Visa:** Visas are required for tourist/business stays up to 30 days.
- **HIV Test:** Required for all applicants for employment passes, work permits, and permanent resident status (except spouses and children of Singapore citizens).
- **Vaccinations:** A yellow fever vaccination certificate is required of any traveler older than 1 year of age arriving from, or having transited, a country within the preceding 6 days, any part of which is infected, and also of travelers arriving from, or transiting, countries in the endemic zones.
EMBASSIES/CONSULATES
- **U.S. Embassy:** 27 Napier Road, Singapore; Tel: 476-9100 or 65-476-9100; Fax: 65-476-9340; Website: www.usembassysingapore.org.sg.
- **Canadian Embassy:** IBM Towers, 80 Anson Road, Singapore; Tel: 325-3200; Fax: 325-3297; e-mail: spore@dfait-maeci.gc.ca.
- **British High Commission:** Tanglin Road, Singapore 247919; Commercial Section: Tanglin PO Box 19, Singapore 247919; Tel: 65-6424-4200; Fax: 65-6424-4218; e-mail: Commercial.Singapore@fco.gov.uk; Website: www.britain.org.sg.

HOSPITALS/DOCTORS:
Medical care in Singapore is of very high quality, and most physicians speak English. Travelers are advised to obtain, before departure, supplemental travel health insurance with specific overseas coverage. The policy should provide for direct payment to the overseas hospital and/or physician at the time of service and include a medical evacuation benefit.

- SingHealth Polyclinics, 3 Second Hospital Avenue, Singapore; Tel: 6236-4800; Website: http://polyclinic.singhealth.com.sg. Family practice and preventive care.
- Mt. Elizabeth Hospital (485 beds); Tel: 6737-2666. All specialties; emergency, burn, trauma units; considered one of the best hospitals in Southeast Asia.
- Gleneagles Hospital (375 beds); Tel: 6473-7222. Used by U.S. Embassy personnel.
- International SOS: International SOS Pte Ltd., 331 North Bridge Road, #17-00, Odeon Towers, Singapore 188720; Alarm Center Eng Tel: 65-6338-7800; Alarm Center Eng Fax: 65-6338-7611

Current Advisories and Health Risks

CHOLERA: This disease is not reported as active at this time.

DENGUE FEVER: Seasonal outbreaks occur countrywide, with risk elevated from May through September. All travelers should take protective measures against daytime mosquito bites.

FILARIASIS: Low risk; both the bancroftian and Malayan forms may occur and are transmitted by a variety of mosquitoes.

HEPATITIS: Hepatitis A vaccine is recommended for all travelers. Hepatitis E and hepatitis C are endemic, but no vaccines are available. The hepatitis B carrier rate in the general population is estimated at 5%. Hepatitis B is spread by infected blood, contaminated needles, and unsafe sex. Vaccination is recommended for stays longer than 3 months; for persons at occupational or social risk; and for any traveler desiring maximum protection.

INFLUENZA: Influenza is transmitted year-round in the tropics. The flu vaccine is recommended for all travelers.

JAPANESE ENCEPHALITIS: There is no significant risk of Japanese encephalitis (JE), and the JE vaccine is not recommended for anyone living or working in Singapore.

MALARIA: There is no risk of malaria in Singapore.

TRAVELERS' DIARRHEA: Low risk. Tap water in Singapore is potable. A quinolone antibiotic is recommended for the treatment of acute diarrhea. Persistent diarrhea may be due to a parasitic disease such as giardiasis, amebiasis, or cryptosporidiosis.

OTHER DISEASES/HAZARDS: Helminthic infections (low incidence). Stingrays, poisonous fish, sea anemones, the Indo-China man-of-war, and the very dangerous sea wasp are found along the coral reefs that fringe Singapore. Swimmers should take sensible precautions to avoid these hazards.

Slovak Republic

BRATISLAVA

CAPITAL:
Bratislava
EMBASSY (IN THE U.S.):
202-965-5160
GMT:
+1 hour
TELEPHONE COUNTRY CODE:
421
USADIRECT:
0-800-000-101
ENTRY REQUIREMENTS
- **Passport/Visa:** Passport and proof of health insurance coverage required. Visa not required for stays of less than 90 days.
- **HIV Test:** Not required.
- **Vaccinations:** None required.

EMBASSIES/CONSULATES
- **U.S. Embassy:** Bratislava; Tel: 421-7-330-0861.
- **Canadian Embassy:** Carlton Court Yard & Savoy Buildings, Mostova 2, 811 02 Bratislava, Slovakia; Tel: 421-2-5920-4031; Fax: 421-2-5443-4227; e-mail: brslva@ international.gc.ca.
- **British Embassy:** Panska 16, 811 01 Bratislava; Tel: 421-2-5998-2000; Fax: 421-2-5998-2237.

HOSPITALS/DOCTORS:
Vladimir Strakrle, M.D., Outpatient Department for Infectious Diseases, Travel Medicine and Hepatology, Ponavka 2, Brno; Tel: 42-055240743.

Current Advisories and Health Risks

IMMUNIZATIONS: All travelers to Europe and Russia should be up-to-date on their routine immunizations: tetanus-diphtheria (Td), measles-mumps-rubella (MMR), influenza, and varicella (chickenpox). Hepatitis A and hepatitis B vaccines are strongly recommended for all travelers. Typhoid fever, rabies, and tick-borne encephalitis vaccines are recommended on an individual basis, according to the traveler's itinerary and possible disease exposure.

AIDS/HIV: The countries with the highest incidences of AIDS and HIV are the Russian Federation, the Baltic States (Estonia, Latvia, and Lithuania), Bulgaria, Belarus, Moldova, Romania, and Ukraine. Injecting drug use and unsafe sex are driving the spread of HIV, but the virus is also moving from high-risk groups into the general population, where heterosexual contact is the main route of transmission. In Eastern Europe and Russia travelers should avoid unprotected sex with new partners, as well as unscreened blood transfusions and medical injections. (Many travelers now carry their own packets of sterile needles and syringes.) Blood supplies are reportedly screened in Czechoslovakia, Hungary, and Poland, but lack of public health funding may hamper complete screening for HIV and hepatitis B and C. Travelers should consider evacuation to a Western European medical facility when surgical care or blood transfusion is needed.

DIPHTHERIA: Since the epidemic in the early nineties diphtheria has come under good control through improved childhood vaccination programs.

EHRLICHIOSIS: Cases of human granulocytic ehrlichiosis have been reported from Slovenia and the Netherlands.

EUROPEAN TICK-BORNE ENCEPHALITIS (TBE): The tick, *Ixodes ricinus*, is the vector for this disease, (the same tick that transmits Lyme disease). Ticks are widely distributed in brushy and forested areas at elevations up to 1,500 meters. TBE occurs in all European countries (especially Austria, Germany, Switzerland, the Czech Republic, Hungary, the Balkans, and Eastern Europe) except the Benelux countries and the Iberian Peninsula. Transmission is maximal during spring and fall months. A vaccine is available in Europe and Canada.

HEMORRHAGIC FEVER WITH RENAL SYNDROME (HFRS): Cases of Hantavirus illness are reported in the Balkans and in eastern Europe. A milder form of HFRS (caused by Puumala virus) occurs in Scandinavia, other European countries, and European Russia. Travelers should avoid contact with rodent urine and rodent feces, which transmit the virus.

HEPATITIS A: Hepatitis A vaccine is recommended for all travelers. There is increased risk of hepatitis A in Spain, Greece, the Balkans, Eastern Europe, and Russia.

HEPATITIS B: The hepatitis B carrier rate in the general population of Europe varies, but is less than 1% in most western European countries. The carrier rate increases to 1% to 4% in Spain, Greece, Eastern Europe, and Russia. Hepatitis B is spread by infected blood, contaminated needles, and unprotected sex. Vaccination is recommended for stays longer than 3 months; for anyone at occupational or social risk; for anyone desiring maximal protection.

LEISHMANIASIS: Cutaneous and visceral leishmaniasis is present in the countries bordering the Mediterranean. Risk areas include Portugal, Spain, southern France, the Naples area, Majorca, the suburbs of Athens, and the Greek Isles. Travelers to these areas should take measures to prevent sand fly bites.

LYME DISEASE: Risk of transmission occurs throughout Europe in rural brushy, wooded, and forested areas up to elevations of 1,500 meters, especially in Scandinavia, Austria,

Switzerland, southern Germany, and northern Italy. The ticks that transmit Lyme disease are most abundant and active April through September.

MALARIA: There is no risk of malaria in Europe or Russia.

MEDITERRANEAN SPOTTED FEVER (BOUTONNEUSE FEVER): Occurs in southern France and in the coastal regions of other Mediterranean countries, and also along the Black Sea coast, in brushy and/or forested areas below 1,000 meters elevation. Peak transmission period is July through September. Disease may be acquired in and around tick-infested houses and terrain, but more than 95% of cases are associated with contact with tick-carrying dogs.

PERTUSSIS (WHOOPING COUGH): Reported in the Netherlands. The new strain of *Bordetella pertussis* bacterium is resistant to a leading vaccine and attacks adults as well as children.

RABIES: Occurs primarily in wild animals, especially foxes, in many rural areas of Europe. Countries free of human rabies include: Albania, Cyprus, Denmark, the Faeroe Islands, Finland, Gibraltar, Greece, Iceland, Ireland, Italy, the Isle of Man, Italy, Macedonia, Malta, Monaco, Norway, Portugal, Spain, Sweden, and the United Kingdom.

SAND FLY FEVER AND WEST NILE FEVER: Cases are reported from Albania and the Adriatic area.

TRAVELERS' DIARRHEA: Low risk in most western European countries. Higher risk occurs in Spain, Greece, the Balkans, and Eastern Europe, especially Bulgaria, Hungary, and Romania. Giardiasis is a threat in Russia. Travelers to higher risk areas should drink only bottled, boiled, or treated water and avoid undercooked food. A quinolone antibiotic is recommended for the treatment of diarrhea.

TYPHOID FEVER: Persons traveling extensively in Spain, Greece, Yugoslavia, and the Balkans, or the eastern European countries, especially Bulgaria, Hungary, and Romania, should consider typhoid vaccination.

OTHER ILLNESSES/HAZARDS: Brucellosis, echinococcosis (southern Europe), Legionnaire's disease (legionellosis outbreaks have been reported in tourists on package tours to Spain and Naples, Italy; contaminated water is the probable source), leptospirosis, listeriosis (from contaminated soft cheeses and meat; reported from France), tick-borne relapsing fever (risk in rocky, rural livestock areas), and soil-transmitted helminthic infections (roundworm, hookworm, and whipworm infections; reported in southern Europe). Raw cod ("lutefish") in Scandinavia may contain the fish tapeworm, *Diphyllobothrium latum*, a cause of anemia.

ROAD SAFETY: Pedestrians should use extra caution when crossing the street in countries where there is left-sided traffic. There is a higher incidence of motor vehicle fatalities in Spain, Portugal, Yugoslavia, Greece, and eastern Europe. Seat belts should be worn at all times.

Slovenia

CAPITAL:
Ljubljana
EMBASSY (IN U.S.):
202-667-5363
GMT:
+1 hour
TELEPHONE COUNTRY CODE:
386
USADIRECT:
None
ENTRY REQUIREMENTS
- **Passport/Visa:** Passport required. Visa not required for business/tourist stays up to 90 days.
- **HIV Test:** Not required.
- **Vaccinations:** None required.

EMBASSIES/CONSULATES
- **U.S. Embassy:** Presernova 31, Ljubljana; Tel: 1-200-5500; Fax: 1-200-5535; Website: www.usembassy.si.
- **Canadian Embassy:** c/o Triglav Insurance Company Ltd., Miklosiceva 19, Ljubljana; Tel: 1-430-3570; Fax: 386-1-430-3575.
- **British Embassy:** 4th Floor Trg Republike 3, 1000 Ljubljana; Tel: 386-1-200-3910; Fax: 386-1-425-0174; e-mail: info@british-embassy.si; Website: www.british-embassy.si.

HOSPITALS/DOCTORS:
Medical care in Slovenia generally is of high quality, but many physicians may not speak English. Travelers are advised to obtain, before departure, supplemental travel health insurance with specific overseas coverage. The policy should provide for direct payment to the overseas hospital and/or physician at the time of service and include a medical evacuation benefit. Travelers should consider evacuation to Vienna, Austria, or other European center, in case of more serious illness.
- University Medical Centre, Ljubljana; Tel: 61-143-1450.
- General Hospital, Maribor; Tel: 62-315-181.
- In Slovenia, there are 26 hospitals and maternity hospitals. The most important Slovene health institution is the Central Teaching Hospital in Ljubljana.

Current Advisories and Health Risks

See the Disease Risk Summary for Europe on page 300 for additional information.

Solomon Islands

CAPITAL:
Honiara
EMBASSY (IN U.S.):
Not applicable
GMT:
+11 hours
TELEPHONE COUNTRY CODE:
677
USADIRECT:
0811

ENTRY REQUIREMENTS
- **Passport/Visa:** Passport, onward/return ticket, and proof of sufficient funds are required. Contact Solomon Islands Mission to the UN, 820 2nd Ave., Suite 800A, New York, NY 10017; Tel: 212-599-6192 or 6193.
- **HIV Test:** Not required.
- **Vaccinations:** *Required*: A yellow fever vaccination certificate is required for travelers older than 1 year of age arriving from infected areas. *Recommended*: All travelers should be up to date on tetanus-diphtheria, measles-mumps-rubella, polio, hepatitis A, and varicella immunizations.

EMBASSIES/CONSULATES
There is no U.S. Embassy or diplomatic post in the Solomon Islands. Consular assistance for U.S. citizens is provided by the U.S. Embassy in Port Moresby, Papua New Guinea; Tel: 675-321-1455.
- **Canadian Embassy:** Accredited to the Australian High Commission. Corner Hibiscus Avenue and Mud Alley, Honiara, Solomon Islands; Tel: 677-21561; Fax: 677-23691.
- **British High Commission:** Telekom House, Mendana Avenue, Honiara, Postal Address: PO Box 676; Tel: 677-21705, 21706; Fax: 677-21549.

HOSPITALS/DOCTORS:
Medical care in the Solomon Islands is rudimentary by Western standards. There are six governmental hospitals and many missionary hospitals that provide basic medical care for a population of 400,000. Travelers are advised to obtain, before departure, supplemental travel health insurance with specific overseas coverage. The policy should provide for direct payment to the overseas hospital and/or physician at the time of service and include a medical evacuation benefit.
- Central Hospital (Numbaneen)/National Referral Hospital, Guadalcanal; Tel: 23-600. This 280-bed hospital is the main referral facility for this country.

Current Advisories and Health Risks

MOSQUITO-TRANSMITTED DISEASES: Dengue fever (present in both urban areas and rural areas), filariasis, and Japanese encephalitis, all occur in this country. Travelers should take measures to prevent both daytime and nighttime mosquito bites. Insect-bite prevention measures include a DEET-containing repellent applied to exposed skin, insecticide (permethrin) spray applied to clothing, and sleeping under a permethrin-treated bed net. Malaria occurs countrywide, except for the southern province of Rennell and Bellona, the eastern province of Temotu, and the outer islands of Tikopia, Anuta, and Fatutaka. Multidrug-resistant falciparum malaria is reported. Atovaquone/proguanil (Malarone), mefloquine (Lariam), or doxycycline is recommended for prophylaxis.

HEPATITIS: Hepatitis A vaccine is recommended for all travelers. Hepatitis B is hyperendemic in this country, with a carrier rate of 20% in certain population groups. Hepatitis B is spread by infected blood, contaminated needles, and unsafe sex. Vaccination is recommended for stays longer than 3 months; for persons at occupational or social risk; and for any traveler desiring maximum protection.

INFLUENZA: Transmitted year-round in the tropics; flu vaccine is recommended for all travelers to this country.

MARINE HAZARDS: Swimming-related hazards include jellyfish, spiny sea urchins, and coral. Ciguatera poisoning is prevalent and can result from eating coral reef fish such as grouper, snapper, sea bass, jack, and barracuda. The ciguatoxin is not destroyed by cooking.

TRAVELERS' DIARRHEA: All tap water should be considered unsafe. Travelers are advised to drink only bottled, boiled, or treated water. A quinolone antibiotic is recommended for the treatment of acute diarrhea. Persistent diarrhea may be due to a parasitic infection such as giardiasis, amebiasis, or cryptosporidiosis.

TUBERCULOSIS: Travelers planning an extended stay should have a pre-departure TB skin test (PPD test) and be retested after returning from this country.

TYPHOID FEVER: Typhoid vaccine is recommended for all travelers, with the exception of short-term visitors who restrict their meals to major restaurants and hotels, such as business travelers and cruise passengers. Because the typhoid vaccines are only 60% to 70% effective, safe food and drink selection remains important.

OTHER DISEASES/HAZARDS: Travelers are advised to wear shoes or sandals to prevent transmission of hookworm. There is a low risk of scrub typhus during the rainy seasons. Travelers walking through grassy areas should protect themselves from the bite of chigger mites. Centipedes, scorpions, and large black ants may be encountered by hikers and "bush walkers."

Somalia

CAPITAL:
Mogadishu
EMBASSY (IN U.S.):
202-342-1575

GMT:

+3 hours

TELEPHONE COUNTRY CODE:

252

USADIRECT:

None

ENTRY REQUIREMENTS

- **Passport/Visa:** Valid passport and visa are required.
- **HIV Test:** Not required.
- **Vaccinations:** A yellow fever vaccination certificate is required for all travelers arriving from infected areas. *Cholera:* A vaccination certificate is required for travelers arriving from infected areas.

EMBASSIES/CONSULATES

- **U.S. Embassy:** Corso Primo Luglio, Mogadishu; Tel: 20811.
- **Canadian High Commission:** Accredited to the Canadian High Commission in Kenya. Limuru Road, Gigiri, Nairobi, Kenya; Tel: 254-20-366-3000; Fax: 254-20-366-3900; e-mail: nrobi@international.gc.ca; Website: www.nairobi.gc.ca.
- **British Embassy:** Waddada Xasan Geedd Abtoow 7/8, (PO Box 1036), Mogadishu; Tel: 252-1-20288/9, 21472/3.

HOSPITALS/DOCTORS:

The local medical facilities are inadequate. The U.S. State Department recommends evacuating personnel to Nairobi, Kenya, in lieu of using Somali hospitals.

Current Advisories and Health Risks

ARBOVIRAL FEVERS: Chikungunya fever, Rift Valley fever, West Nile fever, and sand fly fever may occur. Rift Valley fever outbreak reported in 1998.

CHOLERA: This disease is active in this country. The risk of cholera, however, is extremely low in international travelers from developed countries, such as the United States and Canada. Cholera vaccine (no longer available in the United States) is recommended only for persons at high risk who work and live in highly endemic areas under less than adequate sanitary conditions.

- The oral cholera vaccine (Dukoral) provides up to 60% crossover protection against ETEC diarrhea.
- Many countries, including Canada, license an oral cholera vaccine.
- Cholera vaccine is not "officially" required for entry into, or exit from, any country. Despite this, some countries, on occasion, require proof of cholera immunization from travelers coming from cholera-infected countries. Anticipating such a situation, travelers may wish to carry a medical exemption letter from their health-care provider. If possible, it is advisable to contact the embassy or consulate at the destination country to confirm the requirement for cholera vaccination (if any) and the acceptability of a medical exemption letter.

DENGUE FEVER: Moderate risk. Thirty-three cases of dengue were reported in American personnel in Somalia in 1992; the virus is estimated to have caused 17% of febrile illnesses in U.S. troops previously stationed in this country.

HEPATITIS: High risk. All nonimmune travelers should receive hepatitis A vaccine. The hepatitis B carrier rate in the general population is estimated to be as high as 19%. Vaccination against hepatitis B is recommended for health-care workers and all long-term visitors to this country. Hepatitis E outbreaks have been reported in refugee camps, and the disease is a hazard for health-care and relief workers.

LEISHMANIASIS: A hyperendemic focus of visceral leishmaniasis (kala-azar) persists along the Shabeelle River in the Giohar District in southern Somalia. Cutaneous leishmaniasis has not been reported but may occur in southern Somalia near the borders with Kenya and Ethiopia.

MALARIA: Risk is present year-round throughout this country, including urban areas. Risk of transmission is highest in July and December, after the semi-annual rains. The risk of malaria is greater in the south, particularly along the Shabeelle and Juba River valleys. There is limited malaria risk in the city center of Mogadishu. Falciparum malaria accounts for 95% of cases countrywide, but in 106 U.S. marines returning from Somalia in 1993, *P. vivax* accounted for 87% of cases. Prophylaxis with atovaquone/proguanil (Malarone), mefloquine (Lariam), or doxycycline is currently recommended for travel to malarious areas. (*Note:* Two cases of mefloquine-resistant *P. falciparum* malaria were reported in U.S. troops stationed in Somalia.)

SCHISTOSOMIASIS: Year-round risk of urinary schistosomiasis, primarily in the valleys of the Giuba and Shabeelle rivers in southern Somalia. Travelers to these areas should avoid bathing, wading, or swimming in freshwater lakes, ponds, or streams.

TRAVELERS' DIARRHEA: High risk. All water supplies are potentially contaminated. Travelers should observe all food and drink safety precautions. A quinolone antibiotic is recommended for the treatment of acute diarrhea. Diarrhea not responding to antibiotic treatment may be due to a parasitic disease such as giardiasis or amebiasis.

YELLOW FEVER: This country lies within the Yellow Fever Endemic Zone. Although yellow fever has not been reported, vaccination is recommended.

OTHER DISEASES/HAZARDS: African tick typhus, brucellosis, echinococcosis, filariasis (occurs in southern Somalia, in the area between Kenya and the Indian Ocean), histoplasmosis (common), leptospirosis (high incidence), meningitis, Q fever, rabies (transmitted primarily by dogs but also by foxes, cats, camels, donkeys, hyenas, badgers, and jackals), tick-borne relapsing fever (endemic), tuberculosis (a major health problem), trachoma, typhoid fever, epidemic typhus (louse-borne; increased risk in persons having contact with refugees), murine typhus (flea-borne), and intestinal worms.

South Africa

CAPITAL:
Pretoria
EMBASSY (IN U.S.):
202-966-1650; Embassy of South Africa,
3201 New Mexico Ave. NW, Washington, DC 20016
GMT:
+2 hours
TELEPHONE COUNTRY CODE:
27
USADIRECT:
0-800-99-0123

ENTRY REQUIREMENTS

Travelers should check with this country's embassy (or a consulate) in the United States, Canada, or the United Kingdom for any changes in these requirements.

• **Passport/Visa:** Tourist or business visa not required for stays of up to 90 days.

• **HIV Test:** Not required for tourists.

• **Vaccinations:** A yellow fever vaccination certificate is required of all travelers older than 1 year of age arriving from a country any part of which is infected or from any country in the Yellow Fever Endemic Zones.

EMBASSIES/CONSULATES

• **U.S. Embassy:** *Pretoria:* 877 Pretorius Street, Arcadia; Tel: 12-342-1048; Fax: 12-342-5504. *Johannesburg:* Tel: 11-644-8000; Fax: 11-646-6916.

• **Canadian Embassy:** 19th Floor, South African Reserve Bank Building, 60 St., George's Mall, Cape Town; Tel: 21-423-5240; Fax: 27-21-423-4893; e-mail: cptwn@dfait-maeci.gc.ca.

• **British High Commission:** 255 Hill Street, Arcadia 0002, Pretoria; Tel: 27-12-421-7500; Fax: 27-12-421-7555; e-mail: bhc@icon.co.za; Website: http://www.britain.org.za.

HOSPITALS/DOCTORS:

Medical facilities are good in urban areas and in the vicinity of game parks and beaches, but limited elsewhere. Travelers should consult a doctor if entering malarious areas such as Kruger National Park, northern KwaZulu/Natal, parts of Swaziland, Mozambique, and northern Zimbabwe, and take necessary antimalarial prophylactics.

CAPE TOWN

• Milnerton Medi-Clinic, Koeberg and Racecourse Roads, Cape Town (Milnerton) 7441.

DURBAN

• Entabeni Hospital, 148 South Ridge Rd. This 273-bed private hospital has emergency services available 24 hours a day.

• St. Augustine's Hospital, 107 Chelmsford Rd. This 418-bed private hospital is a major trauma center with emergency services available 24 hours a day.

George
- Lamprecht Clinic, York and Gloucester Avenues. This is the preferred facility for expatriates and travelers in the South Cape. The hospital does not have an emergency unit.

Johannesburg
- The Glynnwood Hospital, 33 Harrison St. Telephone: This 290-bed private general hospital provides emergency services 24 hours a day, but it is not a major trauma center.
- The Mayo Clinic of South Africa is located west of Johannesburg, Gauteng, in the suburb of Constantia Kloof. The Flora Clinic is situated alongside.
- Arwyp Medical Centre; this 250-bed hospital and trauma center provides emergency services 24 hours a day.
- International SOS: International SOS Assistance (Pty) Ltd., Stand 72 (adjoining Grand Central Airport), New Road, Midrand 1685, South Africa; Alarm Center Tel: 27-11-541-1350; Alarm Center Fax: 27-11-541-1058

Current Advisories and Health Risks

ACCIDENTS/ILLNESSES: Accidents, especially motor vehicle crashes, are the leading cause of death among travelers younger than 55 years of age; cardiovascular disease causes most fatalities in older travelers. Infections cause less than 1% of fatalities but are responsible for most of the illnesses experienced by travelers.

AFRICAN TICK TYPHUS: African tick typhus is focally distributed, including periurban areas near Johannesburg. Cases are often reported among travelers, usually after visiting game parks.

AIDS/HIV: Heterosexual contact is now the predominant mode of transmission. In some provinces, 35% of the adult population is HIV-positive; this is the highest incidence in Africa. South Africa has an estimated 5 million people living with HIV—more than any other nation except India. All travelers are cautioned against unsafe sex, medical or dental injections (which may not be sterile), and blood transfusions.

AIR POLLUTION: High levels of photochemical pollutants from coal-fired power stations are present in the high veld east of Pretoria.

ANIMAL HAZARDS: Animal hazards include snakes (cobras, mambas, adders, vipers) and spiders (black and brown widow).

ARBOVIRAL FEVER: Sporadic outbreaks of West Nile fever and Chikungunya fever occur primarily in Central Cape Province and eastern and southern Transvaal during warmer months. Travelers should take measures to prevent insect (mosquito) bites.

CHOLERA: This disease is reported active in this country, but the threat to tourists is very low. Cholera vaccine is recommended primarily for people at high risk (e.g., health-care, relief workers) who work and live in highly endemic areas under less than adequate sanitary conditions.

DENGUE FEVER: Low risk; dengue fever is currently not endemic.

HEPATITIS: The hepatitis A vaccine is recommended for all travelers. Hepatitis E is endemic at low levels. The hepatitis B carrier rate in the general population is variable and is as high as 15% in some population groups. Hepatitis B is spread by infected blood, contaminated needles, and unprotected sex. Vaccination is recommended for long-stay (longer than 3 months) travelers; persons who may be at occupational or social risk; and anybody desiring maximum protection.

INFLUENZA: Influenza is transmitted from April through September in the Southern Hemisphere. The flu vaccine is recommended for all travelers during the flu season.

MALARIA: This disease is present year-round in lowland areas of Mpumalanga Province, Northern Province, and northeastern KwaZulu-Natal as far south as the Tugela River. Risk (relatively low for tourists who take mosquito precautions) is present in Kruger National Park, especially during April. Falciparum malaria accounts for up to 99% of cases. Prophylaxis with atovaquone/proguanil (Malarone), mefloquine (Lariam), or doxycycline is recommended. All travelers should take measures to prevent evening and nighttime mosquito bites.

MARINE HAZARDS: Stingrays, jellyfish, and several species of poisonous fish are common in the country's coastal waters and are potential hazards to unprotected swimmers.

MENINGITIS: Low risk. South Africa is south of the sub-Saharan "meningitis belt." Long-term visitors who expect to have close contact with the indigenous population may consider vaccination against meningococcal disease.

POLIO: This disease is endemic. All travelers should be fully immunized.

RABIES: Rabies is endemic in South Africa, although only a few human cases are reported annually. Most human rabies cases are attributed to an increasing stray and wild dog population. All animal bites or scratches, especially from a dog, should be taken seriously and require immediate medical evaluation.

SCHISTOSOMIASIS: Risk is present primarily in the warmer months (October through April) in the northeast and the eastern coastal area, generally below 1,500 meters elevation. Urinary schistosomiasis is present in large areas of the northeast (including Kruger National Park), KwaZulu-Natal Province, and along the coastal areas of Eastern Cape Province as far south as Humansdorp. Risk areas for intestinal schistosomiasis occur in the low veld of Eastern and Northern Transvaal Provinces and sporadically in coastal areas of KwaZulu-Natal Province. Travelers to these areas should avoid swimming, bathing, or wading in freshwater lakes, ponds, or streams.

TRAVELERS' DIARRHEA: Low to moderate risk in urban areas. Cities and townships have municipal water systems that supply water to hotels and homes. Tap water safety varies. Travelers should observe food and drink precautions, especially outside urban areas. A quinolone antibiotic, combined with loperamide (Imodium), is recommended for the treatment of acute diarrhea. Persistent diarrhea may be due to a parasitic infection such as giardiasis, amebiasis, or cryptosporidiosis.

TUBERCULOSIS: Tuberculosis (TB) is a major health problem in this country. Travelers planning an extended stay should have a pre-departure TB skin test (PPD test) and be retested after leaving this country or returning home.

TYPHOID FEVER: Typhoid vaccine is recommended for those traveling off the usual tourist routes, for those visiting friends or relatives, and for long-stay visitors. Because the typhoid vaccines are only 60% to 70% effective, safe food and drink selection remains important.

OTHER DISEASES/HAZARDS: Brucellosis (usually from the ingestion of unpasteurized dairy products), leishmaniasis (low to negligible risk), leptospirosis, tuberculosis (highly endemic in Western Cape), typhoid fever, and helminthic disease (roundworm disease, hookworm disease, strongyloidiasis in lower socioeconomic populations) are reported.

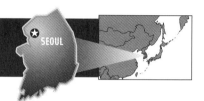

South Korea (Korea, Republic of)

CAPITAL:
Seoul

EMBASSY (IN U.S.):
202-939-5660

GMT:
+9 hours

TELEPHONE COUNTRY CODE:
82

USADIRECT:
00-729-11 to place calls using Korea Telecom; 00-369-11 to place calls using ONSE; 00-309-11 to place calls using Dacom

ENTRY REQUIREMENTS

- **Passport/Visa:** *U.S. citizens:* Passport but no visas required for tourist or business stays up to 15 days. For longer stays and other types of travel, visas must be obtained in advance. Changes of status (from tourism to teaching, for example) not normally granted. Applicants must depart and apply for new visas at an embassy or consulate outside Korea.
- **HIV Test:** Required for stays longer than 90 days by foreigners working as entertainers.
- **Vaccinations:** None required.

EMBASSIES/CONSULATES

- **U.S. Embassy:** 82 Sejong-Ro Chongro-Ku, Seoul; Tel: 82-2-397-4114; Fax: 82-2-738-8845; Website: usembassy.state.gov/seoul.

- **Canadian Embassy:** 10th Floor, Kolon Building, 45 Mugyo-Dong, Chung-Ku, Seoul; Tel: 82-2-3455-6000; Fax: 82-2-3455-6123; e-mail: seoul@dfait-maeci.gc.ca, Website: www.cec.or.kr/canada.
- **British Embassy:** Taepyeongno 40, 4 Jeong-dong, Jung-gu, Seoul 100-120; Tel: 82-2-3210-5500; Fax: 82-2-725-1738; Website: www.uk.or.kr.

HOSPITALS/DOCTORS:

Medical facilities are of high quality. The U.S. Embassy in Seoul and the U.S. Consulate in Pusan have lists of hospitals and medical specialists who speak English. Travelers to Korea are advised to obtain, before departure, supplemental travel health insurance with specific overseas coverage. The policy should provide for direct payment to the overseas hospital and/or physician at the time of service and include a medical evacuation benefit.

- International Clinic–Asan Medical Center, Seoul; Tel: 2-224-5001 or 5002. Largest medical center in South Korea, with more than 220 medical and surgical specialists, many of them U.S. and Canadian board-certified. VIP suites are available.
- International Clinic, Samsung Medical Center, Seoul; Tel: 2-3410-0200. Modern, with English-speaking staff; used by the expatriate community.
- AEA International Korea Ltd. provides 24-hour emergency service for foreigners, acting as a link between patient and Korean hospitals for a fee; Tel: 02-790-7561.
- International SOS: International SOS Korea Ltd., 5th Floor, Shindong Building, 726-164 Hannam-Dong, Yongsan-Ku, Seoul 140-210, South Korea; Alarm Center Tel: 72-2-3140-1700; Alarm Center Fax: 72-790-6785

Current Advisories and Health Risks

ANIMAL HAZARDS: Animal hazards include centipedes and black widow spiders. Lynxes, bears, and wild boars may be encountered in remote areas.

DENGUE FEVER: No apparent risk.

HELMINTHIC INFECTIONS: Low risk of ascariasis (roundworm) and hookworm disease. Anisakiasis, fascioliasis, fasciolopsiasis, paragonimiasis, and clonorchiasis are endemic. Travelers should avoid eating uncooked water plants and raw or undercooked seafood and shellfish, including Ke Jang (raw crab in soy sauce).

HEMORRHAGIC FEVER WITH RENAL SYNDROME: Risk of hemorrhagic fever with renal syndrome (HFRS) is present year-round, countrywide. Elevated risk is associated with dusty, dry conditions and peak rodent populations. The virus (hantavirus) that causes HFRS is transmitted by infected rodent secretions (e.g., excreta) and virus-carrying dust particles. Most cases occur from October through December, associated with peak human activity in rodent-infested areas during harvest.

HEPATITIS: Hepatitis A vaccine is recommended for all travelers. The hepatitis B carrier rate in the general population is estimated at 6% to 9%. Hepatitis B is spread by infected blood, contaminated needles, and unprotected sex. Vaccination is recommended for stays longer than 3 months; for persons at occupational or social risk; and for anyone desiring maximum protection.

JAPANESE ENCEPHALITIS: Risk of Japanese encephalitis (JE) is present, but at low levels. There is no risk of JE in Seoul. Cases of Japanese encephalitis have been reported in the southwest during the peak transmission season, June through October. Vaccination is recommended for travelers who will be staying in rural-agricultural endemic areas longer than 2 to 3 weeks during the peak transmission season. All travelers to rural areas should take measures to prevent mosquito bites.

MALARIA: Low risk, but cases of vivax malaria have increased annually in counties bordering the DMZ and have spread as far as 40 km south of the DMZ. The U.S. military has also reported cases of vivax malaria in soldiers stationed near the DMZ. Limited risk exists for overnight stays in these regions during spring (starting in April) and summer months. Malaria prophylaxis is not currently recommended for travelers, but travelers should be aware of the possibility of infection. All travelers should take measures to prevent evening and nighttime mosquito bites.

TRAVELERS' DIARRHEA: Medium to high risk outside of first-class hotels and resorts. Travelers are advised to drink only bottled, boiled, filtered, or treated water and to consume only well-cooked food. A quinolone antibiotic, combined with loperamide (Imodium), is recommended for the treatment of acute diarrhea. Persistent diarrhea may be due to a parasitic disease such as giardiasis, amebiasis, or cryptosporidiosis.

TUBERCULOSIS: Tuberculosis (TB) is a major health problem in this country. Travelers planning an extended stay should have a pre-departure TB skin test (PPD test) and be retested after returning home.

TYPHOID FEVER: Typhoid vaccine is recommended for all travelers, with the exception of short-term visitors who restrict their meals to major restaurants and hotels. Because the typhoid vaccines are only 60% to 70% effective, safe food and drink selection remains important.

OTHER DISEASES/HAZARDS: Filariasis (low risk occurs in southern coastal provinces, especially Chejudo), leptospirosis (elevated risk associated with areas of stagnant water and muddy soils), rabies (extremely rare), murine typhus (flea-borne), scrub typhus (mite-borne; risk elevated in grassy rural areas; 90% of cases occur October through December), tuberculosis (highly endemic), typhoid fever, and acute hemorrhagic conjunctivitis.

Spain

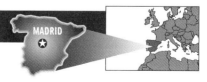

MADRID

CAPITAL:
Madrid
EMBASSY (IN U.S.):
202-728-2330; Embassy of Spain, 2375 Pennsylvania Avenue NW, Washington, DC 20037

GMT:
+1 hour
TELEPHONE COUNTRY CODE:
34
USADIRECT:
900-99-0011

ENTRY REQUIREMENTS
- **Passport/Visa:** No visa required for stays of up to 3 months.
- **HIV Test:** Not required.
- **Vaccinations:** None required.

EMBASSIES/CONSULATES
- **U.S. Embassy:** Serrano 75, Madrid; Tel: 91-587-2200; Fax: 34-91-587-2303; Website: www.embusa.es/indexbis.html.
- **Canadian Embassy:** Goya Building, 35 Nuñez de Balboa, Madrid; Tel: 91-423-3250; Fax: 91-423-3251; e-mail: mdrid@dfait-maeci.gc.ca; Website: www.canada-es.org.
- **British Embassy:** Calle de Fernando el Santo 16, 28010 Madrid; Tel: 34-91-700-82-00; Fax: 34-91-700-83-09; Website: www.ukinspain.com.

HOSPITALS/DOCTORS:
Medical care in Western Europe is of high quality, and many physicians speak English. Travelers are advised to obtain, before departure, supplemental travel health insurance with specific overseas coverage. The policy should provide for direct payment to the overseas hospital and/or physician at the time of service and include a medical evacuation benefit.
- Unidad Medico Anglo Americana, Conde de Aranda 1, Madrid; Tel: 91-435-1823.
- Unidad Medica Anglo-Americana. Hospital Clinico y Provincal, Barcelona (1,001 beds); all specialties, including cardiology.
- International SOS:
  - SOS Seguros Y Reaseguros, S.A., Ribera del Loira 4-6, 28042 Madrid, Spain; Alarm Center Tel: 34-91-572-4363; Alarm Center Fax: 34-91-345-1908
  - SOS, Seguros y Reaseguros, S.A., Avda. Diagonal, 436 - 2°-1a, 08037 Barcelona, Spain; Admin Tel: 34-93-238-8510; Admin Fax: 34-93-292-0100

Current Advisories and Health Risks

ACCIDENTS/ILLNESSES: Motor vehicle accidents, injuries, and drownings are the leading cause of death among travelers younger than 55 years of age. Cardiovascular disease causes most fatalities in older travelers. Infections cause less than 1% of fatalities in overseas travelers but overall are the most common cause of travel-related illness.

HEPATITIS: Hepatitis A vaccine is recommended for nonimmune travelers. Hepatitis E is endemic, but levels are unclear. The hepatitis B carrier rate in the general population varies, ranging from approximately 1% in the northwest to more than 3% in the southeast Mediterranean areas. Hepatitis B vaccine is recommended for stays longer than 3 months and for short-term travelers wanting increased protection. Travelers should be aware that the risk of hepatitis B is increased by unsafe sex and the use of unsterile needles and syringes.

INFLUENZA: Influenza is transmitted from November through March. Flu vaccine is recommended for travelers who visit this country.

LEISHMANIASIS: Risk of cutaneous and visceral leishmaniasis exists in rural areas of central Spain, the south (Andalucia), the east (Catalonia and Valencia), and the Balearic Islands. Travelers should take measures to prevent sand fly bites, which are most common during the evening and at night.

LYME DISEASE: Lyme disease occurs in northern Spain, but the risk is low. Travelers to rural areas should take precautions against tick bites. In southern Spain, an atypical form of Lyme disease occurs and is caused by a related *Borrelia* organism.

MEDITERRANEAN SPOTTED (BOUTONNEUSE) FEVER: Risk areas include the southern Mediterranean coast, the west-central and northern provinces (except areas bordering the Bay of Biscay), and the Balearic Islands (Majorca, Menorca, and Ibiza). The Canary Islands are risk free. Most cases result from contact with tick-carrying dogs.

RABIES: Spain is currently rabies free.

TRAVELERS' DIARRHEA: Medium risk. Urban water supplies are considered potable, but travelers are advised to consume only bottled, boiled, or treated water. A quinolone antibiotic, combined with loperamide (Imodium), is recommended for the treatment of acute diarrhea. Persistent diarrhea may be due to a parasitic infection such as giardiasis, amebiasis, or cryptosporidiosis.

TYPHOID FEVER: There is a higher risk of typhoid fever than in other major European countries. Typhoid vaccine is recommended for those traveling off the usual tourist routes, for those visiting friends or relatives, and for long-stay visitors. Because the typhoid vaccines are only 60% to 70% effective, safe food and drink selection remains important.

OTHER DISEASES/HAZARDS: Brucellosis (risk associated with consumption of unpasteurized dairy and goat cheese products), echinococcosis, fascioliasis, legionellosis (outbreaks associated with resort hotel spas and hot tubs; reported in Granada and Majorca), leptospirosis, trichinosis, tick-borne relapsing fever, tuberculosis, and intestinal helminth infections are reported.

Sri Lanka

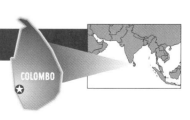

CAPITAL:
Colombo
EMBASSY (IN U.S.):
202-483-4025
GMT:
+5 hours

ENTRY REQUIREMENTS
- **Passport/Visa:** Passport, onward/return ticket and proof of sufficient funds ($15 U.S. per day) required. Tourist visa granted at entry valid for 90 days.
- **HIV Test:** Not required.
- **Vaccinations:** A yellow fever vaccination certificate is required for all travelers older than 1 year arriving from infected areas.

EMBASSIES/CONSULATES
- **U.S. Embassy:** 210 Galle Road, Colombo; Tel: 1-448-007 or 1-447-355; Fax: 94-1-437-345; e-mail: consularcolombo@state.gov; Website: usembassy.state.gov/srilanka.
- **Canadian Embassy:** 6 Gregory's Road, Cinnamon Gardens, Colombo; Tel: 1-69-58-41; Fax: 94-1-68-70-49; e-mail: clmbo-cs@dfait-maeci.gc.ca.
- **British High Commission:** 190 Galle Road, Kollupitiya, (PO Box 1433), Colombo 3; Tel: 94-11-2-437336/43; Fax: 94-11-2-430308; e-mail: bhc@eureka.lk.

HOSPITALS/DOCTORS:
The U.S. Embassy in Colombo maintains referral lists of doctors and hospitals. Medical care in Sri Lanka is below Western standards. Serious illness or injury may require evacuation to another country. Supplemental medical insurance with specific overseas coverage, including medical evacuation coverage, is recommended.
- Asiri Hospitals Limited, 181 Kirula Rd., Colombo; Tel: 500608 to 500612.
- Durdans Hospital, 3 Alfred Place, Colombo; Tel: 575205 to 575207.
- General Hospital, Regent St., Colombo; Tel: 691111. Emergency trauma service.

Current Advisories and Health Risks

ANIMAL HAZARDS: Animal hazards include snakes (kraits, cobras, coral snakes, vipers), spiders (black widow and red-backed), leopards, bears, and wild pigs. Stingrays, sea wasps, starfish, and marine invertebrates (sea cones, jellyfish, sea nettles, sea urchins, sea anemones) are common in the country's coastal waters and are potential hazards to unprotected swimmers.

CHOLERA: This disease is reported active in this country, but the threat to tourists is very low. Vaccination is recommended only for people at increased risk, such as relief or health-care workers.

DENGUE FEVER: Risk is year-round below 1,000 meters elevation, especially in urban areas. All travelers should take measures to prevent daytime mosquito bites.

FILARIASIS: Mosquito-borne; bancroftian filariasis is endemic in both urban and rural areas of the southwestern coast.

HEPATITIS: Hepatitis A vaccination is recommended for all travelers. Hepatitis E is likely endemic, but incidence is unclear. The carrier rate of the hepatitis B virus in the general population is estimated at 1%. Hepatitis B is spread by infected blood, contaminated needles, and unsafe sex. Vaccination is recommended for stays longer than 3 months; for persons at occupational or social risk; and for any traveler desiring maximum protection.

INFLUENZA: Influenza is transmitted year-round in the tropics. The flu vaccine is recommended for all travelers at risk.

JAPANESE ENCEPHALITIS: Sporadic cases of Japanese encephlitis (JE) occur year-round, but there have also been recent explosive epidemics in the region around Anuradhapura, as a result of increased mosquito breeding sites. JE vaccination is recommended for extended travel (longer than 4 weeks) in rural-agricultural areas, especially during the peak transmissions seasons, October through January and May through June.

MALARIA: Malaria occurs countrywide, including urban areas, below 800 meters elevation. The districts of Colombo, Kalutara, and Nuwara Eliya, however, are free of malaria. The northern half and southeastern quadrant of Sri Lanka are highly malarious, especially around Anuradhapura. Falciparum malaria accounts for up to 30% of cases, vivax the rest. Prophylaxis with atovaquone/proguanil (Malarone), mefloquine (Lariam), or doxycycline is recommended in malarious areas.

RABIES: Risk is present but declining. Sporadic cases of human rabies are reported countrywide. Rabies vaccine is recommended for travel longer than 3 months; for shorter stays for travelers who plan to venture off the usual tourist routes, where they may be more exposed to the stray dog population; or when travelers desire extra protection.

TRAVELERS' DIARRHEA: All water supplies in Sri Lanka, including piped city water supplies, are potentially contaminated. Travelers should observe strict food and drink safety precautions. A quinolone antibiotic, combined with loperamide (Imodium), is recommended for the treatment of acute diarrhea. Persistent diarrhea may be due to a parasitic diseases, such as giardiasis, amebiasis, or cryptosporidiosis.

TUBERCULOSIS: Tuberculosis (TB) is a major health problem in this country. Travelers planning an extended stay should have a pre-departure TB skin test (PPD test) and be retested after returning from this country.

TYPHOID FEVER: Typhoid vaccine is recommended for all travelers, with the exception of short-term visitors who restrict their meals to major restaurants and hotels. Because the typhoid vaccines are only 60% to 70% effective, safe food and drink selection remains important.

Sudan

CAPITAL:
Khartoum
EMBASSY (IN U.S.):
202-338-8565
GMT:
+2 hours
TELEPHONE COUNTRY CODE:
Operator assistance required.
USADIRECT:
800-001.

ENTRY REQUIREMENTS

- **Passport/Visa:** Passport and visa required. Visa must be obtained in advance, and visas are issued only at the Consulate General in New York. Transit visa valid up to 7 days; requires $50 fee (cash or money order), onward/return ticket, and visa for next destination, if appropriate. Tourist/business visa for single entry up to 1 month (extendible) requires $50 fee, 1 application form, 2 photos, proof of sufficient funds for stay, and SASE for return passport. Business visa requires company letter stating purpose of visit and invitation from Sudanese officials. Visas not granted to passports showing Israeli visas. Allow 4 weeks for processing. Travelers must declare currency on arrival and departure. Check additional currency regulations for stays longer than 2 months.
- **HIV Test:** Not required.
- **Vaccinations:** A valid yellow fever vaccination certificate is required for all travelers older than 1 year of age arriving from infected areas or from any country in the yellow fever endemic zones.

EMBASSIES/CONSULATES

- **U.S. Embassy:** Sharia Ali Abdul Latif, Khartoum; Tel: 11-74700.
- **Canadian Embassy:** Ethiopia; Tel: 251-1-151-100.
- **British Embassy:** Off Sharia Al Baladia, Khartoum East (PO Box No 801); Tel: 249-11-777105; Fax: 249-11-776457; e-mail: british@sudanmail.net.

HOSPITALS/DOCTORS:
Medical care in Sudan is substandard. Travelers to this country are advised to obtain, before departure, supplemental travel health insurance with specific overseas coverage. The policy should provide for direct payment to the overseas hospital and/or physician at the time of service and include a medical evacuation benefit. In case of serious accident or illness, medical evacuation to another country is strongly advised.
- Khartoum Civil Hospital (795 beds); general medical facility; some specialty services.

Current Advisories and Health Risks

AFRICAN SLEEPING SICKNESS (TRYPANOSOMIASIS): The Gambian form of this illness occurs in southern Sudan, primarily in Western and Equatoria provinces. Rhodesian sleeping sickness may occur in areas adjacent to Ethiopia and in areas adjacent to

Uganda. Increased risk occurs during the dry season. Travelers should take measures to prevent tsetse fly bites.

CHOLERA: This disease is active in this country. Immunization is recommended primarily for health-care and relief workers.

DENGUE FEVER: Mosquito-borne. Reported primarily from the coastal regions. Other arboviral infections include sand fly fever (widespread), Rift Valley fever, Crimean-Congo hemorrhagic fever (tick-borne), and West Nile fever.

HEPATITIS: Hepatitis A vaccine is recommended for all travelers. The hepatitis B carrier rate in the general population is estimated at 12% to 19%. Hepatitis B is spread by infected blood, contaminated needles, and unsafe sex. Vaccination is recommended for stays longer than 3 months; for persons at occupational or social risk; and for any traveler desiring maximum protection. Because the risk of illness or injury during travel cannot be predicted, some experts believe that *all* travelers should be immunized against hepatitis B, because of the risk of receiving a medical injection with an unsterile needle or syringe. Hepatitis E outbreaks have been reported from Khartoum, but endemic levels are unclear.

LEISHMANIASIS: An epidemic of visceral leishmaniasis (kala-azar) is afflicting the Nuer and Dinka tribes in southern Sudan. Kala-azar also reported from the Upper Blue Nile, Blue Nile, and Kassala provinces, and the Eastern Equatoria, Darfur, and Kordofan districts. Outbreaks also have occurred north of Khartoum along the Nile River. Endemic areas for cutaneous leishmaniasis include Darfur, Kordofan, and other provinces of central Sudan, and north of Khartoum, along the Nile River. Travelers to all regions should take measures to prevent insect (sand fly) bites.

MALARIA: Risk is present year-round throughout this country, including all urban areas. Increased incidence exists during and after the rainy season, June through October, especially in southern Sudan. There is less malaria risk in the desert areas of the extreme north and northwest. Chloroquine-resistant falciparum malaria is reported. Prophylaxis with atovaquone/proguanil (Malarone), mefloquine (Lariam), or doxycycline is currently recommended for travel to malarious areas.

MENINGITIS: Sudan lies within the sub-Saharan "meningitis belt." Quadrivalent meningococcal vaccine is recommended for travelers staying longer than 1 month during the dry season, December through June, and should be considered for shorter stays, any time of the year if extensive, close contact with the local populace is anticipated.

POLIOMYELITIS (POLIO): This disease is active. All travelers should be fully immunized. The WHO has also reported recent cases of poliomyelitis in Benin, Botswana, Burkina Faso, Central African Republic, Chad, Côte d'Ivoire, and Guinea that have been linked to outbreaks of polio originating in northern Nigeria.

RABIES: Risk of dog-transmitted rabies in Khartoum and elsewhere, including rural areas. Rabies vaccination is recommended before long-term travel (longer than 4 weeks) to this country.

SCHISTOSOMIASIS: Risk is widespread, especially in the major irrigation systems in the Gezira area between the Blue Nile and White Nile rivers. Travelers should avoid swimming, bathing, or wading in freshwater lakes, ponds, or streams.

TRAVELERS' DIARRHEA: Drinking water is untreated and may be bacterially contaminated. A quinolone antibiotic is recommended for the treatment of acute diarrhea. Persistent diarrhea may be due to a parasitic disease such as giardiasis, amebiasis, or cryptosporidiosis.

TUBERCULOSIS: Tuberculosis (TB) is a major health problem in this country. Travelers planning an extended stay should have a pre-departure TB skin test (PPD test) and be retested after returning home.

TYPHOID FEVER: Typhoid vaccine is recommended for all travelers. Because the typhoid vaccines are only 60% to 70% effective, safe food and drink selection remains important.

YELLOW FEVER: Vaccination is recommended for all travelers older than 9 months of age. Sudan is in the Yellow Fever Endemic Zone. A valid vaccination certificate may be required for ongoing travel to other countries.

OTHER DISEASES/HAZARDS: AIDS/HIV (lower incidence than in other countries in sub-Saharan Africa), African tick typhus, brucellosis, dracunculiasis, echinococcosis (high prevalence in the south), filariasis (mosquito-borne; reported from the Nuba Mountains around Kadogli in Kurdufan Province), loiasis (deer-fly-borne), leprosy, leptospirosis, onchocerciasis (high prevalence along rivers in southwestern Sudan), relapsing fever (louse-borne and tick-borne), toxoplasmosis, tuberculosis (a major health problem), trachoma, typhoid fever, typhus (flea-borne and louse-borne), and helminthic infections (intestinal worms; very common). Animal hazards include snakes (vipers, cobras), centipedes, scorpions, and black widow spiders.

Suriname

PARAMARIBO

CAPITAL:
Paramaribo
EMBASSY (IN U.S.):
202-244-7488
GMT:
−3 hours
TELEPHONE COUNTRY CODE:
597

USADIRECT:

156

ENTRY REQUIREMENTS

- **Passport/Visa:** Passport, visa, and onward/return ticket are required. Multiple-entry visa requires 2 application forms, 2 photos, and appropriate fee. Business visa requires company letter explaining purpose of trip, name of institution to be visited and its address and telephone number in Suriname, and expected duration of visit. Processing fee: $45 (money order only). For return of passport by mail, include $10 for registered mail or $18 for Express Mail (money order only), or enclose SASE. Allow 10 working days for processing.
- **HIV Test:** Not required.
- **Vaccinations:** A yellow fever vaccination certificate is required of all travelers arriving from infected areas.

EMBASSIES/CONSULATES

- **U.S. Embassy:** Dr. Sophie Redmondstraat 129, Paramaribo; Tel: 477-881.
- **Consulate of Canada:** Wagenwegstraat 50, boven, Paramaribo, Suriname; Tel: 59-7-424-527; Fax: 59-7-425-962; e-mail: cantim@sr.net.
- **British High Commission:** Accredited to the British High Commission in Guyana. 44 Main Street, (PO Box 10849), Georgetown; Tel: 592-22-65881/2/3/4; e-mail: firstname.surname@fco.gov.uk.
- **British Consulate:** c/o VSH United Buildings, Van't Hogerhuysstraat, 9-11, PO Box 1860, Paramaribo; Tel: 597-402558, 402870; Fax: 597-403515, 403824; e-mail: united@sr.net.

HOSPITALS/DOCTORS:

Medical care in Suriname is below Western standards. Travelers to this country are advised to obtain, before departure, supplemental travel health insurance with specific overseas coverage. The policy should provide for direct payment to the overseas hospital and/or physician at the time of service and include a medical evacuation benefit.

- St. Vincentius, Paramaribo (320 beds); private hospital; 4-bed ICU.
- University Hospital, Paramaribo (425 beds); government hospital; 5-bed ICU.
- Medical Clinic, Paramaribo.

Current Advisories and Health Risks

ANIMAL HAZARDS: Snakes (vipers), centipedes, scorpions, black widow spiders, brown recluse spiders, banana spiders, and wolf spiders. Electric eels and piranha may be found in the country's fresh waters. Portuguese man-of-war, sea wasps, and stingrays are found in the coastal waters of Suriname and could be a hazard to swimmers.

ARBOVIRAL ENCEPHALITIS: At least six distinct viruses causing encephalitis have been detected in Suriname. The area of greatest risk occurs in the savanna region located 20 to 40 km inland from the coastal strip. All travelers to these inland regions should take measures to prevent mosquito bites.

DENGUE FEVER: Limited dengue transmission occurs, primarily in the Paramaribo area. Outbreaks occur at irregular intervals, particularly in urban areas. The mosquitoes that transmit dengue fever bite primarily during the daytime and are present in populous urban areas as well as resort and rural areas.

HEPATITIS: Hepatitis A vaccine is recommended for all travelers. The hepatitis B carrier rate in the general population is estimated at 2% to 3%. Hepatitis B is spread by infected blood, contaminated needles, and unprotected sex. Vaccination is recommended for stays longer than 3 months; for persons at occupational or social risk; and for anyone desiring maximum protection.

LEISHMANIASIS: Cutaneous leishmaniasis ("bush yaws"), as well as mucocutaneous leishmaniasis, occurs primarily in the forested areas of the interior. Travelers should take measures to prevent insect (sand fly) bites.

MALARIA: Risk is present year-round. Elevated risk is present along the upper Marowijne River in the east, and in the southern interior. Only the city of Paramaribo, a narrow strip along the Atlantic coast, and areas of the interior above 1,300 meters elevation are considered risk free. Falciparum malaria accounts for 80% to 90% of cases; the remainder are caused by *P. vivax*. Chemoprophylaxis with atovaquone/proguanil (Malarone), mefloquine (Lariam), or doxycycline is currently recommended in malarious areas.

RABIES: Reported in animals, especially dogs and cats, but cases of human rabies cases appear to be infrequent. Travelers should seek medical evaluation of any animal bite. Rabies vaccination is usually indicated following the unprovoked bite of a dog, cat, bat, or monkey.

SCHISTOSOMIASIS: Risk is present year-round, but elevated during the height of the rainy season, May and June. Infected areas are found in the northern coastal strip from the Commewijne River west to the Nickerie River, with risk of infection apparently highest in the Suriname and Saramacca districts. Travelers should avoid swimming in freshwater lakes, ponds, or streams.

TRAVELERS' DIARRHEA: All water sources outside of Paramaribo should be considered contaminated. A quinolone antibiotic is recommended for the treatment of acute diarrhea. Persistent diarrhea may be due to a parasitic disease such as giardiasis, amebiasis, or cryptosporidiosis, or an intestinal virus.

TUBERCULOSIS: Tuberculosis (TB) is a major health problem in this country. Travelers planning an extended stay should have a pre-departure TB skin test (PPD test) and be retested after returning home.

TYPHOID FEVER: Typhoid vaccine is recommended for all travelers, with the exception of short-term visitors who restrict their meals to major restaurants and hotels. Because the typhoid vaccines are only 60% to 70% effective, safe food and drink selection remains important.

YELLOW FEVER: Vaccination is recommended for all travelers to this country.

OTHER DISEASES/HAZARDS: Filariasis (risk may occur in urbanized areas of Brokopondo, Commewijne, and Suriname Districts and in the city of Paramaribo), brucellosis, fungal infections (histoplasmosis, coccidiomycosis), leptospirosis, AIDS (incidence data lacking because of inadequate surveillance), tuberculosis (moderately endemic), and strongyloidiasis and other helminthic infections. Incidence of hookworm disease is reported to be as high as 40%.

Sweden

STOCKHOLM

CAPITAL:
Stockholm
EMBASSY (IN U.S.):
202-944-5600
GMT:
+1 hour
TELEPHONE COUNTRY CODE:
46
USADIRECT:
020-799-111
ENTRY REQUIREMENTS
• **Passport/Visa:** A valid passport is required.
• **HIV Test:** Not required.
• **Vaccinations:** None required.
EMBASSIES/CONSULATES
• **U.S. Embassy:** Dag Hammerskjoldsvag 31, Stockholm. Tel: 8-783-5300 or 8-783-5310; Fax: 46-8-660-5879; Website: www.usemb.se.
• **Canadian Embassy:** Tegelbacken 4, Stockholm. Tel: 8-453-3000; Fax: 8-24-24-91; e-mail: stkhm@dfait-maeci.gc.ca; Website: www.canadaemb.se.
• **British Embassy:** Skarpögatan 6-8, Box 27819, 115 93 Stockholm; Tel: 46-8-671-3000; Fax: 46-8-662-9989; Website: www.britishembassy.se.
HOSPITALS/DOCTORS
• Karolinska Hospital, Stockholm (1,654 beds); Tel: 8-729-2000. All specialties.
• Sahlgrenska Hospital, Goteborg (1,979 beds); Tel: 31-60-1000. All specialties.

Current Advisories and Health Risks

See the Disease Risk Summary for Europe on page 300.

Switzerland

 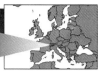

CAPITAL:
Bern

EMBASSY (IN U.S.):
202-745-7900

GMT:
+1 hour

TELEPHONE COUNTRY CODE:
41

USADIRECT:
0-800-89-0010

ENTRY REQUIREMENTS
- **Passport/Visa:** A valid passport is required.
- **HIV Test:** Not required.
- **Vaccinations:** None required.

EMBASSIES/CONSULATES
- **U.S. Embassy:** Jubilaeumstrasse 93, Bern; Tel: 31-357-7011 or 31-357-7218; Website: www.us-embassy.ch.
- **U.S. Consulates:** American Center of Zurich, Dufourstrasse 101; Tel: 1-422-2566. American Center of Geneva, World Trade Center IBC-Building, Geneva Airport, Route de Prebois 29; Tel: 22-798-1605 or 798-1615.
- **Canadian Embassy:** Kirchenfeldstrasse 88, Bern; Tel: 31-357-3200; Fax: 31-357-3210; e-mail: bern@dfait-maeci.gc.ca; Website: www.canada-ambassade.ch.
- **British Embassy:** Thunstrasse 50, 3005 Berne; Tel: 41-31-359-7700; Fax: 41-31-359-7701; Website: www.britain-in-switzerland.ch.

HOSPITALS/DOCTORS:
Medical care in Switzerland is of high quality, and many physicians speak English. Travelers are advised to obtain, before departure, supplemental travel health insurance with specific overseas coverage. The policy should provide for direct payment to the overseas hospital and/or physician at the time of service and include a medical evacuation benefit.

- Hopital Cantonal, 24 Rue Michel-du-Crest, Geneva (1,800 beds); major university teaching hospital; all specialties.
- University Hospital, Zurich (1,200 beds); Tel: 1-257-1111. All specialties.
- In Geneva, telephone 144 for any medical problem. The emergency center can summon an ambulance, if necessary, or send a doctor. The emergency center also can give a referral to the closest 24-hour walk-in clinic (called "permanence medical" in French). One such clinic is Permanence Medical Vermont at 9A, Rue de Vermont; Tel: 734-5150.
- International SOS:
  - SOS Assistance SA, Zweigniederlassung Basel, Steinenbachgässlein 49, 4051 Basel, Switzerland, Tel. 41-61-271-66-14, Fax: 41-61-271-62-30

- SOS Assistance S.A., 12 Chemin Riantbosson, 1217 Meyrin 1, Geneva, Switzerland; Alarm Center Tel: 41-22-785-6464; Alarm Center Fax: 41-22-785-6424

Current Advisories and Health Risks

ALTITUDE SICKNESS (AMS): Travelers ascending rapidly to alpine elevations over 8,000 feet are subject to altitude sickness, or acute mountain sickness (AMS). Diamox (acetazolamide) may be useful for prevention or treatment, especially for persons who will be climbing and sleeping at high altitudes. Immediate descent is the best treatment for moderate to severe AMS.

See also the Disease Risk Summary for Europe on page 300.

Syria (Syrian Arab Republic)

CAPITAL:
Damascus

EMBASSY (IN U.S.):
202-232-6313

GMT:
+2 hours

TELEPHONE COUNTRY CODE:
963

USADIRECT:
0-801

ENTRY REQUIREMENTS
- **Passport/Visa:** Valid passport and visa required.
- **HIV Test:** Testing required for students and anyone staying longer than 1 year. Contact the Syrian Embassy (Tel: 202-232-6313) for further details.
- **Vaccinations:** A yellow fever vaccination certificate is required for all travelers arriving from infected areas.

EMBASSIES/CONSULATES
- **U.S. Embassy:** Damascus. Abu Rumaneh, Al Mansur Street, No. 2; Tel: 11-333-052 or 332-557.
- **Canadian Embassy:** Lot 12, Mezzeh Autostrade, Damascus, Syria; Tel: 963-11-611-6692, 611-6851; Fax: 963-11-611-4000; e-mail: dmcus@international.gc.ca; Website: www.damascus.gc.ca.
- **British Embassy:** Kotob Building, 11 Mohammad Kurd Ali Street, Malki, PO Box 37, Damascus; Tel: 963-11-373-9241/2/3/7; Fax: 963-11-373-1600.

HOSPITALS/DOCTORS
- Mu'assat University Hospital, Damascus (850 beds); all specialties; emergency and trauma services.

- Social Insurance Foundation Hospital, Damascus (400 beds); specializes in emergency, trauma, and occupational medicine.
- National Hospital, Aleppo (482 beds); general medical facility.

Current Advisories and Health Risks

MALARIA: Transmission occurs from May through October, peaking in July and August, below 1,100 meters elevation in rural areas (except the As Suwayda and Dayr az Zawr provinces), particularly in the northern provinces bordering Turkey and Iraq. Urban areas are generally risk free. Ninety-nine percent of malaria cases are due to *P. vivax*, 1% to *P. falciparum*. Low level of risk in endemic areas. Chloroquine prophylaxis is recommended for travel to the lower river valleys of northeast Syria.

TRAVELERS' DIARRHEA: Medium to high risk outside of first-class hotels. Cases of amebiasis and giardiasis occur, even among the higher socioeconomic classes. A quinolone antibiotic is recommended for the treatment of acute diarrhea. Persistent diarrhea may be due to a parasitic disease such as giardiasis or amebiasis, or an intestinal virus.

HEPATITIS: Hepatitis A vaccine is recommended for all travelers. The hepatitis B carrier rate in the general population is estimated at 3% to 4%. Vaccination against hepatitis B is recommended for health-care workers and should be considered by long-term visitors to this country.

LEISHMANIASIS: Cases of cutaneous leishmaniasis occur in the steppe region, which is the transitional area between the fertile river valleys and the southeastern desert area. There is no apparent risk of visceral leishmaniasis. Travelers to this country should take measures to prevent insect (sand fly) bites.

SCHISTOSOMIASIS: Urinary schistosomiasis is found in the basins of the Euphrates and Bolikh Rivers to the Iraqi border in the northeast. Travelers should avoid swimming or wading in freshwater streams, ponds, or irrigated areas.

RABIES: Human cases occur sporadically (about 10 cases per year). Jackals, foxes, and stray dogs constitute the main animal reservoir of rabies in this country. Travelers should avoid stray animals and seek immediate medical attention of any animal bite.

OTHER DISEASES: Boutonneuse fever, brucellosis, echinococcosis (carried by stray dogs; reported sporadically), relapsing fever (tick-borne; reported frequently), sand fly fever (may occur), tuberculosis, typhoid fever, and helminthic infections (roundworm, whipworm, and dwarf tapeworm infections are common in rural areas; estimated prevalence is low).

Taiwan

CAPITAL:

Taipei

EMBASSY (IN U.S.):

202-895-1800

GMT:

+8 hours

TELEPHONE COUNTRY CODE:

886

USADIRECT:

00-801-102-880

ENTRY REQUIREMENTS

- **Passport/Visa:** Passport, onward/return ticket, and valid visa for next destination, if applicable, are required. Visa not required for stays of up to 14 days.
- **HIV Test:** Health certificate, including AIDS test, is mandatory for anyone staying longer than 3 months.
- **Vaccinations:** A yellow fever vaccination certificate is required from all travelers older than 1 year arriving from infected areas.

EMBASSIES/CONSULATES

- **U.S. Embassy:** No.7 Lane 134, Hsin Yi Road Section 3, Taipei; Tel: 2-2709-2000; Fax: 2-2709-0908.
- **U.S. Consulate:** No. 2 Chung Cheng 3rd Road, 5th Floor, Kaohsiung. Tel: 7-238-7744; Fax: 886-7-238-5237; e-mail: aitamcit@mail.ait.org.tw.
- **Canadian Embassy:** 365 Fu Hsing North Road, Taipei. Tel: 2-2544-3000; Fax: 2-2544-3592; e-mail: tapei@dfait-maeci.gc.ca; Website: www.canada.org.tw.
- **British Embassy:** None.

HOSPITALS/DOCTORS:

Medical care in Taiwan is of high quality, and most physicians speak English. Travelers are advised to obtain, before departure, supplemental travel health insurance with specific overseas coverage. The policy should provide for direct payment to the overseas hospital and/or physician at the time of service and include a medical evacuation benefit.

- Jen-Ai Hospital (Tali, Taichung). Jen-Ai Hospital is a not-for-profit organization with two separate branches located in Taichung, the central part of Taiwan: Jen-Ai Hospital (Tali) is a 746-bed, tertiary-care community hospital; Jen-Ai Hospital (Taichung) is a 146-bed secondary-care hospital. Jen-Ai Hospital, Tali, is recognized as the biggest regional teaching hospital in the Tali area; it is also the location of the Jen-Ai Hospital International Patient Center; Tel: 04-2481-9900, ext. 2911 or 1995.
- Chang Gung Memorial Hospital, Taipei; Tel: 02-2713-5211. General medical/surgical facility with ICU, 24-hour emergency services.
- International SOS: International SOS (Taiwan) Ltd., Rm 405, 4F, No. 96, Chong Shan N. Road, Sec. 2, Taipei, Taiwan; Alarm Center Tel: 786-2-2523-2220; Alarm Center Fax: 786-2-2523-9897.

Current Advisories and Health Risks

ANIMAL HAZARDS: Animal hazards include snakes (coral, krait, viper), centipedes, scorpions, and black widow spiders.

DENGUE FEVER: Countrywide risk, year-round. The incidence of dengue is higher in the warmer, wetter months, April through October, especially in the southwestern coastal counties and islands. The mosquitoes which transmit dengue are most active during the day in populous urban areas, as well as resort and rural areas. Prevention of dengue consists of taking protective measures against daytime mosquito bites.

HELMINTHIC INFECTIONS (FLUKES AND WORMS): Liver fluke diseases (clonorchiasis and fascioliasis), intestinal fluke disease (fasciolopsiasis), lung fluke disease (paragonimiasis), and intestinal worm disease (capillariasis and angiostrongyliasis) are reported throughout this country. Other intestinal helminthic infections include ascariasis (roundworms), ancylostomiasis (hookworms), enterobiasis (pinworms), trichuriasis (whipworms) and beef and pork tapeworm disease. Travelers should avoid eating undercooked pork or beef; raw, undercooked, pickled, or smoked freshwater fish; aquatic plants, such as watercress and water chestnuts; raw, salted, or wine-soaked crustacea (freshwater crabs, crayfish, shrimp); and raw freshwater fish, snails, prawns, crabs, planarians, vegetables that may be contaminated by the mucus of infected slugs, land snails, or aquatic snails. Hookworm disease is prevented by not walking barefoot outdoors.

HEPATITIS: All travelers should receive hepatitis A vaccine. Hepatitis E is endemic, but the levels are unclear. The hepatitis B carrier rate in the general population is estimated to be over 10%. Hepatitis B is spread by infected blood, contaminated needles, and unsafe sex. Vaccination is recommended for stays longer than 3 months; for persons at occupational or social risk; and for any traveler desiring maximum protection.

INFLUENZA: Influenza is transmitted from November through March. Flu vaccine is recommended for all travelers at risk.

JAPANESE ENCEPHALITIS: Japanese encephalitis (JE) is a mosquito-borne viral illness that occurs year-round, countrywide, in both urban and rural areas. Transmission of disease is elevated during the warmer, wetter months, usually April through October, with a higher incidence likely occurring in the southwestern coastal counties and islands. Vaccination is recommended for travelers who will be staying in rural-agricultural areas longer than 3 to 4 weeks, especially during the peak transmission season.

MALARIA: There is currently no risk of malaria on Taiwan. This disease was officially eradicated in 1965.

MARINE HAZARDS: Several species of poisonous fishes (stone, puffer, scorpion, zebra), as well as jellyfish, sea anemones, sea nettles, sea urchins, and sea cucumbers, are found in the coastal waters around Taiwan and are potential hazards to swimmers.

TRAVELERS' DIARRHEA: Medium to high risk outside of first-class hotels. Acute diarrhea should be treated with a quinolone antibiotic, combined with loperamide (Imodium). Persistent diarrhea may be due to a parasitic disease such as giardiasis, amebiasis, or cryptosporidiosis.

TUBERCULOSIS: Tuberculosis (TB) is a major health problem in this country. Travelers planning an extended stay should have a pre-departure TB skin test (PPD test) and be retested after returning from this country.

TYPHOID FEVER: Typhoid vaccine is recommended for all travelers, with the exception of short-term visitors who restrict their meals to major restaurants and hotels. Because the typhoid vaccines are only 60% to 70% effective, safe food and drink selection remains important.

OTHER DISEASES/HAZARDS: Filariasis (bancroftian variety; mosquito-borne; endemic on the Pescadores, Kinmen, and Matsu islands), leptospirosis, scrub typhus (countrywide; risk may be elevated on Penghu, Kinmen, Matsu, and Orchid islands; transmitted primarily in mountainous, wooded, grassy areas, or cleared forest and scrub brush-type areas).

Tajikistan

CAPITAL:
Dushanbe
EMBASSY (IN U.S.):
202-223-6090
GMT:
+5 hours
TELEPHONE COUNTRY CODE:
992
USADIRECT:
None
ENTRY REQUIREMENTS
• **Passport/Visa:** A passport and visa are required.
• **HIV Test:** Not required.
• **Vaccinations:** None required.
EMBASSIES/CONSULATES
Visa issued by Russian Embassy, Consular Division: 202-939-8907.
• **U.S. Embassy:** Dushanbe; Tel: 7-3772-210-356.
• **Canadian Embassy:** Accredited to the Canadian Embassy in Kazakhstan. 34 Karasai Batir Street (Vinogradov Street), Almaty, 480100, Kazakhstan; Tel: 7-3272-501151; Fax: 7-3272-582493; e-mail: almat@international.gc.ca; Website: www.dfait-maeci.gc.ca/canadaeuropa/kazakhstan.

• **British Embassy:** 43 Lutfi Street, Dushanbe; Tel: 992-91-901-5079; Fax: 992-91-901-5078; e-mail: reception@britishembassy-tj.com; Website: www.britishembassy.gov.uk/tajikistan.

HOSPITALS/DOCTORS:

• Travelers should contact the U.S. Embassy for medical referrals.

Current Advisories and Health Risks

ARBOVIRAL DISEASES: Tahjna virus fever (mosquito-borne; virus circulates through much of the former U.S.S.R.), sand fly fever (sand fly-borne; limited to regions of southern central Asia, April through October), West Nile fever (mosquito-borne; cases have occurred in the Tadzikstan), North Asian tick fever (occurs wherever tick vectors are found).

CRIMEAN-CONGO HEMORRHAGIC FEVER: Also known as Central Asian hemorrhagic fever. Risk areas are rural steppe, savannah, semi-desert, and foothill/low mountain habitats below 2,000 meters elevation. Outbreaks occurred in south-central Kazakhstan during 1989.

HEPATITIS: All nonimmune travelers should receive hepatitis A vaccine before visiting these regions. The hepatitis B carrier rate in the general population of the countries in these regions is estimated to be as high as 8%.

LEISHMANIASIS: Risk for cutaneous leishmaniasis is primarily limited to Uzbekistan, Kazakhstan, and Turkmenistan. Travelers to these regions should take measures to prevent sand fly bites.

LYME DISEASE: Occurs focally in rural forested areas below 1,500 meters elevation.

MALARIA: Limited foci of vivax malaria exist in Kazakhstan and Uzbekstan. Tajikistan has reported an increase in malaria following the civil war (1992-1996), with *P. vivax* identified in 84% of cases, *P. falciparum* in 16%. Most cases of malaria in Tajikistan are reported from the region of Khatlon Oblast. Information on chloroquine resistance is not available. Travelers are advised to consult with a travel medicine specialist about the need for prophylaxis.

TICK-BORNE ENCEPHALITIS: Peak transmission period for tick-borne encephalitis (TBE) is April through June. Risk is present primarily in rural brushy and forested areas below 1,500 meters elevation. TBE is usually known as "Central European tick-borne encephalitis" or "Russian spring-summer encephalitis" west of the Urals.

TRAVELERS' DIARRHEA: All water supplies are suspect, including municipal tap water, which may be untreated and grossly contaminated.

OTHER DISEASES/HAZARDS: Boutonneuse fever (tick-borne; reported most commonly along the shores of the Black and Caspian Seas), brucellosis, echinococcosis (dog feces are infective), legionellosis, leptospirosis, rabies, rickettsialpox, tick-borne relapsing fever (reported from Kirghizstan, Turkmenistan, and Uzbekistan), trichinosis, typhoid fever, tularemia, tuberculosis, and soil-transmitted and helminthic infections (roundworm, hookworm, and whipworm infections and strongyloidiasis).

Tanzania

DAR ES SALAAM ★

CAPITAL:
Dar es Salaam

EMBASSY (IN U.S.):
202-939-6125; Tanzanian Embassy at 2139 R St. NW, Washington, DC 20008; or 212-972-9160; Mission to UN, 205 East 42nd St., 13th Floor, New York, NY 10017

GMT:
+3 hours

TELEPHONE COUNTRY CODE:
255

USADIRECT:
None

ENTRY REQUIREMENTS
Travelers should check with this country's embassy (or a consulate) in the United States, Canada, or the United Kingdom for any changes in requirements.

- **Passport/Visa:** Visas for mainland Tanzania are valid for Zanzibar. Business/tourist visas are valid 6 months from date of issuance.
- **HIV Test:** Not required.
- **Vaccinations:** *Yellow fever:* A vaccination certificate is required for all travelers older than 1 year of age arriving from infected areas. This includes travelers arriving from Kenya and Uganda. The Centers for Disease Control and Prevention (CDC) recommends yellow fever vaccine for all travelers older than 9 months of age arriving from any country.

EMBASSIES/CONSULATES
- **U.S. Embassy:** 140 Msese Road, Kinondoni District Street, Dar es Salaam; Tel: 255-22-266-6010 through 5; e-mail: consulardx@state.gov.
- **Canadian Embassy:** 38 Mirambo Street, Corner Garden Avenue, Dar es Salaam; Tel: 255-22-211-2831/5 or 211-2837 or 211-2863 or 211-2865/6; e-mail: dslam@ dfait-maeci.gc.ca.
- **British High Commission:** Umoja House, Garden Avenue, PO Box 9200, Dar es Salaam; Tel: 255-22-211-0101; Fax: 255-22-211-0102; e-mail: bhc.dar@fco.gov.uk; Website: www.britishhighcommission.gov.uk/tanzania.

HOSPITALS/DOCTORS:
Medical facilities are limited. Essential medicines often are in short supply or unavailable. Mission hospitals provide about 40% of medical care countrywide.
- Tanzania Heart Institute.
- Muhimbili Hospital, Dar es Salaam (1,000 beds); general medical/surgical facility; orthopedics.

Current Advisories and Health Risks

ALTITUDE SICKNESS (AMS): Acetozolamide (Diamox) prophylaxis for altitude sickness, or acute mountain sickness (AMS), should be considered by all travelers climbing Mt. Kilimanjaro (19,000 feet; 6,000 meters). Rapid descent remains the best treatment for AMS.

AFRICAN SLEEPING SICKNESS (TRYPANOSOMIASIS): Sleeping sickness occurs country-wide, and the incidence is increasing. Disease risk is most prevalent in a region from Kigoma at Lake Tanganyika to Arusha in the northern part of the country. Cases of sleeping sickness continue to be reported in tourists, many of whom have been in or near Serengeti. Areas of disease transmission persist in Arusha, Kigoma, Lindi, Mtwara, Rukwa, Tabora, and Ziwa Magharibi Regions. There may be risk in Mbeya. Travelers to these regions should take protective measures against insect (tsetse fly) bites.

AIDS/HIV: Heterosexual transmission is the predominant means of transmission. HIV prevalence is estimated at 50% of the high-risk and 16% of the general urban populations. All travelers are cautioned against unsafe sex, medical or dental injections (which may not be sterile), and blood transfusions.

ANIMAL HAZARDS: Animal hazards include snakes (vipers, cobras), centipedes, scorpions, and black widow spiders.

CHOLERA: This disease is reported active in this country, but the threat to tourists is very low. Cholera vaccine is recommended primarily for people at high risk (e.g., relief workers) who work and live in highly endemic areas under less than adequate sanitary conditions.

FILARIASIS: Bancroftian filariasis (mosquito-borne) is reported along the coast, including Pemba and Zanzibar, and also reported south of Lake Victoria, north of Lake Nyasa, and in the vicinity of Lake Tanganyika.

HEPATITIS: All nonimmune travelers should receive hepatitis A vaccine. Hepatitis E is endemic, likely at high levels. The hepatitis B carrier rate in the general population is estimated at 4%. Vaccination against hepatitis B is recommended for health-care workers and all long-term visitors to this country. Hepatitis B is spread by infected blood, contaminated needles, and unprotected sex. Vaccination is recommended for long-stay (longer than 3 months) travelers; persons who may be at occupational or social risk; and anybody desiring maximum protection.

INFLUENZA: Influenza is transmitted year-round in the tropics. The flu vaccine is recommended for all travelers.

INSECTS: All travelers should take measures to prevent both daytime and nighttime insect bites. Insect-bite prevention measures include a DEET-containing repellent applied to exposed skin, insecticide (permethrin) spray applied to clothing and gear, and use of a permethrin-treated bed net at night.

LEISHMANIASIS: Risk is estimated to be low. A few cases of cutaneous leishmaniasis have been reported from northern areas.

MALARIA: High risk is present below 2,000 meters elevation throughout this country, including urban areas, and the islands of Zanzibar and Pemba. Risk of malaria is increased during and just after the rainy seasons, November through December and March through May. Risk has also been increasing in high plateau areas, previously considered areas of limited risk. *P. falciparum* accounts for greater than 90% of cases. Prophylaxis with atovaquone/proguanil (Malarone), mefloquine (Lariam), or doxycycline is recommended.

MENINGITIS: The Centers for Disease Control and Prevention (CDC) does not currently recommend vaccination. Travelers who expect close, long-term contact with the local populace, however, may consider immunization with the quadrivalent meningococcal vaccine.

ONCHOCERCIASIS: Black fly–borne; risk area extends from the Usambara mountains in the northeast to Lake Nyasa in the south. Travelers to these areas should take measures to prevent insect (black fly) bites.

POLIO: This disease is endemic. All travelers should be fully immunized.

RABIES: Sporadic cases of human rabies are reported countrywide. All animal bites or scratches, especially from a dog, should be taken seriously, and immediate medical attention sought.

ROAD SAFETY: Travelers should exercise caution and avoid intercity travel at night. Roads often are poorly maintained and lack shoulders; during rainy season, many are passable only with four-wheel-drive vehicles. Excessive speed, unpredictable driving habits, and lack of basic safety equipment on many vehicles present additional hazards. Drivers frequently have unexpected encounters with cyclists, pedestrians, livestock, and wild animals. Emergency service and first aid are unavailable outside major cities and tourist areas.

SCHISTOSOMIASIS: This disease is focally distributed countrywide. Major risk areas include the shores of Lake Victoria, the Tanga and Kigoma districts, and the Lake Rukwa area. Urban transmission occurs in Dar es Salaam. Schistosomiasis is transmitted on Zanzibar and Pemba islands. Travelers should avoid swimming or wading in freshwater lakes, ponds, or streams.

TRAVELERS' DIARRHEA: Potential high risk in all areas. Several cities have water treatment facilities, but piped water supplies are frequently untreated and may be contaminated. Travelers should observe food and drink safety precautions. A quinolone antibiotic, combined with loparamide (Imodium), is recommended for the treatment of acute diarrhea. Persistent diarrhea may be due to a parasitic infection such as giardiasis, amebiasis, or cryptosporidiosis.

TUBERCULOSIS: Tuberculosis (TB) is a major health problem in this country. Travelers planning an extended stay should have a pre-departure TB skin test (PPD test) and be retested after leaving this country or returning home.

TYPHOID FEVER: Typhoid vaccine is recommended for those traveling off the usual tourist routes, those visiting friends or relatives, and for long-stay visitors. Because the typhoid vaccines are only 60% to 70% effective, safe food and drink selection remains important.

YELLOW FEVER: Vaccination is recommended for all travelers older than 9 months of age arriving from any country.

OTHER DISEASES/HAZARDS: Anthrax (cutaneous; usually from contact with freshly slaughtered infected animals), African tick typhus, brucellosis (from unpasteurized dairy products), Chikungunya fever (explosive urban outbreaks have occurred), dengue (no recent reports), echinococcosis (high incidence in the Masai of northern areas), leptospirosis, leprosy, plague (hundreds of cases reported annually, mostly from the Lushoto District), relapsing fever (louse- and tick-borne; mainly in central Tanzania), toxoplasmosis, tuberculosis (a major health problem), trachoma, typhoid fever (endemic at moderate to high levels), and intestinal worms (very common).

Thailand

BANGKOK

CAPITAL:
Bangkok
EMBASSY (IN U.S.):
202-4944-3600
GMT:
+7 hours
TELEPHONE COUNTRY CODE:
66
USADIRECT:
1-800-001-33
001-999-111-11
ENTRY REQUIREMENTS
- **Passport/Visa:** A valid passport is required.
- **HIV Test:** "Those suspected of carrying AIDS" may be denied entry. Travelers should contact the Thai Embassy in Washington for further information and advice.
- **Vaccinations:** A yellow fever vaccination certificate is required if arriving from infected areas or from countries in the Yellow Fever Endemic Zones in Africa and South America.
EMBASSIES/CONSULATES
- **U.S. Embassy:** Consular Section, 95 Wireless Road, Bangkok; Tel: 2-205-4000.
- **U.S. Consulate:** 387 Vidhayanond Road, Chiang Mai; Tel: 53-252-629.

- **Canadian Embassy:** 15th Floor, Abdulrahim Place, 990 Rama IV, Bangrak, Bangkok 10500, Thailand; Tel: 66-2-636-0540; Fax: 66-2-636-0555: e-mail: bngkk@international.gc.ca; Website: www.dfait-maeci.gc.ca/bangkok.
- **British Embassy:** Wireless Road, Bangkok, 10330; Tel: 66-2-305-8333; Fax: 66-2-305-8372, 8380; Website: www.britishemb.or.th.

HOSPITALS/DOCTORS

- International Travel Medicine Clinic, BNH Hospital, Bangkok; this clinic provides all routine and tropical vaccinations and can provide referral advice and counseling regarding health-related matters.
- Queen Saovabha Memorial Institute (Thai Red Cross Society); this facility operates a snake farm (with daily lectures and demonstrations in English), an animal bite clinic, and a "Travelers' Advisory" bulletin board listing current health hazards and preventive medicine recommendations for tourists.
- Bangkok General Hospital & Heart Institute.
- Phyathai Hospital; often used by expatriates.
- University Hospital, Bangkok; Tel: 252-0570. Extensive neurosurgical, cardiovascular, and trauma capability.
- Samitivej Hospital; this is a luxurious hospital located in an expatriate neighborhood; highly recommended for its excellent care.
- Bangkok/Pattaya Hospital (southeast of Bangkok).
- Bangkla Baptist Hospital (Bangkla Chacheungsao).
- Chiang Mai-McCormick Hospital; well equipped to treat foreigners.
- Chiang Mai Ram Hospital; the most modern of all hospitals in Chiang Mai, with many U.S.-trained physicians.
- Lanna Hospital; especially well known for its ob/gyn services.
- International SOS: International SOS Services (Thailand) Ltd., 11th floor - Diethelm Towers, 93/1 Wireless Road, Lumpini, Pathumwan, Bangkok 10330, Thailand; Alarm Center Tel: 66-2-205-7777; Alarm Center Fax: 66-2-256-7151/0

Current Advisories and Health Risks

ACCIDENTS AND INJURIES

- *Note:* Bangkok is sometimes called "the gridlock city" because of its chaotic traffic. The traffic is left handed (as in England), and there is a high incidence of accidents and pedestrian injuries. All drivers should be alert, and seat belts should be worn at all times.

AIDS/HIV: An explosive increase of HIV infection has occurred in commercial sex workers, of whom 14% to 72% are now seropositive. a majority of patients are heterosexual. Thailand now has the highest number of officially reported AIDS cases in Southeast Asia. Blood used for transfusion in Thailand is checked for the AIDS virus.

ANIMAL HAZARDS: Animal hazards include snakes (kraits, vipers, cobras), centipedes, scorpions, and black widow spiders. (Snake bite antivenin is available from the Thai Red Cross.) Other possible hazards include tigers, leopards, crocodiles, pythons, poisonous toads and frogs, and large, aggressive lizards. Stingrays, jellyfish, and several species of poisonous fish (puffer, goblin, stone, toad, scorpion, pig, porcupine, and box jellyfish) are common in the country's coastal waters and are potentially hazardous to unprotected or careless swimmers. Large sharks are common on the Andaman (Indian Ocean) side. There are no saltwater crocodiles in Thailand.

AVIAN INFLUENZA:

- After a period of quiescence in Southeast Asia, outbreaks of highly pathogenic avian influenza (A/H5N1) are again being reported in chickens and ducks in China, Indonesia, Thailand, and Vietnam. In Thailand, outbreaks have been reported in 21 of 76 provinces.
- Human cases, some fatal, have occurred after contact with infected poultry.

CHOLERA: Sporadic cases may occur. Cholera is an extremely rare disease in travelers from developed countries. Cholera vaccine is recommended primarily for people at high risk (e.g., relief workers) who work and live in highly endemic areas under less than adequate sanitary conditions.

- The oral cholera vaccine (Dukoral) provides up to 60% crossover protection against ETEC diarrhea.
- Many countries, including Canada, license an oral cholera vaccine. The oral vaccine is not available in the United States.

DENGUE FEVER: Highly endemic, and a risk for travelers. Peak infection rates occur in the rainy season, between June and August, countrywide, but particularly in northeastern Thailand. Dengue and dengue hemorrhagic fever are major health problems both in Thailand and throughout SE Asia. Prevention is by avoiding daytime mosquito bites.

FILARIASIS: Both the Malayan and bancroftian varieties occur in scattered areas, primarily the southern peninsular coastal provinces, the central provinces of Sisaket and Surin, and the forested areas along the Thailand-Burma border. Travelers should prevent mosquito bites.

HEPATITIS: Hepatitis A vaccine is recommended for all nonimmune travelers. Hepatitis E is endemic, with seropositivity rates of 22% in adults. There is no vaccine for hepatitis E. The hepatitis B carrier rate in the adult general population is about 9%. The usual traveler without lifestyle problems is at virtually no risk of acquiring hepatitis B virus (HBV), but vaccination is recommended for sexual tourists, long-term visitors, and anybody wanting increased protection. Hepatitis C is endemic and is largely transmitted by blood products and body fluids. Like HBV, hepatitis C carries no increased risk for travelers who have a normal lifestyle.

INFLUENZA: Influenza is transmitted year-round in the tropics. The flu vaccine is recommended for all travelers older than 50 years of age; all travelers with any chronic disease or weakened immune system; travelers of any age wishing to decrease the risk of this illness; and pregnant women after the first trimester.

JAPANESE ENCEPHALITIS: Japanese encephalitis (JE) is highly endemic nationwide, especially in the central and northern provinces; sporadic cases occur in the south. There is risk of infection in the suburban areas of major cities, except Bangkok, where JE is uncommon. Highest risk in the south occurs during the rainy and early dry seasons; in the north, during late summer and autumn. Vaccination is recommended for travelers who will be staying in rural-agricultural areas longer than 2 weeks during the peak transmission season. In addition, all travelers should take measures to prevent mosquito bites, especially in the evening. The Regional Medical Officer of the American Embassy currently recommends JE vaccination for all expatriate Americans.

LEPTOSPIROSIS: Leptospirosis is an endemic disease in Thailand, with most cases occurring during the rainy season, June through December. Epidemics and common-source outbreaks (from contaminated drinking and swiming water) are reported, the last outbreak being in the northeastern province of Nakhornratchasrima.

MALARIA: This disease rarely occurs in people visiting the usual tourist sites in Thailand. In the past 2 decades, malaria-endemic regions have been shrinking, now involving mostly land near the borders with Myanmar and Cambodia. There are small pockets on a few islands and along the Malaysian border.

- There is no risk of malaria in Bangkok and other major urban areas (Chiangmai, Chiangrai) or the large coastal resort cities (Phuket, Pattaya, Haadya, and Sonkhla). Prophylaxis is recommended for Koh Chang island. The central part of Thailand and the cities usually visited by tourists have been free of malaria for more than 10 years, with the exception of Kanchanaburi Province and the River Kwai region.
- Although malaria is mostly eradicated from urban areas and the plains, there is some risk of malaria in the forested foothills, jungles, rubber plantations, and fruit orchards. The northern part of the country contributes 44% of all malaria cases in Thailand, with Tak and Mae Hongsorn leading the list. In northeast Thailand, most cases come from Ubon Ratchathani and Srisaket. Southern Thailand has an increasing incidence of malaria, in contrast to the rest of the country, where it is decreasing.
- Countrywide, *Plasmodium falciparum* causes about 60% of cases of malaria, *P. vivax* about 40%. *P. malariae* causes less than 1% of cases. There is a high incidence of multidrug-resistant falciparum malaria. *P. falciparum* resistance to standard treatment doses of mefloquine runs as high as 50%.
- The Thai Ministry of Health currently recommends no prophylaxis because the incidence of malaria in tourists is so low.
- Travelers to malarious areas, however, are advised to take an antimalarial prophylactic drug, either atovaquone/proguanil (Malarone) or doxycycline. Atovaquone/proguanil is also useful for the treatment of malaria if it has not been taken for prophylaxis, or it could be carried as a standby treatment if no prophylaxis is used. Currently, a 3-day regimen of artesunate plus mefloquine has been the preferred treatment for malaria in Thailand.
- Protection against insect bites, especially between dusk and dawn, is a high priority.

RABIES: There is a high incidence of dog rabies in Thailand, and about 60 cases of human rabies were reported in 2000. Dogs account for about 95% of rabid animals, cats about 3.5%. Cases in other mammals and wildlife have been reported (cattle, monkeys, gibbons, bears, civets, bats, and large rats). Rabid, stray dogs are common in Bangkok, as well as in other urban and rural areas. Although rabies is rare among tourists, there is risk. No one should pet or pick up any stray animals. All children should be warned to avoid contact with unknown animals. Human diploid cell rabies vaccine is available but is very expensive and no more effective than the newer "second generation" tissue culture vaccines. These include the Vero cell and purified chick and duck embryo cell vaccines. Human and equine rabies immune globulin (HRIG and ERIG) are manufactured by the Thai Red Cross in limited quantity for local use only. Since the European manufacturers of ERIG have ceased production, immune globulin for post-exposure treatment is in very short supply. Rabies pre-exposure vaccination is recommended for long-term residents, particularly children, and for travelers who plan to venture off the five-star hotel trail and expose themselves to the large stray dog population. Vaccination is strongly recommended for travelers who plan extensive touring to neighboring countries including India, Cambodia, Laos, Myanmar, and Vietnam, where tissue culture vaccines, and particularly rabies immune globulin, may not be available. The U.S. State Department recommends vaccination for all expatriate corporate employees and their families, especially the children. A rabies clinic is operated by the Queen Saovabha Institute/Thai Red Cross Society Hospital in Bangkok.

SCHISTOSOMIASIS: There is potential risk of schistosomiasis, albeit minimal, in the southern province of Nakhon Si Thammarat, where intermediate snail hosts exist. To be safe, travelers should avoid swimming or wading in freshwater lakes, ponds, or streams in these areas.

TRAVELERS' DIARRHEA: Moderate risk. *Campylobacter* bacteria cause greater than 50% of cases of traveler's diarrhea in Thailand, and greater than 90% of *Campylobacter* species are now reported to be resistant to quinolone antibiotics. Quinolones, however, are still recommended as the first choice for the treatment of acute diarrhea, because a good clinical response may still be obtained. Azithromycin (Zithromax) is the best alternative antibiotic. Persistent diarrhea may be due to a parasitic disease such as giardiasis or amebiasis, but these infections rarely affect tourists.

TUBERCULOSIS: The clinical incidence of tuberculosis (TB) in Thailand has been increasing since 1987, because of in part to the high incidence of HIV infection. TB in this country has a prevalence of greater than 100 cases per 100,000 population—the highest WHO risk category. Travelers planning to stay longer than 3 months should have a pre-departure PPD skin test and a repeat PPD after leaving. Domestic help should be screened for TB.

TYPHOID FEVER: Typhoid is reported countrywide, with the highest incidence in the northern and the southern regions, and the incidence greater in the summer and during the rainy seasons (between March and October). Typhoid vaccine is recommended for those traveling off the usual tourist routes, those visiting friends or relatives, and for long-stay visitors. Typhoid vaccines are 60% to 70% effective; safe food and drink precautions should continue to be observed.

OTHER DISEASES/HAZARDS: Angiostrongyliasis (primarily in north-northeastern provinces; associated with eating raw seafood, snails, or vegetables), anisakias (from raw seafood) reported in 1993, anthrax (an unlikely hazard for tourists, who should avoid uncooked or poorly cooked meat), capillariasis (associated with eating raw fish), gnathostomiasis (associated with eating raw freshwater fish such as eels, frogs, birds, or snakes), cestode infections (roundworm and hookworm disease), fascioliasis (liver fluke disease; transmitted by eating contaminated water vegetables), leptospirosis (high rates during the rainy season), melioidosis (highest risk in northeastern Thailand; may cause a variety of infections, such as pneumonia or an abscess, or be the source of an obscure fever), opisthorchiasis and clonorchiasis (liver fluke diseases; transmitted by raw seafood; travelers should especially avoid "koi pla"—uncooked, pickled freshwater fish), paragonimiasis (lung fluke disease; endemic in central, north, and northeastern Thailand, including Chiang Rai; travelers should avoid raw freshwater crabs), pinworms (*E. vermicularis* infection has a prevalence of 41.6% among children in hill tribe villages of the Mae Suk District, Chiangmai Province), trichinosis (avoid undercooked pork sausages), and typhus (both tick-borne and murine).

Togo

CAPITAL:
Lomé
EMBASSY (IN U.S.):
202-234-4212
GMT:
+0 hours
TELEPHONE COUNTRY CODE:
228
USADIRECT:
None
ENTRY REQUIREMENTS

- **Passport/Visa:** Short-stay visas: up to 90 days. Long-stay visas: from 3 months to 2 years. Visas can be extended on arrival in Lomé at the Sûreté Nationale for visits not exceeding 6 months.
- **HIV Test:** Not required.
- **Vaccinations:** A yellow fever vaccination certificate is required for all travelers older than 1 year of age arriving from *all* countries.

EMBASSIES/CONSULATES

- **U.S. Embassy:** Intersection of Rue Kouenou and Rue Tokmake, Lomé: Tel: 228-21-29-92 or 228-21-29-93; Fax: 228-21-79-52.

- **Consulate of Canada:** 101 Boulevard des Armées, Maison N 311, projet Sida 3, Quartier Tokoin Habitat, Lomé, Togo; Tel: 228-2-21-32-99; Fax: 228-2-20-30-01; e-mail: honcontogo@laposte.tg.
- **British High Commission:** Accredited to the British High Commission in Ghana. Osu Link, off Gamel Abdul Nasser Avenue, (PO Box 296), Accra; Tel: 233-21-7010650, 221665; Fax: 233-21-7010655; e-mail: high.commission.accra@fco.gov.uk; Website: www.britishhighcommission.gov.uk/ghana.

HOSPITALS/DOCTORS:

Medical services are provided by the state. Most towns have either a hospital or a dispensary, but these are usually overcrowded and lack adequate supplies. Visitors who get seriously ill are advised to contact their embassy, which can refer them to a specialist or arrange evacuation. Health insurance and a good supply of personal medical provisions are recommended. There is no reciprocal health agreement with the United Kingdom or Canada. It is important to carry a basic first aid kit.

- Tokoin National Hospital, Lomé (650 beds); general medical/surgical facility; trauma unit.
- Hospital Baptiste Biblique Adeta; well-equipped medical/surgical facility. Travelers should contact the U.S. Embassy for additional physician referrals.

Current Advisories and Health Risks

IMMUNIZATIONS: All travelers should be up to date on their routine immunizations: tetanus-diphtheria (Td), measles-mumps-rubella (MMR), polio, influenza, and varicella (chickenpox). Immunizations against hepatitis A, hepatitis B, meningitis, rabies, and typhoid fever are recommended.

MALARIA: All travelers to Togo including infants, children, and former residents of this country should take one of the following antimalarial drugs: atovaquone/proguanil, doxycycline, mefloquine, or (in special circumstances) primaquine. Travelers should also take measures to prevent evening and nighttime mosquito bites. Insect bite prevention measures include a DEET-containing repellent applied to exposed skin, insecticide (permethrin) spray applied to clothing, and use of a permethrin-treated bed net at night.

For additional information, consult the Disease Risk Summary for Sub-Saharan Africa on page 307.

Tonga

CAPITAL:
Nuku'alofa
EMBASSY (IN U.S.):
415-781-0365
GMT:
+13 hours

TELEPHONE COUNTRY CODE:
676
USADIRECT:
None
ENTRY REQUIREMENTS
- **Passport/Visa:** A visa is required only for visits exceeding 30 days.
- **HIV Test:** Not required.
- **Vaccinations:** A yellow fever vaccination certificate is required for all travelers coming from infected or endemic areas.

EMBASSIES/CONSULATES
- **U.S. Consulate:** Tel: 415-781-0365.
- **U.S. Embassy:** The nearest U.S. Embassy is in Suva, Fiji; Tel: 679-314-466.
- **Canadian Embassy:** Accredited to the Australian High Commission. Salote Road, Nuku'Alofa, Tonga; Tel: 676-23-244; Fax: 676-23-243.
- **British High Commission:** PO Box 56, Nuku'alofa, Tonga; Tel: 676-24285/24395; Fax: 676-24109; e-mail: britcomt@kalianet.to.

HOSPITALS/DOCTORS:
Local residents and visitors with serious medical problems often are referred to New Zealand for treatment. Government provides comprehensive medical and dental facilities for residents and visitors. All doctors, dentists, and senior nursing staff have extensive overseas training and offer standard of medical service equal to that of most developing countries. Private medical practitioners are also available to visitors. Doctors and hospitals often expect immediate cash payments. U.S. medical insurance is not always valid outside the United States. Two hospitals with emergency and outpatient facilities are:
- Vaiola Hospital, Nuku'alofa (202 beds); general medical/surgical facility; emergency room.
- Ngu Hospital, Neiafu (61 beds); limited medical and surgical services.

Current Advisories and Health Risks

ACCIDENTS/ILLNESSES AND MEDICAL INSURANCE
- Accidents and injuries are the leading cause of death among travelers younger than 55 years of age and most often are caused by motor vehicle and motorcycle crashes; drownings, aircraft crashes, homicides, and burns are less common causes.
- Heart attacks cause most fatalities in older travelers.
- Infections cause only 1% of fatalities in overseas travelers, but overall, infections are the most common cause of travel-related illness.
- Travelers are advised to obtain, before departure, supplemental travel health insurance with specific overseas coverage. The policy should provide for direct payment to the overseas hospital and/or physician at the time of service and include a medical evacuation benefit. The policy should also provide 24-hour hotline access to a multilingual assistance center that can help arrange and monitor delivery of medical care and determine if medical evacuation or air ambulance services are required.

ANIMAL HAZARDS: Stingrays, poisonous fish, various sharks, sea anemones, corals and jellyfish are hazards to swimmers. Tropical centipedes can inflict painful stings if touched. Common sense is usually adequate to avoid these hazards.

CHOLERA: This water-borne diarrheal disease occurs sporadically in Oceania. Rare cases of cholera have occurred in this country but there is little, if any, danger to tourists.

- Cholera is an extremely rare disease in travelers from developed countries. Cholera vaccine is recommended primarily for people at high risk (e.g., relief workers) who work and live in highly endemic areas under less than adequate sanitary conditions.
- The oral cholera vaccine (Dukoral) provides up to 60% crossover protection against ETEC diarrhea.
- Many countries, including Canada, license an oral cholera vaccine. The oral vaccine is not available in the United States.
- Cholera vaccine is not "officially" required for entry into, or exit from, any country. Despite this, some countries, on occasion, require proof of cholera vaccination from travelers coming from cholera-infected countries. Anticipating such a situation, certain travelers may wish to carry a medical exemption letter from their health-care provider. Travel Medicine, Inc., recommends that travelers use the International Certificate of Vaccination (Yellow Card) for this purpose, having their health-care provider affirm that they are "exempt from cholera vaccine" and validate the exemption with both the provider's signature and the appropriate official stamp (the "Uniform Stamp" in the United States).

DENGUE FEVER: Sporadic cases and outbreaks are reported. Travelers should take protective measures against mosquito bites.

FILARIASIS: Sporadic cases and outbreaks are reported. Travelers should take protective measures against mosquito bites.

HEPATITIS: All nonimmune travelers should receive hepatitis A vaccine. The hepatitis B carrier rate in the general population exceeds 10%. Vaccination against hepatitis B should be considered for stays for longer than 3 months and by short-term travelers desiring maximum protection. Travelers should be aware that hepatitis B can be transmitted by unsafe sex and the use of contaminated needles and syringes.

JAPANESE ENCEPHALITIS: Sporadic cases and outbreaks of Japanese encephalitis (JE) are reported. Travelers should take protective measures against mosquito bites.

MALARIA: No risk.

ROAD SAFETY: Traffic moves on the left. Although roads in Nuku'alofa are paved, most other roads are not. Animals and unwary pedestrians walking in the road make night driving on unlit secondary roads hazardous.

ROSS RIVER FEVER: Sporadic cases and outbreaks are reported. Travelers should take protective measures against mosquito bites.

TRAVELERS' DIARRHEA: Low to medium risk: The tap water in Nuku'alofa is potable, but travelers are advised to consume only boiled or bottled water unless assured the water has been adequately treated. A quinolone antibiotic, combined with loperamide (Imodium), is recommended for the treatment of diarrhea.

TYPHOID FEVER: Typhoid vaccine is recommended, especially for long-term travelers, adventure travelers, and those wishing maximum disease protection. Because the typhoid vaccines are only 60% to 70% effective, safe food and drink guidelines should continue to be observed.

Trinidad and Tobago

PORT-OF-SPAIN

CAPITAL:
Port-of-Spain
EMBASSY (IN U.S.):
202-467-6490
GMT:
−4 hours
TELEPHONE COUNTRY CODE:
809
USADIRECT:
1-800-872-2881
ENTRY REQUIREMENTS
• **Passport/Visa:** Passport and onward/return ticket required. Visa not required for tourist/business stay of up to 90 days.
• **HIV Test:** Not required.
• **Vaccinations:** A yellow fever vaccination certificate is required for travelers older than 1 year of age arriving from infected areas.
EMBASSIES/CONSULATES
• **U.S. Embassy:** 15 Queen's Park West in Port-of-Spain; Tel: 1-868-622-6371; Fax: 1-868-628-5462.
• **Canadian Embassy:** Maple House, Tatil Centre, Sweet Briar Road, St. Clair, Port-of-Spain; Tel: 1-868-622-6232; Fax: 1-868-628-2581; e-mail: pspan@dfait-maeci.gc.ca.
• **British High Commission:** 19 St Clair Avenue, St Clair, Trinidad; Tel: 1-868-622-2748, 628-1234, 628-1068, 622-8985/86, 622-8960/61/62; Fax: 1-868-622-4555; e-mail: csbhc@opus.co.tt; Website: www.britain-in-trinidad.org.
HOSPITALS/DOCTORS:
Port-of-Spain General Hospital (882 beds); general medical and surgical facility; neurosurgery, orthopedics.

Current Advisories and Health Risks

DENGUE FEVER: This mosquito-transmitted viral disease is prevalent throughout the Caribbean. Major outbreaks of dengue have previously occurred on Trinidad. Travelers should take measures to prevent daytime mosquito bites.

HEPATITIS: Hepatitis A vaccine is recommended for all travelers. Hepatitis B vaccine is recommended for stays longer than 3 months and for short-term travelers wanting increased protection. Travelers should be aware that the risk of hepatitis B is increased by unsafe sex and the use of unsterile needles and syringes.

INFLUENZA: Influenza is transmitted year-round in the tropics. The flu vaccine is recommended for all travelers older than 50 years of age; all travelers with any chronic disease or weakened immune system; travelers of any age wishing to decrease the risk of this illness; and pregnant women after the first trimester.

LEPTOSPIROSIS: There have been reports of leptospirosis from this country. Travelers should avoid contact with animal urine or water potentially contaminated with animal urine.

MALARIA: No malaria is present at this time.

MARINE HAZARDS:
- Swimming-related hazards include jellyfish, spiny sea urchins, and coral.
- Ciguatera poisoning is prevalent and can result from eating coral reef fish such as grouper, snapper, sea bass, jack, and barracuda. The ciguatoxin is not destroyed by cooking.

RABIES: Animal rabies was reported in 1987. The potential of transmission to humans exists. Travelers should especially avoid stray dogs and seek immediate treatment of any wild animal bite. Rabies vaccination is usually indicated following the unprovoked bite of a dog, cat, bat, or monkey.

TRAVELERS' DIARRHEA: Low to moderate risk. In urban and resort areas, the hotels and restaurants generally serve reliable food and potable water. Elsewhere, travelers should observe all food and drink safety precautions. A quinolone antibiotic, combined with loperamide (Imodium), is recommended for the treatment of acute diarrhea. Diarrhea not responding to antibiotic treatment may be due to a parasitic disease such as giardiasis.

TYPHOID FEVER: Typhoid vaccine is recommended for extended travel outside of tourist areas. The typhoid vacccine is 60% to 70% effective. Food and drink precautions should continue to be observed.

YELLOW FEVER: This disease has been reported active in the jungle regions of Trinidad. Yellow fever vaccine is recommended only for those who plan travel outside of urban areas. No human cases of yellow fever have been reported since 1980, but there is potential risk.

OTHER DISEASES/HAZARDS: Brucellosis, filariasis (bancroftian variety; mosquito-borne; may occur in the Lesser Antilles from Trinidad north to Guadeloupe), histoplasmosis, intestinal helminthic infections (hookworm, roundworm, and whipworm infections and strongyloidiasis), sexually transmitted diseases, HIV/AIDS, tuberculosis, and viral encephalitis.

Tunisia

CAPITAL:
Tunis
EMBASSY (IN U.S.):
202-862-1850
GMT:
+1 hour
TELEPHONE COUNTRY CODE:
216
USADIRECT:
None
ENTRY REQUIREMENTS
- **Passport/Visa:** Passport and onward/return ticket are required. Visas not required for tourist/business stay of up to 4 months.
- **HIV Test:** Not required.
- **Vaccinations:** A yellow fever vaccination certificate is required for all travelers arriving from infected areas.

EMBASSIES/CONSULATES
- **U.S. Embassy:** 144 Avenue de la Liberte, Tunis-Belvedere, Tunis; Tel: 216-1-782-566; Fax: 216-1-789-719 or 216-1-789-923; Website: usembassy.state.gov/posts/ts1/wwwhmain.html.
- **Canadian Embassy:** 3, rue du Sénégal, Place d'Afrique, Tunis-Belvédère; Tel: 216-1-796-577; Fax: 216-1-792-37; e-mail: tunis@dfait-maeci.gc.ca.
- **British Embassy:** Rue du Lac Windermere, Berges du Lac, Tunis 1053; Tel: 216-71-108-700; Fax: 216-71-108-703-Chancery; e-mail: TunisConsular@tunis.mail.fco.gov.uk (Consular).

HOSPITALS/DOCTORS:
Medical care in Tunisia is below Western standards. Travelers to this country are advised to obtain, before departure, supplemental travel health insurance with specific overseas coverage. The policy should provide for direct payment to the overseas hospital and/or physician at the time of service and include a medical evacuation benefit.
- Clinique Carthage, Carthage. e-mail: jneina@gnet.tn.
- Clinique Carthage, La Marsa.
- Charles Nicolle Hospital, Tunis (756 beds); general medical/surgical facility.
- Hadi Chakar Hospital, Tunis (870 beds); general medical/surgical facility.
- Tunis Medical Center (private).
- Centre Hospitalo, Sousse.

Current Advisories and Health Risks

HEPATITIS: Hepatitis A vaccine is recommended for all travelers. The hepatitis B carrier rate in the general population is estimated at 4.6%. Hepatitis B is spread by infected blood, contaminated needles, and unprotected sex. Vaccination is recommended for stays longer than 3 months; for persons at occupational or social risk; and for anyone desiring maximum protection.

INFLUENZA: Influenza is transmitted from November through March. The flu vaccine is recommended for all travelers at risk.

LEISHMANIASIS: Cutaneous leishmaniasis is reported from northern, central (primarily Qafsah, Sidi Bu Zayd, and Safaqis governorates), and the southeastern areas. Visceral leishmaniasis (kala-azar) occurs in the northern half of Tunisia, primarily the northeast, including the outskirts of Tunis. All travelers should take measures to prevent insect (sand fly) bites.

MALARIA: Low risk. Indigenous malaria has not occurred since 1978, but foci of vivax malaria activity may still remain. Travelers should take measures to prevent insect bites. Prophylaxis is not recommended.

RABIES: Sporadic cases of human rabies are reported countrywide. All animal bites or scratches, especially from a dog, should be medically evaluated without delay.

SAND FLY FEVER: Disease risk is present in the northern, central, and southeastern areas of the country. Transmission occurs primarily in April through October, when sand fly activity is highest.

SCHISTOSOMIASIS: Risk areas include the oases in Qafsah and Qabis governorates and in the village of Hadjeb El Aioun, 120 miles south of Tunis. Other areas may be involved. Travelers should avoid swimming or wading in freshwater lakes, ponds, irrigation ditches, or streams in these areas.

TRAVELERS' DIARRHEA: A quinolone antibiotic, combined with loperamide (Imodium), is recommended for the treatment of acute diarrhea. Persistent diarrhea may be due to a parasitic disease such as giardiasis or amebiasis.

TYPHOID FEVER: Typhoid vaccine is recommended. Because the typhoid vaccines are only 60% to 70% effective, safe food and drink guidelines should continue to be observed.

OTHER DISEASES/HAZARDS: Boutonneuse fever (African tick typhus; distribution is widespread; contracted from dog ticks, often in suburban areas), brucellosis (risk from raw goat/sheep milk and cheese), echinococcosis (a major health problem in central Tunisia), leptospirosis, trachoma, soil-transmitted helminthic infections (roundworm, hookworm inections) are common in rural areas.

Turkey

★ ANKARA

CAPITAL:
Ankara

EMBASSY (IN U.S.):
202-659-8200

GMT:
+2 hours

TELEPHONE COUNTRY CODE:
90

USADIRECT:
00-800-122-77

ENTRY REQUIREMENTS
- **Passport/Visa:** Tourist visa can be obtained at the airport on arrival.
- **HIV Test:** Not required.
- **Vaccinations:** None required.

EMBASSIES/CONSULATES
- **U.S. Embassy:** 110 Ataturk Boulevard, Ankara; Tel: 312-468-6110; Fax: 312-467-0019; e-mail: ca-ankara@state.gov; Website: www.usemb-ankara.org.tr.
- **U.S. Consulates:** 104-108 Mesrutiyet Caddesi, Istanbul. Tel: 212-251-3602; Fax: 90-212-252-7851; e-mail: ca_istanbul@state.gov; Website: www.usisist.org.tr.
- **Canadian Embassy:** Nenehatun Caddesi No. 75, Gaziosmanpasa 06700, Ankara; Tel: 90-312-459-9200, Fax: 90-312-459-9363, e-mail: ankra@dfait-maeci.gc.ca, Website: www.dfait-maeci.gc.ca/ankara).
- **Canadian Consulates:** Istiklal Caddesi No 373/5, Beyoglu, 80050 Istanbul; Tel: 90-212-251-9838, Fax: 90-212-251-9888.
- **British Embassy:** Sehit Ersan Caddesi 46/A, Cankaya, Ankara; Tel: 90-312-455-3344; e-mail: britembank@fco.gov.uk (check Firecrest for individuals); Website: www.britishembassy.org.tr.

HOSPITALS/DOCTORS
- American Hospital, Istanbul (325-beds); private facility; most specialties, including trauma; 24-hour emergency services; often used by expatriates.
- International Hospital, Istanbul (140 beds); private; most specialties.
- Volkan Korten, MD, Director of Travel Medicine and Infectious Diseases, Academic Hospital, Istanbul; Tel: 216-651-0000 or 216-327-4142. Practice includes most specialties, including travel medicine.
- Hacettepe University Hospital; Tel: 312-310-3545. Considered the best health center in Ankara.
- Bayindir Hospital, Ankara; private; most specialties; preferred private hospital in Ankara.

Current Advisories and Health Risks

CHOLERA: This disease is reported active in this country, but the threat to tourists is very low. Cholera vaccine is recommended primarily for people at high risk (e.g., relief workers) who work and live in highly endemic areas under less than adequate sanitary conditions.

HEPATITIS: Hepatitis A vaccine is recommended for all nonimmune travelers. Water-borne epidemics of hepatitis E are endemic, but levels are unclear. The hepatitis B carrier rate in the general population is estimated at 6% to 10%. Hepatitis B is spread by infected blood, contaminated needles, and unsafe sex. Vaccination is recommended for stays longer than 3 months; for persons at occupational or social risk; and for any traveler desiring maximum protection. Because the risk of illness or injury during travel cannot be predicted, some experts believe that *all* travelers should be immunized against hepatitis B because of the risk of receiving a medical injection with an unsterile needle or syringe.

INFLUENZA: Influenza is transmitted from November through March. The flu vaccine is recommended for all travelers to this country.

LEISHMANIASIS: Cutaneous leishmaniasis is common in the southeastern region of Turkey and the Tigris-Euphrates Basin. Visceral leishmaniasis (kala-azar) occurs along the Aegean coast, the Mediterranean coast, the Sea of Marmara coast, and the Black Sea coast. Travelers should take measures to prevent insect (sand fly) bites.

MALARIA: There is no current threat of malaria in Turkey.

RABIES: Human cases are reported and are usually due to contact with rabid stray dogs. Travelers should seek immediate treatment following the unprovoked bite of a dog, cat, or fox. Bites by other animals should be considered on an individual basis.

TRAVELERS' DIARRHEA: Moderate risk outside of resorts and first-class hotels. Contamination of existing municipal water systems is common. A quinolone antibiotic, combined with loperamide (Imodium), is recommended for the treatment of acute diarrhea. Persistent diarrhea may be due to a parasitic infection such as giardiasis, amebiasis, or cryptosporidiosis.

TYPHOID FEVER: Typhoid vaccine is recommended for those traveling off the usual tourist routes, for those visiting friends or relatives, and for long-stay visitors. Because the typhoid vaccines are only 60% to 70% effective, safe food and drink selection remains important.

OTHER DISEASES/HAZARDS: Brucellosis (usually transmitted by raw goat or sheep milk), Mediterranean spotted fever (boutonneuse fever; this tick-borne illness occurs in the western and southern regions), cutaneous larva migrans ("creeping eruption," caused by the larvae of dog or cat hookworms; usually contracted by walking barefoot on moist soil or wet sand, where animals have defecated), echinococcosis (human cases reported sporadically, especially in northern and northeastern areas), North Asian tick typhus (in areas bordering the former Soviet Union), sand fly fever (transmission occurs predominantly from April through October), tick-borne encephalitis (sporadic cases reported;

presumed risk in brushy, forested western and northern regions), tuberculosis, typhoid fever (endemic, with frequent outbreaks), and helminthic infections (roundworm, hookworm, and whipworm infections) are common in rural areas.

Turkmenistan

CAPITAL:
Ashgabat

EMBASSY (IN U.S.):
202-588-1500

GMT:
+5 hours

TELEPHONE COUNTRY CODE:
993

USADIRECT:
None

ENTRY REQUIREMENTS
- **Passport/Visa:** A passport and visa are required.
- **HIV Test:** Not required.
- **Vaccinations:** None required.

EMBASSIES/CONSULATES
- **U.S. Embassy:** 9 Pushkin Street, Ashgabat; Tel: 993-12-511-306 or 350-045; Fax: 993-12-511-305; Website: www.usemb-ashgabat.usia.co.at.
- **Canadian Embassy:** Accredited to the Canadian Embassy in Turkey. Cinnah Caddesi No. 58, Çankaya 06690, Ankara, Turkey; Tel: 90-312-409-2700; Fax: 90-312-409-2810; e-mail: ankra@international.gc.ca; Website: www.dfait-maeci.gc.ca/ankara.
- **British Embassy:** 3rd Floor, Office Building, Four Points Ak Altin Hotel, Ashgabat; Tel: 993-12-363462, 363463, 363464, 363466, 363498; Fax: 993-12-363465; e-mail: beasbppa@online.tm; Website: www.britishembassy.gov.uk/turkmenistan.

HOSPITALS/DOCTORS:
Medical care is substandard throughout the country including in Ashgabat. Adequate medical evacuation coverage for all travelers is a high priority. For serious medical conditions, every effort should be made to go to Western Europe. Hospital accommodations are inadequate throughout the country.

Current Advisories and Health Risks
See the Disease Risk Summaries for Central Asia on page 302.

Turks and Caicos

CAPITAL:
Grand Turk

EMBASSY (IN U.S.):
202-462-1340

GMT:
−5 hours

TELEPHONE COUNTRY CODE:
809

USADIRECT:
01-800-872-2881

ENTRY REQUIREMENTS

- **Passport/Visa:** Overseas Territory of the United Kingdom. Islands include Anguilla, Montserrat, Cayman Islands, Turks and Caicos. Proof of U.S. citizenship, photo ID, onward/return ticket and sufficient funds are required for tourist stays up to 6 months. Consult the British Embassy for further information (Tel: 202-588-7800).
- **HIV Test:** Not required.
- **Vaccinations:** None required.

EMBASSIES/CONSULATES

- **U.S. Embassy:** Next to the McDonald's Restaurant on Queen Street in downtown Nassau; Tel: 242-322-1181 or 242-328-2206; Fax: 242-356-7174.
- **Canadian Embassy:** 2001 Leeward Highway, Providenciales; Tel: 1-649-941-5245; Fax: 1-649-946-4484; e-mail: ewing@mcleanmcnally.com.
- **British Governor's Office:** Turks and Caicos Islands, Waterloo, Grand Turk; Tel: 649-946-2309; Fax: 649-946-2903.

HOSPITALS/DOCTORS

- General Hospital, Cockburn Town (32 beds); limited medical and surgical services.
- Adequate, but limited, medical care by English-speaking physicians is available in this country.

Current Advisories and Health Risks

ACCIDENTS/ILLNESSES AND MEDICAL INSURANCE

- Accidents and injuries are the leading cause of death among travelers younger than 55 years of age and most often are caused by motor vehicle and motorcycle crashes; drownings, aircraft crashes, homicides, and burns are less common causes.
- Heart attacks cause most fatalities in older travelers.
- Infections cause only 1% of fatalities in overseas travelers, but overall, infections are the most common cause of travel-related illness.
- **Medical Insurance:** Travelers are advised to obtain, before departure, supplemental travel health insurance with specific overseas coverage. The policy should provide for direct payment to the overseas hospital and/or physician at the time of service and include a medical evacuation benefit. The policy should also provide 24-hour hotline access to a

multilingual assistance center that can help arrange and monitor delivery of medical care and determine if medical evacuation or air ambulance services are required.

DENGUE FEVER: This mosquito-transmitted viral disease is prevalent throughout the Caribbean. Travelers should take measures to prevent daytime insect bites.

HEPATITIS: Hepatitis A vaccine is recommended. Vaccination against hepatitis B should be considered for stays longer than 3 months and by short-term travelers desiring maximum protection. Travelers should be aware that hepatitis B can be transmitted by unsafe sex and the use of contaminated needles and syringes.

INFLUENZA: Influenza is transmitted year-round in the tropics. The flu vaccine is recommended for all travelers older than 50; all travelers with chronic disease or a weakened immune system; travelers of any age wishing to decrease the risk of this illness; and pregnant women after the first trimester.

MARINE HAZARDS:

• Swimming-related hazards include jellyfish, spiny sea urchins, and coral.

• Ciguatera poisoning is prevalent and can result from eating coral reef fish such as grouper, snapper, sea bass, jack, and barracuda. The ciguatoxin is not destroyed by cooking.

• For scuba diving hyperbaric chamber referral: The Divers' Alert Network (DAN) maintains an up-to-date list of all functioning hyperbaric chambers in North America and the Caribbean. DAN does not publish this list, because at any one time a given chamber may be nonfunctioning, or its operator(s) may be away or otherwise unavailable. Through Duke University, DAN operates a 24-hour emergency phone line for anyone (members and nonmembers) to call and ask for diving accident assistance. Dive medicine physicians at Duke University Medical Center carry beepers, so someone is always on call to answer questions and, if necessary, make referrals to the closest functioning hyperbaric chamber. In a diving emergency, or for the location of the nearest decompression chamber, call 919-684-8111.

TRAVELERS' DIARRHEA: Low to medium risk. A quinolone antibiotic, combined with loperamide (Imodium), is recommended for the treatment of acute diarrhea.

Uganda

KAMPALA

CAPITAL:
Kampala
EMBASSY (IN U.S.):
202-726-7100
GMT:
+3 hours

256
800-001

ENTRY REQUIREMENTS

- **Passport/Visa:** Valid passport and visa are required.
- **HIV Test:** Not required.
- **Vaccinations:** Yellow fever vaccine is required for travelers coming from endemic countries. Recommended for all travelers going outside urban areas. Uganda is designated as a yellow fever endemic zone. Although no human cases have been reported since 1964, current surveillance is unreliable.

EMBASSIES/CONSULATES

- **U.S. Embassy:** Gaba Road, Kansanga, Kampala; Tel: 256-41-234-142; Fax: 256-41-258-451; e-mail: uscons@infocom.co.ug
- **Canadian Embassy:** IPS Building, Parliament Road, Kampala; Tel: 256-41-258-141 or 235-768; Fax: 256-41-234-518; e-mail: canada.consulate@infocom.co.ug
- **British High Commission:** 10/12 Parliament Avenue, PO Box 7070, Kampala; Tel: 256-31-312000; Fax: 256-41-257304; e-mail: bhcimm@infocom.co.ug.

HOSPITALS/DOCTORS

- Mulago General Hospital, Kampala (1,080 beds); general medical facility; no anesthesiology.
- Nsambya Hospital, Kampala (370 beds); general medical/surgical facility.

Current Advisories and Health Risks

ACCIDENTS/ILLNESSES AND MEDICAL INSURANCE

- Accidents and injuries are the leading cause of death among travelers younger than 55 years of age and most often are caused by motor vehicle and motorcycle crashes; drownings, aircraft crashes, homicides, and burns are less common causes.
- Heart attacks cause most fatalities in older travelers.
- Infections cause only 1% of fatalities in overseas travelers, but overall, infections are the most common cause of travel-related illness.
- Travelers are advised to obtain, before departure, supplemental travel health insurance with specific overseas coverage. The policy should provide for direct payment to the overseas hospital and/or physician at the time of service and include a medical evacuation benefit. The policy should also provide 24-hour hotline access to a multilingual assistance center that can help arrange and monitor delivery of medical care and determine if medical evacuation or air ambulance services are required. Health insurance is essential.
- East African Flying Doctor Services, based in Nairobi, has introduced a special Tourist Membership, which guarantees that any member injured or ill while on safari can call on a flying doctor for free air transport.

AFRICAN SLEEPING SICKNESS (TRYPANOSOMIASIS): Prevalent in scattered areas countrywide. Major risk of disease presumably persists in the southeast (extending from the northern shores of Lake Victoria and Lake Kyoga), with foci of Gambiense disease primarily in northwestern and north central areas (along the White Nile and the Sudanese border). All travelers to these regions should take measures to prevent tsetse fly bites.

AIDS/HIV: Promiscuous heterosexual contact is the predominant mode of transmission. HIV-1 prevalence is estimated at up to 86% of the high-risk urban population. All travelers are cautioned against unsafe sex, unsterile medical or dental injections, and unnecessary blood transfusions. It is advisable to take a kit of sterilized syringes and needles for any possible injections needed.

ANIMAL HAZARDS: Animal hazards include snakes (vipers, cobras), centipedes, scorpions, and black widow spiders. Crocodiles are known to attack boats and people on shore.

CHOLERA: This disease is active in this country. Cholera is an extremely rare disease in travelers from developed countries. Cholera vaccine is recommended primarily for people at high risk (e.g., relief workers) who work and live in highly endemic areas under less than adequate sanitary conditions.

• The oral cholera vaccine (Dukoral) provides up to 60% crossover protection against ETEC diarrhea.

• Many countries, including Canada, license an oral cholera vaccine. The oral vaccine is not available in the United States.

• Cholera vaccine is not "officially" required for entry into, or exit from, any country. Despite this, some countries, on occasion, require proof of cholera vaccination from travelers coming from cholera-infected countries. Anticipating such a situation, certain travelers may wish to carry a medical exemption letter from their health-care provider. Travel Medicine, Inc., recommends that travelers use the International Certificate of Vaccination (Yellow Card) for this purpose, having their health-care provider affirm that they are "exempt from cholera vaccine" and validate the exemption with both the provider's signature and the appropriate official stamp (the "Uniform Stamp" in the United States).

EBOLA VIRUS HEMORRHAGIC FEVER: Sporadic, rare Ebola virus disease activity occurs. Transmission is via direct contact with blood or body fluids of acutely ill patients.

FILARIASIS: Sporadic cases are reported. Travelers to this country are advised to take protective measures against black fly bites.

HEPATITIS: High risk. All nonimmune travelers should receive hepatitis A vaccine. The hepatitis B carrier rate in the general population is estimated at 10%. Hepatitis B vaccine is recommended for stays longer than 3 months, frequent short stays, adventure travelers, and any traveler desiring increased protection; and also with the possibility of unsafe sex with a new partner, or of receiving a medical or dental injection. Hepatitis C is endemic.

INFLUENZA: Influenza is transmitted year-round in the tropics. The flu vaccine is recommended for all travelers over age 50; all travelers with any chronic or immunocompromising conditions; travelers of any age wishing to decrease the risk of this illness; and pregnant women after the first trimester.

LASSA FEVER: Sporadic, rare Lassa fever activity occurs. Transmission is via contact with infected rodents.

LEISHMANIASIS: Visceral leishmaniasis occurs in the northeast province of Karamoja. Sporadic cases of cutaneous leishmaniasis are reported from the Mt. Elgon vicinity. Travelers should take protective measures against insect (sand fly) bites.

LOIASIS: Sporadic cases are reported. Travelers to this country are advised to take protective measures against black fly bites.

MALARIA: Risk is present year-round throughout this country, including urban areas. Falciparum malaria accounts for approximately 80% of cases. Other cases of malaria are due to the *P. malariae* species, followed by *P. ovale* and (rarely) *P. vivax.* Chloroquine-resistant falciparum malaria is reported.
- Prophylaxis with atovaquone/proguanil (Malarone), mefloquine (Lariam), or doxycycline is recommended.
- All travelers should take measures to prevent evening and nighttime mosquito bites. Insect bite prevention measures include a DEET-containing repellent applied to exposed skin, insecticide (permethrin) spray applied to clothing and gear, and use of a permethrin-treated bed net at night while sleeping.

MENINGITIS: Risk is present. An outbreak of meningococcal meningitis began in Kampala in 1989 and extended to other provinces. Vaccination against meningococcal disease is advised, especially for travelers who expect close, prolonged contact with the indigenous population.

ONCHOCERCIASIS: Sporadic cases are reported. Travelers to this country are advised to take protective measures against black fly bites.

POLIO: This disease is endemic in sub-saharan Africa. All travelers should be fully immunized.

RABIES: Increased incidence of rabies is reported in Kampala and Karamoja Provinces. Rabies vaccine is recommended for all stays longer than 3 months and shorter stays at locations more than 24 hours' travel from a reliable source of postexposure rabies vaccine. Consider for shorter stays in travelers desiring maximum protection. All dog bites or scratches incurred in this country should be medically evaluated.

SCHISTOSOMIASIS: Intestinal schistosomiasis occurs primarily in the northwest and along the northern shore of Lake Victoria. Urinary schistosomiasis is confined to northern central Uganda, north of Lake Kyoga. Travelers should avoid swimming or wading in freshwater lakes, ponds, or streams.

TRAVELERS' DIARRHEA: High risk. Supplies of potable water are inadequate to meet the needs of the population. Piped water supplies may be grossly contaminated. Travelers should observe food and drink safety precautions. A quinolone antibiotic, combined with loperamide (Imodium), is recommended for the treatment of acute diarrhea. Diarrhea not responding to treatment with an antibiotic, or chronic diarrhea, may be due to a parasitic disease such as giardiasis or amebiasis.

TUBERCULOSIS: Tuberculosis (TB) is a major public health problem in this country and is related in part to the high incidence of HIV infection and AIDS. Travelers planning an extended stay should have a pre-departure TB skin test (PPD test) and be retested after leaving this country.

TYPHOID FEVER: Typhoid vaccine is recommended. The typhoid vacccines are 60% to 70% effective. Food and drink precautions should continue to be observed.

YELLOW FEVER: Vaccination is recommended. No cases have been reported recently, but this country is in the Yellow Fever Endemic Zone. A valid yellow fever vaccination certificate will be required of travelers arriving from Kenya (where yellow fever is active).

OTHER DISEASES/HAZARDS: African tick typhus (contracted from dog ticks—often in urban areas and from bush ticks), brucellosis, chikungunya fever (mosquito-transmitted), Crimean-Congo hemorrhagic fever (tick-borne; cases reported from Entebbe), dengue (not reported recently), echinococcosis, leprosy, leptospirosis, louse-borne typhus, toxoplasmosis, syphilis, tuberculosis (a major health problem), trachoma, typhoid fever, and intestinal worms (very common).

Ukraine

CAPITAL:
Kiev
EMBASSY (IN U.S.):
202-333-0606
GMT:
+3 hours
TELEPHONE COUNTRY CODE:
380
USADIRECT:
8-100-11

ENTRY REQUIREMENTS

• **Passport/Visa:** A passport and visa are required. Visa requires one application form, one photo, a letter of invitation, and a fee of $100 to $165 (money order only), depending on whether you apply for a single-, double-, or multiple-entry visa. Transit visa requires onward/return ticket. Anyone applying for a visa for a stay of 3 months or longer is required to present a certificate showing HIV-negative status; U.S. test results are sometimes accepted. For additional information, contact the Consular Office of the Embassy of Ukraine, 3350 M St. NW, Washington, DC 20007: Tel: 202-333-7507 or 7508 or 7509.

- **HIV Test:** Testing is required for foreigners staying longer than 3 months. U.S. test result is currently acceptable.
- **Vaccinations:** None required. Tetanus/diphtheria immunization is recommended.

EMBASSIES/CONSULATES

- **U.S. Embassy:** 10 Vulitsa Yuria Kotsubinskoho, Kiev; Tel: 380-44-490-4000 or 240-0856; Fax: 244-7350; Website: www.usemb.kiev.ua.
- **Canadian Embassy:** 31 Yaroslaviv Val Street, Kiev; Tel: 380-44-464-1144; Fax: 380-44-464-0598; e-mail: kyiv@dfait-maeci.gc.ca.
- **British Embassy:** 01025 Kiev Desyatinna 9; Tel: 380-44-490-3660; Fax: 380-44-490-3662; e-mail: ukembinf@sovamua.com.

HOSPITALS/DOCTORS:

Medical care in Ukraine is below Western standards, although some private clinics are adequately equipped and staffed with English-speaking doctors. Travelers to Ukraine are advised to obtain, before departure, supplemental travel health insurance with specific overseas coverage. The policy should provide for direct payment to the overseas hospital and/or physician at the time of service and include a medical evacuation benefit. In cases of serious illness or injury, foreign diplomats and their dependents usually travel to Frankfurt, Germany, for medical care. Travelers may seek medical care in Germany or any Western European country with the understanding that pre-payment in the national currency is often necessary and that a local physician must authorize a hospital admission.

- Assist Ukraine (SOS), Kiev; Tel: 044-221 8203.
- American Medical Center, 1 Berdychivska Street, Kiev; Tel: 044-490-7600; e-mail: kiev@amcenters.com.
- LifeLine Medical Clinic, Beresneki Region; Tel: 044-553-9787 or 553-7416. Western-trained physicians.
- St. Luke American-Ukrainian Medical Center, 150a vul. Gorkogo; Tel: 044-252-8552.

Current Advisories and Health Risks

AIDS/HIV: The incidence of AIDS/HIV is rapidly increasing and an epidemic appears to be in the making in this country, as is happening in Russia. The reasons include (1) an increase in injecting drug use, (2) increases in commercial sex and sexual promiscuity, (3) an increase in sexually transmitted diseases, (4) decreased availability of sterile needles and syringes for safe medical injections, and (5) inadequate puplic health education and prevention programs.

BOUTONNEUSE FEVER: Tick-borne; reported most commonly in the Black Sea coastal areas of the Caucasus, Transcaucasus, and Crimea, and along the Caspian Sea coastline.

CRIMEAN-CONGO HEMORRHAGIC FEVER: Also known as Central Asian hemorrhagic fever. Tick-borne; reported mostly from southern areas, but outbreaks have occurred in some areas of Rostov Oblast (near the sea of Azov), April through November. Risk areas are rural steppe, savannah, semi-desert, and foothill/low mountain habitats below 2,000 meters elevation.

DIPHTHERIA: An epidemic diphtheria that began in 1990 in the Russian Federation has spread extensively, involving all countries of the former Soviet Union. Seventy percent of cases have occurred in persons older than 15 years. All travelers to Ukraine, especially adults, should be fully immunized. Diphtheria vaccine is administered in combination with the tetanus toxoid vaccine (Td vaccine).

HEPATITIS: All travelers should receive hepatitis A vaccine. Hepatitis E accounts for up to 18% of hepatitis in the Volga Delta region, but less than 1% regionwide. The hepatitis B carrier rate in the general population is estimated at 5% to 7%. Hepatitis B is spread by infected blood, contaminated needles, and unsafe sex. Vaccination is recommended for stays longer than 3 months; for persons at occupational or social risk; and for any traveler desiring maximum protection. Because the risk of illness or injury during travel cannot be predicted, some experts believe that *all* travelers should be immunized against hepatitis B because of the risk of receiving a medical injection with an unsterile needle or syringe.

INFLUENZA: Influenza is transmitted from November to April. The flu vaccine is recommended for all travelers at risk.

LEISHMANIASIS: Risk for cutaneous leishmaniasis primarily limited to southern regions, including portions of Georgia Republic and the southern Ukraine, below 1,300 meters elevation. Visceral leishmaniasis is confined to areas of the Transcaucasus. Travelers to these regions should take measures to prevent sand fly bites.

LYME DISEASE: Occurs focally in rural forested areas primarily in the mid-south to the Baltic region eastward. The vector ticks are most abundant and active from May through August.

MALARIA: There is no risk of malaria in Ukraine.

TICK-BORNE ENCEPHALITIS (TBE): Tick-borne encephalitis (TBE) is transmitted from the Baltics to the Crimea by ixodid ticks. Peak transmission period is April through October. Risk is present primarily in rural brushy and forested areas below 1,500 meters elevation, especially in suburban "forests" bordering large cities. TBE is usually known as "Central European tick-borne encephalitis" west of the Urals. Increased incidence reported in the Perm-Sverlovsk areas (central Urals) in the 1990s. The TBE vaccine should be considered for stays longer than 3 weeks for those who will be hiking or camping in wooded or grassland areas. The vaccine is available only in Europe and by special release in Canada. Travelers to rural areas should take measures to prevent tick bites.

TYPHOID FEVER: Typhoid vaccine is recommended for all travelers, with the exception of short-term visitors who restrict their meals to major restaurants and hotels. Because the typhoid vaccines are only 60% to 70% effective, safe food and drink selection remains important.

OTHER DISEASES/HAZARDS: Brucellosis, echinococcosis (sheep and reindeer are hosts; dog feces are infective), legionellosis, leptospirosis (a particular problem in fish-breeding areas of Rostov Province; extensive outbreaks have occurred in east central areas), North Asian (Siberian) tick typhus (occurs in the steppe areas bordering Kazakhstan, Georgia, and Azerbaijan; risk elevated in May and June), rabies, rickettsialpox, tick-borne relapsing fever, trichinosis (greatest risk in western Belarus and the Ukraine), tularemia ("rabbit fever"; risk may be elevated in the north), tuberculosis (40% rise in cases since 1995), and helminthic infections (roundworm, hookworm, and whipworm infections and strongyloidiasis) reported, especially from the Transcaucaus, and especially Azerbaijan.

United Arab Emirates (UAE)

ABU DHABI

CAPITAL:
Abu Dhabi

EMBASSY (IN U.S.):
202-338-6500

GMT:
+4 hours

TELEPHONE COUNTRY CODE:
971

USADIRECT:
0-800-121, or 0-800-151 for placing calls from U.S. military bases

ENTRY REQUIREMENTS

- **Passport/Visa:** Passport and visa required. Tourist visa requires a typed letter from the applicant's employer indicating type and length of position held or, for students/homemakers/retirees, bank statement proving sufficient funds for stay. Business visas issued only by the UAE Embassy and require company letter and sponsor in UAE to send a fax or telex to UAE Embassy confirming trip and accepting financial responsibility. Single-entry visa, valid within 2 months from the date of issuance, for stays of up to 30 days. Multiple-entry visa (for business only), valid up to 10 years from date of issue for maximum stay of 6 months per entry, no fee. Transit visa must be obtained in advance (through travel agency, hotel, or company in UAE), valid for a stay of up to 15 days. For further information, contact the Embassy of the United Arab Emirates, 3522 International Court NW, Suite 100, Washington, DC 20008; Tel: 202-243-2400; Website: UAE-embassy.org.
- **HIV Test:** AIDS test required for residency permits; test performed on arrival in the UAE.
- **Vaccinations:** A yellow fever vaccination certificate is required of all travelers arriving from infected areas.

EMBASSIES/CONSULATES

- **U.S. Embassy:** 11th St., also known as Al-Sudan St., Abu Dhabi; Tel: 971-2-443-6691 or 971-2-443-4457; Fax: 971-2-443-5786; Website: www.usembabu.gov.ae.
- **Canadian Embassy:** 440 26th St. (corner of 26th St. and Dalma St., between German and French embassies), Abu Dhabi; Tel: 971-2-445-6969; Fax: 971-2-445-8787; e-mail: abdbi@dfait-maeci.gc.ca.
- **British Embassy:** PO Box 248, Abu Dhabi; Tel: 971-2-6101100; Fax: 971-2-6101518; e-mail: chancery.abudhabi@fco.gov.uk; Website: www.britain-uae.org.

HOSPITALS/DOCTORS

- Dubai Hospital (635 beds); major referral facility; ambulance service; helipad.
- Raship Hospital, Dubai (500 beds); emergency/trauma facility; ambulance; helipad.
- Al Baraha Hospital, Dubai (208 beds); Tel: 971-4-71-0000. 24-hour emergency services available.
- Dr. J.P.R. McCulloch Clinic, Abu Dhabi; Tel: 2-633-3900.

Current Advisories and Health Risks

See the Disease Risk Summary for the Middle East on page 310.

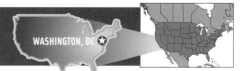

United States of America

WASHINGTON, DC ★

CAPITAL:
Washington, DC

EMBASSY (IN U.S.):
Not applicable.

GMT:
−5 hours

TELEPHONE COUNTRY CODE:
1

USADIRECT:
1-800-CALL ATT

ENTRY REQUIREMENTS

- **Passport/Visa:** A passport is required. Travelers should check visa requirements with a U.S. embassy or consulate.
- **HIV Test:** HIV-positive visitors must apply at the U.S. Embassy for a waiver of ineligibility before entry.
- **Vaccinations:** None required.

EMBASSIES/CONSULATES

- **Canadian Embassy:** 501 Pennsylvania Ave. NW, Washington, DC; Tel: 1-202-682-1740; Fax: 1-202-682-7726; e-mail: wshdc-outpack@dfait-maeci.gc.ca; Website: canadianembassy.org/splash.

- **British Embassy:** 3100 Massachusetts Avenue, NW, Washington, DC 20008; Tel: 1-202-588-6500; Fax: 1-202-588-6511.

HOSPITALS/DOCTORS:

Medical facilities generally are of a high standard, but medical care is expensive, and adequate insurance coverage is essential. Foreigners residing in the United States with school-age children should be aware that school entry requirements include proof of immunization against diphtheria, measles, poliomyelitis, and rubella; schools in some states require immunization against tetanus, pertussis, and mumps.

- International SOS:
  - International SOS Assistance, Inc., 3600 Horizon Boulevard, Suite 300, Trevose, PA 19053; Alarm Center Tel: 1-215-942-7226; Alarm Center Fax: 1-215-942-7297
  - International SOS Assistance, Inc, 2211 Norfolk, Suite 517, USA, Houston, TX 77098; Admin Tel: 1-713-521-7611; Admin Fax: 1-713-521-7655

Current Advisories and Health Risks

DENGUE FEVER: Confirmed cases of dengue fever have been reported in Hawaii, but the risk to travelers is minimal; mosquito bite prevention measures should be observed. Locally acquired cases of dengue fever are occasionally reported in southern Texas.

FOOD AND WATER SAFETY: There is very low risk of food- and drink-related illness nationwide. Tap water is potable. Sporadic cases of food-borne illness, usually due to *Salmonella* or *Campylobacter*, are reported. Undercooked or raw eggs and undercooked chicken are often the sources of outbreaks, usually confined to institutions, such as nursing homes, or to gatherings such as picnics. Gastroenteritis, caused by *Vibrio* species, *Salmonella*, or *Campylobacter*, has been reported after the consumption of contaminated oysters in Louisiana, Maryland, North Carolina, Florida, and Mississippi. *Vibrio cholerae* infections, transmitted by contaminated shellfish (crab, shrimp, raw oysters), occur sporadically along the Gulf of Mexico (Texas, Louisiana). Ciguatera fish poisoning is occasionally reported from Hawaii and Florida.

INTESTINAL PARASITES: Giardiasis occurs primarily in the wilderness areas of the Rocky Mountains and the Pacific Northwest but the distribution of risk, nationwide, is not clearly defined. Campers and hikers are advised to boil or filter drinking water obtained from lakes, streams, or ponds. Outbreaks of giardiasis and cryptosporidiosis have occurred after breakdowns in municipal water treatment plants. Chlorine or iodine should not be relied on to remove parasites from drinking water.

HEPATITIS: Low risk nationwide of hepatitis A, but the vaccine is recommended for all travelers. Hepatitis B is spread by infected blood, contaminated needles, and unprotected sex. Vaccination is recommended for stays longer than 3 months; for persons at occupational or social risk; and for anyone desiring maximum protection.

INFLUENZA: Influenza is transmitted from November through March. Flu vaccine is recommended for all travelers at potential risk.

VIRAL GASTROENTERITIS: Outbreaks of Norwalk virus–related vomiting and diarrhea occur sporadically on cruise ships departing U.S. ports. Personal hygiene and hand washing help limit the spread of illness.

LEPTOSPIROSIS: Reported from Hawaii and Puerto Rico. Most transmission occurs from immersion in freshwater streams or in association with surface water sports.

LYME DISEASE: Lyme disease occurs in the Northeast (from Maryland to Maine), the Middle Atlantic states, the upper Midwest (Wisconsin and Minnesota), and the northern Pacific Coast region (Oregon and northern California). Travelers should take precautions against tick bites in these regions.

RABIES: Almost all cases of human rabies in the United States are transmitted by bats. The number of cases of animal rabies (raccoons, skunks) in the United States is increasing. Along the U.S.-Mexican border, rabies transmitted by dogs and coyotes is a potential threat to humans. In Alaska, the arctic fox and red fox are primarily infected. Bats anywhere in the United States should be considered potentially rabid. Other wild animals that rarely transmit rabies include groundhogs, wolves, bobcats, and black bears. No cases of wild animal rabies have been reported from the states of Washington, Idaho, Utah, Nevada, and Colorado.

TICK-BORNE DISEASES: Lyme disease occurs in the Middle Atlantic States, the Northeast, the upper Midwest, and the northern Pacific Coast region. Babesiosis occurs in the Nantucket region and was recently reported in Wisconsin. A new *Babesia* strain has appeared in Washington State. Human monocytic ehrlichiosis occurs in the south-central and southeastern United States. Human granulocytic ehrlichiosis is reported from Minnesota, Wisconsin, California, and the northeastern United States. Other tick-borne infections include Rocky Mountain spotted fever (occurs mostly in the Southeast), Coloroado tick fever (Western states), relapsing fever (Western states), tularemia (all states; more cases reported in Arkansas, Missouri, and Oklahoma), tick paralysis (Western states and Pacific coast) and Q fever (can also be acquired by inhalation).

VIRAL ENCEPHALITIS (OTHER THAN FROM WEST NILE VIRUS):
- St. Louis encephalitis (SLE), named for the city where the first cases were recognized in 1933, is the most common variety of viral encephalitis in the United States. It occurs along the Gulf Coast and in the Ohio and Mississippi river valleys, Florida, and the Western states.
- Eastern equine encephalitis (also a mosquito-borne disease with a fatality rate of up to 60%) occurs in the eastern and north-central United States and Canada.
- Western equine encephalitis (a milder disease with a fatality rate of 3%) is endemic in central and western United States and in Canada.
- Viral encephalitis is commonly spread by *Culex* mosquitoes, but the *Aedes albopictus* mosquito ("Asian tiger mosquito") is also known to transmit encephalitis viruses.

WEST NILE VIRUS ENCEPHALITIS: West Nile virus is a mosquito-transmitted virus that was most likely imported to the United States by air travelers from Europe. In 2002, almost 3,000 cases of encephalitis were reported in the United States, but in 2004 the total number of cases declined to 741. The disease is now moving from the East Coast across the country to the west. Almost one-third of the cases of neuroinvasive disease in 2004 occurred in Arizona and California; the other cases occurred throughout the rest of the country. No vaccine is currently available.

Uruguay

CAPITAL:
Montevideo
EMBASSY (IN U.S.):
202-331-1313
GMT:
-3 hours
TELEPHONE COUNTRY CODE:
598
USADIRECT:
000-410
ENTRY REQUIREMENTS
- **Passport/Visa:** Passport required. Visa not required for tourist/business stays of up to 90 days. For additional information, consult the Embassy of Uruguay, 1913 I St. NW, 3rd Floor, Washington, DC 20006; Tel: 202-331-4219; or the nearest consulate: California (310-394-5777), Florida (305-443-7453 or 9764), or New York (212-753-8191 or 8192); Website: www.embassy.org/uruguay.
- **HIV Test:** Not required.
- **Vaccinations:** None required.
EMBASSIES/CONSULATES
- **U.S. Embassy:** Lauro Muller 1776; Tel: 598-2-203-6061 or 598-2-408-7777; Fax: 598-2-408-4110; Website: www.embeeuu.gub.uy
- **Canadian Embassy:** 749 Plaza Independencia app.102, Montevideo; Tel: 598-2-902-2030; Fax: 598-2-902-2029; e-mail: mvdeo@dfait-maeci.gc.ca.
- **British Embassy:** Calle Marco Bruto 1073, 11300 Montevideo, PO Box 16024; Tel: 598-2-622-3630, 622-3650; Fax: 598-2-622-7815; e-mail: bemonte@internet.com.uy
HOSPITALS/DOCTORS:
Medical care in Uruguay is mostly of high quality, and many physicians speak English. Travelers to this country are advised to obtain, before departure, supplemental travel health insurance with specific overseas coverage. The policy should provide for direct payment to the overseas hospital and/or physician at the time of service and include a medical evacuation benefit.
- Hospital Britanico (British Hospital), Montevideo (120 beds); Tel: 2-487-1020. Frequently used by U.S. Embassy personnel; 24-hour emergency services.

Current Advisories and Health Risks

CHAGAS DISEASE: Reported in all rural areas of Uruguay except the Atlantic coast areas. Areas with high incidence include the departments of Artigas, Rivera, Salto, and Tacuarembo. Risk occurs in those rural-agricultural areas where there are adobe-style huts and houses that potentially harbor the night-biting triatomid (assassin) bugs. Travelers sleeping in such structures should take precautions against nighttime bites.

CHOLERA: Not officially reported, but sporadic cases may occur. There is little risk to travelers, and vaccination is not recommended.

HEPATITIS: All travelers should receive hepatitis A vaccine. The carrier rate for the hepatitis B virus in the general population is less than 1%; vaccination against hepatitis B should be considered for stays longer than 3 months and by short-term travelers desiring maximum protection.

MALARIA: There is no risk of malaria in Uruguay.

RABIES: There is no risk of rabies in Uruguay.

TRAVELERS' DIARRHEA: Low to moderate risk. Travelers should observe food and drink precautions. A quinolone antibiotic, combined with loperamide (Imodium), is recommended for the treatment of diarrhea. Persistent diarrhea may be due to a parasitic disease such as giardiasis, amebiasis, or cryptosporidiosis.

TYPHOID FEVER: Typhoid vaccine is recommended for all travelers, with the exception of short-term visitors who restrict their meals to major restaurants and hotels. Because the typhoid vaccines are only 60% to 70% effective, safe food and drink selection remains important.

YELLOW FEVER: No risk.

OTHER DISEASES/HAZARDS: Brucellosis, echinococcosis (up to 1.4% of the rural human population may be infected), AIDS/HIV (relatively low incidence), measles (extensive outbreaks have occurred), tuberculosis (low incidence), strongyloidiasis and other helminthic infections, and trichinosis (3% of the population may be infected).

Uzbekistan

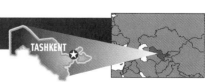

CAPITAL:
Tashkent
EMBASSY (IN U.S.):
202-887-5300
GMT:
+5 hours

998
8^641-744-0010. ^ indicates a second dial tone.
ENTRY REQUIREMENTS
- **Passport/Visa:** Required. Visa applicants may need to meet specific requirements.
- **HIV Test:** HIV testing is required of anyone staying more than 15 days. (Long-term visitors must renew HIV certificate after the first 3 months in Uzbekistan and annually thereafter.) Foreign test results are accepted under certain conditions.
- **Vaccinations:** None required.

EMBASSIES/CONSULATES
- **U.S. Embassy:** Ulitsa Chilanzarskaya, 82; Tel: 998-71-120-5450; Fax: 998-71-120-6335; Website: www.usis.uz/wwwhcon.htm.
- **Canadian Embassy:** Center 5, No. 64, Apt. 21, Tashkent; Tel: 998-71-137-67-28; Fax: 998-71-120-72-70; e-mail: antal@online.ru.
- **British Embassy:** Ul. Gulyamova 67, Tashkent 700000; Tel: 99871-1206451, 1206288, 1207852, 1207853, 1207854; Fax: 99871-1206549; e-mail: brit@emb.uz.

HOSPITALS/DOCTORS:
Medical care in Uzbekistan is below Western standards. Travelers are advised to obtain, before departure, supplemental travel health insurance with specific overseas coverage. The policy should provide for direct payment to the overseas hospital and/or physician at the time of service and include a medical evacuation benefit.
- Tashkent International Medical Clinic; Tel: 998-71-2545595. Carries all the features of a traditional family practice Western clinic. This clinic was founded in 1994 by the U.S., German, U.K., and Japanese embassies for the sole purpose of providing quality Western standard health care to the expatriate population living and working in Tashkent.

Current Advisories and Health Risks

See the Disease Risk Summary for Central Asia on page 302.

Vanuatu

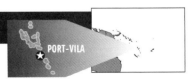

PORT-VILA

CAPITAL:
Port-Vila
EMBASSY (IN U.S.):
212-425-9652
GMT:
+11 hours
TELEPHONE COUNTRY CODE:
678

USADIRECT:

None

ENTRY REQUIREMENTS

• **Passport/Visa:** Passport and onward/return ticket required. A visa not required for stay of up to 30 days. Travelers should consult the Vanuatu Mission to the UN (Tel: 1-212/593-0144 or 0215) for further information.

• **HIV Test:** Not required.

• **Vaccinations:** None required.

EMBASSIES/CONSULATES

• **UN Mission:** Tel: 212-593-0144 or 0215.

• **U.S. Embassy:** There is no U.S. Embassy in Vanuatu. Assistance for U.S. citizens is provided by the American Embassy in Port Moresby, Papua New Guinea; Tel: 675-321-1445; Fax: 675-321-1593.

• **Canadian Embassy:** Australian High Commission, KPMG House, Port Vila; Tel: 678-22-777; Fax: 678-23-948.

• **British High Commission:** Port Vila, Vanuatu, PO Box 567, Port Vila; Tel: 678-23100; e-mail: bhcvila@vanuatu.com.vu.

HOSPITALS/DOCTORS:

Medical care in Vanuatu is rudimentary by Western standards. Travelers are advised to obtain, before departure, supplemental travel health insurance with specific overseas coverage. The policy should provide for direct payment to the overseas hospital and/or physician at the time of service and include a medical evacuation benefit. The nearest reliable medical facilities are in Australia and New Zealand. Emergency transport to Australia should be considered for any serious medical problem.

• The Luganville Hospital, Luganville, Espirito Santo Island, has a hyperbaric chamber and five wards for medicine, surgery, maternity, pediatrics, and tuberculosis.

Current Advisories and Health Risks

HEPATITIS: Hepatitis A vaccine is recommended for all travelers. The hepatitis B carrier rate in the general population is estimated to exceed 10%. Hepatitis B is spread by infected blood, contaminated needles, and unsafe sex. Vaccination is recommended for stays longer than 3 months; for persons at occupational or social risk; and for any traveler desiring maximum protection.

INFLUENZA: Influenza is transmitted year-round in the tropics; flu vaccine is recommended for all travelers.

INSECT-BORNE DISEASES: Dengue fever, filariasis, and Japanese encephalitis (JE) occur sporadically, with occasional outbreaks. The JE vaccine is indicated for stays longer than 3 to 4 weeks; adventure travelers; expatriates; and, particularly, anybody working outside in rural areas during the peak transmission season. Travelers who make shorter, repeat visits to rural agricultural areas should also consider vaccination against JE. All travelers should take measures to prevent both daytime and nighttime insect bites.

Insect bite prevention measures include a DEET-containing repellent applied to exposed skin, insecticide (permethrin) spray applied to clothing, and sleeping under a permethrin-treated bed net.

MALARIA: There is a generally high risk of malaria throughout this country, including urban areas. Falciparum malaria accounts for 60% of cases. Both chloroquine-resistant vivax and chloroquine-resistant falciparum malaria are reported. Atovaquone/proguanil (Malarone), mefloquine (Lariam), or doxycycline is recommended for malaria prophylaxis.

MARINE HAZARDS:
• Swimming-related hazards include jellyfish, spiny sea urchins, and coral.
• Ciguatera poisoning is prevalent and can result from eating coral reef fish such as grouper, snapper, sea bass, jack, and barracuda. The ciguatoxin is not destroyed by cooking.

TRAVELERS' DIARRHEA: The drinking water in this country is collected in ground catchment systems, and water supplies should be considered potentially contaminated. The tap water in Vila is considered safe. A quinolone antibiotic, combined with loperamide (Imodium), is recommended for the treatment of acute diarrhea. Persistent diarrhea may be due to a parasitic infection such as giardiasis, amebiasis, or cryptosporidiosis.

TUBERCULOSIS: Tuberculosis (TB) is a major health problem in this country. Travelers planning an extended stay should have a pre-departure TB skin test (PPD test) and be retested after returning from this country.

TYPHOID FEVER: Typhoid vaccine is recommended for all travelers, with the exception of short-term visitors who restrict their meals to major restaurants and hotels, such as business travelers and cruise passengers. Because the typhoid vaccines are only 60% to 70% effective, safe food and drink selection remains important.

Venezuela

CARACAS

CAPITAL:
Caracas
EMBASSY (IN U.S.):
202-342-2214
GMT:
−4 hours
TELEPHONE COUNTRY CODE:
58
USADIRECT:
0800-225-5288

ENTRY REQUIREMENTS
- **Passport/Visa:** A tourist card and multiple-entry visa are available.
- **HIV Test:** Not required.
- **Vaccinations:** No vaccinations are required to visit this country.

EMBASSIES/CONSULATES
- **U.S. Embassy:** Calle Suapure and Calle F, Colinas de Valle Arriba, Caracas; Tel: 2975-6411 or 2-975-9821; Website: usembassy.state.gov/caracas.
- **Canadian Embassy:** Avenida Francisco de Miranda con Avenida Sur Altamira, Altamira, Caracas ; Tel: 212-263-4666 or 263-1414 or 263-3270, Fax: 212-263-8326; e-mail: crcas@dfait-maeci.gc.ca.
- **British Embassy:** Torre La Castellana, Piso 11, Avenida La Principal de la Castellana, La Castellana, Caracas 1061; Tel: 58-212-263-8411; Fax: 58-212-267-1275; e-mail: britishembassy@internet.ve.

HOSPITALS/DOCTORS
- Centro Medico de Caracas (145 beds); Avenida Los Erasos, San Bernardino, Caracas; modern, high-quality private facility; most specialties, including trauma.
- Hospital Universitario de Caracas (1,200 beds); most specialties; emergency services.
- Hospital de Clinicas Caracas (170 beds); Avenida Panteoin, Caracas; general medical/surgical facility featuring high-quality care.
- International SOS: International SOS Assistance, Inc, Av. Eugenio Mendoza, con 1ª Transversal La Castellana, Edif. Banco Lara, Mezz., Ofic. D-1, Caracas, Venezuela 1066; Admin Tel: 58-212-263-7591 /3009 /1495; Admin Fax: 58-212-266-7727

Current Advisories and Health Risks

ACCIDENTS/ILLNESSES: Motor vehicle accidents, injuries, and drownings are the leading cause of death among travelers under the age of 55. Cardiovascular disease causes most fatalities in older travelers. Infections cause less than 1% of fatalities in overseas travelers but overall are the most common cause of travel-related illness.

ANIMAL HAZARDS: Animal hazards include snakes (vipers), centipedes, scorpions, black widow spiders, brown recluse spiders, banana spiders, and wolf spiders.

CHAGAS DISEASE: This disease is endemic to rural areas in the northern one half of Venezuela. In some areas, up to 50% of the population has been exposed. Chagas disease is among the top 10 causes of death in Venezuelans older than 45 years of age. Risk occurs in those rural-agricultural areas where there are adobe-style huts and houses that potentially harbor the night-biting triatomid (assassin) bugs. Travelers sleeping in such structures should take precautions against nighttime bites. Contaminated food and unscreened blood transfusions are also sources of infection.

CHOLERA: This disease is reported active in this country, but the threat to tourists is very low. Cholera vaccine is recommended primarily for people at high risk (e.g., relief workers) who work and live in highly endemic areas under less than adequate sanitary conditions.

DENGUE FEVER: Year-round risk is present in coastal and lowland urban areas. Outbreaks of dengue occur regularly in central and northern Venezuela, including Caracas. Higher risk occurs in Miranda, Sucre, Merida, and Nueva Esparta (Margarita Island). All travelers should take protective measures against daytime mosquito bites.

FILARIASIS: Limited risk of mosquito-transmitted bancroftian filariasis in coastal areas. Mansonellosis, another type of filariasis, transmitted by black flies, is endemic in Amazonas Federal Territory. Travelers to these regions should take measures to prevent insect bites.

HEPATITIS: All nonimmune travelers should receive hepatitis A vaccine before visiting this country. Hepatitis E is endemic, but levels are unclear. The carrier rate for the hepatitis B virus in the general population is estimated at 2% to 3%, but rates as high as 31% have been found in some aboriginal populations (e.g., the Yucpa Indians in Zulia State). Hepatitis B is spread by infected blood, contaminated needles, and unprotected sex. Vaccination is recommended for stays longer than 3 months; for persons at occupational or social risk; and for anyone desiring maximum protection.

INFLUENZA: Influenza is transmitted year-round in the tropics. The flu vaccine is recommended for all travelers to this country.

LEISHMANIASIS: Cutaneous leishmaniasis (CL) is widespread in rural areas below 2,000 meters elevation, especially in rural west-central areas. Transmission of CL has been reported at elevations as high as 2,500 meters in the Andes. Except for a focus in northern Bolivar State, visceral leishmaniasis is limited primarily to northwestern and northern areas below 500 meters elevation. All travelers to risk areas should take measures to prevent insect (sand fly) bites, which occur primarily during the night.

MALARIA: Risk is present year-round in most rural areas below 600 meters elevation. Risk of malaria is highest in rural areas of the following states: Apure, Amazonas, Barinas, Bolivar, Sucre, Tachira, and Delta Amacuro. There is risk of malaria in Angel Falls. Most north-central areas, including the Federal District and the states of Aragua, Carabobo, Cojedes, Miranda, and Yaracuy, are free of malaria. These areas include the major cities and resort areas of northern Venezuela. Chloroquine-resistant falciparum malaria probably occurs in most malarious areas. Prophylaxis with atovaquone/proguanil (Malarone), mefloquine (Lariam), or doxycycline is recommended. All travelers should take measures to prevent evening and nighttime mosquito bites.

MARINE HAZARDS

- Portuguese man-of-war, sea wasps, and stingrays are found in the coastal waters of Venezuela and could be a hazard to swimmers.
- Ciguatera poisoning is prevalent and can result from eating coral reef fish such as grouper, snapper, sea bass, jack, and barracuda. The ciguatoxin is not destroyed by cooking.
- Scuba diving hyperbaric chamber listing: Divers' Alert Network (DAN) maintains an up-to-date list of all hyperbaric chambers in North America and the Caribbean. In as-

sociation with Duke University Medical Center in North Carolina, DAN operates a 24-hour emergency phone number (919-684-8111) for members and nonmembers to call, and their staff is available to answer questions and, if necessary, make referral to the closest functioning hyperbaric chamber.

ONCHOCERCIASIS: Risk occurs along fast-flowing rivers at elevations up to 1,000 meters elevation in the northcentral, northeast, and southern regions. Up to 90% of the population is infected in some southern regions. Travelers to these areas should take measures to prevent insect (black fly) bites.

RABIES: Sporadic cases of human rabies are reported countrywide. All animal bites or scratches, especially from a dog, should be evaluated medically.

SCHISTOSOMIASIS: Risk is present year-round. Risk areas are limited to north-central Venezuela, including the Federal District (but not Caracas) and the surrounding states of Aragua, Carabobo, Guarico, and Miranda. Travelers should avoid swimming in freshwater lakes, ponds, or streams. Risk may be elevated in periurban areas.

TRAVELERS' DIARRHEA: High risk outside of Merida, Caracas, Maracaibo, and resort areas. Water supplies in most urban areas are filtered and chlorinated but may be contaminated within the distribution system. Travelers should follow food and drink precautions. A quinolone antibiotic, combined with loperamide (Imodium), is recommended for the treatment of acute diarrhea. Persistent diarrhea may be due to a parasitic infection such as giardiasis, amebiasis, or cryptosporidiosis.

TUBERCULOSIS: Tuberculosis (TB) is a major health problem in this country. Travelers planning an extended stay should have a pre-departure TB skin test (PPD test) and be retested after returning from this country.

TYPHOID FEVER: Typhoid vaccine is recommended for those traveling off the usual tourist routes, for those visiting friends or relatives, and for long-stay visitors. Because the typhoid vaccines are only 60% to 70% effective, safe food and drink selection remains important.

YELLOW FEVER: Vaccination is recommended for all travelers older than 9 months of age arriving from *all* countries. Greatest risk of yellow fever exists in Merida State. Although a vaccination certificate is not required to enter this country, one may be required for ongoing travel to other countries in Latin America, Africa, the Middle East, and Asia.

OTHER DISEASES/HAZARDS: AIDS/HIV (endemic; seroprevalence increasing rapidly among women), angiostrongyliasis, brucellosis, echinococcosis, fascioliasis, leptospirosis, mansonellosis, paragonimiasis, tuberculosis, typhoid fever, Venezuelan hemorrhagic fever, Venezuelan equine encephalitis (mosquito-borne; highest risk in northwestern areas, primarily Zulia State), and helminthic diseases (due to hookworm, roundworm, whipworm, and *Strongyloides*) are reported.

Vietnam

HANOI

CAPITAL:
Hanoi
EMBASSY (IN U.S.):
202-861-0737
GMT:
+7 hours
TELEPHONE COUNTRY CODE:
84
USADIRECT:
None

ENTRY REQUIREMENTS
- **Passport/Visa:** Passport and visa are required.
- **HIV Test:** Not required.
- **Vaccinations:** A yellow fever vaccination certificate is required of all travelers older than 1 year arriving from infected areas.

EMBASSIES/CONSULATES
- **U.S. Embassy:** 6 Ngoc Khanh, Ba Dinh District, Hanoi; Tel: 84-4-831-4590 or 84-4-772-1500; Website: www.usembassy.state.gov/vietnam.
- **Canadian Embassy:** 31 Hung Vuong St., Hanoi; Tel: 84-4-823-5500; e-mail: hanoi@dfait-maeci.gc.ca.
- **British Embassy:** Central Building, 4th floor, 31 Hai Ba Trung, Hanoi, Vietnam; Tel: 84-4-936-0500.

HOSPITALS/DOCTORS
- Bach Mai Hospital, Hanoi (1,200 beds); general medical facility.
- Hanoi Family Medical Practice, Kim Ma Road, Van Phuc, Hanoi.
- Ho Chi Minh City Hospital, Saigon.
- Czech Friendship Hospital, Haiphong.
- International SOS:
  - OSCAT/AEA Vietnam Company Ltd., Representative Office, 65 Nguyen Du Street, District 1, Ho Chi Minh City, S.R. Vietnam; Alarm Center Tel: 74-7-729-7520; Alarm Center Fax: 74-7-729-7551; Clinic Tel: 74-7-729-7424, Dental Clinic Tel: 74-7-723-0498; Clinic Fax: 74-7-729-7551
  - OSCAT/AEA Vietnam Company Ltd., Representative Office, Hanoi Branch, Central Building, 31 Hai Ba Trung, Hoan Kiem District, Hanoi, S.R. Vietnam; Clinic Tel: 74-4-934-0666; Clinic Fax: 74-4-934-0556
  - OSCAT/AEA Vietnam Company Ltd., 1 Le Ngoc Han Street, Vung Tau, S.R. Vietnam; Clinic Tel: 74-64-758-776; Clinic Fax: 74-64-758-779
  - OSCAT/AEA Vietnam Company Ltd., Representative Office, Hanoi Branch, Central Building, 31 Hai Ba Trung, Hoan Kiem District, Hanoi, S.R. Vietnam; Alarm Center Tel: 74-4-934-0555; Alarm Center Fax: 74-4-934-0556; Clinic Tel: 74-4-934-0666; Clinic Fax: 74-4-934-0556

- OSCAT/AEA Vietnam Company Ltd., 1 Le Ngoc Han Street, Vung Tau, S.R. Vietnam; Clinic Tel: 74-64-758-776; Clinic Fax: 74-64-758-779

Current Advisories and Health Risks

ANIMAL HAZARDS: Animal hazards include snakes (vipers, cobras, kraits), scorpions, and black widow spiders. Other hazards include crocodiles, pythons, and large, aggressive lizards, as well as poisonous frogs and toads, all abundant in and near swamps and rivers. Tigers, leopards, bears, and wild pigs are found in the forested and hilly regions of the country. Stingrays, jellyfish, and several species of poisonous fish are common in the country's coastal waters and are potentially hazardous to swimmers.

CHOLERA: This disease is active in this country. The risk of cholera, however, is extremely low in international travelers from developed countries, such as the United States and Canada. Cholera vaccine is recommended primarily for persons at high risk who work and live in highly endemic areas under less than adequate sanitary conditions.

DENGUE FEVER: Epidemic outbreaks occur sporadically. Dengue occurs year-round, with peak transmission in the warmer rainy season, April through October in the north and June through December in the south. Elevated risk exists throughout the Red River Delta and Mekong Delta, and in the coastal district and provincial capitals of central Vietnam. Incidence is low in remote, mountainous regions. All travelers are advised to take precautions against mosquito bites.

HEPATITIS: All nonimmune travelers should receive hepatitis A vaccine before visiting this country. Outbreaks of hepatitis E have been reported, related to sewage-contaminated water. The overall hepatitis B carrier rate in the general population is estimated to exceed 12%. Hepatitis B is spread by infected blood, contaminated needles, and unprotected sex. Vaccination is recommended for long-stay (more than 3 months) travelers; persons who may be at occupational or social risk; and anybody desiring maximum protection.

INFLUENZA: Influenza is transmitted year-round in the tropics. Vaccination is recommended.

JAPANESE ENCEPHALITIS: Risk of Japanese encephalitis (JE) is present in rural and peri-urban lowland areas countrywide, except for Ho Chi Minh City and Hanoi. Peak transmission in the subtropical north occurs during the monsoon season, June through July. In the tropical south, disease risk is present year-round, but peak levels occur in June through July. Travelers to rural areas (especially with pig rearing and rice farming) should consider vaccination if duration of trip exceeds 3 to 4 weeks.

MALARIA: Countrywide risk occurs below 1,400 meters elevation. Rural only, except no risk in the Red River delta and the coastal plain north of the Nha Trang. There is no risk in Hanoi, Ho Chi Minh City (Saigon), Da Nang, Nha Trang, Qui Nhon, and Haiphong. Malaria rates are highest in the rural mountainous areas, followed by the central plains and the lowland deltas, respectively. Elevated risk occurs during the warmer rainy months, May through October. The risk of malaria in urban areas is low. *P. falciparum* causes 70% to 75% of cases countrywide, but *P. vivax* may cause 75% of cases in some coastal areas. Chloroquine-resistant falciparum malaria is reported. Prophylaxis with atovaquone/proguanil (Malarone), mefloquine (Lariam), or doxycycline prophylaxis is advised for travel to malarious areas.

MARINE HAZARDS: Stingrays, jellyfish, and several species of poisonous fish are common in the country's coastal waters and are potentially hazardous to swimmers.

RABIES: Sporadic cases of human rabies are reported countrywide. All animal bites or scratches, especially from a dog, should be taken seriously, and immediate medical attention sought. Rabies vaccination may be required. Although rabies is rare among tourists, there is risk. No one should pet or pick up any stray animals. All children should be warned to avoid contact with unknown animals. Rabies vaccine is recommended for travel longer than 3 months and for shorter stays for travelers who plan to venture off the usual tourist routes, where they may be more exposed to the stray dog population.

SCHISTOSOMIASIS: Endemic status unclear. Risk may exist along the Mekong Delta. Travelers should avoid swimming or wading in freshwater lakes, ponds, streams, or irrigation ditches.

TRAVELERS' DIARRHEA: All water supplies should be considered potentially contaminated. Travelers should observe food and drink safety precautions. A quinolone antibiotic is recommended for the treatment of diarrhea. Persistent diarrhea may be due to a parasitic disease such as giardiasis, amebiasis, or cryptosporidiosis.

TUBERCULOSIS: Tuberculosis (TB) is a major health problem in this country. Travelers planning an extended stay should have a pre-departure TB skin test (PPD test) and be retested after leaving this country or returning home.

TYPHOID FEVER: Typhoid vaccine is recommended for those traveling off the usual tourist routes, for those visiting friends or relatives, and for long-stay visitors. Typhoid vaccines are 60% to 70% effective; safe food and drink precautions should continue to be observed.

OTHER DISEASES/HAZARDS: AIDS/HIV (endemic at low, but increasing, levels), anthrax, angiostrongyliasis (from eating raw snails, slugs, or vegetables), helminthic (worm) infections (ascariasis, hookworm disease, strongyloidiasis, clonorchiasis, fasciolopsiasis, and paragonimiasis), filariasis (bancroftian filariasis is endemic throughout southern Vietnam; Malayan filariasis is endemic in the Red River Delta in northern Vietnam), leptospirosis, leprosy (moderately high levels), melioidosis (endemic countrywide), meningitis (endemic), plague (especially in the central highlands, but may occur countrywide), rabies (transmitted by dogs), typhus (louse-borne and flea-borne), scrub typhus (mite-borne; risk elevated in mountainous, wooded southeastern areas), tuberculosis (highly endemic), and trachoma (widespread).

Wallis and Futuna (France)

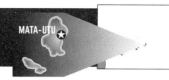

MATA-UTU

CAPITAL:
Mata-Utu
EMBASSY (IN U.S.):
202-944-6000
GMT:
+12 hours
TELEPHONE COUNTRY CODE:
681
USADIRECT:
None
ENTRY REQUIREMENTS
• **Passport/Visa:** Passport and visa required.
• **HIV Test:** Not required.
• **Vaccinations:** None required.
EMBASSIES/CONSULATES:
Not applicable.
HOSPITALS/DOCTORS
• Wallis Hospital (85 beds); general medical facility; pharmacy, x-ray, laboratory.

Current Advisories and Health Risks

HEPATITIS: All nonimmune travelers should receive hepatitis A vaccine. The hepatitis B carrier rate in the general population exceeds 10%. Vaccination against hepatitis B should be considered for stays longer than 3 months and by short-term travelers desiring maximum protection. Travelers should be aware that hepatitis B can be transmitted by unsafe sex and the use of contaminated needles and syringes.

INSECT-BORNE DISEASES: Filariasis, Japanese encephalitis, Ross River fever, and dengue are potential risks. All travelers should take personal protective measures against mosquito and insect bites. Long-term visitors should consider vaccination against Japanese encephalitis.

MALARIA: No risk.

TRAVELERS' DIARRHEA: Medium risk. Water supplies should be considered potentially contaminated, and travelers are advised to drink only bottled, boiled, or treated water, unless assured that the local water is safe. Standard safe food precautions should also be observed.

TYPHOID FEVER: Risk is low, but long-term travelers should consider vaccination. All travelers should observe safe food and water guidelines.

Yemen (Republic of Yemen)

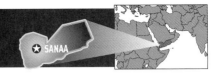

CAPITAL:
Sanaa
EMBASSY (IN U.S.):
202-965-4760
GMT:
+3 hours
TELEPHONE COUNTRY CODE:
967
USADIRECT:
00-800-101
ENTRY REQUIREMENTS
• **Passport/Visa:** A 30-day visa is available. Visitor's visa requires letter of invitation.
• **HIV Test:** Not required.
• **Vaccinations:** A yellow fever vaccination certificate is recommended and is required of all travelers arriving from infected areas.
EMBASSIES/CONSULATES
• **U.S. Embassy:** Dhahr Himyar Zone, Sheraton Hotel District, Sanaa; Tel: 967-1-303-155 ext. 118 or 265 or 266; Fax: 967-1-303-175.
• **Canadian Embassy:** Yemen Computer Co. Ltd., Building 4, 11th Street off Haddah Street, Sanaa; Tel: 967-1-20-88-14; Fax: 967-1-20-95-23; e-mail: yccnet@y.net.ye.
• **British Embassy:** 129 Haddah Road, Sana'a; Postal address: PO Box 1287; Tel: 967-1-264081/82/83/84; Fax: 967-1-263059.
HOSPITALS/DOCTORS
• *Caution*: Travelers should use hospitals for emergency situations only; care is well below Western standards.

Current Advisories and Health Risks

ACCIDENTS/ILLNESSES AND MEDICAL INSURANCE
• Accidents and injuries are the leading cause of death among travelers younger than 55 years of age and most often are caused by motor vehicle and motorcycle crashes; drownings, aircraft crashes, homicides, and burns are less common causes.
• Heart attacks cause most fatalities in older travelers.
• Infections cause only 1% of fatalities in overseas travelers, but overall, infections are the most common cause of travel-related illness.
• Travelers are advised to obtain, before departure, supplemental travel health insurance with specific overseas coverage. The policy should provide for direct payment to the overseas hospital and/or physician at the time of service and include a medical evacuation benefit. The policy should also provide 24-hour hotline access to a multilingual as-

sistance center that can help arrange and monitor delivery of medical care and determine if medical evacuation or air ambulance services are required.

CHOLERA: Sporadic cases may occur. Cholera is an extremely rare disease in travelers from developed countries. Cholera vaccine is recommended primarily for people at high risk (e.g., relief workers) who work and live in highly endemic areas under less than adequate sanitary conditions.

- The manufacture and availability of the injectable cholera vaccine in the United States ceased in June 2000.
- Many countries, including Canada, license an oral cholera vaccine. The oral vaccine is not available in the United States.
- Cholera vaccine is not "officially" required for entry into, or exit from, any country. Despite this, some countries, on occasion, require proof of cholera vaccination from travelers coming from cholera-infected countries. Anticipating such a situation, certain travelers may wish to carry a medical exemption letter from their health-care provider. Travel Medicine, Inc., recommends that travelers use the International Certificate of Vaccination (Yellow Card) for this purpose, having their health-care provider affirm that they are "exempt from cholera vaccine" and validate the exemption with both the provider's signature and the appropriate official stamp (the "Uniform Stamp" in the United States).

HEPATITIS: Hepatitis A vaccine is recommended for all nonimmune travelers. Hepatitis E has not been reported but likely occurs. The hepatitis B carrier rate in the general population is estimated at 10% to 15%. Vaccination against hepatitis B should be considered for stays longer than 3 months and by short-term travelers desiring maximum protection. Travelers should be aware that hepatitis B can be transmitted by unsafe sex and the use of contaminated needles and syringes.

INFLUENZA: Influenza is transmitted from November through March. The flu vaccine is recommended for all travelers older than 50 years of age; all travelers with chronic disease or a weakened immune system; travelers of any age wishing to decrease the risk of this illness; and pregnant women after the first trimester.

INSECTS: Insect-bite precautions are recommended for rural travel and include use of a DEET-containing repellent applied to exposed skin; permethrin insecticide spray applied to clothing, gear, and mosquito nets; and use of a mosquito bed net at night while sleeping.

LEISHMANIASIS: Cutaneous leishmaniasis commonly occurs in semirural villages of the Asir mountains. Visceral leishmaniasis occurs sporadically in rural areas, usually in the foothill region or the Asir mountains, at elevations between 400 and 1,500 meters. Travelers to these areas should take measures to prevent insect (sand fly) bites.

MALARIA: Transmission occurs year-round, with risk elevated in October through March in endemic areas up to 2,000 meters elevation. Risk areas include rural and urban locales in foothill and coastal areas, including Socotra. Elevated risk occurs in irrigated agricultural areas and near wadis. The high mountain areas (above 2,000 meters elevation), northern and eastern desert regions, including Sanaa and Aden City, are risk-free.

- Prophylaxis with atovaquone/proguanil (Malarone), mefloquine (Lariam), or doxycycline is recommended.
- All travelers should take measures to prevent evening and nighttime mosquito bites. Insect bite prevention measures include a DEET-containing repellent applied to exposed skin, insecticide (permethrin) spray applied to clothing and gear, and use of a permethrin-treated bed net at night while sleeping.

ONCHOCERCIASIS: Black fly-borne. Probably occurs throughout Yemen, in wadis flowing into the Gulf of Aden and the Red Sea; known to be endemic in all westward-flowing permanent streams (wadis) between the northern Wadi Surdud (Al Hudaydah Province) and the southern Wadi Ghayl (Taiz Province) at elevations of 300 to 1,200 meters; cases have been reported from Al Hudafdah to Taiz, mostly in Al Barh between Mokha and Taiz. All travelers to these regions should take measures to prevent insect (black fly) bites.

POLIO: This disease is active. All travelers should be fully immunized.

RABIES: High potential risk due to large population of stray dogs. All animal bites or scratches, especially from a dog, should be taken seriously, and immediate medical attention sought. Rabies vaccination is indicated following the unprovoked bite of a dog, cat, jackal, or fox. Access to rabies vaccine or rabies immune globulin may require emergency travel to another country. No one should pet or pick up any stray animals. All children should be warned to avoid contact with unknown animals. Rabies vaccine is recommended for travel longer than 3 months; for shorter stays for travelers who plan to venture off the usual tourist routes, where they may be more exposed to the stray dog population.

SCHISTOSOMIASIS: High potential risk. Transmission occurs year-round. Focally distributed (commonly associated with wadis, oases, aqueducts, cisterns, and irrigation canals) in urban and rural locales, particularly in foothill and highland areas; only Marib and Al Bayda are risk free. Primary recognized risk areas occur in Ibb, Taiz, and Sanaa Provinces. Travelers should avoid freshwater exposure.

TRAVELERS' DIARRHEA: High risk. Well water usually is contaminated. Piped water supplies are potentially contaminated. Bottled water or carbonated soft drinks are available and generally safe. Travelers should observe food and drink safety precautions. A quinolone antibiotic, combined with loperamide (Imodium), is recommended for the treatment of acute diarrhea. Giardiasis and amebiasis are reported.

TUBERCULOSIS: Tuberculosis (TB) is a major public health problem in this country. Travelers planning an extended stay should have a pre-departure TB skin test (PPD test) and be retested after leaving this country.

TYPHOID FEVER: Typhoid vaccine is recommended. Because the typhoid vaccines are only 60% to 70% effective, safe food and drink guidelines should continue to be observed.

OTHER DISEASES/HAZARDS: Filariasis (mosquito-borne; sporadically reported), brucellosis (human cases usually related to exposure to unpasteurized dairy products, especially raw goat/sheep milk or milk products), cholera, dengue fever (low-level transmission may occur in coastal regions), dracunculiasis (endemic in Al Hudaydah Province, with cases reported from Sadah Province), echinococcosis (reported sporadically in humans), plague (flea-borne; last outbreak in 1969 in Sadah Province; cases were also reported in the 1980s), flea-borne typhus, louse-borne typhus, louse- and flea-borne relapsing fever, trachoma, tuberculosis, and helminthic infections (roundworm, hookworm, and whipworm infections are common in rural areas).

Zambia

CAPITAL:
Lusaka
EMBASSY (IN U.S.):
202-265-9717
GMT:
+2 hours
TELEPHONE COUNTRY CODE:
260
USADIRECT:
00-899
ENTRY REQUIREMENTS
• **Passport/Visa:** A visa is required.
• **HIV Test:** Not required.
• **Vaccinations:** No vaccinations are required.
EMBASSIES/CONSULATES
• **U.S. Embassy:** Corner of Independence and United Nations Avenue, Lusaka; Tel: 1-250-955, 1-250-955, or 1-250-230; Fax: 260-1-252-225.
• **Canadian Embassy:** 5199 United Nations Avenue, Lusaka; Tel: 1-25-08-33; Fax: 1-25-41-76; e-mail: lsaka@dfait-maeci.gc.ca.
• **British High Commission:** 5210 Independence Avenue, PO Box 50050, 15101 Ridgeway, Lusaka; Tel: 260-1-251133; Fax: 260-1-253798; e-mail: BHC-Lusaka@fco.gov.uk.
HOSPITALS/DOCTORS:
Medical care in Zambia is below Western standards; shortages of routine medications and supplies may be encountered. Travelers to this country are advised to obtain, before departure, supplemental travel health insurance with specific overseas coverage. The policy should provide for direct payment to the overseas hospital and/or physician at the

time of service and include a medical evacuation benefit. In the event of serious medical emergency, every effort should be made to go to Johannesburg, South Africa.
• University Teaching Hospital, Lusaka (1,500 beds).

Current Advisories and Health Risks

AFRICAN SLEEPING SICKNESS (TRYPANOSOMIASIS): Risk of African sleeping sickness persists in the northern areas, particularly in the Luangwa Valley and Kafue National Park. One third of rural areas countrywide are infested with tsetse flies. Travelers should take personal protection measures against insect (tsetse fly) bites.

AIDS/HIV: Heterosexual transmission is the predominant means of transmission. HIV-1 prevalence is estimated at 50% of the high-risk urban population. All travelers are cautioned against unsafe sex, unsterile medical or dental injections, and unnecessary blood transfusions.

ANIMAL HAZARDS: Animal hazards include snakes (vipers, cobras), centipedes, scorpions, and black widow spiders.

ARBOVIRAL FEVERS: Dengue has not been reported recently from this region. Outbreaks of chikungunya fever have been reported from Zambia.

CHOLERA: This disease is reported active at this time. Sporadic cases may occur. Cholera is an extremely rare disease in travelers from developed countries. Cholera vaccine is recommended only for people at high risk (e.g., relief workers) who work and live in highly endemic areas under less than adequate sanitary conditions.

DENGUE FEVER: Dengue has not been reported recently from this region.

FILARIASIS: Risk may occur in northern areas. Travelers should take precautions against mosquito bites.

HEPATITIS: Hepatitis A vaccine is recommended for all travelers. The hepatitis B carrier rate in the general population is estimated at 13% to 14%. Hepatitis B vaccine is recommended for stays longer than 3 months and for short-term travelers wanting increased protection. Travelers should be aware that the risk of hepatitis B is increased by unsafe sex and the use of unsterile needles and syringes.

INFLUENZA: Influenza is transmitted year-round in the tropics. The flu vaccine is recommended for all travelers at risk.

MALARIA: Risk is present year-round in the Zambezi River Valley, including urban areas, but seasonal in the rest of the country, primarily from November through June (during and just after the rainy season). Incidence has been increasing in Copperbelt Province and Southern Province. Chloroquine-resistant falciparum malaria is reported.

Prophylaxis with atovaquone/proguanil (Malarone), mefloquine (Lariam), or doxycycline is recommended.

MENINGITIS: Quadrivalent meningococcal vaccine is recommended for travelers staying longer than 1 month during the dry season, May through October, and should be considered for shorter stays during the dry season if prolonged contact with the local populace is anticipated.

ONCHOCERCIASIS: Cases of onchocerciasis are reported from near Choma in the Southern Province, perhaps the southernmost limit of transmission of this disease in Africa. Travelers to this region should take precautions against insect (black fly) bites.

POLIOMYELITIS (POLIO): This disease continues to be active in Africa. All travelers should be fully immunized.

RABIES: Sporadic cases of human rabies are reported countrywide. All animal bites or scratches, especially from a dog, should be evaluated without delay. Rabies vaccine is recommended for travel longer than 3 months and for shorter stays for travelers who plan to venture off the usual tourist routes.

SCHISTOSOMIASIS: Urinary schistosomiasis is endemic in all provinces. Intestinal schistosomiasis is less widely distributed, with most risk in Northern Province, Luapula Province (including Lake Mweru vicinity), Lusaka vicinity, and Southern Province (including the shores of Lake Kariba). All travelers should avoid swimming, bathing, or wading in freshwater lakes, ponds, or streams.

TRAVELERS' DIARRHEA: Public water supplies are filtered and chlorinated. In Lusaka and Kabwe, water is obtained from deep bore holes and is treated. Water in these cities is considered potable. Travelers should observe all food and drink safety precautions. A quinolone antibiotic, combined with loperamide (Imodium), is recommended for the treatment of acute diarrhea. Persistent diarrhea may be due to a parasitic disease such as giardiasis or amebiasis.

TUBERCULOSIS: Tuberculosis (TB) is a major health problem in this country. Travelers planning an extended stay should have a pre-departure TB skin test (PPD test) and be retested after leaving this country.

TYPHOID FEVER: Typhoid vaccine is recommended. Because the typhoid vaccines are only 60% to 70% effective, safe food and drink selection remains important.

YELLOW FEVER: Risk may be present in northwestern forest areas because the vector mosquito is present. The CDC recommends yellow fever vaccination for all travelers older than 9 months of age arriving from any country.

OTHER DISEASES/HAZARDS: African tick typhus (contracted from dog ticks, often in urban areas, and bush ticks), brucellosis (usually from consumption of unpasteurized dairy products), relapsing fever (tick-borne), toxoplasmosis, tuberculosis (a major health problem), typhoid fever, and intestinal worms (very common).

Zimbabwe

★ HARARE

CAPITAL:
Harare
EMBASSY (IN U.S.):
202-332-7100
GMT:
+2 hours
TELEPHONE COUNTRY CODE:
263
USADIRECT:
110-989-90

ENTRY REQUIREMENTS
- **Passport/Visa:** Passport, visa, onward/return ticket, and proof of sufficient funds are required for a stay of up to 6 months. Visas issued on arrival in Zimbabwe. Travelers should contact the Embassy of Zimbabwe for entry requirements.
- **HIV Test:** Not required.
- **Vaccinations:** A yellow fever vaccination certificate is required for all travelers older than 1 year arriving from an infected area.

EMBASSIES/CONSULATES
- **U.S. Embassy:** 172 Herbert Chitepo Ave., Harare; Tel: 4-250-593, 250-594, or 250-595; Fax: 4-722-618 or 796-488.
- **Canadian Embassy:** 45 Baines Ave., Harare; Tel 4-252-181 through 185; Fax: 263-4-252-186 or 187; e-mail: harare-consular@dfait-maeci.gc.ca.
- **British Embassy:** Corner House, 7th Floor, Samora Machel Avenue/Leopold Takawira Street, (PO Box 4490), Harare; Tel: 263-4-772990, 774700; Fax: 263-4-774617; Website: www.britainzw.org.

HOSPITALS/DOCTORS:
Medical care is substandard throughout the country, including in Harare and Bulawayo. Travelers are advised to obtain, before departure, supplemental travel health insurance with specific overseas coverage. The policy should provide for direct payment to the overseas hospital and/or physician at the time of service and include a medical evacuation benefit. For serious medical conditions, every effort should be made to go to Johannesburg, South Africa.
- Parirenyatwa Hospital, Harare (900 beds); emergency services; intensive care and burn units.
- The Central Harare Hospital, Lobengula Road, Southerton, Harare; Tel: 263-4-664-695 or 690.
- Bulawayo has three main hospitals: the United Bulawayo Hospital (the Central), Mpilo, and the Mater Dei (a private hospital).

Current Advisories and Health Risks

AFRICAN SLEEPING SICKNESS (TRYPANOSOMIASIS): Low-risk; may occur in the northern Zambezi River drainage area, including the Lake Kariba vicinity. Outbreaks along the border with Mozambique were reported in the 1980s. Travelers should take measures to prevent insect (tsetse fly) bites.

AIDS/HIV: Heterosexual contact is the predominant mode of transmission. About 35% of the adult population is HIV-positive, among the highest rates in Africa.

ANIMAL HAZARDS: Animal hazards include snakes (vipers, cobras), centipedes, scorpions, and black widow spiders.

ARBOVIRAL DISEASES: Explosive outbreaks of chikungunya fever have occurred in urban areas, but most cases are in rural regions. West Nile and Sindbis fevers are endemic in neighboring South Africa. Dengue fever is not reported. All travelers should take measures to prevent insect bites.

CHOLERA: This disease is reported active at this time. Cholera is an extremely rare disease in travelers from developed countries; vaccination not routinely recommended, except for health-care workers and others at high risk.

EBOLA VIRUS HEMORRHAGIC FEVER: Sporadic, rare Ebola virus disease activity occurs. Transmission is via direct contact with blood or body fluids of acutely ill patients.

HEPATITIS: Hepatitis A is highly endemic. Vaccination is recommended for all nonimmune travelers. Hepatitis E is endemic, but levels are unclear. The hepatitis B carrier rate in the general population is estimated at 8% to 10%. Hepatitis B is spread by infected blood, contaminated needles, and unsafe sex. Vaccination is recommended for stays longer than 3 months; for persons at occupational or social risk; and for any traveler desiring maximum protection.

INFLUENZA: Influenza is transmitted year-round in the tropics. The flu vaccine is recommended for all travelers.

LASSA FEVER: Sporadic, rare Lassa fever activity occurs. Transmission is via contact with infected rodents.

MALARIA: Year-round transmission occurs countrywide, except that the central plateau (stretching from the southwest to the northeast, with elevations from 1,200 to 1,500 meters, including Harare City) is essentially malaria-free. Malaria is especially endemic in the Zambezi River Valley. Epidemics have occurred in the Matabeleland North and northern Midlands provinces. Prophylaxis with atovaquone/proguanil (Malarone), mefloquine (Lariam), or doxycycline is recommended. All travelers should take measures to prevent evening and nighttime mosquito bites.

MENINGITIS: Low risk. Zimbabwe is south of the sub-Saharan "meningitis belt." Vaccination with the quadrivalent meningococcal vaccine should be considered by long-term visitors who expect to have close contact with the indigenous population.

PLAGUE: Sporadic cases have occurred in the northwest, and north of Harare. Anthropologists, archaeologists, medical personnel, and missionaries may be at higher risk and might consider prophylaxis with doxycycline.

POLIOMYELITIS: Polio is reported active in Botswana and other counties in sub-Saharan Africa. All travelers should be fully immunized against this disease.

RABIES: Sporadic human cases are reported, with dogs and jackals as the primary sources of exposure. Most cases occur in Matabeleland North and South provinces, which have been declared "rabies areas." All animal bites or scratches, especially from a dog, should be evaluated immediately.

RIFT VALLEY FEVER: Explosive outbreaks have occurred in both urban and rural regions. West Nile and Sindbis fevers are endemic in neighboring South Africa. All travelers should take measures to prevent mosquito bites.

SCHISTOSOMIASIS: Peak transmission of urinary schistosomiasis occurs in the northeast during the hot, dry season (September and October). Transmission is year-round in the Zambezi Valley, the shores of Lake Kariba and the southeast low veld. Intestinal schistosomiasis occurs primarily in the north and east. Travelers are advised to avoid swimming or wading in freshwater lakes, ponds, or streams.

TRAVELERS' DIARRHEA: Outside major urban areas, travelers should observe all food and drink safety precautions. A quinolone antibiotic, combined with loperamide (Imodium), is recommended for the treatment of acute diarrhea. Persistent diarrhea may be due to a parasitic infection such as giardiasis, amebiasis, or cryptosporidiosis.

TUBERCULOSIS: Tuberculosis (TB) is a major health problem in this country. Travelers planning an extended stay should have a pre-departure TB skin test (PPD test) and be retested after returning from this country.

TYPHOID FEVER: Typhoid vaccine is recommended for those traveling off the usual tourist routes, those visiting friends or relatives, and for long-stay visitors. Because the typhoid vaccines are only 60% to 70% effective, safe food and drink selection remains important.

OTHER DISEASES/HAZARDS: African tick typhus (contracted from dog ticks—often in urban areas—and bush ticks), brucellosis (from consumption of raw dairy products), leptospirosis, tuberculosis (a major health problem), and intestinal worms (very common).

Diabetes*

Adjusting Insulin Injections and Meal Times While Crossing Time Zones

Frequent blood glucose monitoring is essential for safety during flight. Even individuals who do not test frequently at home should test at least every 4 to 6 hours while traveling. Patients should be cautioned to keep themselves well hydrated with nonalcoholic, caffeine-free beverages throughout their flight.

Diabetes management is usually based on a normal 24-hour medication schedule. When traveling north or south, no adjustments in the 24-hour schedule are needed. However, east or west travel across time zones abbreviates or extends the day depending on the direction of travel.

In general, adjustments to insulin doses are unnecessary if patients are crossing fewer than five time zones. Traveling eastward will shorten one's day, and, in general, may necessitate a reduction in insulin (especially for shorter flights) because insulin doses would be administered closer than normal and thus could cause hypoglycemia. In contrast, westward travel means a longer day, and so insulin doses may need to be increased. However, this seemingly simple and workable rule of "westward = more insulin; eastward = less insulin" may not always hold true. Differing times of departure and prolonged flights may require a more complicated approach.

Patients who are not insulin pump users should be transferred to a "basal-bolus" insulin regimen before traveling if they are not on one already because, short of pump therapy, this is the ideal system to cope with all time zone travel situations. Changing to insulin glargine (Lantus) for basal insulin, with insulin lispro (Humalog) or insulin aspart (Novolog) coverage before each meal, would probably be the most flexible and effective regimen.

In general, patients should be advised to leave their wrist watches unadjusted during travel so that they continue to correspond to the time at their point of embarkation. This will make it easier for patients to judge the timing of their insulin injections and meals.

Advice for Traveling East Across Five Or More Time Zones

An example of an eastward-bound flight would be one from Los Angeles to London, as shown in Table A.1. The flight departs Los Angeles at 8:45 P.M., which is 4:45 A.M. London time. It arrives in London at 7:15 A.M. Los Angeles time, which is 3:15 P.M. London time. Total flight time is 10.5 hours.

Scenario 1 Assume that the patient taking this flight normally takes insulin (basal and rapid-acting) on a twice-daily schedule as follows: neutral protamine Hagedorn (NPH) plus regular insulin, 16 units and 10 units, respectively, before breakfast, and 10 units and 10 units, respectively, before dinner. Assuming the patient will be served two meals and a snack (dinner shortly after take off, a mid-flight snack, and breakfast before landing), the following course can be recommended:

Before departure, the usual evening dose of 10 units NPH plus 10 units regular should be taken. Keeping the wrist watch synchronized to Los Angeles time while in flight, about 11 to 12 hours later, one half of the usual morning dose of NPH (8 units) plus the full complement of regular insulin (10 units) should be taken, followed by a meal (which, in this case, is likely to be breakfast). Because of the long duration of the flight, however, extra short-acting insulin may be necessary for meals or snacks consumed at times that are not similar to the patient's normal routine (e.g., the dinner and the mid-flight snack). That evening in London, just before dinner (London time), the remaining one half of the usual morning dose of NPH insulin (8 units) plus the full complement of regular insulin (10 units) should be taken.

Thus, the total NPH insulin dose has not been altered, but rather has been split to help the patient adjust to the change in time zones. The next morning in London, on local time, the patient's pre-travel regimen can be resumed.

Scenario 2 Assume that the patient taking this flight is instead on a regimen of once-daily insulin glargine (24 units at bedtime) with a pre-meal ultra-rapid-acting insulin analog (10 units of lispro or aspart before each meal). An alternative would be to take the usual dose of glargine at the usual time, say 10:00 P.M. Los Angeles time (this would be on the flight). Twenty-four hours later (i.e., again around 10:00 P.M. Los Angeles time, which would be around 6:00 A.M. London time on the morning of the day after arrival), the patient can take one half the usual glargine dose (12 units). That night at bedtime (London time) the remaining one half of the usual glargine dose (12 units) may be taken, thus keeping the total 24-hour glargine dose the same. Pre-meal coverage using ultra-short-acting insulin would remain the same or be increased if more than the usual amount of food will be eaten or if there are more meals than usual. The pre-travel regimen of 24 units of glargine at bedtime can be resumed on the third night (second night in London).

For shorter stays, especially if patients are on glargine, it might be easier to continue taking the insulin according to the *usual time* in Los Angeles, recognizing that this might involve some inconvenience. For example, the "bedtime dose" of glargine, normally taken at around 10:00 P.M., would have to be taken at around 6:00 A.M. while in London.

Advice for Traveling West Across Five Or More Time Zones

An example of a westward-bound flight would be from New Jersey to Honolulu, Hawaii, as shown in Table A.2. The flight departs New Jersey at 11:40 A.M., which is 6:40 A.M. in Honolulu. It arrives in Honolulu at 10:40 P.M. New Jersey time, which is 5:40 P.M. Honolulu time. Total flight time is 11 hours.

Scenario 1 If this is the same patient as in scenario 1 for eastward travel, i.e., someone who normally takes insulin on a twice-daily schedule of 16 units NPH plus 10 units regular in the morning and 10 units NPH plus 10 units regular in the evening, the following course can be recommended:

The traveler should take the usual morning dose (16 units NPH plus 10 units regular) in the morning before departure. Again, keeping the wrist watch synchronized to New Jersey time, about the time of the usual evening meal (i.e., about 10 hours after the morning dose of insulin), one half of the usual evening NPH plus the full complement of short-acting insulin (i.e., 5 units NPH plus 10 units regular) should be taken, followed by a meal or snack. That evening at dinner (Honolulu time), the remaining one half of the intermediate-acting insulin along with the full dose of short-acting insulin (i.e., 5 units NPH plus 10 units regular) should be taken. The next morning (local time), the usual insulin doses can be resumed.

Scenario 2 Assume, as in scenario 2 for eastward travel, that the patient taking this flight is on a once-daily regimen of glargine (24 units at bedtime) with pre-meal rapid-acting insulin analog (10 units of lispro before each meal). The alternative would be to take the usual dose of glargine (24 units) the night before departure. Twenty-four hours later, which in this case would be just before landing in Honolulu, one half of the usual dose (12 units) should be taken. That night at bedtime (Honolulu time), the remaining one half of the usual bedtime dose of glargine (12 units) may be taken. Again, the 24-hour glargine requirement would remain the same, but the dose would be split to help the patient adjust to the change in time zones. Pre-meal coverage with a rapid-acting insulin analog would also remain the same or, if more than the usual amount of food or number of meals are consumed, extra lispro could be given during the flight, based on carbohydrate content of the food to be consumed and blood glucose values.

Advice for Those Who Use Insulin Pumps

Patients using insulin pumps can continue with their normal routine of basal and bolus doses, and they can change the time setting on their pump once reaching the destination. It may be safer to allow blood glucose levels to run slightly higher than normal for the first day or so rather than to risk hypoglycemia.

Patients on pumps should carry supplies of long-acting insulin (Ultralente or glargine) and regular insulin or a rapid-acting insulin analog (lispro or aspart), along with syringes and extra batteries to use in case of pump malfunction or battery failure. In such cases, patients should be instructed to administer a once-daily dose of glargine equivalent to the total 24-hour basal dose. If the patient has Ultralente, the total dose (which is again equivalent to the total basal rate) should be split between the morning and evening. All doses of short- or rapid-acting insulin should remain the same and should be given before each meal as usual.

Advice for Those on Oral Agents for Diabetes

The timing of oral medications for diabetes is not as crucial as that for insulin. If the patient is on a twice-daily regimen of metformin (Glucophage), a thiazolidinedione, or a sulfonylurea, for instance, it may be easier to skip a dose and have slight hyperglycemia for 6 to 8 hours rather than to take two doses too close together and risk becoming hypoglycemic. Patients on carbohydrate absorption inhibitors (i.e., acarbose [Precose]) or one of the newer nonsulfonylurea secretagogues such as repaglinide (Prandin) or nateglinide (Starlix) can continue their usual regimen of taking it before meals.

Table A.1   Time Differences Between Departure and Destination Points on an Eastward-Bound Flight from Los Angeles to London

	Los Angeles Time	London Time
Departure	8:45 P.M.	4:45 A.M.
Arrival	7:15 A.M.	3:15 P.M

Table A.2   Time Differences Between Departure and Destination Points on a Westward-Bound Flight from New Jersey to Honolulu, Hawaii

	New Jersey Time	Honolulu Time
Departure	11:40 A.M.	6:40 A.M.
Arrival	10:40 A.M.	5:40 P.M

Further Reading

Chapter One: Overview of Travelers' Health

DuPont HL, Steffen R: Textbook of Travel Medicine and Health. Hamilton, Ontario, BC Dekker, 2001. (Tel: 905-522-7017; info@bcdecker.com).

Keystone JS, Kozarsky PE, Freedman DO, et al: Travel Medicine, Philadelphia, Elsevier, 2003.

Chapter Four: Jet Lag and Motion Sickness

Arendt J, Deacon S: Treatment of circadian rhythm disorders—melatonin. Chronobiol Int 1997;14:185-204.

Belcaro G, Cesarone MR, Shah SS, et al: Prevention of edema, flight microangiopathy and venous thrombosis in long flights with elastic stockings. A randomized trial: The LONFLIT 4 Concorde Edema-SSL Study. Angiology 2002;53:635-645.

Benson AJ: Motion sickness. In: Stellman JM: Encyclopaedia of Occupational Health and Safety. 4th ed. Geneva, International Labour Office, 1998;50.12.

Cruickshanks JM, Gorlin R, Jennett B: Air travel and thrombotic episodes: The economy class syndrome. Lancet 1988;2:497-498.

Ferrari E, Chevalier T, Chapelier A, Baudouy: Travel as a risk factor for venous thromboembolic disease: A case-control study. Chest 1999;115:440-444.

Hirsh J, O'Donnell MJ: Venous thrombosis after long flights: Are airlines to blame? Lancet 2001;357:1461-1462.

House of Lords Science and Technology Select Committee: 5th Report. Air Travel and Health. London: House of Lords; 15 November 2000. (An electronic version of this report is available at: www.publications.parliament.uk/pa/ld199900/ldselect/ldsctech/121/12101.htm)

Kozarsky PE: Prevention of Common Travel Ailments. Inf Dis Clin N Am 1998;12:305-324.

Kraaijenhagen RA, Haverkamp D, Koopman MM, et al: Travel and risk of venous thrombosis. Lancet 2000;356:1492-1493.

Morris HH, Estes ML: Traveler's amnesia: Transient global amnesia secondary to triazolam. JAMA 1987;258:945-946.

Penev PD, Zee PC: Melatonin: A clinical perspective. Ann Neurol 1997;42:545-555.

Rees DC, Chapman NH, Webster MT, et al: Born to clot: The European burden. Br J Haematol 1999;105:564-566.

Samana MM: An epidemiologic study of risk factors for deep vein thrombosis in medical outpatients: The Sirius study. Arch Intern Med 2000;160:3415-3420.

Waterhouse J, Reilly T, Atkinson G: Jet-Lag. Lancet 1997;350:1611-1615.

Chapter Five: Food and Drink Safety

Gerba CP, Johnson D, Hasan, MN: Efficacy of iodine water purification tablets against *Cryptosporidium* oöcysts and *Giardia* cysts. Wilderness and Environmental Medicine 1997;8(2):96-100.

Khan LK, Li R, Gootnick D, et al: Thyroid abnormalities related to iodine excess from water purification units. Lancet 1998;352:1519.

Chapter Six: Travelers' Diarrhea

Ericsson CD, DuPont HL, Steffen R: Travelers' Diarrhea. BC Decker, Hamilton, Ontario, pp. 151-183, 2003.

Ericsson CD: Travellers' Diarrhea. Int J Antimicrobial Agents 2003;21:116-124. J Travel Med 2002;9:141-150.

Leggat PA, Goldsmith JM: Travellers' Diarrhea. Trav Med Infect Dis, 2004;2:17-22.

Rao G, Aliwalas MG, Slaymaker E, Brown B: Bismuth revisited: An effective way to prevent travelers' diarrhea. J Travel Med 2004;11:239.

Stauffer WM, Konop RJ, Kamat D: Traveling with infants and young children. Part III: Travelers' diarrhea. J Travel Med 2002;3:141-150.

Steffen R, Castelli F, Nothdurft H, et al: Vaccination against enterotoxigenic Escherichia coli, a cause of travelers' diarrhea. J Travel Med 2005;12:102-107.

Steffen R, Tornieporth N, Costa-Clemens S, et al: Epidemiology of travelers' diarrhea: details of a global survey. J Travel Med 2004;11:231.

Chapter Seven: Malaria

Fischer PR, Bialek R: Prevention of malaria in children. Clin Infect Dis 2002;34:493-498

Hien TT, White NJ: Qinghaosu. Lancet 1993;341:603-608.

Kain KC, Shanks GD, Keystone JS: Malaria chemoprophylaxis in the age of drug resistance. I. Currently recommended drug regimens. Clin Infect Dis. 2001;33:226-234.

McGreadt R, Ashley EA, Nosten F: Malaria and the pregnant traveler. Travel Med Infect Dis 2004;2:127-142.

Newman RD, Parise ME, Barber AM, Steketee RW: Malaria-related deaths among U.S. travelers, 1963-2001. Ann Intern Med 2004;141:547-555.

Shanks GD, Kain KC, Keystone JS: Malaria chemoprophylaxis in the age of drug resistance. II. Drugs that may be available in the future. Clin Infect Dis 2001;33:381-385.

Stauffer W, Fischer PR: Diagnosis and treatment of malaria in children. Clin Infect Dis 2003;37:1340-1348.

Chapter Eight: Insect Bite Prevention

Fradin MS: Comparative efficacy of insect repellents against mosquito bites. N Engl J Med. 2002;347:13-18.

Ginther B: Toxicity of local anesthetics. EMedicine, May 25, 2001.

Goodyer L, Behrens RH: Short report: The safety and toxicity of insect repellents. Am J Trop Med Hyg 1998;59:323-324.

Chapter Nine: Insect-Borne Diseases

Gibbons RV, Vaughn DW: Dengue: An escalating problem. BMJ 2002;324:1563-1566.

Monath TP: Yellow fever: An update. Lancet Infect Dis 2001;1:11-20.

Petersen LR, Hayes EB: Westward ho?—The spread of West Nile Virus. N Engl J Med 2004;351:2257-2259.

Shlim DR, Solomon T: Japanese encephalitis vaccine for travelers: Exploring the limits of risk. Clin Infect Dis 2002;35:183-188.

Tiroumourougane SV, Raghava P, Srinivasan S: Japanese viral encephalitis. Postgrad Med 2002;78:205-215.

Wendi-Wagner P: Risk and prevention of tick-borne encephalitis in travelers. J Travel Med 2004;11:307-315.

Wichmann O, and Jelinek T: Dengue in travelers: A review. J Travel Med 2004;11: 161-175.

Chapter Ten: Travel-Related Diseases

Ali SA, Hill DR: Giardia intestinalis. Curr Opin Infect Dis 2003;16:453-460.

Bharti AR, Nally JE, Ricaldi JN: Leptospirosis: A zoonotic disease of global importance. Lancet Infect Dis 2003;3:757-771.

Gross AGP, Bartley PB, Sleigh AC, et al: N Engl J Med 2002;346:1212-1219.

Jackson AC Warrell MJ, Rupprecht CE, et al: Management of rabies in humans. Clin Infect Dis 2003;36:60-63.

Parry CM, Hien TT, Dougan G, et al: Typhoid fever. N Engl J Med 2002;347: 1770-1782.

Rupprecht CE, Gibbons RV: Prophylaxis against rabies. N Engl J Med 2004;351:2626-2635.

Chapter Eleven: Lyme Disease

Bozler E: Basic and clinic approaches to Lyme disease: A Lyme Disease Foundation Symposium. Clin Infect Dis 1997;25(suppl 1):S1-S75.

Magid DM, Schwartz B, Craft J, et al: Prevention of Lyme Disease after tick bites: A cost-effective analysis. N Engl J Med 1992;327:534-541.

Nowak D, Fedorowski JJ: Current concepts of Lyme disease. Hosp Phys 1997;33:16-35.

Varela AS, Luttrell MP, Howerth EW, et al: First culture isolation of *Borrelia lonestari*, putative agent of southern tick-associated rash illness. J Clin Microbiol 2004;42:1163-1169.

Chapter Twelve: Hepatitis

Chen LH: The emergence of new hepatitis viruses. Travel Medicine Advisor Update 1998;8:9-10.

Janisch TH: Emerging viral pathogens in long-term expatriates (1): Hepatitis E Virus. Trop Med Internatl Health 1997;2:885-891.

Koff RS: Hepatitis A. Lancet 1998;351:1643-1647.

Lee WM: Hepatitis B virus Infection. N Engl J Med 1997;337:1733-1745.

Mast EE, Krawczynski K: Hepatitis E: An overview. Annu Rev Med 1996;47:257-266.

Troisi CL, Hollinger FB, Krause DS, Pickering LK: Immunization of seronegative infants with hepatitis A vaccine (HAVRIX; SKB): A comparative study of two dosing schedules. Vaccine 1997;15:1613-1617.

Chapter Thirteen: Diabetes

Chandran M, Edelman S: Have insulin, will fly: Diabetes management during air travel and time zone adjustment strategies. Clin Diabetes 2003;21:82-85.

Chapter Fourteen: Sexually-Transmitted Diseases (STDs)

Antiretroviral post-exposure prophylaxis after sexual, injection-drug use, or other non-occupational exposure to HIV in the United States. MMWR Jan 21 2005; 54(RR2);1-20.

Cohen MS: HIV and sexually transmitted diseases: Lethal synergy. Top HIV Med 2004;12:104-107.

Haque N, Zafar T, Brahmbhatt H, et al: High-risk sexual behaviours among drug users in Pakistan: Implications for prevention of STDs and HIV/AIDS. J STD AIDS 2004;601-607.

Hearst N, Hulley SB: Preventing the heterosexual spread of AIDS. JAMA 1988;259:2428-2432.

Lalvani A, Shastri JS: HIV epidemic in India: Opportunity to learn from the past. Lancet 1996;347:1349-1350.

Stephenson J: Studies reveal early impact of HIV infection, effects of treatment. JAMA 1998;279:641-642.

Weisfuse IB: Gonorrhea control and antimicrobial resistance. Lancet 1998;351:928.

Chapter Fifteen: Altitude Sickness

Alexander JK: Coronary heart disease at altitude. Tex Heart Inst J 1994;21:261.

Beaumont M, Goldenburg F, Lejeune D, et al. Effect of zolpidem on sleep and ventilatory patterns at simulated altitude of 4,000 meters. Am J Respir Crit Care Med 1996;153:1864-1869.

Burtscher M, Philadelphy M, Likar R: Sudden cardiac death during mountain hiking and downhill skiing (letter). N Engl J Med 1993;29:1738-1739.

Dietz TE: Altitude illness clinical guide for physicians 1999. http://www.gorge.net/hamg/AMS_medical.html.

Dubowitz G: Effect of temazepam on oxygen saturation and sleep quality at high altitude: Randomized placebo controlled crossover trial. BMJ 1998;316:587-589.

Dumont L, Madirosoff C, Tramer MR: Efficacy and harm of pharmacological prevention of acute mountain sickness: Quantitative systematic review. BMJ 2000;321:267-272.

Gertsch JH, Basnyat B, Johnson EW, et al: Randomised, double-blind, placebo-controlled comparison of ginkgo biloba and acetazolamide for prevention of acute mountain sickness among Himalayan trekkers: The prevention of high-altitude illness trial (PHAIT). BMJ 2004;328:797-802.

Hackett PH: The cerebral etiology of high-altitude cerebral edema and acute mountain sickness. Wilderness Environ Med 1999;10:97-109.

Hacket PH: High altitude and common medical conditions. In Hornbein TF, Schoene RB (eds): High Altitude: An Exploration of Human Adaptation, Marcel Dekker, New York, 2001, p 851.

Herbert W, Froelicher V: Exercise tests for coronary and asymptomatic patients. The Physician and Sports Medicine 1991;19:129-133.

Keller HR, Maggiorini M, Bartch P, Oelz O: Simulated descent vs. dexamethasone in treatment of acute mountain sickness: A randomized trial. BMJ 1995;310:1232-1235.

Mittleman A, Maclure M, Tofler G, et al. Triggering of acute myocardial infarction by heavy physical exertion. N Engl J Med 1993;329:1677-1682.

Roach RC, Bartsch P, Oelz O, Hackett PH: Lake Louise AMS Scoring Consensus Committee. The Lake Louise acute mountain sickness scoring system. In Sutton JR Houston CS, Costas G, (eds): Hypoxia and Molecular Medicine. Burlington, Vt., Charles S. Houston, 1999, 23-45.

Rennie D: Will mountain trekkers have heart attacks? (editorial). JAMA 1989;26:1045-1046.

Shlim DR, Houston R: Helicopter rescues and deaths among trekkers in Nepal. JAMA 1989;261:1017.

Chapter Sixteen: Medical Care Abroad

Aldis JW: Healthcare abroad. In Keystone JS, Kozarsky PE, Freedman DO, Nothdurft HD, Connor BA (Eds): Travel Medicine. Philadelphia, 2004, Elsevier, pp 461-467.

Chapter Nineteen: Business Travel and Health

Traveling Healthy Newsletter August 2000, Copyright Travel Medicine, Inc. Occup Environ Med 1999;56:245-252

Chapter Twenty: Travel and Pregnancy

Khan LK, Li R, Gootnick D, et al: Thyroid abnormalities related to iodine excess from water purification units. Lancet 1998;352:1519.

Khan WA, Seas C, Dhar U, et al: Treatment of shigellosis: Comparison of azithromycin and ciprofloxacin. A double-blind, randomized, controlled trial. Ann Int Med 1997;126:697-703.

Koren G, Pastuszak A: Drugs in Pregnancy. N Engl J Med 1998;338:1128-1137.

Nielsen GL, Sorensen HT, Larsen H, Pedersen L: Risk of adverse birth outcome and miscarriage in pregnant users of non-steroidal anti-inflammatory drugs: Population based observational study and case-control study. BMJ 2001;322:266-270.

Nosten F, McReady R, Simpson JA, et al: Effects of *Plasmodium vivax* malaria in pregnancy. Lancet 1999;354:546-549.

Rose, SR: Pregnancy and travel. Emerg Med Clin N Am 1997;15:93-111.

Samuel BU, Barry M: The pregnant traveler. Infect Dis Clinics N Am 1998;12:325-354.

Chapter Twenty-One: Traveling with Children

Figueroa-Quintanilla D, Salazar-Lindo E, Sack RB, et al: A controlled trial of bismuth subsalicylate in infants with acute watery diarrheal disease. N Engl J Med 1993;328:1653-1658.

Troisi CL, Hollinger FB, Krause DS, Pickering LK: Immunization of seronegative infants with hepatitis A vaccine (HAVRIX; SKB): A comparative study of two dosing schedules. Vaccine 1997;15:1613-1617.

Travel Information Online

Passports/Visas Made Simple (and much more)

(http://travel.state.gov)—The Department of State, Bureau of Consular Affairs has established this site not only to help people apply for passports, but also to help find a vast amount of other information related to foreign travel. (You can download the printable passport applications.) Can't find your birth certificate? This site will help.

Getting Your Shots Before You Go

Staying healthy abroad usually means getting immunized against some exotic diseases, but most doctors' offices don't stock the vaccines you'll need. To locate a travel clinic near you, go to one of these sites:

International Society of Travel Medicine—www.istm.org
American Society of Tropical Medicine and Hygiene—www.astmh.org
Travel Health Online—www.tripprep.com
Travel Medicine, Inc.—www.travmed.com
Canadian Travel Clinics—www.phac-aspc.gc.ca/tmp-pmv/travel/clinic_e.html

What Time Is It in Paramaribo?

(www.timeanddate.com)—The World Clock makes it easy to know what time it is in cities and countries around the globe. This source also gives you the GMT/UTC offset, sunrise and sunset, dialing codes, and geographic coordinates.

Health Concerns Answered by the Experts

(http://www.cdc.gov/travel)—Before you head off to the Amazon check to see if there are any epidemics in the area. The CDC website warns about current epidemics and disease outbreaks, as well as giving immunization requirements for yellow fever.

Should You Even Go?

(http://travel.state.gov/index.html) and (www.fco.gov.uk)—Consular information sheets and travel warnings are issued by both the United States and British governments. These sites provide you with detailed safety and security advisories. If you become ill, get arrested, or need emergency funds transferred, they can also help.

What's That Disease?

(http://www.cdc.gov/az.do)—Here is a data base giving you information not just on travel-related diseases, but also on a large number of other medical topics.

What to Leave at Home

(http://www.tsa.gov/public or http://www.tsa.gov/interweb/assetlibrary/Prohibited_ English_4-1-2005_v2.pdf)—Along with tips and other travel security-related information, the U.S. Transportation Security Administration website includes the latest list of items you are prohibited from packing in your carry-on and checked luggage.

Just the Facts...

(http://www.cia.gov/cia/publications/factbook)—If you want to know the capital of Azerbaijan, the population of Bhutan, or the total land area of Crete, the online version of the CIA's annual World Fact Book is the place to go. Searchable by country, the site also features useful reference maps and a gallery of world flags.

Index

Note: Page numbers followed by f refer to figures (illustrations); page numbers followed by t refer to tables.

Malaria *(Continued)*
    in cases of chloroquine sensitivity, 116, 117, 281
    for pregnant travelers, 265
    chloroquine-resistant, prophylaxis against, 113–116, 117
      in child travelers, 113, 114, 115, 282
    chloroquine-sensitive, prophylaxis against, 116–118
      in child travelers, 116, 117, 281
    delayed attacks of, 109
    diagnosis of, 110
    morbidity and mortality associated with, 106f
    Plasmodium species causing, 107
    primaquine-resistant, treatment of, 119
    radical cure of, 118–119
    relapses of, prevention of, 118–119
    symptoms of, 109
      factors affecting severity of, 108–109
    transmission of, 107–108, 108f
    treatment of, 119–127, 122t–123t
      in children, 120, 122t, 283
      in pregnant women, 125, 265
      self-administered treatment, 126t, 127
Malarone (atovaquone/proguanil), for malaria, 113, 119–120, 122t, 126t
    in child travelers, 282
Malawi, 539–542
Malayan filariasis, 148–149
Malaysia, 542–544
Mali, 544–548
Martinique (French West Indies), 548–549
Mauritania, 549–551
Mauritius, 551–554
Measles, 43
    vaccine for, 43–44
      in adult travelers, 58t
      in children, 54f
      in child travelers, 274t
      in HIV-positive travelers, 62t
Meclizine (Antivert), for motion sickness, 69

Medical evacuation, 232, 242. *See also* Medical transport.
Medical kit, for travelers, 20–21, 249
Medical transport, 232, 242–246
    air ambulance services and, 244
      providers of, 244–245
    commercial airliner services and, 243
    eligibility protocols for, 246
Mediterranean spotted fever, 156
Mefloquine (Lariam), for malaria, 114–115, 120, 123t, 126t
    in child travelers, 282
    in pregnant travelers, 265
Melatonin, in management of jet lag, 64
Meningococcal meningitis, 44, 167–168
    areas of distribution of, in central Africa, 167f
    vaccine for, 44–45, 168
      in adult travelers, 58t
      in child travelers, 275
      in HIV-positive travelers, 62t
      in pregnant travelers, 263
Metronidazole (Flagyl), for travelers' diarrhea, 98
Mexico, 554–558
    disease risk summary for Central America and, 295–297
Micronesia, 558–560
Micropur MP 1 (chlorine tablets), in disinfection of water, 85, 86f
Middle East, disease risk summaries for, 310–311
Moldova, 560–562
Mongolia, 562–564
Montenegro, 646–647
Morocco, 564–567
Mosquito bites, 128
    disease transmission via, 129
      malarial, 107–108, 108f. *See also* Malaria.
      non-malarial, 141, 142, 144, 148
    prevention of, 142, 264
    treatment of, 136

People's Republic of China, 402–408

Pepto-Bismol (bismuth subsalicylate), for travelers' diarrhea, 93, 94, 95
  in children, 278–279, 279t

Permethrin, in prevention of insect bites, 22, 135f, 135–136, 137f

Pertussis, 38, 45
  vaccine for, 38, 39, 45
    in children, 54f
    in child travelers, 274t

Peru, 607–610

Phenergan (dimenhydrinate), for motion sickness, 69

Philippines, 610–614

Plague, 155–156

Plaquenil (hydroxychloroquine), for malaria, 117

Plasmodium species, malaria due to infection by. *See* Malaria.

Pneumococcal vaccine
  for adult travelers, 58t
  for children, 54f
  for HIV-positive travelers, 62t
  for pregnant travelers, 263

Poland, 614–616

Poliomyelitis, 45
  vaccine for, 45–46
    in adult travelers, 59t
    in children, 54f
    in child travelers, 274t
    in HIV-positive travelers, 62t
    in pregnant travelers, 263

Polynesia (French), 452–453

Pork tapeworm disease, 175

Portable hyperbaric chamber (Gamow bag), in treatment of altitude illness, 224–225

Portugal, 616–618

Positioning, in management of motion sickness, 68

Pregnancy. *See also* Pregnant travelers.
  exercise during, 268–269
  trauma during, 261–262

Pregnant travelers, 258–272
  diarrhea in, 99, 271
    treatment of, 99, 266–267, 271
  drug use guidelines for, 265–268
  dysentery treatment in, 271–272
  insurers providing assistance services to, 260
  Lyme disease treatment in, 186
  malaria prevention and treatment in, 125, 265
  obstetric emergencies in, 261
  trip supplies needed by, checklist for, 259
  vaccines for, 262–264

Primaquine, for malaria, 115–116, 118, 122t

Primaquine-resistant malaria, treatment of, 119

Principe, 638–640

Pristine (liquid chlorine dioxide), in disinfection of water, 85–86

Proguanil, for malaria, 117, 122t, 126t
  in child travelers, 282

Protective clothing, in prevention of insect bites, 134, 137f

Puerto Rico, 618–619

Pufferfish poisoning, 181

Pulmonary disease, as indication for inflight oxygen, 27

Pulmonary edema, high-altitude, 219–220
  reduction of risk of, 220, 222
  treatment of, 224

Pulmonary embolism, in travelers, 73

Purifiers, in water treatment, 87–88, 88f

Pyrimethamine/sulfadoxine (Fansidar), for malaria, 120

Q

Qatar, 619–621

Qinghaosu, as source of artemisinin, 124

Quinidine, for malaria, 121, 124

Quinine, for malaria, 120–121, 122t, 126t

NOTES

NOTES

NOTES

NOTES

NOTES

NOTES

NOTES

NOTES